# Emergency Management of Skeletal Injuries

## *Editors*

**Ernest Ruiz**
Professor and Head
Emergency Medicine Program
University of Minnesota
Minneapolis, Minnesota

**James J. Cicero**
Chief, Department of Emergency Medicine
Associate Professor of Clinical Emergency Medicine
St. Paul Ramsey Medical Center
St. Paul, Minnesota

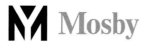 Mosby

St. Louis  Baltimore  Boston  Carlsbad  Chicago  Naples  New York  Philadelphia  Portland
London  Madrid  Mexico City  Singapore  Sydney  Tokyo  Toronto  Wiesbaden

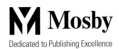

**Mosby**
Dedicated to Publishing Excellence

**A Times Mirror**
**Company**

Editor: Laurel Craven
Associate Developmental Editor: Wendy Buckwalter
Project Manager: Christopher J. Baumle
Production Editor: David Orzechowski
Designer: Jeanne Wolfegeher
Manufacturing Supervisor: Tim Stringham
Cover art: Ellen Dawson

Printed in the United States of America
Composition by Carlisle Communications, Ltd.
Printing/binding by Maple Vail—York

Mosby–Year Book, Inc.
11830 Westline Industrial Drive
St. Louis, Missouri 63146

**Library of Congress Cataloging in Publication Data**
Emergency management of skeletal injuries   /   [edited by] Ernest Ruiz,
    James J. Cicero.— 1st ed.
        p.    cm.
    Includes bibliographical references and index.
    ISBN 0-8016-7243-0 (alk. paper)
    1. Musculoskeletal system—Wounds and injuries. 2. Fractures.
I. Ruiz, Ernest. II. Cicero, James J.
    [DNLM: 1. Bone and Bones—injuries. 2. Emergency Medicine. WE
200 E525 1995]
RD731E44   1995
DNLM/DLC
for Library of Congress

95  96  97  /  9  8  7  6  5  4  3  2  1

# CONTRIBUTORS

**Cheryl D. Adkinson, M.D., F.A.C.E.P.**
Associate Professor of Clinical Emergency Medicine
Medical School, University of Minnesota
Department of Emergency Medicine
Hennepin County Medical Center
Minneapolis, Minnesota

**Douglas D. Brunette, M.D., F.A.C.E.P.**
Associate Professor of Clinical Emergency Medicine
Medical School, University of Minnesota
Department of Emergency Medicine
Hennepin County Medical Center
Minneapolis, Minnesota

**Mary Carr, M.D., F.A.C.E.P.**
Assistant Professor of Clinical Emergency Medicine
Medical School, University of Minnesota
Department of Emergency Medicine
St. Paul Ramsey Medical Center
St. Paul, Minnesota

**James J. Cicero, M.D., F.A.C.E.P.**
Associate Professor of Clinical Emergency Medicine
Medical School, University of Minnesota
Chief of Emergency Medicine
St. Paul Ramsey Medical Center
St. Paul, Minnesota

**Robert Collier, M.D., F.A.C.E.P.**
Assistant Professor of Clinical Emergency Medicine
Medical School, University of Minnesota
Department of Emergency Medicine
Hennepin County Medical Center
Minneapolis, Minnesota

**Timothy J. Crimmins, M.D., F.A.C.E.P.**
Associate Professor of Clinical Emergency Medicine
Medical School, University of Minnesota
Department of Emergency Medicine
Hennepin County Medical Center
Minneapolis, Minnesota

**Ralph J. Frascone, M.D., F.A.C.E.P.**
Assistant Professor of Clinical Emergency Medicine
Medical School, University of Minnesota
Department of Emergency Medicine
St. Paul Ramsey Medical Center
St. Paul, Minnesota

**Paul R. Haller, M.D.**
Assistant Professor of Clinical Emergency Medicine
Medical School, University of Minnesota
Department of Emergency Medicine
St. Paul Ramsey Medical Center
St. Paul, Minnesota

**Carson R. Harris, M.D., F.A.C.E.P.**
Assistant Professor of Clinical Emergency Medicine
Medical School, University of Minnesota
Department of Emergency Medicine
St. Paul Ramsey Medical Center
St. Paul, Minnesota

**Wayne F. Hass, M.D., F.A.C.E.P.**
Associate Professor of Clinical Emergency Medicine
Medical School, University of Minnesota
Assistant Chief of Emergency Medicine
St. Paul Ramsey Medical Center
St. Paul, Minnesota

**Joel S. Holger, M.D., F.A.C.E.P.**
Assistant Professor of Clinical Emergency Medicine
Medical School, University of Minnesota
Department of Emergency Medicine
St. Paul Ramsey Medical Center
St. Paul, Minnesota

**Ross M. Huelster, P.A.**
Department of Emergency Medicine
St. Paul Ramsey Medical Center
St. Paul, Minnesota

**Kevin P. Kilgore, M.D., F.A.C.E.P.**
Assistant Professor of Clinical Emergency Medicine
Medical School, University of Minnesota
Department of Emergency Medicine
St. Paul Ramsey Medical Center
St. Paul, Minnesota

**Jo Ellen Linder, M.D., F.A.C.E.P.**
Assistant Clinical Professor
University of California at San Francisco
Fresno Campus
Huntington Memorial Hospital
Pasadena, California

**Louis J. Ling, M.D., F.A.C.E.P.**
Professor of Clinical Emergency Medicine
Medical School, University of Minnesota
Department of Emergency Medicine
Hennepin County Medical Center
Minneapolis, Minnesota

**Brian Mahoney, M.D., F.A.C.E.P.**
Associate Professor of Clinical Emergency Medicine
Medical School, University of Minnesota
Department of Emergency Medicine
Hennepin County Medical Center
Minneapolis, Minnesota

**Brian D. Patty, M.D.**
Department of Emergency Medicine
Hennepin County Medical Center
Minneapolis, Minnesota

**David W. Plummer, M.D., F.A.C.E.P.**
Associate Professor of Clinical Emergency Medicine
Medical School, University of Minnesota
Department of Emergency Medicine
Hennepin County Medical Center
Minneapolis, Minnesota

*Karen A. Quaday, M.D., F.A.C.E.P.*
Assistant Professor of Clinical Emergency Medicine
Medical School, University of Minnesota
Department of Emergency Medicine
St. Paul Ramsey Medical Center
St. Paul, Minnesota

*Ernest Ruiz, M.D., F.A.C.E.P.*
Professor of Clinical Emergency Medicine
Head, Emergency Medicine Program
Medical School, University of Minnesota
Minneapolis, Minnesota

*Robert A. Rusnak, M.D., F.A.C.E.P.*
Associate Professor of Clinical Emergency Medicine
Medical School, University of Minnesota
Department of Emergency Medicine
Hennepin County Medical Center
Minneapolis, Minnesota

*Stephen W. Smith, M.D.*
Assistant Professor of Clinical Emergency Medicine
Medical School, University of Minnesota
Department of Emergency Medicine
Hennepin County Medical Center
Minneapolis, Minnesota

*Steve Sterner, M.D., F.A.C.E.P.*
Associate Professor of Clinical Emergency Medicine
Medical School, University of Minnesota
Assistant Chief of Emergency Medicine
Hennepin County Medical Center
Minneapolis, Minnesota

*Albert K. Tsai, M.D., F.A.C.E.P.*
Staff, Department of Emergency Medicine
Hennepin County Medical Center
Minneapolis, Minnesota

Dedicated to the understanding families of our contributors

# PREFACE

Out text is intended to provide the emergency physician with an easily read and clearly laid out guide to the management of skeletal injuries. It is our hope that it will be useful in the busy Emergency Department. The authors have tried to include enough information on pathophysiology and anatomy to satisfy our readers' need to know without overdoing it. The authors are all emergency physicians with extensive clinical experience dealing with their subject matter. Although there are treatment plans outlined that not all orthopedists or emergency physicians will agree with, the recommendations are safe.

We would like to thank all of our authors for their scholarly effort. James Kaufmann, Ph.D., Debbie Heiberger, R.N., Carol Klitz, R.N., and our artist, Diane Erickson, were immensely helpful, skilled, and patient in preparing the manuscripts and illustrations. Without their help, this text could not have been produced.

*Ernest Ruiz*
*James J. Cicero*

**A note to the reader**

The treatment plans outlined in the text are safe, although they may differ from those that some emergency physicians and orthopedists may recommend. The authors have made every effort to ensure that drug selection and dosing are accurate. We suggest that the practitioner take due precaution to check the suitability of any drug or drug dose for each patient.

# CONTENTS

# Evaluation, Definitions, and Radiologic Examination

*Douglas D. Brunette*

Almost by definition, a patient with an orthopedic injury has sustained some kind of trauma. The initial approach to any patient with trauma (single or multiple trauma) begins with the ABCs of the primary survey, as described by the Committee on Trauma of the American College of Surgeons.[1] This chapter covers the evaluation of orthopedic injury after the patient has been examined and treated for any life-threatening injuries. The purposes of this chapter are to detail a systematic strategy for evaluating orthopedic injuries in the emergency department, to review the nomenclature and definitions of orthopedic injuries, and to outline a basic approach to radiologic examination.

## EVALUATION

Unlike many clinical problems that emergency physicians face daily, orthopedic injuries usually allow the emergency physician time to take a complete history and perform a thorough physical examination. Although the history and examination must be complete, they can still be concise and goal-directed.

---

**Information needed for the historical evaluation of an orthopedic injury**

Age
Sex
Mechanism
Time of injury
Symptoms
Prior orthopedic treatment
Type of work
Prior orthopedic history
Allergies
Medications
Past medical history
Last meals, drinks, drugs
Tetanus immune status

---

## History

The above box lists the many pieces of information that are essential for the historical evaluation of an orthopedic injury.

**Age.** Age is important in determining not only the course of certain injuries, but also their treatment. It is common practice to treat the same injury by different methods, determined solely by the patient's age. For example, the definitive treatment of Colles' fracture is generally more aggressive in young patients, compared with elderly patients.

**Sex.** Differences between men and women in terms of bone mass and strength often result in differences in injury pattern. Choice of treatment is sometimes affected by the degree of bone mass and strength present. Postmenopausal women, for example, are more likely to have osteoporosis complicating the orthopedic injury.

**Mechanism.** Identifying the exact mechanism of injury is particularly important. This information typically leads the emergency physician to suspect another injury; for example, a calcaneal fracture caused by a fall is clearly associated with axial skeletal fractures, notably in the lumbar region. Knowledge of the mechanism also provides insight into the degree of force associated with the injury and the likelihood of additional significant injury.

**Time of injury.** In many patients with orthopedic injuries, the treatment and prognosis depend on the time elapsed between injury and definitive management. In hip dislocations, for example, the risk of subsequent avascular necrosis increases as the time from dislocation to reduction increases.

**Symptoms.** Asking the orthopedically injured patient about any other symptoms that may be associated with the injury is essential. Questions regarding muscle strength, range of motion, and sensation are appropriate. Unless specifically prompted, patients will not report certain symptoms, such as areas of skin anesthesia. Although subjective, the patient's answers to such questions usually establish the focus for the examination.

**Prior orthopedic treatment.** This information is significant when the patient has been transferred (from either the injury scene or another health care facility) to the examining physician's place of practice. The examining physician should be aware of prior attempts at reduction and the medications administered.

**Type of work.** Although it is probably not as important, the patient's work can play a role in certain management decisions. Patients with injuries that might affect their livelihood considerably require treatment plans that address this issue. The handedness of the patient must also be ascertained.

**Prior orthopedic history.** Ask the patient if this injury has ever occurred before the current episode. For example, recurrent shoulder dislocations are managed differently from first-time dislocations. It is prudent to ascertain the patient's complete orthopedic history.

**Allergies.** Antibiotics, anesthetics, and muscle relaxants are frequently used in the emergency department management of patients with acute orthopedic injuries. Ask the patient about any previous allergic reaction to such drugs.

**Medications.** Whenever providing any type of medical care, inquire about all the medications the patient is currently taking. This information not only determines present health status and past medical history, but may also predict possible drug interactions.

**Past medical history.** Many orthopedic treatment decisions are affected by the patient's past medical history. Systemic conditions, such as significant cardiac or pulmonary disease, diabetes, or peripheral vascular disease, greatly influence orthopedic decision-making.

**Last meals, drinks, drugs.** Last meals, drinks, or drugs are very important and frequently overlooked in the patient's history. The presence of alcohol, illicit drugs, or a full stomach may complicate treatment considerably. Neither "conscious sedation" for fracture or dislocation reduction nor an elective orthopedic procedure should be attempted until this information is obtained and considered. An elective orthopedic procedure, for example, should never be performed on a patient who is not adequately prepared for general anesthesia.

**Tetanus immune status.** In cases of open wounds, the patient's tetanus immune status must be obtained from either the patient or the patient's previous medical records. If no information on the patient's tetanus immune status is available, a tetanus booster should be administered; in the case of gross contamination, human tetanus immune globulin should be administered.

## Physical examination

A thorough physical examination (see box on page 3) should be conducted before treatment or even manipulation of the orthopedically injured patient. Vascular, motor, and sensory function must be ascertained prior to manipulation, especially in injuries where there is a high likelihood of neurovascular damage from the injury itself.

---

### The physical examination

**Simple inspection**

Swelling
Color
Deformity

**Palpation**

Point of maximal tenderness
Hematoma
Crepitus from air
Compartment finger-pressure assessment

**Range of motion**

Passive
Active

**Motor strength**

Class 1-5

**Sensation**

Two-point discrimination
Light touch/pinprick discrimination

**Vascular assessment**
Capillary refill
Skin temperature
Pulses

**Specific examination techniques**

---

**Simple inspection.** Simply inspecting the involved site provides important information. This should be done before palpation of the injured area, range-of-motion testing, strength testing, and sensory examination. Almost invariably, the involved area is tender. Taking the time to simply inspect without laying on hands instills confidence in the patient that the examining physician is concerned about the patient's pain and will attend to the patient's needs.

The area of injury should be inspected for swelling, redness, and deformity. It is important to examine the uninvolved, contralateral extremity because this helps define subtle changes. Bone is a vascular organ and bleeds when fractured. Swelling almost always accompanies a fracture.

**Palpation.** The uninvolved, contralateral extremity is palpated first to gain comparative information and to ensure the patient's acceptance of the physical examination technique. The injury should be palpated for skin temperature, hematoma, crepitus from subcutaneous air, compartment finger-pressure assessment, and points of maximal tenderness. Care should be taken to minimize patient suffering during this process. Except in patients with altered mental status (due, for example, to alcohol, drugs, head injury, or diversion of attention to other sites of major injury), palpation of a fracture

is usually painful. In patients with an obvious major deformity, delay palpation, range-of-motion testing, and strength testing until after the patient's pain has been controlled and radiographs have defined the injury. Testing for bony crepitus in the conscious patient should never be done; eliciting bony crepitus when there are adequate clinical grounds for suspecting fracture only causes unnecessary pain and provides no information beyond that available from a radiograph of an unstable fracture.

**Range of motion, motor strength.** Testing range of motion, armed with a working knowledge of the normal values for a given joint, is essential. The patient's affected side can usually be compared with the unaffected side. Range of motion can be assessed by both passive and active methods. Passive range-of-motion testing is critical in the evaluation of compartment syndrome.

Strength testing is important and should be done carefully. The rating scale below is the one most commonly used.[2]

0 = no evidence of contractility or motion
1 = slight contractility, but no joint motion
2 = complete motion without gravity
3 = complete motion against gravity; no resistance
4 = resistance present, but not normal strength
5 = full resistance present

**Sensation.** Determining sensation, particularly that distal to the site of injury, is an important part of the physical examination. Light-touch, pinprick discrimination, and two-point discrimination should be tested fully. This examination requires anatomic knowledge of which nerves are being tested as well as which nerves are likely involved.

**Vascular assessment.** The vascular integrity of an extremity, particularly distal to the site of injury, must also be ascertained. This can be done by examining skin color, skin temperature, and capillary refill, and by palpating distal pulses. When a distal pulse cannot be palpated on the affected side, vascular Doppler ultrasound can frequently locate a pulse that is not palpable with the fingers. To appreciate subtle differences and compromises, compare the affected side with the unaffected side.

**Specific examination techniques.** Specific examination techniques are appropriate for certain types of injury or areas of injury. For example, examination of the knee requires the pivot-shift test, which is specific to knee examination. A working knowledge of which tests should routinely be conducted for certain types or areas of injury is important. Such tests are discussed throughout this book.

## DEFINITIONS

To diagnose and treat orthopedic injury, five major areas are considered: joint movement, limb deformity, fracture, subluxation and dislocation, and soft-tissue injury. Each of these areas has terminology that will help the examining physician understand and document the injury and discuss it with orthopedic specialists when necessary. Key terms are defined in this section.

**Joint movement**

**Active and passive movement.** Active movement results from the patient's own muscular action; passive movement, from the examiner's action on the involved body part.

**Abduction and adduction.** Abduction is movement of a body part away from the midline of the body; adduction is movement of the body part toward the midline.

**Dorsiflexion, palmar flexion, and plantar flexion.** Dorsiflexion is movement of the hands/fingers or feet/toes in the direction of the dorsal surface. Palmar flexion is movement of the fingers or hands toward the palmar surface of the hand. Plantar flexion is movement of the toes/feet toward the plantar surface of the foot.

**Eversion and inversion.** Eversion is a turning of the plantar surface of the foot in an outward direction; inversion, an inward turning of the plantar surface.

**Internal and external rotation.** Internal rotation is a turning of the anterior surface of the limb medially; external rotation, a turning of this surface laterally.

**Pronation and supination.** Pronation is a turning of the palmar surface of the hand either downward or posteriorly; supination, a turning of this surface upward or posteriorly.

**Limb deformity**

The terms *valgus* and *varus* refer to the direction of the deformity. Valgus refers to deformity away from the midline of the body; varus, toward the midline. An easy way to remember is to associate the *l* in valgus with the word "lateral," or away from the midline.

The term *torsion* refers to a twist (internal or external) in the longitudinal axis of the extremity.

**Fracture**

Simply defined, a fracture is a break in the contiguity of bone.

**Clinical signs and fracture types.** The clinical signs of fracture are swelling, pain, deformity, and crepitus. In a *closed* fracture, there is no break in the skin or mucosa overlying the bone. In an *open* fracture, such disruption is present. There are three types of open fracture[3]:

Type I:  Fracture with an associated clean wound less than 1 cm in length

Type II:  Fracture with an associated wound longer than 1 cm, and no extensive soft-tissue damage, flaps, or avulsions

Type III:  Subtypes:
—open fracture with extensive soft-tissue damage
—open fracture with vascular injury requiring repair
—open segmental fracture
—traumatic amputation involving bone
—gunshot wound involving bone
—open fractures from farming accidents

**Radiographic findings.** The radiograph reveals whether the fracture is complete or incomplete. A complete fracture has breaks in both cortices of the involved bone,

whereas an incomplete fracture involves only one cortex.

The radiograph also provides an accurate anatomic description of the fracture (Fig. 1-1). A *transverse* fracture is one that is at right angles to the long axis of the bone. An *oblique* fracture runs diagonally to the long axis of the bone. In a *spiral* fracture, the fracture line is coiled around the long axis in a helical fashion, indicating a rotational force. In a "comminuted" fracture, more than two fracture fragments are present.

The position and alignment of the fracture is also revealed by the radiograph in Fig. 1-2. In a *displaced* fracture, the fracture fragments have diverged from their normal anatomic relationship with each other. In an *angulated* fracture, the fragments have moved, relative to the longitudinal axis of the bone. In an *avulsion* fracture, the bone fragment has been pulled from its normal position by muscle action on tendons or ligaments. *Impaction* occurs when bony fragments collapse, forming a depression (indentation) or *compression* (compacted bony fragments). *Rotation* occurs when the fragments have twisted in relation to each other since fracture.

Articular surface involvement is shown on the radiograph in Fig. 1-3. It is important to approximate the amount of articular surface involved. This is usually performed by measuring the percentage of articular surface interrupted by a fracture. A fracture that splits the articular surface into two equal fragments is said to involve 50% of the articular surface.

Pediatric fractures include some distinctive types of injury (Figs. 1-4 and 1-5). A *greenstick* fracture is an incomplete, angulated fracture of a long bone. A *torus* fracture is an incomplete fracture with a small fold in the cortex. *Salter-Harris* fractures are fractures that involve the epiphyseal growth plate. While not a fracture, bowing may also appear in the pediatric patient.

**Subluxation and dislocation**

When the facing articular surfaces of a joint are not in normal anatomic relationship with each other, either subluxation or dislocation exists (Fig. 1-6). Subluxation is the partial loss of the normal anatomic relationship between joint surfaces; dislocation, the total loss.

Subluxations and dislocations should be named according to the major joint involved. The subluxation or dislocation is described by the direction of the distal segment relative to the proximal segment. When a dislocation is complicated by fracture, the injury should be termed a fracture-dislocation.

**Soft-tissue injury**

**Sprain.** A sprain is an injury to a ligament. A first-degree sprain is a minor stretching of a ligament that results in minimal swelling and hemorrhage. A second-degree sprain is a partial tear of a ligament and is clinically manifested with swelling, painful joint movement, and loss of function. A third-degree sprain is a complete tear of a ligament. Clinical signs are similar to those of the second-

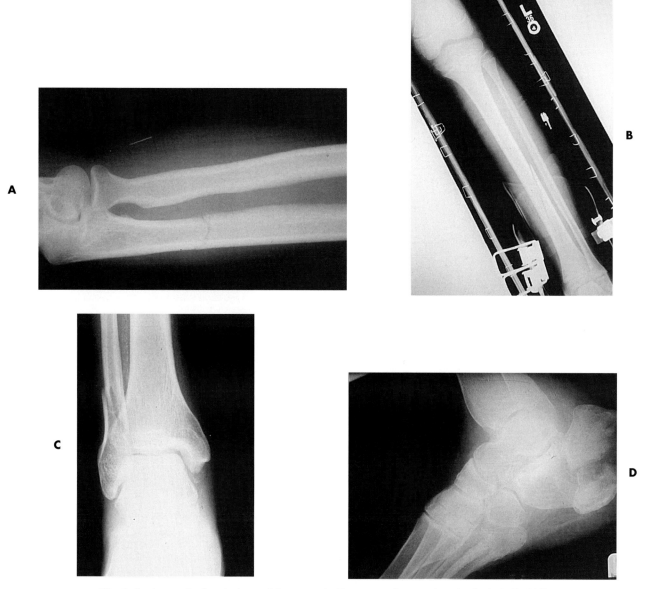

**Fig. 1-1.** Anatomic descriptions of fractures. **A,** Transverse fracture (proximal ulna). **B,** Oblique fracture (tibia). **C,** Spiral oblique fracture (distal fibula). **D,** Comminuted fracture (calcaneus).

degree sprain, with the added feature of joint instability, either spontaneously or on stress testing.

**Strain.** A strain is an injury to a muscle or tendon. A first-degree strain is a minor stretching of the muscle or tendon that causes swelling, tenderness or palpation, and minimal or no loss of function. A second-degree strain is a partial tearing of a muscle or tendon; clinical signs are swelling, bruising, muscle spasm, and functional loss with decreased strength. A third-degree strain is a complete tear of a muscle or tendon. The clinical signs and symptoms are similar to those of a second-degree strain, but they are more severe. Loss of function is typical with a third-degree strain.

**Tendonitis.** Tendonitis is an inflammatory condition marked by pain along the involved tendon. Clinical signs include pain with movement and various degrees of loss of function. Frequently, palpable crepitus along the involved tendon during movement is elicited by the examiner. Common sites include the wrist (de Quervain's disease) and elbow (tennis elbow).

**Bursitis.** Bursitis is an inflammatory process involving a bursa and is usually caused by trauma or infection. The patient has local pain, swelling, and usually warmth and redness, especially when infection is present. Bursas commonly affected include the olecranon and greater trochanteric.

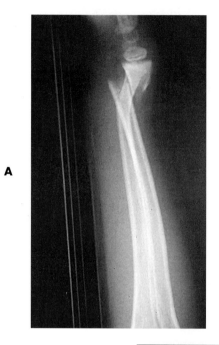
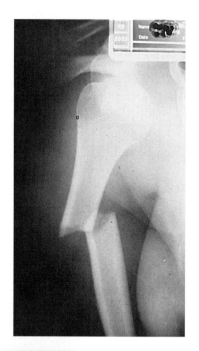
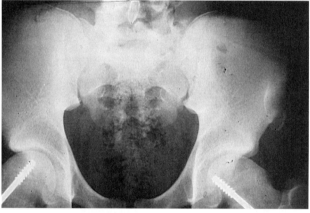

**Fig. 1-2.** Position and alignment of fractures. **A,** Displacement (distal radial fracture). **B,** Displacement and angulation (proximal humerus). **C,** Avulsion (anterior superior iliac spine).

## RADIOLOGY

Medical imaging plays a vital part in the evaluation of acute orthopedic injuries. The examining physician should have a good working knowledge of general radiologic principles and techniques.

### General concepts and practicalities

Many of the methods used by physicians to evaluate orthopedic injury involve exposing the patient to radiation. The examining physician must understand certain principles about radiation exposure and be familiar with the generally accepted protocols.

X-rays are a form of electromagnetic energy emitted by photons and fall into the category of ionizing radiation. Ionizing radiation has significant biological effects that are dose-dependent. *Rad* and *rem* are two of the more common terms used to denote units of radiation. Rad (acronym for *r*adiation *a*bsorbed *d*ose) is simply a unit dose of radiation,

while rem (acronym of *r*oentgen *e*quivalent in *m*an) refers to a unit dose radiation with a certain biological effect. In practical terms, a dose of 1 rad equals 1 rem. Table 1-1 lists the approximate doses for ten radiographic examinations commonly performed in the author's emergency department radiology area.

The maximal permissible dose of radiation for occupational workers is 5 rems in any one year, whereas the annual dose limit for the public is 0.5 rem.[4] Table 1-1 shows that a patient with multiple orthopedic injuries can quickly exceed the recommended yearly dose limit. There is a general consensus that low-dose radiation poses a small, albeit real, long-term risk. For example, the lifetime risk of 1 rad whole-body exposure, weighted according to life tables, is 56.6 leukemias in males and 38.4 leukemias in females per one million individuals exposed.[5] Infants and smaller children are considered at higher risk because they

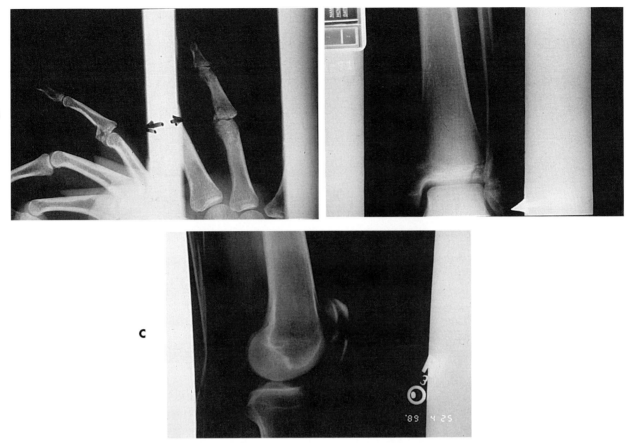

**Fig. 1-3.** Articular surface involvement. **A,** Fracture of the middle phalanx involving the articular surface. **B,** Fracture of the distal tibia involving the articular surface. **C,** Displaced fracture of the patella involving the articular surface.

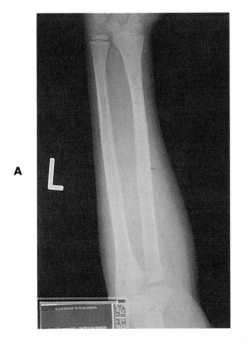
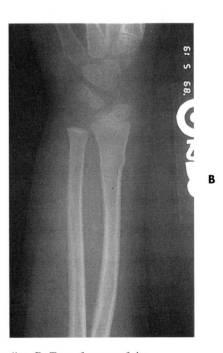

**Fig. 1-4.** Pediatric fractures. **A,** Greenstick fracture of the distal radius. **B,** Torus fracture of the distal radius.

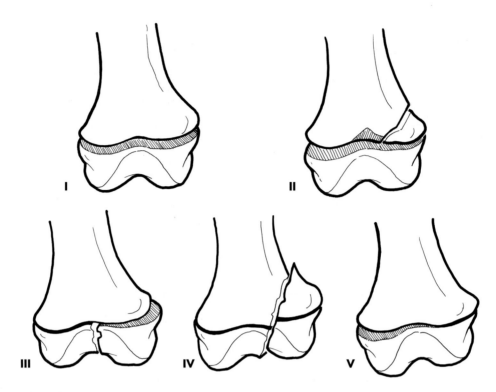

**Fig. 1-5.** Salter-Harris fracture classification.

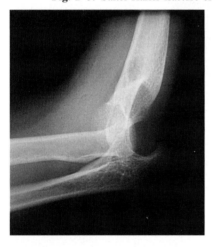

**Fig. 1-6.** Dislocation (posterior elbow).

**Table 1-1.** Approximate doses for commonly performed radiographic examinations

| Radiographic examination | Radiation dose (mR) |
|---|---|
| PA chest | 6 |
| Femur (one view) | 15 |
| Foot (one view) | 25 |
| AP wrist/hand | 29 |
| Lateral C-spine | 47 |
| Lateral skull | 82 |
| AP hip | 154 |
| AP abdomen | 230 |
| Lateral thoracic spine | 743 |
| Lateral lumbar spine | 1325 |

Key: AP = Anteroposterior
C = Cervical
mR = Milliroentgen

have increased time available for expressing any radiation injury, as well as increased susceptibility caused by rapid growth of organ systems.

The medical imaging department at our facility employs a "10-day rule," which states that elective nuclear medicine procedures involving the internal administration of radionuclides and elective x-ray examinations of the abdomen and pelvis are to be performed only during the 10 days following the first day of the menstrual cycle in women of childbearing age. Exceptions to this rule are women who have been taking oral contraceptives or have had an intrauterine device in place for at least three months, or who have undergone sterilization.

Medical imaging that will expose a fetus to ionizing radiation involves special considerations. Fetuses are most susceptible to teratogenic effects of radiation during the first trimester. The teratogenic threshold is thought to be between 5 and 10 rads.[6] The risk is considered negligible if the dose is less than 5 rads.[7]

During imaging studies, patients, especially younger patients, should routinely have gonadal shielding. Many of the newer, plain radiographic imaging devices are so well collimated that scatter is limited; thus, shielding may not be absolutely necessary. However, shielding costs very little, alleviates patient concerns about radiation exposure, and probably does limit gonadal exposure.

**Specific radiographic imaging techniques**

**Conventional radiography.** The emergency physician should know the standard views for conventional radio-

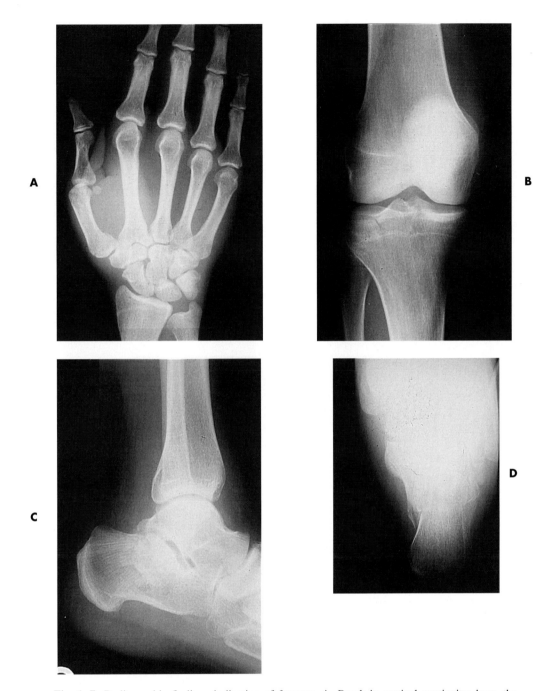

**Fig. 1-7.** Radiographic findings indicative of fracture. **A,** Break in cortical continuity; here, the break is seen in the base of the first metacarpal bone. **B,** Radiolucent line; the line here indicates a fracture of the tibial plateau. **C,** Increased density caused by overlapping cortical bone, here indicating a fracture of the calcaneus. **D,** Bony fragments, evident on calcaneal view and indicating a fracture of the calcaneus.

graphs, how they are taken, and how the normal radiograph appears. Generally, most series of films are comprised of an anteroposterior (AP), a lateral, and an oblique view. Three views are required when evaluating for possible fracture or dislocation. It is common for a significant fracture to be missed on a single, plain-radiographic view. The information obtained from conventional radiographs depends considerably on positioning and radiographic technique. A poorly positioned lateral radiograph of the wrist,

for example, is not helpful and may be misleading in diagnosing a distal dorsal ulnar dislocation. The emergency physician should never settle for radiographs that are incomplete or suboptimal due to poor technique. Clinical circumstances may, on occasion, preclude the use of proper technique, but such occurrences should be rare.

In the vast majority of cases, it is the emergency physician who is responsible for the initial interpretation of plain radiographs. Initial diagnosis and management decisions are

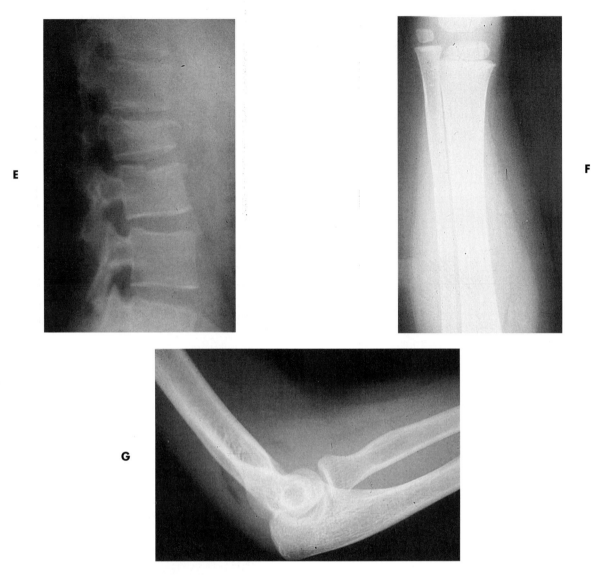

**Fig. 1-7, cont'd. E,** Increased density secondary to impaction, indicating here a lumbar spine fracture. **F,** Marked soft-tissue swelling observed in the lower leg of a child (result of poorly visualized tibial fracture). **G,** Joint effusion; here, significant anterior and posterior fat-pad signs indicate elbow joint effusion secondary to probable radial head fracture.

typically based on initial radiographic interpretation. A common medicolegal problem is the failure to identify fractures. The following radiographic findings indicate fracture: breaks in cortical continuity, radiolucent lines, increased density caused by overriding cortical bone, bony fragments in the absence of obvious fracture, increased density caused by impacted spongy bone, soft-tissue swelling, and joint effusion. The emergency physician should be familiar with the appearance of each of these findings (Fig. 1-7).

**Conventional tomography.** In plain radiographs, overlapping soft-tissue and bone can obscure a fracture line, making the diagnosis difficult or impossible. When this occurs, conventional tomography is useful for better delineating the fracture line. Conventional tomographic examinations of the cervical, thoracic, and lumbar spine, as well as of the knee (specifically, for tibial plateau fractures),

are commonly performed to supplement the plain radiographic views of these areas.

**Nuclide bone scanning.** This radiographic technique is useful when plain radiographic examinations are negative for fracture, but a strong clinical suspicion for fracture remains. Nuclide bone scans of the hip and carpal scaphoid and for suspected stress fractures are the most common uses. Technetium 99m phosphate or disphosphonate is used. Although it is a sensitive examination for fracture, this scan is nonspecific. Other bone problems, such as infection, will result in a positive scan. Finally, nuclide bone scanning is sometimes useful in diagnosing avascular necrosis.

**Computed tomography.** Computed tomography (CT) has greatly reduced the usefulness of conventional tomography. CT scanning has the advantage of giving the examining physician critical information on the spatial relationships in fractures. CT is particularly useful for examining the pelvis, axial spine, skull base, facial bones, and calcaneus.

**Magnetic resonance imaging.** At present, magnetic resonance imaging (MRI) plays a limited role in the diagnosis and management of fracture, with the possible exception of Salter-Harris injuries in children. However, MRI can be useful for examining soft-tissue injuries. MRI of the knee joint, for example, can effectively evaluate meniscal and cruciate integrity. This method is apparently a sensitive imaging modality for the diagnosis of avascular necrosis. The major contraindications to MRI include the presence of magnetically active cardiac pacemakers and intracranial aneurysm clips. Most orthopedic appliances are not significantly ferromagnetic and usually do not represent an absolute contraindication to MRI scanning. Claustrophobia is occasionally experienced in patients undergoing MRI scanning; such patients tend to tolerate the procedure better if they lie prone in the scanner. If this is not possible, or if the patient still has disabling claustrophobia, sedation, typically with an anxiolytic, may be necessary.

### Special considerations

**Portable versus standard medical imaging.** As a general rule, patients can be sent to the medical imaging department for the majority of orthopedic radiographic examinations. Portable radiographs should be obtained in the emergency department only if the patient is considered unstable from other traumatic injuries.

**Pediatric and elderly patients.** These two patient groups frequently have other conditions that complicate an acute orthopedic injury. For example, these patients typically have a diminished capacity for self-care. Children, who by definition need routine adult care and supervision, may have these needs increased as a result of orthopedic injury. Crutch walking may represent a major obstacle for children. Elderly patients may need a caregiver's help to perform chores of living that younger adults manage without assistance. Any disposition from the emergency department must consider the physical, social, and psychological support needed for effective living during orthopedic healing.

**Difficult-to-interpret radiographs.** Uncommon bony pathologic disease, certain incidental bony abnormalities, and normal pediatric skeletal development can make the interpretation of orthopedic radiographs difficult. It is very useful for the emergency physician to have reference textbooks that address these radiologic problems available in the department.[8,9]

## DISCUSSION

Orthopedic injuries are treated frequently in the emergency department setting. The practicing emergency physician must use a systematic approach for the evaluation of orthopedic injury, understand the nomenclature and definitions of orthopedic injuries, and utilize radiographic examinations efficiently.

## REFERENCES

1. Degowin EL, Degowin RL: The neuropsychiatric examination. Bedside diagnostic examination, ed 4, New York, Macmillan, 1981.
2. Gustilo RB, Anderson JT: Prevention of infection in the treatment of one thousand and twenty-five open fractures of long bones, *J Bone Joint Surg* 58A:453, 1976.
3. National Commission on Radiological Protection (NCRP): Basic radiation protection criteria, report no. 39, Washington, DC, National Commission on Radiological Protection, 1971.
4. National Commission on Radiological Protection: Medical radiation exposure of pregnant and potentially pregnant women, report no 54, Washington, DC, National Commission on Radiological Protection, 1977.
5. Committee on Trauma of the American College of Surgeons: Advanced trauma life support instructor's manual. Chicago, American College of Surgeons, 1993.
6. Keats TE, Smith TH: An Atlas of Normal Developmental Roentgen Anatomy, ed 2, Chicago, 1988, Year Book Medical Publishers.
7. Keats TE: An Atlas of Normal Roentgen Variants That May Simulate Disease, ed 3, Chicago, 1984, Year Book Medical Publishers.
8. Committee on the biologic effects of ionizing radiation (BIER III): The effects on population of exposure to low levels of ionizing radiation. Washington, DC, 1980, National Academy Press.
9. Russell LB: Irradiation damage to embryo, fetus, and neonates. In: Biological risks of medical irradiations, AAPM monograph no 5:33, New York, American Institute of Physics, 1980.

# 2

# Prehospital Orthopedic Treatment

*Ralph J. Frascone*
*Brian D. Patty*

Prehospital caregivers include first responders, basic emergency medical technicians (EMTs), intermediate EMTs, paramedics, and nurses. The stabilization procedures used by different emergency medical services (EMS) vary because of the differences among prehospital environments, training levels of prehospital personnel, and local medical direction policies.

Orthopedic injuries are rarely life-threatening. (Notable exceptions are axial skeletal, pelvic, and femur fractures.) Patients with orthopedic injuries, however, often have associated life-threatening injuries. The transportation and resuscitation of an otherwise critically injured patient should never be delayed to perform extensive field treatment of non–life-threatening fractures. The old adage "Life before limb" is still valid.

EMS personnel must treat the patient in a logical sequence. This sequence is identical to that used by the emergency physician. The sequence includes: the primary survey, stabilization, the secondary survey, history, and extrication.

## STABILIZATION, SURVEYS, AND HISTORY
### Primary survey and stabilization

The first duty of all EMS personnel is to protect themselves and their crews.[1,2] Securing the scene involves an immediate survey of the situation. This survey should be quick

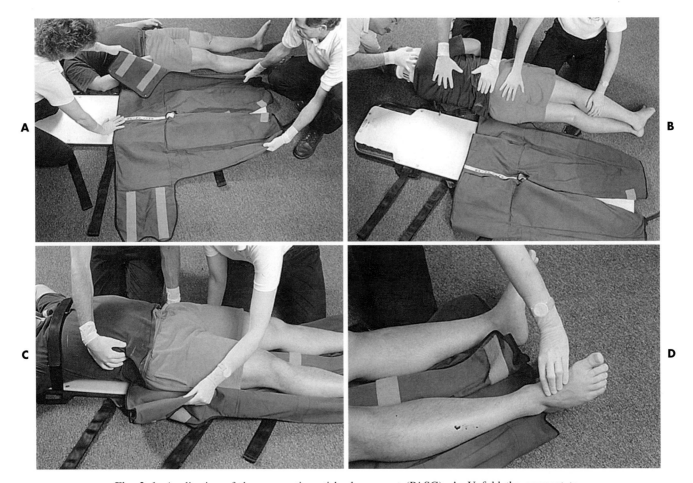

**Fig. 2-1.** Application of the pneumatic antishock garment (PASG). **A,** Unfold the garment to identify and free all the straps. Preferably, the garment is on a backboard at this time. **B,** Logroll the patient onto the garment and backboard. **C,** Place the patient on the garment with the abdominal portion placed at a level right below the costal margin. **D,** Check circulation, motor response, and sensory response (*CMS*). **E,** Wrap the abdomen and legs with the garment and secure with Velcro. **F,** With the abdominal valve closed, inflate the lower-extremity portion and close the valves. **G,** If indicated, close the leg valves, open the abdominal valve, and inflate the abdominal portion. **H,** Recheck CMS. Notes: 1) Before applying PASG, conduct a thorough secondary survey from the xiphoid process to the toes. 2) Do a CMS check before and after applying the PASG. Typically, foot pulses will diminish or be absent following inflation secondary to the pressure of the suit. 3) Check blood pressure before and after inflating each section. 4) Should respiratory compromise develop following the inflation of the abdominal portion, deflate it immediately. 5) Deflation of the PASG should only be done following establishment of two large bore IV lines. Deflate the PASG slowly and sequentially, from the abdominal portion to the leg portion. Should the patient develop hypotension, maintain fluid resuscitation until the patient stabilizes. Once the patient has been stabilized, resume deflation.

but thorough. Immediate dangers to the crew and patients, such as explosion hazards, downed wires, spilled chemicals, fires, and other potential hazards, must be noted. The number and the location of victims must also be determined. Armed with this information, a decision can be made as to whether the number of personnel is adequate. If it is not, additional resources must be requested immediately. Appropriate precautions against infectious diseases must be taken, for example, gloves, masks, goggles, and gowns.[3]

Time spent at the scene should be as brief as possible when life-threatening injuries are indicated either by initial patient assessment or by the mechanism of injury. As many interventions as are safely possible should be performed while en route to the hospital.

After approaching the patient, the prehospital provider establishes the patient's level of consciousness (LOC). The next priority is to evaluate the patient following a series of steps: the primary survey, the resuscitation phase, the secondary survey, and the definitive care stage. The primary survey is meant to identify and treat problems that may be life-threatening. The correction of the problems discovered in the primary survey is undertaken in the resuscitation phase.

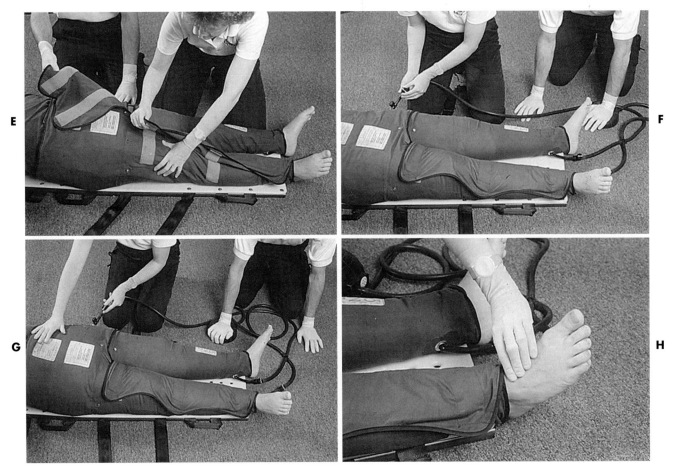

**Fig. 2-1, cont'd.** For legend see opposite page.

The primary survey can be remembered through use of the mnemonic "ABCDE," which represents the sequence of events that constitute the primary survey:[4,5]

A = *a*irway and cervical-spine control

B = *b*reathing

C = *c*irculation and vital signs

D = *d*isability

E = *e*xposure

The procedures used to stabilize abnormalities discovered during the primary survey are also performed in a logical sequence. While the patient is being evaluated, such problems are corrected by the available means. Severely injured patients should be treated with airway support (including intubation if necessary), spinal immobilization, IV fluids and, perhaps, the pneumatic antishock garment (PASG) (Fig. 2-1).

The timing, and even the use of some of the above treatments, has sparked some controversy. The order in which various interventions are performed is determined by the immediacy of the life-threatening problem that they are meant to correct. With a coordinated team effort, however, it is possible to conduct a complete primary survey and, at the same time, resuscitate and stabilize the patient. Once again, the goal in this earliest stage should be to minimize time spent at the scene by performing as many of the interventions as possible while en route to the hospital.[6]

### Secondary survey and definitive care

After the primary survey and resuscitation, the prehospital personnel proceed to the secondary survey.[2,4] The purpose of the secondary survey is to uncover previously unrecognized life-threatening problems and to assess the patient for other injuries. It is during this time that musculoskeletal injuries are often discovered.

The secondary survey consists of a head-to-toe examination. The spine and the extremities are assessed for the following:[7]

- Deformity
- Swelling
- Tenderness
- Open versus closed fracture or dislocation
- Crepitus
- Ecchymosis
- Discoloration
- Instability
- Circulation
- Motor response
- Sensory response

The above problems, of course, can represent a variety of orthopedic injures, including sprain, strain, dislocation, subluxation, and fracture. Generally, the EMS crew need not distinguish these five categories of injuries because treatment is driven by the location, not the type, of the injury.

It is important to note that while en route the patient is reevaluated at frequent intervals. A high index of suspicion for previously undiscovered or new problems must be maintained.

The definitive care phase follows the secondary survey. During this phase, most musculoskeletal injuries are splinted and otherwise treated. In some EMS systems, prehospital providers are allowed to administer pain control medications (see "Special Considerations: Pain Control").

### History

Details about the mechanism of injury can provide the prehospital personnel as well as the physician with valuable clues about possible injuries. It is essential for the crew to obtain as much information about the accident as possible.[8-10] This information can be obtained from observation as well as from the patient, witnesses, police, and others. In the case of motor-vehicle accidents, details about the location of the patient, speed of the vehicles, seat-belt usage, windshield damage, air-bag deployment, amount of body and bumper incursion, interior damage, presence or absence of skid marks, deaths at the scene, and direction of force, among others, are invaluable. Other important facts may include the patient's loss of consciousness, estimated blood loss, and alcohol or drug use. Fractures must always be suspected in a trauma victim who has an altered LOC.

Many crews are taught to take a history using the mnemonic "AMPLE":[2]

A = *a*llergies
M = *m*edications
P = *p*ast medical history or pregnancy
L = *l*ast meal
E = *e*vents preceding the accident

Of course, any treatment the patient receives while under the care of the EMS crew is also significant and must be reported to the receiving center and recorded on the run sheet.

A wise emergency physician takes the time to discuss the case with the prehospital worker and to carefully review the written EMS record.[4]

The use of instant photography at scenes is becoming an increasingly popular way to communicate the mechanism of injury to the physician. This results in a better understanding of what happened and has some value in predicting the types of injuries that the patient may have suffered. In some EMS systems, diagnostic protocols are partially based on scene descriptions and the mechanism of injury, for example, the speed of the accident, bumper incursion, interior damage, and height of fall.[4]

### Extrication and scene management

Extricating patients from difficult places, including the inside of automobiles, is a skill which requires specialized equipment and training. In general, the role of EMS personnel is limited to patient care. In some systems, however, prehospital caregivers are trained to participate in extrication and search-and-rescue. Always, the patient is the first priority after the scene is deemed safe.

If EMS personnel will be involved in extrication and search-and-rescue activities, they must be thoroughly trained and familiar with the use and operation of the necessary specialized equipment. Appropriate protective gear must be worn at all times. Failure to do so is the primary cause of accidents at rescue scenes.[3] Of course, all EMS personnel must use universal precautions when dealing with patients to avoid inadvertent contamination.

## GENERAL PRINCIPLES OF PREHOSPITAL FRACTURE TREATMENT

Prehospital personnel are taught to prioritize fractures.[2] The first priority is spinal fracture; the second, fracture of the head, rib cage, or pelvis; and third, fractures of the extremities with lower extremity fractures and those of joints being the most important.

They are also taught to move patients with orthopedic injuries as little as possible and to always monitor circulation, motor response, and sensory response (CMS) before and after splinting.

In general, prehospital workers are not permitted to reduce dislocations on any angulated fracture that is not severe. They are also told, "When in doubt, splint" (Table 2-1) (see exception below).

The physician must keep in mind that the backboard is the ultimate splint and that, under many circumstances, the use of one part of the body to splint another is perfectly acceptable care for the prehospital critical patient.

### Prehospital reduction of fractures and dislocations

As stated above, in general, prehospital crews are not allowed to reduce fractures and dislocations. The only exception to this rule is in systems where travel time is long and care will be delayed, prehospital crews are allowed to reduce certain injuries if the patient's CMS status is compromised. This should occur rarely and when transport time would exceed one hour. In general, it is best to "splint the patient as he lies." Some fractures and dislocations unintentionally "self-reduce" with standard care measures.

Except for fractures involving joints, prehospital personnel should be allowed to straighten most badly angulated long-bone fractures prior to splinting and transport. One attempt should be made, and it should be done with minimal force. All realignment attempts should be preceded and followed by CMS checks, and no attempt should be made in the face of strong patient resistance. This "straightening" should not be considered reduction of the fracture or dislocation.

Should the patient's pulse disappear with splint application, we recommend a single attempt to adjust or remove the splint and reapply it while maintaining fracture stabili-

**Table 2-1.** Splints

| Injury | Splint |
| --- | --- |
| Clavicle fracture | Sling or sling and swath |
| A-C separation | Sling or sling and swath |
| Shoulder dislocation | |
| *Adducted position* | Sling and swath |
| *Abducted position* | Airplane, vacuum, or ladder splint |
| Proximal humerus fracture | Sling or sling and swath |
| Midshaft humerus fracture | Pillow splint or sling and swath with board splint |
| Elbow fracture/dislocation | Pillow, ladder, or sling and swath with board splint |
| Forearm and wrist fracture/dislocation | Pillow, board, plastic foam, SAM, or air or Robert Jones splint |
| Hand fracture/dislocation | Roller or self-adhering gauze |
| Finger fracture/dislocation | Rigid aluminum, SAM, or tongue blade splint or "buddy taping" |
| Pelvic fracture | PASG |
| Hip fracture | Traction splint or pillow and backboard |
| Hip dislocation | Pillows and backboard |
| Femur fracture | Traction splint or PASG |
| Knee fracture/dislocation | Vacuum, pillow, cardboard or padded board splint |
| Lower leg fracture/dislocation | Vacuum, pillow, air, SAM, board, or traction or Robert Jones splint |
| Ankle and foot fracture/dislocation | Vacuum, air, pillow, or Robert Jones splint |
| Toe fracture/dislocation | "Buddy taping" |

Key: A-C = Acromial-clavicular
PASG = Pneumatic antishock garment
SAM = Neoprene-covered malleable aluminum splint

zation and alignment. If this effort does not restore circulation, we recommend splinting the extremity and alerting the receiving physician to the problem.

**Rationale for splint application**

There are several reasons to apply a splint.[1,11] The first is to avoid movement of the fracture site. This immobilization in turn often decreases pain, bleeding, and damage to the surrounding soft tissues, including muscles, nerves and vessels. Additionally, splinting may prevent a closed fracture from becoming an open one. Finally, splinting allows for easier patient transfer.

A splint should be applied in such a manner as to immobilize the joint above and below the injury site. All rigid splints must be generously padded to prevent further injury, such as nerve or skin damage.

If the fracture is open, sterile dressings should be applied to prevent further contamination, the extremity should be elevated, and cold packs should be applied whenever possible. In the rare circumstance that severe bleeding is associated with an open fracture, direct pressure should be applied. During repositioning of a fracture for transfer or when applying a traction splint, the ends of an open fracture may inadvertently recede into the wound. This should be noted and reported to the receiving physician.

Thorough splinting should be done before moving any stable patient. Conversely, complicated, time-consuming splinting should not be done on critical or unstable patients.

Humankind has been treating fractures and dislocations for thousands of years. There are many different approaches to splinting, some of which are archaic and, as such, are either no longer used or used so sporadically so as to be beyond the scope of this text. This chapter covers only those techniques which would typically be in use today. For the purposes of this chapter, specific recommendations as to which of several choices of appropriate splints for a given injury will be avoided unless there is a clear-cut advantage of one splint over the other.

## SPECIFIC TREATMENT OF SKELETAL INJURIES BY ANATOMY
### Cervical, thoracic, and lumbosacral spine injuries

Prehospital workers must always be alert for the possibility of spinal injuries. History consistent with neck injury, intoxication-associated closed-head injury, midline neck tenderness, neck pain, a direct blow to the neck, and neurologic findings are all important factors that can lead one to suspect that the patient has sustained a spinal injury.

The backboard serves as an excellent total-body splint. With the appropriate securing straps applied, it adequately immobilizes the thoracic and lumbosacral (L) spine. For the cervical (C)-spine injuries, however, additional splinting measures are needed due to the C-spine's increased mobility and vulnerability. For extrication purposes, the short-board technique is used for cervical immobilization.[12]

The most common form of splinting in use today for the cervical spine is probably that of lateral or *V blocks*. These can be used alone or in combination with the *C-collar* (Figs. 2-2 to 2-4). The physician must understand that C-collars are *not* intended to be immobilization devices; they are extrication devices. Even when properly applied, C-collars allow significant movement of the C-spine.[12-16] The patient must not be considered adequately immobilized with the use of a C-collar alone. The patient should be

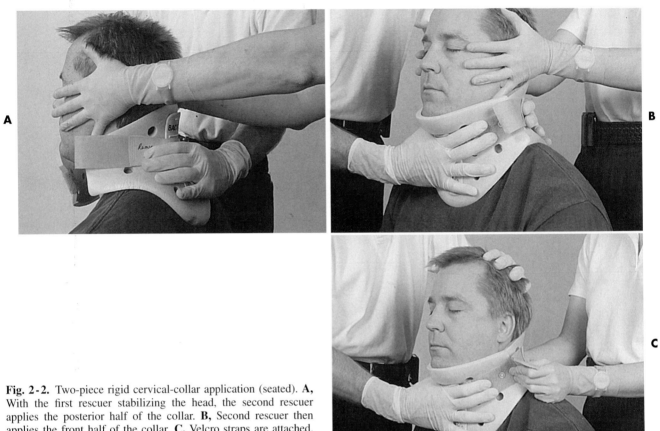

**Fig. 2-2.** Two-piece rigid cervical-collar application (seated). **A,** With the first rescuer stabilizing the head, the second rescuer applies the posterior half of the collar. **B,** Second rescuer then applies the front half of the collar. **C,** Velcro straps are attached. Note: Maintain in line cervical-spine stabilization throughout the application process.

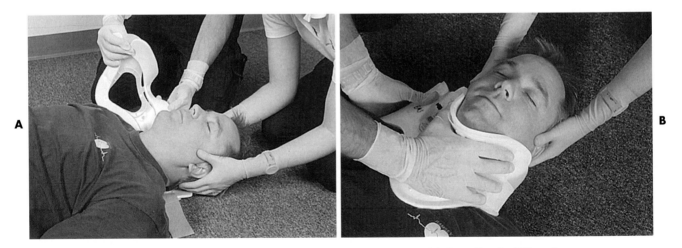

**Fig. 2-3.** Application of one-piece cervical-collar (Stifneck—Laerdal, Long Beach, CA), patient supine. **A,** Slide the back portion of the collar behind the patient's neck. Fold the Velcro loop inward on top of the foam padding to prevent it from collecting debris. Once the loop is visible, position the chin piece and attach the strap. **B,** An alternative method is to start by positioning the chin piece and then sliding the back portion of the collar behind the patient's neck.

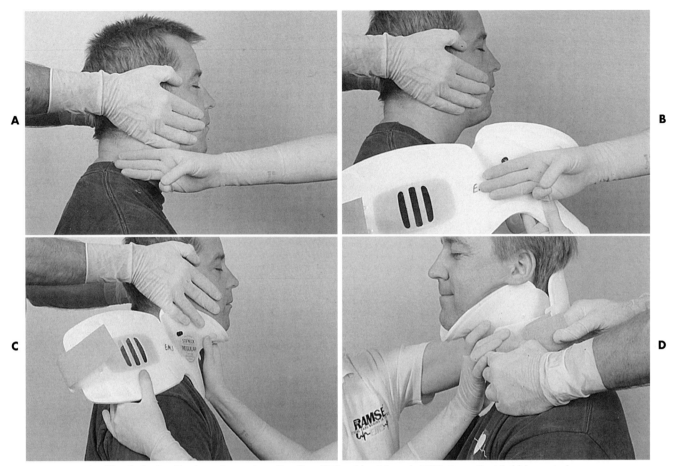

**Fig. 2-4.** Application of one piece C-collar (Stifneck), sitting. **A,** With the patient held in neutral position by the first rescuer, the second rescuer uses the fingers to visually measure the distance from the shoulder to the chin. **B,** The key dimension on the collar is the distance between the sizing post (black fastener) and the lower edge of the rigid plastic encircling band (not the foam padding). **C,** With the patient's head held in neutral alignment, position the chin piece by sliding the collar up the chest wall. Make sure the chin is well supported by the chin piece and that the chin extends far enough onto the chin piece to cover at least the central fastener. Difficulty in positioning the chin piece may indicate the need for a shorter collar. **D,** Recheck the position of the patient's head and collar for proper alignment. Make sure that the patient's chin covers at least the central fastener in the chin piece. If it doesn't, tighten the collar further until proper support is obtained. Select the next-smallest size collar if further tightening of the collar may cause the patient's neck to become extended.

considered to have optimal stabilization only when properly secured to a backboard with an accepted form of lateral protection (Fig. 2-5).

Many brands of C-collars are available, but there are only two types, the one-piece and the two-piece collar. The former is gaining popularity for several reasons primarily because it is thought to provide better immobilization. Other advantages of a one-piece collar include its availability in a wide range of sizes that can be more specific for the patient. In addition, it can be stored flat and, at the scene, nested on a rescuer's arm (multiple sizes carried around the arm by wrapping the devices concentrically around each other) thereby giving the rescuer many choices of sizes to apply to the patient.

Besides V-blocks, patients can also be adequately secured with *horseshoe blankets* and disposable cardboard lateral blocks (Fig. 2-6). These techniques require banding of the forehead to the lateral supports. This can be done with Velcro or two-inch-wide adhesive tape. Chin straps are also used in some EMS systems. With their use, prehospital personnel must be aware of the increased potential for aspiration, should the patient vomit. Training for this possibility must include loosening the chin strap, turning the patient to the side, and applying suction. Body-length vacuum splints may also be used as backboards and have the added advantage of being able to splint the patient as he lies (Fig. 2-7). They are easy to transport but are somewhat expensive and fragile.

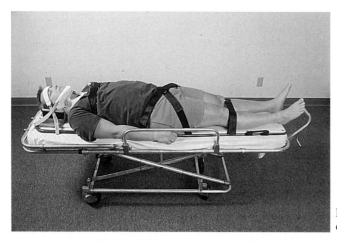

**Fig. 2-5.** Patient properly immobilized using a backboard, cervical collar, V-block, and straps.

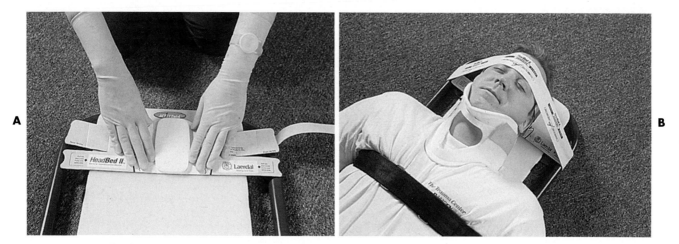

**Fig. 2-6.** Disposable V-Block (Headbed II—Laerdal, Long Beach, CA). **A,** Device is applied to backboard. **B,** Patient properly secured to backboard and device.

Whatever method of immobilization is selected by the EMS caregivers, they must remember that manual stabilization must be applied until the C-collar, V-block, and backboard are secured. These devices must not be removed until it is determined by the receiving physician that the patient does not have a spinal injury. This determination by the physician should include, at the very minimum, an examination of the patient and, if necessary, the obtaining of radiographs while the patient is still immobilized.

There are many different ways to place a patient on a backboard. These include the logroll (Fig. 2-8), scoop stretcher, and various lifts. The logroll has recently been questioned because it may cause movement of the lower thoracic and upper L-spine.[15] It remains the procedure most commonly used today because an acceptable alternative has not yet been developed.

Spinal immobilization with items such as the short backboard (Fig. 2-9) and the Kendrick Extrication Device (KED) (Fig. 2-10) has proved invaluable in many extrication circumstances. The KED also allows the patient's extrication through the roof of a vehicle while the spine

remains immobilized. We recommend that a short backboard, KED, or similar device be used whenever possible during motor-vehicle extrications.

Most EMS systems routinely apply spinal immobilization, including backboards. Many teams, for instance, will automatically apply a backboard on any patient involved in high-speed motor vehicle accidents or falls greater than a specific height. Some EMS systems have begun using more specific indicators for spinal management.[17] If the patient has no neck pain or tenderness, has normal vital signs, is not intoxicated, is not at the extremes of age, has no focal neurologic signs, and has no altered LOC, then a backboard may not be necessary.

Backboard application and C-spine immobilization should not be considered benign procedures. Possible complications include excessive neck extension in adults and excessive neck flexion in children (Figs. 2-11 and 2-12).[18,19] Additional complications may include impaired pulmonary function, motion during application, patient discomfort, missed posterior injuries, prolonged scene times and increased emergency department times and expense.

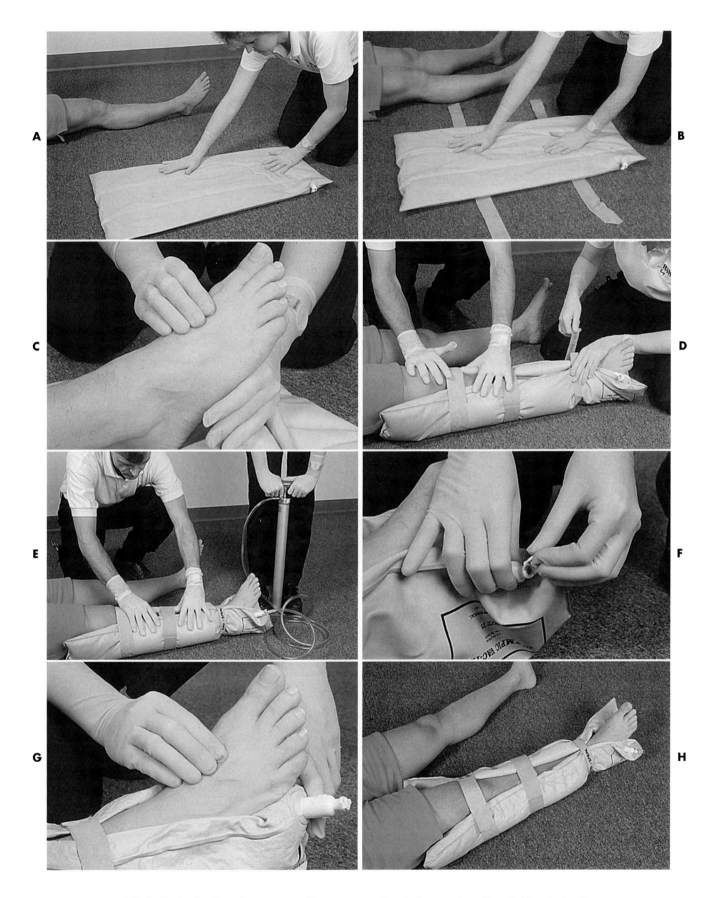

**Fig. 2-7.** Application of a vacuum splint to an extremity. **A,** Lay out the splint, shaking the beads to a uniform layer. **B,** Place Velcro straps under the splint. **C,** Check circulation, motor response, and sensory response (CMS). **D,** Mold the splint around the extremity while attaching the Velcro straps. **E,** Remove the valve cover and insert the connector into the valve and begin operating the vacuum pump. The second rescuer continues to mold the splint during pumping action. **F,** Disconnect the pump and reinsert the valve cap. **G,** Recheck CMS. **H,** Properly applied vacuum splint.

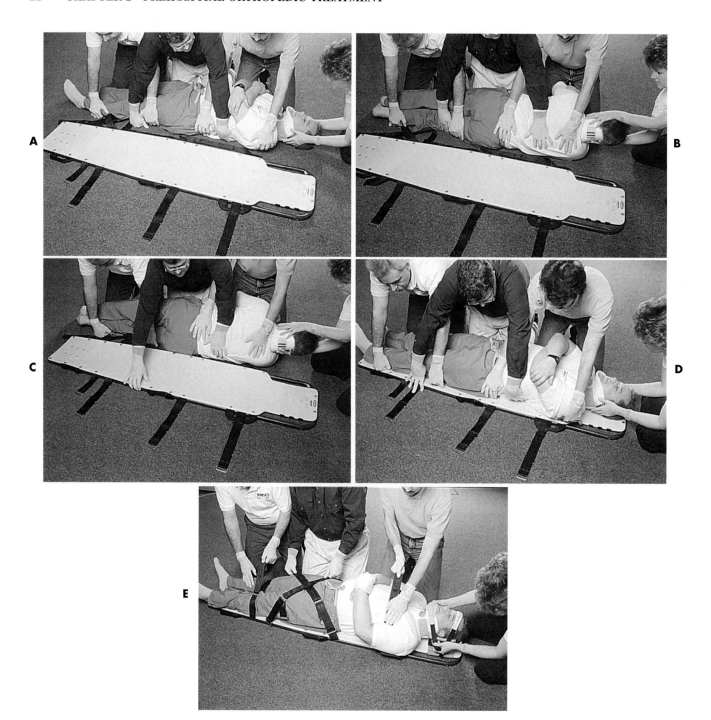

**Fig. 2-8.** Application of backboard by logroll. **A,** Apply a cervical collar. Caregiver at head maintains proper C-spine alignment and control. Remaining caregivers prepare for roll. **B,** On the command of the caregiver at the head, roll the patient to one side. **C,** The backboard is moved into place. **D,** Again, on command of the caregiver at the head, lower the patient onto the board. **E,** Patient properly secured to the backboard.

### General management of upper extremity fractures and dislocations

Prehospital personnel may find it difficult to distinguish one upper extremity injury from another. For example, without a radiograph, it can be difficult to distinguish a clavicle fracture from an acromial-clavicular (A-C) separation from a shoulder dislocation. Fortunately, the prehospital treat-

ment of these injuries varies little. Likewise, the complication rates tend to be low and are not generally affected by different prehospital splinting techniques.

**Clavicle.** These fractures are splinted primarily for pain relief. A simple sling or a sling and swath are the preferred methods. The older technique of applying a *figure-of-eight* or a *clavicular strap* is used less frequently and is no longer recommended by many authorities.

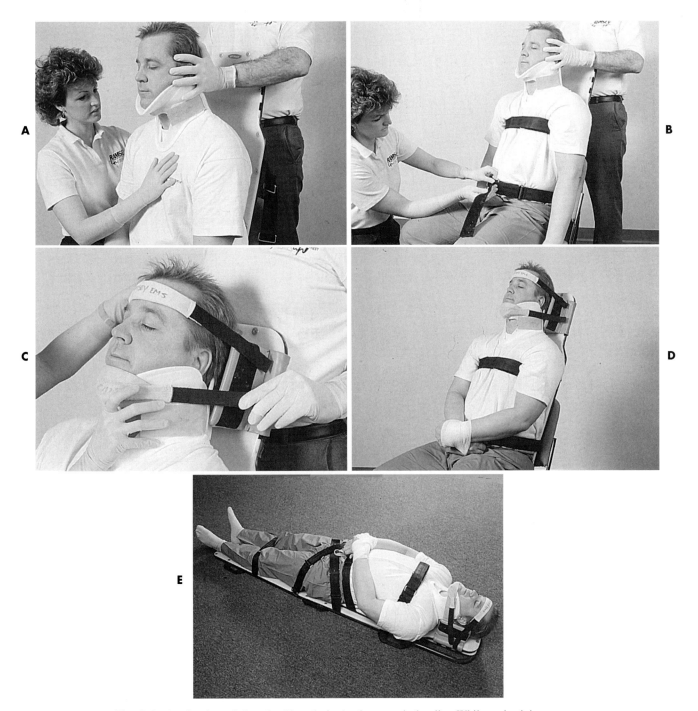

**Fig. 2-9.** Application of short backboard. **A,** Apply a cervical collar. While maintaining proper stabilization by rescuer 1, rescuer 2 moves the short board into place. **B,** Rescuer 2 applies the straps. **C,** The head and chin are secured to the spine board and V-block. The patient and the short backboard are moved as a unit to a long spine board. **D,** Patient properly secured to the short board. **E,** The patient and short board properly secured to a long backboard.

**Acromial-clavicular separation.** These injuries are particularly confusing to prehospital personnel. They are frequently mistaken for shoulder dislocations, particularly when the A-C separation is of the Grade 3 variety. Again, the exact identification of this injury is not important in the prehospital arena; the injury can be adequately treated with a sling or a sling and swath.

**Shoulder dislocations and fractures.** The treatment of a shoulder dislocation depends on whether the arm can be adducted to the body. If it can, then a sling and swath is the preferred method of treatment. However, if adduction is not possible, the use of an *airplane splint* is appropriate. Several types of airplane splints are in current use. The older, padded-board splint is being replaced by the newer

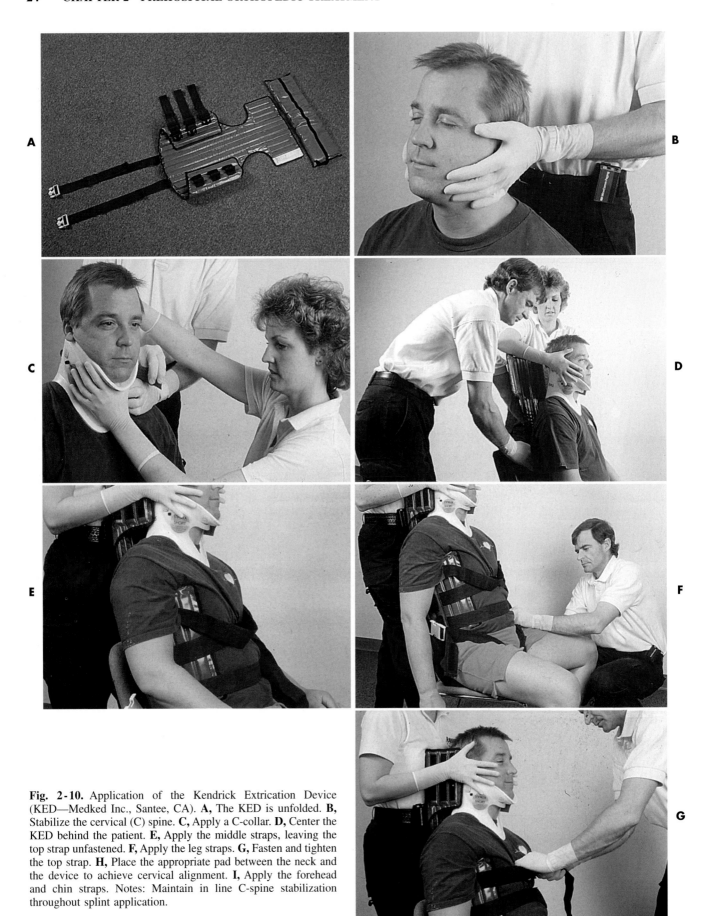

**Fig. 2-10.** Application of the Kendrick Extrication Device (KED—Medked Inc., Santee, CA). **A,** The KED is unfolded. **B,** Stabilize the cervical (C) spine. **C,** Apply a C-collar. **D,** Center the KED behind the patient. **E,** Apply the middle straps, leaving the top strap unfastened. **F,** Apply the leg straps. **G,** Fasten and tighten the top strap. **H,** Place the appropriate pad between the neck and the device to achieve cervical alignment. **I,** Apply the forehead and chin straps. Notes: Maintain in line C-spine stabilization throughout splint application.

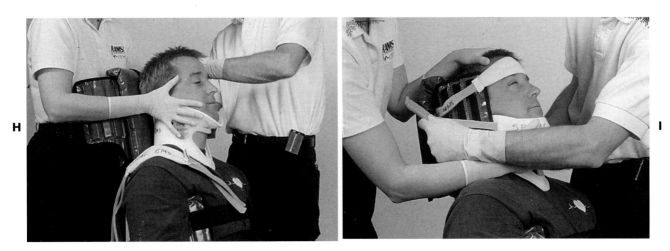

**Fig. 2-10, cont'd.** For legend see opposite page.

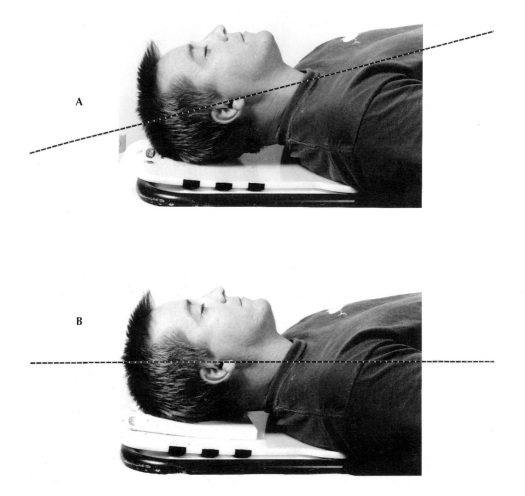

**Fig. 2-11.** Demonstration of backboard-caused malalignment problems. **A,** Hyperextension of the neck caused by a backboard in an adult. **B,** Correction of hyperextension by utilizing an occipital pad.

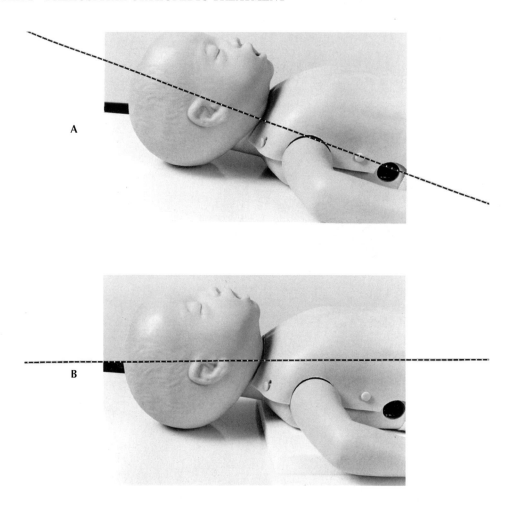

**Fig. 2-12. A,** Hyperflexion of the neck caused by a backboard in a child. **B,** Correction of hyperflexion by utilizing a pad beneath the shoulders.

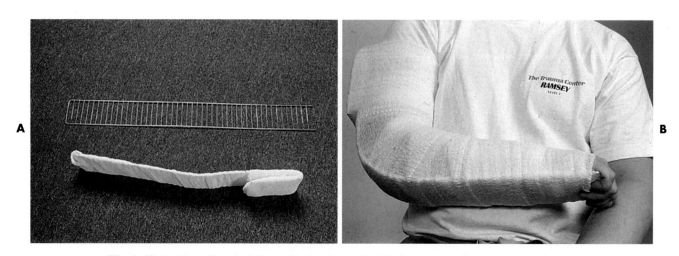

**Fig. 2-13.** Ladder splint. **A,** Splint padded and unpadded. **B,** Long arm splint properly applied to patient.

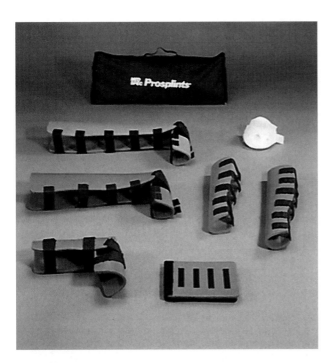

**Fig. 2-14.** Molded closed foam splints (Prosplint—MedSpec Emergency Products Group, Charlotte, NC) (From Emergency Medical Supplies and Vehicle Parts. St. Paul: Road Rescue, Inc., 1991.)

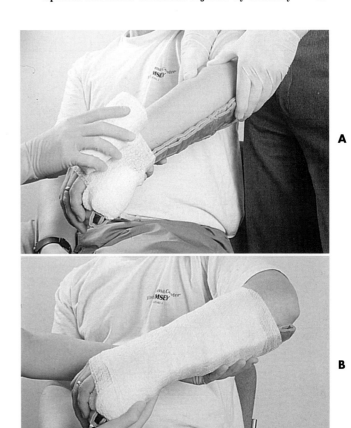

**Fig. 2-15.** Malleable neoprene-covered splints (SAM splint). **A,** Examples of SAM splint. **B,** Typical application.

vacuum splint, which can be shaped to maintain comfortable adduction. Wire ladder splints can also be used to achieve a similar result. Shoulder or proximal humerus fractures are best treated with a simple sling or a sling and swath.

**Humerus fractures (midshaft).** Midshaft humerus fractures are typically treated with a sling and swath. Distal humerus fractures can be adequately treated by first placing a pillow or pad between the lower arm and the body and then splinting the arm against the body. A sling and swath with well-padded board splints is an acceptable alternative. Because of common vascular complications, it is especially important for prehospital personnel to document CMS checks before and after splinting when this injury is suspected.

**Elbow fractures and dislocations.** The elbow is best splinted with the pillow method described above for the treatment of distal humerus fracture. Alternatively, a well-padded board splint with a sling and swath or a wire ladder splint may be used effectively (Fig. 2-13). Again, good documentation of CMS before and after splinting is important.

**Forearm and wrist fractures and dislocations.** There are many different approaches to the splinting of forearm fractures. One of the best is simply to place the forearm on a pillow and then secure the pillow to the body. Rigid wood, rigid foam splints (such as Prosplints) (Fig. 2-14), vacuum splints, and neoprene-covered malleable aluminum (SAM) splints (Seaberg Co., Inc., South Beach, Oregon) (Fig. 2-15) have also been used. Cotton batting secured with elastic bandages (Robert Jones splint) is also used on occasion. Some services employ inflatable air splints (Fig. 2-16). There are several problems associated with the use of these splints, such as over- and underinflation.[7,11] The former can result in CMS

compromise. The latter often results secondary to leaking. Overheating and sweating can also occur. The reuse of these splints introduces the possibility of mouthpiece contamination. For this reason, a disposable extension, such as a piece of suction canister connection tubing, should be used routinely when inflating these splints. For obvious reasons, oxygen should never be used to inflate these splints. There is the additional concern of spontaneous overinflation when a patient is brought to altitude (see "Air Transport" later in this chapter). They are also inherently difficult to use in cold climates as they are made of plastic, which stiffens as the temperature falls.[20]

**Hand and finger fractures and dislocations.** The best and most common way to deal with metacarpal fractures is to pack the palm of the hand with a ball of roller gauze and then use a roll of self-adhering strip gauze or an elastic bandage to wrap the hand in the appropriate position of function. Rigid aluminum, wood (tongue blade), and SAM splints, as well as buddy taping (taping the injured finger to an adjacent finger), are all used for splinting finger injuries. Whenever possible, jewelry should be removed from the fingers.

### General management of lower extremity fractures and dislocations

Lower extremity injuries are typically more serious than upper extremity injuries. Pelvic and femur fractures may in

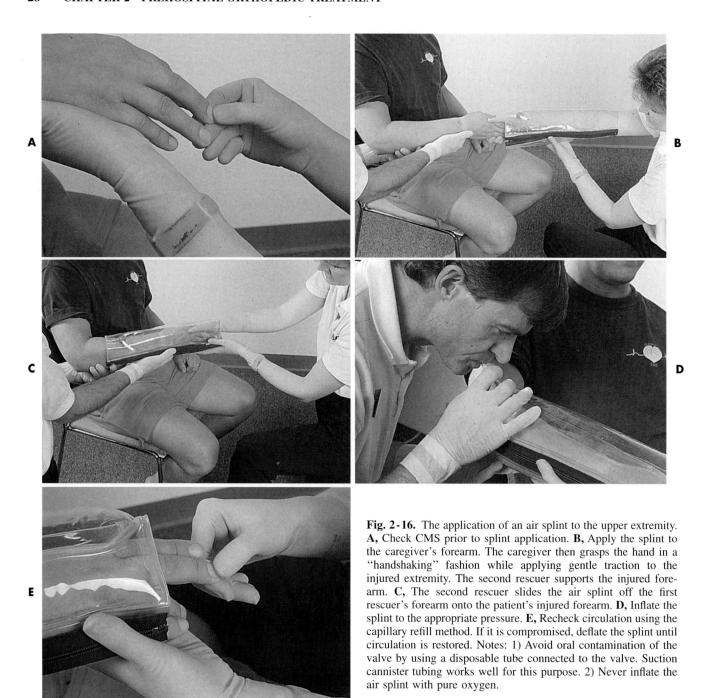

**Fig. 2-16.** The application of an air splint to the upper extremity. **A,** Check CMS prior to splint application. **B,** Apply the splint to the caregiver's forearm. The caregiver then grasps the hand in a "handshaking" fashion while applying gentle traction to the injured extremity. The second rescuer supports the injured forearm. **C,** The second rescuer slides the air splint off the first rescuer's forearm onto the patient's injured forearm. **D,** Inflate the splint to the appropriate pressure. **E,** Recheck circulation using the capillary refill method. If it is compromised, deflate the splint until circulation is restored. Notes: 1) Avoid oral contamination of the valve by using a disposable tube connected to the valve. Suction cannister tubing works well for this purpose. 2) Never inflate the air splint with pure oxygen.

fact be life-threatening. This must always be remembered when choosing a splinting technique. In unstable patients with short transfer times, prolonged meticulous splinting at the scene is inappropriate in a patient who is properly secured to a backboard.

**Pelvic fractures.** A pelvic fracture is one of the most life-threatening orthopedic injuries seen in the emergency department. Great force is usually required to fracture the pelvis, and since the pelvis is near so many vulnerable soft tissue structures, including the bladder, major blood vessels, and kidneys, pelvic fractures are often associated with other life-threatening injuries. Also, pelvic bones themselves, when fractured, can develop bleeding that is difficult to control. The most immediate concern of prehospital personnel is the treatment of shock or potential shock.[20] Along with other necessary stabilization maneuvers, patients with suspected pelvic fractures should have two large bore IV lines placed and fluid resuscitation begun en route. Immediate extrication, application of a backboard, and rapid transportation are the key to survival.

Besides the backboard, the most commonly used splint for this type of injury is the PASG (Fig. 2-1). Many training centers teach EMS personnel to consider the backboard and PASG as a unit; that is, whenever a backboard is applied, the PASG should be applied at the same time. This policy may conserve time spent at the scene and also prevent having to apply the PASG while enroute in an ambulance after the patient suddenly develops shock. Of course, the PASG is not inflated unless indicated.

**Hip fractures.** This injury is usually apparent from the characteristic foreshortening and external rotation of the extremity, which every prehospital caregiver should be able to recognize. They are most often treated by application of backboard. If there are no contraindications, patients with hip fractures should be transported in a position that makes them most comfortable, with pillows used as padding.

Some EMS systems allow the application of traction splints (see "Femur Fractures" below). Patients with hip fractures often report pain relief with the use of these splints. This appears to be especially true in young patients with hip fractures secondary to violent trauma.

**Hip dislocations.** In and of themselves, hip dislocations are orthopedic emergencies that require relatively rapid reduction. Because of the force required to dislocate the hip, these fractures are often associated with life-threatening injuries.

The most common form of hip dislocation a prehospital worker is likely to see is the posterior type secondary to the distal femur striking the dashboard and the resultant force driving the hip posteriorly out of the acetabulum. Generally, this dislocation is readily distinguishable, with characteristic flexion of the hip and knee and internal rotation of the leg. Hip dislocations are usually treated by applying a backboard and splinting of the affected leg to the unaffected leg, using the pillows as pads, and trying to make the patient as comfortable as possible. It is important to get such patients to the hospital in a timely fashion.

**Femur fractures.** As with pelvic and hip fractures, midshaft femur fractures can be life-threatening. These are also typically high impact injuries. Several units of blood can hemorrhage into the thigh without noticeable increase in circumference.[20] These fractures appear to be particularly hazardous in children. Bilateral midshaft fractures are especially dangerous. Whenever possible, midshaft femur fractures should have IV lines established and fluid resuscitation begun in a manner that does not delay the transportation of the patient. Many EMS services apply the PASG more or less routinely for stabilization of femur fractures.

Traction splinting is the preferred method of treating stable patients with femur fractures. Because a patient with a femur fracture may present to the emergency department untreated, all emergency departments should be equipped with a traction splint, and emergency physicians and their staff should be thoroughly trained in its application. Inappropriately applied, the device can cause soft-tissue damage, severe pain and further aggravate the injury.

The HARE traction splint (Fig. 2-17) is the traction device most commonly used today. It is a refinement of the outdated Thomas half-ring splint that is still used by some services. Another modern version of the traction splint is the Sager splint (Fig. 2-18), which is quite popular in some areas of the country. Older techniques, such as single and double padded-board splinting of the affected leg to the unaffected leg, are outdated and are rarely used except in extreme emergency or wilderness settings.

In unstable patients, it is appropriate to employ the PASG alone to stabilize femur fractures. In this type of patient, the additional time required to place traction splints is not warranted.

A frequently asked question is whether a traction splint and the PASG can be used together. This is rarely necessary. The PASG, although inferior to the traction device, is an adequate splint for femur stabilization. If used with the PASG, the traction splint must always be applied over the PASG, never under it. It is often observed that when both are used in combination, neither is optimally effective. For this reason, we recommend that they not be used together.

**Knee fractures and dislocations.** Distinguishing the various types of knee injuries seems particularly problematic for EMS personnel. Knee dislocations are obviously limb-threatening; as such, they require rapid field treatment and transport. Typically, these injuries are treated by applying a backboard in combination with a variety of other splinting techniques, including vacuum, pillow and padded rigid splints. Splinting of the injured leg to the uninjured leg is also used occasionally. Skiers are often treated with disposable cardboard splints or nondisposable, padded, foldable wood splints (Jiffy splints).[21] The latter are usually applied with lacing or Velcro straps. Prehospital personnel are taught to splint knees injuries "as they lie" to avoid further injury, especially to the popliteal artery.

**Patellar subluxations and dislocations.** Patellar subluxation requires special mention because prehospital personnel frequently mistake this injury for a knee dislocation. A patellar subluxation, of course, is a relatively minor problem, whereas a knee dislocation is potentially catastrophic. As stated elsewhere in this text, the maneuver for the reduction of patellar subluxation consists of extending the leg to 0° while applying lateral pressure to the patella. Often, the patella relocates with simple leg extension.[20] Thus, this injury is often inadvertently reduced at the scene.

It is important for the emergency physician to thoroughly examine a patient suspected of having a patellar subluxation. The *apprehension sign* (moving the patella in the direction of the subluxation) is particularly helpful at delineating the patient who may have had a subluxation inadvertently reduced by prehospital personnel. The diagnosis is also aided if the history supplied by the patient or prehospital caregivers includes mention of a "bump" that was out of place on the patient's leg and immediate pain relief upon straightening of the leg.

**Lower leg fractures.** Severely angulated tibia-fibula fractures must be straightened prior to patient transfer.

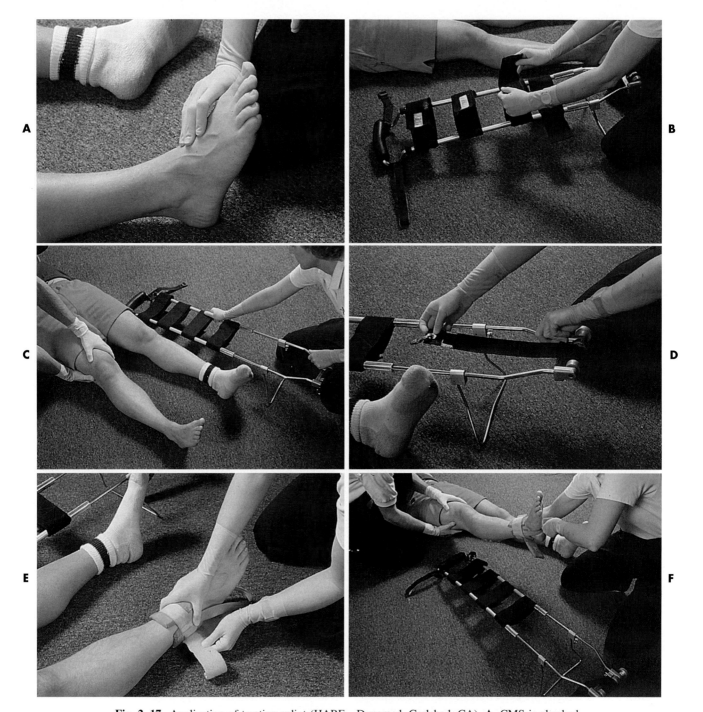

**Fig. 2-17.** Application of traction splint (HARE—Dynamed, Carlsbad, CA). **A,** CMS is checked prior to application of the splint. **B,** Properly prepare the splint by loosening the locking devices and preparing the straps for placement. **C,** Measure the appropriate length of the splint on the opposite side of the fracture. Place the ischial bar directly against the ischium (not the buttocks). The splint should extend approximately six inches beyond the foot. Lock the splint again and bring it to the side of the injury. **D,** The stand is extended and approximately 12 inches of the traction strap is released. **E,** Apply the ankle hitch with the comfort pillows adjusted as necessary. **F,** With an assistant stabilizing the fracture site, apply traction to the limb, and lift the leg approximately 20° to 30° off the horizontal plane. **G,** Place the splint under the leg tightly against the ischium. **H,** Secure the ischial strap but not so tightly as to impair circulation. **I,** Attach the ankle hitch to the traction strap. **J,** Apply traction until the patient experiences relief of pain or the splint traction equals that of the manual traction. **K,** Apply the securing straps. **L,** Recheck CMS. If compromised, the straps are readjusted with particular attention being paid to the ischial strap.

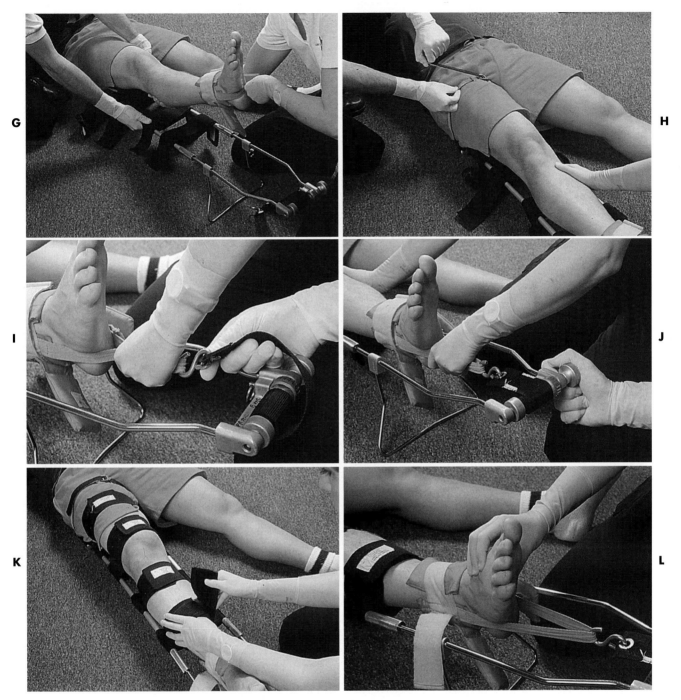

**Fig. 2-17, cont'd.** For legend see opposite page.

Then, the fracture is splinted using a variety of techniques (alone or in combination), such as pillow, air, vacuum, rigid formed aluminum and rigid foam splints. The aforementioned Jiffy splint, a disposable cardboard splint, or a Robert Jones splint may also be used.[21] While the splint was clearly not designed for this purpose, some EMS systems allow the use of traction splints to stabilize mid-shaft tibial-fibular fractures. If used in this manner, the amount of traction applied should be significantly less than when used for femur traction. Traction splinting may be particularly useful when both the femur and the tibia are fractured. Many prehospital personnel report success with the technique.

As previously stated, an open fracture should be dressed with a sterile dressing and straightened as necessary. On straightening, it is not uncommon that the protruding bone fragments will recede into the wound. If this should occur, the EMS caregivers must inform the receiving physician that bone was initially protruding from the wound.

**Ankle, foot and toe fractures, dislocations, and sprains.** Most of these injuries are best treated with pillow splints (Fig. 2-19). Air splints, rigid splinting,

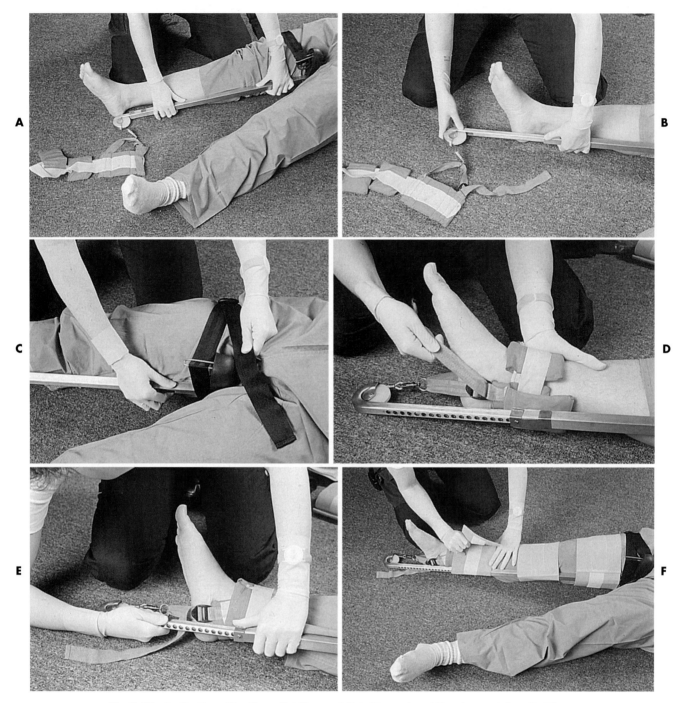

**Fig. 2-18.** Application of traction splint (Sager—Minto Research and Development, Inc., Redding, CA). **A,** Place the splint medially with the top of the splint resting against the ischial tuberosity. **B,** Unlock and lengthen the splint to a point four inches beyond the heel. **C,** Fasten and tighten the thigh strap. **D,** Apply the ankle hitch. **E,** Unlock and extend the splint again to achieve the desired traction as read on the pulley wheel. **F,** Apply the securing straps at the thigh, lower thigh, knee, and lower leg. Notes: After application, strap the patient's ankles and feet together and secure the patient to the spine board.

and Robert Jones splints (cotton batting secured with elastic bandages) may also be used. An isolated toe fracture can be splinted by "buddy taping" it to the adjacent toe with adequate padding between them.

## SPECIAL CONSIDERATIONS
### Airway versus cervical spine management

"Open the airway while maintaining C-spine immobilization" is a phrase heard everyday in EMS education. Clearly, C-spine stabilization is important, but it is possible to be so

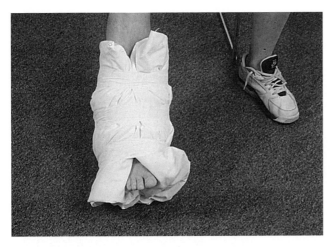

**Fig. 2-19.** Properly applied pillow splint.

concerned about C-spine immobilization that airway management is compromised.[1]

Given all trauma scenes, a very small number of patients will have C-spine injuries. Of those, a smaller proportion will have C-spine injuries with neurologic deficit. A still smaller fraction will have C-spine injuries, initially without neurologic deficit and later with neurologic deficit. The effect that a prehospital caregiver has on the development of neurologic deficit in a patient with C-spine injury is unclear. In fact, it has never been shown conclusively that any action of a prehospital caregiver, with regard to C-spine management, has any effect whatsoever on neurologic outcome. Conversely, a very significant number of patients suffering loss of consciousness from trauma will have some element of airway compromise. Whether or not this airway compromise is properly handled in the field often makes the difference between a dead or severely brain damaged patient and a healthy, functioning member of society.

A good rule of thumb is to manage C-spine injuries as carefully as possible, but to remember that the airway *must* be established and maintained. All commonly employed airway maneuvers cause some degree of C-spine displacement.[22] Accepting that there should be no *unnecessary* movement of the C-spine, it must be emphasized that patients with inadequately managed airways will often be permanently brain damaged and those with unestablished airways will die.

Physicians must be careful not to overemphasize C-spine immobilization to EMS personnel to the detriment of appropriate airway management.

## Amputations

Amputations can be life-threatening, but they rarely are.[1] The immediate concern in the field is to stop the bleeding. Most of the time, this has been done by the time EMS arrives. If it has not, hemorrhage control can almost universally be accomplished by applying direct pressure. Once the bleeding has been controlled, pressure dressings

may be applied. These dressings must be checked frequently because they are often ineffective. Tourniquets should almost always be avoided; their use should be reserved for the very rare case in which bleeding cannot be controlled by direct pressure or when the scarcity of caregivers demands their use. If a tourniquet is applied, it must be clearly marked, and the time it was applied must be indicated. Tourniquets should be released every 15 minutes to allow for tissue perfusion.

The amputated part should be cleaned of gross contamination by flushing with sterile saline and then wrapping in saline-moistened sterile gauze.[23,24] Take care not to soak the gauze so as to not cause tissue maceration. The wrapped part should then be placed in a plastic bag or rigid container (sterile if possible). For small parts, sterile urinalysis containers work for this purpose. This container, in turn, is placed in a larger container of an ice water solution. Under no circumstances should the part be allowed to come into direct contact with the solution or the ice. Dry ice should never be used.

The stump should be likewise cleaned of gross contamination by flushing with sterile saline. It should then be dressed with saline-moistened sterile gauze.

The time the amputation occurred as well as the total warm and cold ischemic times should be recorded and relayed to the emergency physician.

Recent advances in microsurgical technique have greatly improved the chances for replantation of many amputated parts.[25] In general, an amputated part can withstand up to six hours of warm ischemia or up to 24 hours of cold ischemia and still possibly be successfully replanted. All amputated parts should be found and transported to the hospital whenever possible. Parts that would typically not be replanted include single digits in adults (with the exception of the thumb), lower extremities, burned or frostbitten parts, parts suffering prolonged ischemia, proximal forearm amputations, and crush injuries.

## Backboards

The use of standard backboards for maintaining neutral C-spine alignment has recently been the subject of concern in both adults and children.

In adults, application of a backboard tends to cause a few degrees of neck extension (Fig. 2-11). To prevent this, some EMS systems use padding at the occiput, allowing field workers to visually gauge whether the neck is in neutral position.

Young children, by contrast, tend to experience neck flexion when lying flat on a backboard (Fig. 2-12).[18] This is because a young child's head is relatively large when compared with the rest of the body. Two approaches have been proposed for applying backboards in children. One is to place the patient's occiput in a 1.5-inch deep cutout at the head of the backboard. The other approach is to put foam padding or blankets under the shoulders or the entire body of the patient and again allowing field personnel to determine when neutral position is attained. The latter solution seems more practical and is beginning to be employed by some services.

### Football helmet removal

The removal of the football helmet results in significant neck extension when the patient is also wearing shoulder pads (Fig. 2-20). Recent literature strongly condemns the removal of football helmets in the field.[26,27] A helmet should be removed in the field *only* if the patient is not wearing shoulder pads or is experiencing respiratory difficulty. In the latter event, removal of the face mask should be attempted first. This can be accomplished by cutting the

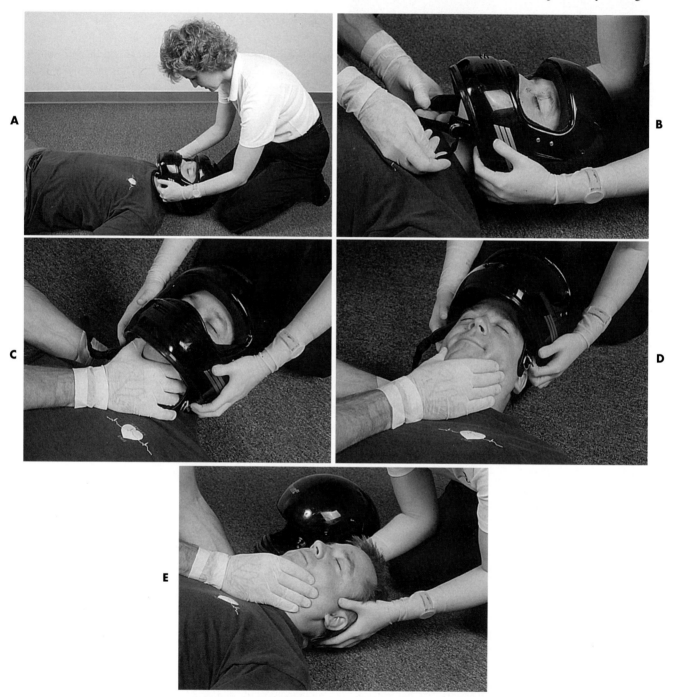

**Fig. 2-20.** Motorcycle helmet removal. **A**, First rescuer stabilizes helmet and neck. **B**, Second rescuer cuts or unfastens the neck strap. **C**, Second rescuer places one hand on the mandible and the other on the occiput. **D**, First rescuer removes helmet spreading it laterally. **E**, After the helmet is removed, the first rescuer takes over stabilization by placing hands on both sides of head. Notes: 1) Full-faced helmets require removal of glasses and the tilting of the helmet backward to clear the nose.

plastic clips that keep many modern face masks in place or by using a bolt cutter to cut the mask itself. It is further recommended that a patient suspected of having neck fractures should have a helmet removed only by the appropriate specialist and under radiographic guidance.

### Air transport

The modern use of emergency air transport services makes it necessary for the physician to understand special considerations regarding altitude physiology, altitude physics, and the special equipment used by these services. This section deals with those considerations specific to the orthopedic care of patients transported by air.

**Air splints.** Standard extremity air splints can be hazardous in nonpressurized aircraft.[5] They are sometimes hazardous in pressurized aircraft. These splints are not equipped with pressure relief valves and can therefore cause neurovascular compromise due to spontaneous overinflation at altitude. This is especially dangerous in an unconscious patient. Air should be released from these splints prior to takeoff; the splint should then be closely observed during the flight. Upon descent these splints may also spontaneously lose pressure and require reinflation.

**Pneumatic anti-shock garment.** PASGs are equipped with pressure relief valves generally set at 105 mm Hg. However, inflation pressures greater than that originally intended are possible.[5] These pressures can cause pain as well as neurovascular or respiratory compromise. Again, upon descent the splint may lose pressure and require reinflation.

**HARE traction splints.** Because of the additional length required, most helicopters used in medical transport today cannot accept HARE traction splints. There are some exceptions to this rule. Some helicopters can accept Sager traction splints but not the HARE traction splint. This must be kept in mind when choosing a splint. The PASG may be an acceptable alternative. If a patient is to be transported by helicopter, it is inadvisable to apply a traction device and then remove it to apply the PASG. Instead, the PASG should be applied as the initial splinting technique and maintained during flight.

**Pain control.** Splinting itself is the mainstay of pain management in the prehospital setting. A 50:50 mixture of nitrous oxide and oxygen is also used by some EMS systems,[28] which is safe and effective. Morphine can also provide excellent prehospital pain control. If the latter is used, it should be given in small increments and always IV and with close monitoring of blood pressure, respirations, and oxygenation. Ideally, both nitrous oxide and morphine should be given only after consulting with a physician.

### Pneumatic anti-shock garment

The PASG is a highly controversial device. However, it is widely held that it is useful in pelvic fractures and, possibly, in femur fractures.[29] Theoretically, with inflation of the abdominal portion of the PASG, pelvic and perhaps con-

comitant abdominal bleeding is tamponaded.[30,31] It was originally thought the garment worked by autotransfusion of blood from the lower extremities to the core. Now, it is understood that this is not the mechanism.[32] Present thought is that the increase in systemic vascular resistance seen with the use of the PASG accounts for most of any blood pressure rise observed. It is possible (though somewhat difficult) to control external bleeding by application of the PASG.

There is concern that elevating the blood pressure in an exsanguinating patient may lead to increased blood loss through secondary hemorrhage. Likewise, using the PASG in penetrating chest trauma is contraindicated.[33] Inflation of the abdominal portion in known diaphragmatic hernia is also contraindicated.

Relative contraindications include congestive heart failure and the third trimester of pregnancy. If inflation of the abdominal portion results in respiratory compromise, then that portion should be deflated immediately. Potential hazards of the PASG, when used long term, include neurovascular impairment with or without compartment syndrome and acidosis. The use of PASG in air transport can be complicated (see Air transport above).

### DISCUSSION

The emergency physician must have a clear understanding of the history and the treatment administered by the prehospital care providers prior to the patient's arrival at the emergency department.

The priorities for the prehospital care of orthopedic patients are the same for the EMS provider as they are for the emergency physician; that is, the primary survey with C-spine control, resuscitation, secondary survey and, finally, definitive care. With few exceptions, fracture management lies in the secondary survey and definitive care phases. The old adage "life before limb" is still applicable. Unnecessary delay caused by overtreatment of musculoskeletal injuries in multiply traumatized critical patients must be avoided. Conversely, in stable patients, fractures should be thoroughly immobilized prior to transport.

A wise emergency physician takes the time to discuss the case with the prehospital caregiver and to carefully review the written EMS record.

### REFERENCES

1. Caroline NL: *Emergency care in the streets,* ed 4, Boston, Little, Brown, 1991, pp 361–387.
2. Grant HD, Murray RH, Bergeron JD: *Emergency care,* ed 6, Englewood Cliffs, 1994, Prentice-Hall, pp. 48-99.
3. Grant HD, Murray RH, Bergeron JD: *Emergency care,* ed 6, Englewood Cliffs, 1994, Prentice-Hall, pp. 706-729.
4. Alexander R, et al: *Advanced trauma life support,* ed 5, Chicago, American College of Surgeons, 1993, pp 11–24.
5. Eichelberger MR, et al: *Pediatric emergencies,* Englewood Cliffs, 1992, Prentice-Hall, pp. 147-159.
6. Heckman JD, et al: Emergency care and transportation of the sick and injured, ed 5, Park Ridge, American Academy of Orthopaedic Surgeons, 1992, pp 65–95.

7. Hafen BQ, Karren KJ: *Prehospital emergency care & crisis intervention,* ed 2, Englewood, Morton, 1983, pp 225–291.

8. Bledsoe BE et al: *Paramedic emergency care,* ed 2, Englewood Cliffs, Prentice-Hall, 1991, pp 400–439.

9. Jones SA, et al: *Advanced emergency care,* Philadelphia, Lippincott, 1992.

10. Simon JE, Goldberg AT: Prehospital pediatric life support, St. Louis, 1983, C. V. Mosby Co., pp. 70-81.

11. Grant HD, Murray RH, Bergeron JD: *Emergency care,* ed 6, Englewood Cliffs, 1994, Prentice-Hall, pp. 258-289.

12. Howell JM, et al: A practical radiographic comparison of short board technique and Kendrick extrication device, *Ann Emerg Med* 18:943-946, 1989.

13. Cline JR, et al: A comparison of methods of cervical immobilization used in patient extrication and transport, *J Trauma* 25:649, 1985.

14. Graziano AF, et al: A radiographic comparison of prehospital cervical immobilization methods, *Ann Emerg Med* 16:1127-1131, 1987.

15. McGuire RA: Spinal instability and the log-rolling maneuver, *J Trauma* 27:525-531, 1987.

16. Podolsky S, et al: Efficacy of cervical spine immobilization methods, *J Trauma* 23:461-465, 1983.

17. Hoffman JR, et al: Low-risk criteria for cervical-spine radiography in blunt trauma: a prospective study, *Ann Emerg Med* 21:1454-1460, 1992.

18. Herzenberg JE: Emergency transport and positioning of young children who have an injury of the cervical spine, *J Bone Joint Surg* 71A:15-22, 1989.

19. Schriger DL, et al: Spinal immobilization on a flat backboard: Does it result in neutral position of the cervical spine? *Ann Emerg Med* 20:878-881, 1991.

20. Heckman JD, et al: Emergency care and transportation of the sick and injured, ed 5, Park Ridge, American Academy of Orthopaedic Surgeons, 1992, pp 260–311.

21. Bowman WD: *Outdoor emergency care,* Denver, National Ski Patrol, 1988, pp 361–387.

22. Hauswald M, et al: Cervical spine movement during airway management: Cinefluoroscopic appraisal in human cadavers, *Am J Emerg Med* 9:535-542, 1991.

23. Kleinert HE, et al: Replantation, *Clinical Symposia* 43:2-32, 1991.

24. Sood R, et al: Extremity replantation, *Surg Clin North Am* 71:317-329, 1991.

25. Feller AM, et al: Replantation surgery, *World J Surg* 15:477-485, 1991.

26. Vegso JJ: Field evaluation and management of head and neck injuries, *Clin Sports Med* 6:1-15, 1987.

27. Watkins RG: Neck injuries in football players, *Clin Sports Med* 5:215-46, 1986.

28. Pons PT: Nitrous oxide analgesia, *Emerg Med Clin North Am* 6:777-782, 1988.

29. Flint LM, et al: Definitive control of bleeding from severe pelvic fractures, *Ann Surg* 189:709-716, 1979.

30. Ali J, Duke K: Pneumatic antishock garment decreases hemorrhage and mortality from splenic injury, *Can J Surg* 34:496-501, 1991.

31. McSwain NE: Pneumatic antishock garment: state of the art 1988, *Ann Emerg Med* 17:506-525, 1988.

32. Bivins HG, et al: Blood volume displacement with inflation of antishock trousers, *Ann Emerg Med* 11:409-412.

33. Ali J, Vanderby B, Purcell C: The effect of the pneumatic antishock garment (PASG) on hemodynamics, hemorrhage, and survival in penetrating thoracic aortic injury, *J Trauma* 31:846-851, 1991.

34. Huerta C, Griffith R, Joyce SM: Cervical spine stabilization in pediatric patients: Evaluation of current techniques, *Ann Emerg Med* 16:1121-1126, 1987.

# Pain and Pain Relief

*Jo Linder*

Pain is an emergency for the person who experiences it, regardless of the urgency of the underlying pathology. I believe we must apply the science and art of pain relief as though a life depended upon it. Certainly the quality of life does.

    *Judith Spross*

Pain has been described as a subjective, irritating sensation associated with tissue damage or pain-inducing neural transmission. Tissue trauma causes release of potent inflammatory and pain mediators. These substances from injured tissue promote tissue breakdown; increase the rate of metabolism, coagulation, and water retention; impair immune function; and trigger sympathetic autonomic features and negative emotions.[1] In the clinical setting, pain is often described as *acute* or *chronic.* Determining whether pain is emanating from a damaged or intact nervous system is also important. *Nociceptive* pain is the term for pain due to tissue damage when the nervous system is normal; if nerve damage is present, the pain is called *neuropathic* pain.[2]

Pain may exacerbate posttraumatic and postoperative complications due to a variety of responses, including retained pulmonary secretions and delayed return of gastrointestinal (GI) function. Additional benefits of pain management include earlier mobilization and decreased length of hospitalization.

All patients deserve effective management of pain and relief of suffering. Anything harmful to the patient, including postoperative pain, should be prevented whenever possible. Pain is more difficult to suppress the longer it is present. Early intervention with analgesics and education of the patient about nonpharmacologic methods of pain control have been shown effective in the prevention of pain.

In patients with acute multiple trauma, pain from a serious injury can mask other injuries. Due to the intensity of the pain stimuli from a serious injury, the patient may not notice pain from other parts of the body. It is important to systematically assess and reassess the patient after the more serious injury has been attended to.

No matter how carefully a procedure is performed, tissue trauma occurs. Therefore, before a so-called painless procedure is attempted, the patient should be informed of the potential for pain and sedation. After the procedure, adequate analgesia should be provided.

To achieve effective pain control, all members on the health care team must be involved. The informed patient who is aware of the reasons for pain as well as the methods available for managing it can also assume the primary responsibility for ensuring that pain is minimized. Written policies help to minimize confusion for health care professionals, especially when individualized patient care plans are communicated via the medical record or a centralized pain-management file. With a method of communicating

---

**Clinical features of neuropathic pain**

Pain onset is delayed after damage
Pain persists in absence of ongoing, obvious stimulus
Pain sensation is frequently described as burning, electric shock–like, pressure, twisting or torquelike, paroxysmal, brief, shooting or stabbing, or other unfamiliar sensation
Pain is present in an area of numbness
Stimulus that does not ordinarily cause pain, for example, touch, now causes pain in affected area (allodynia)
Repetitive stimuli produce pronounced summation and reaction

From Hill CS: Pain. In Rakel RE, ed. Conn's Current Therapy, Philadelphia: WB Saunders, 1992.

---

pain management plans, health care team members will be prepared for a patient who presents with a complaint of pain to the emergency department.

## ASSESSMENT OF PAIN
### Causes: physiologic factors

Whenever possible, the best method for relieving pain is to treat the underlying cause. In the case of a fractured hip, for example, reduction and fixation of the fracture stabilize the bone and ultimately reduce or remove painful stimuli. Nociceptive pain usually responds to commonly used non-narcotic and narcotic analgesics; however, neuropathic pain may be further relieved by the addition of antidepressant and anticonvulsant drugs (see box above).[2]

The primary class of drugs used to treat all types of pain is the nonsteroidal anti-inflammatory drugs (NSAIDs). Several mediators have been recognized in the inflammatory process. Histamine was one of the first identified; however, the $H_1$-antagonists are useful only for the stabilization of vascular effects during the early phase of inflammation. The antagonists of bradykinin and 5-hydroxytryptamine (5-HT) also ameliorate only certain types of inflammatory responses. Other culprits identified in the inflammatory process include leukotrienes and platelet-activating factor (PAF); inhibitors of their synthesis and action are under development.

Prostaglandins have been shown to produce inflammation in several studies and are thought to be associated with the development of pain due to the injury of inflammation. The capacity of prostaglandins to sensitize pain receptors to mechanical and chemical stimulation has been confirmed by electrophysiologic measurements and appears to result from a lowering of the threshold of the polymodal nociceptors of C fibers.[3] Prostaglandins, thromboxanes, and leukotriene $B_4$ are known to cause vasodilation, increased vascular permeability, increased platelet aggregation, and pain. By-products of prostaglandin synthesis, also identified as mediators in the inflammatory process, include free oxygen radicals.

Although the process of inflammation is not the sole cause of pain in any individual, many components of the inflammatory process can contribute to a patient's pain.

### Causes: psychological factors

The patient's complaint of pain must be taken seriously. In the setting of acute pain, treatment should be aggressive enough to prevent prolonged discomfort. When pain fibers become sensitized, the patient may get caught in a cycle of feeling pain, experiencing limited relief of that pain, having anxiety that the pain will return even stronger, feeling that pain, experiencing more limited relief of the pain, and so on. An organized, multidisciplinary approach to treatment is best to prevent the development of chronic pain and to avoid acute exacerbations of patient discomfort.

It is important to assess the expectations of the patient and their families. Preparing the patient to expect some level of pain from an injury or a procedure helps to alleviate anxiety. Previous experience may influence the amount of distress the patient feels. Determining the level of anxiety associated with the current sensation of pain helps physicians prescribe appropriate therapy. Later in this chapter, objective tools for measuring pain are discussed. To assist in the assessment of associated anxiety, have the patient use a separate rating scale to describe emotional suffering.

### Pain threshold variations

Each patient is unique. An individual may respond to pain and to the treatment plan differently than expected. It is important to recognize that physician and patient tolerance may vary. In some cases, high doses of medication may be needed to provide pain relief. In other instances, little medication may be necessary, but the patient may require frequent visits by psychosocial services. If conflict arises because of a difference between the expected and the actual response to treatment, alternative therapy (and possibly a psychotherapist) may be needed. Again, it is invaluable to adopt a team approach to treating pain and to have well-defined policies in place.

### Acute pain

Acute pain is described as "pain following injury or disease" and lasting less than six months. The three classes of pain, with examples of each, are shown in Table 3-1.[4]

As mentioned, it is important to give the patient an idea of how much pain to expect and the duration of the pain. The long-term pain associated with a fracture, for example, may last for several weeks to months. Acute pain in this setting is exacerbated by swelling and movement of bony fragments if the cast or splint loosens. Short-term acute pain is usually relieved after joint reduction with some mild discomfort due to swelling or early mobilization following the procedure.

### Chronic pain

Patients with long-standing pain present a common clinical challenge to the practicing physician. A thorough history

**Table 3-1.** Types of pain

| Type | Definition | Examples |
|------|-----------|----------|
| Acute | Pain following injury or disease | Fractured bone Postoperative pain |
| Chronic malignant | Pain associated with cancer or other progressive disorders | Osteosarcoma Rheumatoid arthritis Sickle cell crises |
| Chronic nonmalignant | Pain in patients whose tissue injury is nonprogressive or healed | Low-back pain Migraine headaches |

From Mooney NE: Nursing Clin North Am 26:73-87,1991. By permission.

from the patient with chronic pain regarding the onset and course of their symptoms is vital to understanding their current disability and prescribing a successful treatment plan. A report on pain and disability from the Institute of Medicine in 1987 found that the term *chronic pain syndrome* was ill-defined and that the epidemiology of chronic pain was deficient.[5] What differentiates chronic pain from acute pain? In a study by Deathe and Helmes, admission to a multidisciplinary pain center required at least three to six months of severe continuing disability.[6] Other researchers vary on the definitions of chronic pain, but all include the element of "persistent pain" described by the patient.

It is believed that chronic pain syndromes are complex, with inflammation contributing little to the underlying discomfort. Returning to a review of the neuroanatomy, nociceptive and mechanoreceptive neural fibers transmit information perceived as pain in the dorsal root ganglia of the spinal cord. The neurons then send stimuli on to the substantia gelatinosa in the dorsal horn of the spinal cord. From the spinal cord via the contralateral spinothalamic tract, the information is projected to the brain-stem reticular formation or to the thalamus. The sensitized brain-stem reticular formation arouses the patient to the presence of pain. From the thalamus, painful stimuli are sent to the cerebral cortex where the patient perceives the quality and location of the discomfort. There is also an emotional component to pain that is determined by the response of the limbic system. How much a patient suffers is linked to the overall well-being of the individual. When patients experience difficulty sleeping, depression, or loss of productivity, they "hurt" more.

The best therapy for patients suffering from chronic pain is to return them to a productive life as soon as possible. This may require rehabilitation with both physical therapy and occupational therapy. It is important to determine whether the pain is associated with a terminal condition or progressive debilitating disease (often called *malignant pain*). Although many patients and caregivers become

frustrated with persistent pain, there is hope. Recent studies have shown that patients can improve and that their use of health services can decrease over time with comprehensive pain management.[6,7]

**Objective means of measuring pain levels**

Physicians lost the ability to "see" pain at the end of the eighteenth century when pain lost its standing as a disease entity. Tumors and fractures were treatable, and diagnosis took precedence over relief of symptoms. Recently, clinicians in several specialties have regained an interest in pain relief, and tools have been developed to make pain "visible."[1,8,9]

Changes in vital signs provide important information regarding the patient's physiologic response to acute pain. The patient should be observed for signs of discomfort including abnormal gait or body position; restlessness, splinting at the site of injury; and altered behavior, including anxiety, mood swings, and dependency.

The best indicator of a patient's discomfort is a description of the pain. The patient may describe the pain in terms of location, type (sharp, dull, boring, and so on), intensity or severity, radiation, changes with movement, what makes it better or worse, and how the pain makes them feel (Fig. 3-1). Rating scales have been developed to obtain objective, descriptive information from the patient (Fig. 3-2). Special attention must be paid when the patient complains of new pain. In the patient with acute trauma or following a postoperative procedure, abrupt changes in pain associated with increases in temperature or pulse rate, or a drop in blood pressure or urine output, require investigation and immediate treatment.

There may be times when the patient's complaints of pain do not fit expected behaviors. Some patients may exaggerate their complaints and others may deny discomfort when they are suffering. The latter patient may be easier to detect (e.g., obvious tachycardia or diaphoresis). The patient who requests increasing amounts of narcotics with little or no objective signs of discomfort may be suspected of malingering. In both cases, the discrepancies should be communicated to the patient and the pain management adjusted accordingly.

**PATIENTS WITH SPECIAL NEEDS**
**Elderly patients**

In general, special care should be given to elderly patients, who typically have diminished sensory input. They may sustain multiple injuries due to their poor vision or unstable gait. Their pain tolerance may increase because of this decreased sensation or a stoic attitude, but studies have failed to confirm this assumption. Some elderly patients may be constant complainers, especially when they have experienced pain for years without adequate relief. Older patients may have multiple-organ system disease and may be taking several medications as a result. The clinician must be cognizant of all these distinguishing characteristics when managing pain in the elderly.

**Initial Pain Assessment Tool**

Date _____

Patient's Name _____ Age _____ Room _____

Diagnosis _____ Physician _____

Nurse _____

I. Location: Patient or nurse mark drawing.

II. Intensity:    Patient rates the pain. Scale used _____

                  Present: _____

                  Worst pain gets: _____

                  Best pain gets: _____

                  Acceptable level of pain: _____

III. Quality: (Use patient's own words, e.g. prick, ache, burn, throb, pull, sharp)

_____

_____

IV. Onset, duration variations, rhythms: _____

_____

V. Manner of expressing pain: _____

_____

VI. What relieves the pain? _____

_____

VII. What causes or increases the pain? _____

_____

VIII. Effects of pain: (Note decreases function, devreased quality of life.)
           Accompanying system (e.g. nausea)

_____

      Sleep

_____

      Appetite

_____

      Physical activity

_____

      Relationsh with others (e.g. irratability)

_____

      Emotions (e.g. anger, suicidal, crying)

_____

      Concentration

_____

      Other

_____

IX. Other comments:

_____

_____

X. Plan

_____

_____

Acute Pain Management Guideline Panel. Acute Pain Management: operative or Medical Procedures and Trauma. Clinical Practive Guideline. AHCPR Pub. No. 92-0032. Rockville, MD: Agency for Health Care Policy and Research, Public Health Service, U.S. Department of Health and Human Services. Feb. 1992. Pg. 118.

**Fig. 3-1.** Initial pain assessment tool.

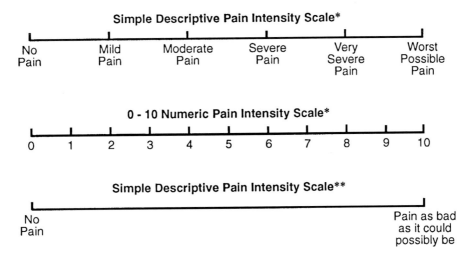

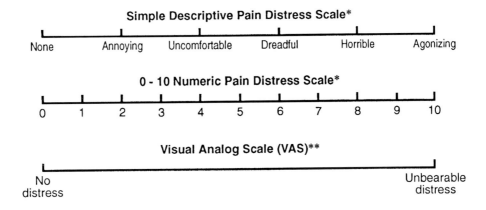

\*   If used as a graphic rating scale, a 10-cm baseline is recommended.
\*\* A 10-cm baseline is recommended for VAS scales.

**Fig. 3-2.** Rating scales for patient use in describing pain.

Pain is experienced by nearly all patients over the age of 60 at some time during the remainder of their lives. Unfortunately, it can be difficult to elicit complaints of pain in these patients. Scales for measuring emotional and descriptive components of pain are often inadequate in this population. Agitation or moaning in a demented patient may be interpreted as a complaint, whether as a response to pain or not.

When prescribing medication for elderly patients, one must take into consideration altered pharmacokinetics due to diminished renal and hepatic metabolism. Postoperative pain studies have found that these patients tended to respond more to analgesics, and that their duration of pain relief was increased.[10] In addition, patients over age 85 are at risk of GI complications and renal toxicity from such agents as acetaminophen and NSAIDs. When opioids are used, dosage should be adjusted to maximize the analgesic effect and to minimize unwanted side effects. These patients should be monitored closely for signs of lethargy, respiratory depression, and constipation due to medication. Of course, these may also be signs of impending multisystem failure or sepsis, which may be masked by narcotics.

As a general rule, analgesic therapy in elderly patients must be carefully managed, with special attention paid to the use of pharmaceutical agents. Whenever possible, the use of other therapeutic modalities to increase the patient's level of activity and decrease reliance on medication is preferred.

**Table 3-2.** Explanations for undertreatment of pain in children

| Incorrect assumptions | Attitudes | Complexity of pain assessment | Research and training inadequacy |
|---|---|---|---|
| There is a correct amount of pain for a given injury. | Pain is necessary because of its religious implications. | Pain is difficult to assess in children because they often cannot or will not tell us, in ways we can understand, the extent of their discomfort. | *Research* Research is limited by inadequate assessment techniques. |
| Children's nervous systems are too immature to experience pain. | Pain is necessary because it is character building. | There is no single universally accepted, well-standardized measure of pain assessment in children. | Research is complicated by ethical constraints. |
| Children metabolize opioids differently. | The use of analgesics is evidence of a weak character. | Inadequate assessment techniques foster undertreatment because PRN dosing is based on patient's report of need for analgesics. | *Training* There are few sources of information regarding pain management in children. |
| Children have no memory of pain. | Some families have attitudes which denigrate the open discussion of pain and its treatment. | Inadequate assessment techniques complicate research on pain and its management. | Faculty discomfort with pain management transmits a lack of concern for this problem to trainers. |
| Children become easily addicted to narcotics. | Physicians and nurses tend to have attitudes about pain in children minimizing their role as causers of pain. | | There is limited information on pain management in the medical school curriculum. |

From Schechter NL: Ped Clin North Am 36(4):785, 1989. By permission.

## Pediatric patients

Recently the undertreatment of pain in children has received a great deal of attention. Several reasons have been put forth to explain this undertreatment (Table 3-2).

The assessment of pain in the pediatric patient is difficult. Currently, there is no widely accepted evaluation method; however, three types of pain assessment procedures are under development and study: 1) observed behaviors that are thought to be associated with pain, 2) physiologic measurements that may correlate with pain or stress, and 3) modified visual analog scales that may be used in the toddler and older child.

Several factors are involved in understanding pain and discomfort in each child. The patient's behavior, physiologic and emotional response, and the patient's previous experience with pain should be determined. Other factors to consider include the source of the pain, the duration of the patient's complaints, the psychosocial environment and parental support, and the reaction of the child to previous painful episodes. In general, children seem ill-equipped to cope with pain and its significance, regardless of their developmental level.[11] One of the greatest challenges to the emergency physician is establishing rapport and interacting positively with any child in a brief period of time. This is especially difficult and even more important in the child experiencing pain (Table 3-3).

The emergency physician is often faced with the issue of whether to have parents remain at the child's bedside during a painful procedure, for example, a fracture reduction. Some studies have suggested that children become more distressed when parents are nearby; others support teaching parents coping strategies to help the child through the procedure. In a survey of school-aged children by Ross and Ross, 99% said the most helpful element during a procedure is the presence of a parent in the room.[11]

A few comments about specific analgesic agents are relevant here (a more thorough discussion of medications is presented later in this chapter). Some of the best agents for pain control and sedation during procedures in the emergency department are short-acting agents.

Fentanyl, a potent synthetic opioid, is not recommended for children under the age of 2. The recommended dose is 2 to 3 µg/kg. Monitoring for respiratory depression and bradycardia is essential and reversible with naloxone.

Ketamine hydrochloride is a short-acting anesthetic that is effective during painful procedures in the emergency department. Ketamine produces a trancelike state via the IM route (five minutes) or the IV route (one minute) at a dose of 0.5 to 1 mg/kg. A benzodiazepine should be used with ketamine to reduce the likelihood of night terrors or hallucinatory effects.

Midazolam may be used in combination with fentanyl and ketamine to assist in sedation. The dose of midazolam is 0.07 mg/kg and may be administered via the nasal, rectal,

**Table 3-3.** Methods used for pediatric pain assessment

|  | Self-Report | Behavioral | Physiological |
|---|---|---|---|
| Infant/Toddler |  | Cry characteristics<br>Cry time<br>Facial expression<br>Visual tracking<br>Body movement<br>Response time to stimulus<br>Behavioral state | Heart rate<br>Blood pressure<br>Respiratory rate<br>Diaphoresis |
| Preschooler | Faces drawings<br>Oucher<br>Poker chip tool<br>Ladder scale<br>Color scales<br>Pediatric Pain Questionnaire | Children's Hospital of Eastern Ontario Pain Scale<br>Procedure Behavior Rating Scale<br>Procedure Behavior Check List<br>Observation Scale of Behavioral Distress<br>Gauvain-Piquard *et al.* scale |  |
| School-Age/Adolescent | Visual analogue scales<br>Numerical rating scales<br>Word scales<br>Pediatric Pain Questionnaire | Objective Pain Scale<br>Procedure Behavior Rating Scale<br>Procedure Behavior Check List |  |

From Beyer JE, Wels N: Ped Clin North Am 36(4):850, 1989. By permission.

IM, or IV route. A positive side effect of midazolam is amnesia of the procedure. Respiratory depression, which is usually brief, may be potentiated with the combination.[12] Assisted ventilation for a few breaths may be all that is necessary to resolve the problem.

Nitrous oxide is another analgesic agent that has been used for painful procedures in children. Children remain awake and experience a dissociative, euphoric sensation. The gas is administered as a nitrous oxide/oxygen mixture via nasal mask or a mask that the child holds so that if the child becomes too drowsy, the mask falls off and ends the gas flow. The gas mixture is easily titrated to provide analgesia, and the child wakes up quickly after the nitrous oxide is discontinued, producing amnesia of the event.

### Patients with other medical conditions

Because of the potential for increased side effects and undesirable drug interactions, it is important to be aware of the patient's concurrent medical conditions. Alcohol and central nervous system (CNS) depressants can potentiate the sedative effects of opioid analgesics. Patients with chronic pain conditions such as metastatic cancer may require higher doses because they develop tolerance, and they may react adversely to opioid agonist-antagonists. Complications due to bleeding at the site of injections may be seen in patients on anticoagulation therapy or with bleeding dyscrasias. In the immunocompromised patient, the risk of infection may outweigh the benefits of certain modes of pain control, such as epidural analgesia. Consideration of pharmacokinetics is important in patients with renal or hepatic insufficiency. Opioids can increase the symptoms of neurologic disorders, and doses should be adjusted accordingly. Meperidine is metabolized faster in patients taking phenytoin, requiring higher, more frequent dosing. Psychotropic medications and opioids have an additive effect, causing increased sedation when taken together. Patients receiving meperidine and monoamine oxidase (MAO) inhibitors have reportedly experienced severe adverse reactions similar to malignant hyperthermia with seizures and death.

### Patients with multiple trauma

Analgesic therapy in the multiple-trauma patient should be used judiciously and should be administered only when close monitoring of respiratory and cardiovascular status is available. Agents that can be rapidly reversed with naloxone or flumazenil are safest in these patients.

### Patients with known or suspected addictive disorders or substance abuse

The patient with a known or suspected history of substance abuse who complains of pain presents an increasingly common dilemma for the clinician. Six recommendations for postoperative pain management in patients with a history of substance abuse have recently been outlined to help physicians recognize and treat pain in such patients appropriately (see box on page 44).

The treatment plan for substance abuse patients must be clear and incorporate limits. The patient should be included in the pain-management planning whenever possible. It is important to select opioid medication at a dosage sufficient to provide pain relief without precipitating withdrawal. The patient who is experiencing ongoing discomfort due to undertreatment may become adamant in requesting more narcotics. Every attempt should be made to include the primary pain management team members in prescribing pain control for these patients when they arrive at the emergency department. Allowing potential substance-abusing patients to manipulate their pain-management plan through episodic caregivers in the emergency department can create a cycle that harms the patient.

---

### Opioid use recommendations in substance abuse patients

Define the mechanism of pain and treat the primary problem whenever possible

Determine the current substance abuse activity or how long it has been since the patient has actively abused drugs

Follow relevant pharmacologic principles of opioid use (i.e., do not give agonist-antagonist opioids to a patient on methadone therapy)

Use all modes of pain reducing therapies including nonopioid medication

Recognized specific drug abuse behaviors should be confirmed and the patient confronted appropriately

Set limits to avoid excessive bargaining about choice of pain management

---

## PAIN MANAGEMENT OPTIONS

This chapter is based in large part on the document *Acute Pain Management: Operative or Medical Procedures and Trauma,* published in March 1992, by the Department of Health and Human Services. In these clinical practice guidelines, the focus is on the recognition of pain and the establishment of systems to ensure a prompt response to the patient in pain. The following approaches regarding treatment are highly recommended: 1) NSAIDs should be used routinely (unless specifically contraindicated); 2) opioid orders should allow a wide range for titration and provide for "rescue doses"; and 3) intraspinal opioids, patient-controlled opioid infusions, and other advanced technologies must be governed by explicit procedures and staff training, generally under the control of a pain management team.[12] Quality assurance guidelines have been developed to formally review pain management programs.[13]

In the emergency department, relief of pain is often secondary to recognizing and treating a potentially life-threatening problem. Acute pain is a human survival response. The relief of pain should not lead to deterioration of the patient's condition. Hypotension and respiratory depression caused by narcotics can be managed in the emergency department when the patient is closely monitored. The judicious use of IV narcotic analgesics titrated for relief of pain while keeping a watchful eye on vital signs, should be a given in emergency care. The effects of narcotic analgesics and benzodiazepines can be reversed if necessary with naloxone and flumazinal.

### Pharmacologic management

Medications should be selected based on their pharmacokinetics (onset and duration), reversibility, side effects, cost, analgesic effect, and addiction potential (Table 3-4). A 15-minute computer instruction session is available on how to interchange equivalent doses of opioid analgesics, based on a study done by Grossman and Sheidler.[14]

The current mainstay medications for pain management are the NSAIDs. Commonly referred to as "aspirin-like," NSAIDs are a large group of compounds that relieve pain, presumably through anti-inflammatory effects. For management of mild to moderate pain, an NSAID should be used unless a contraindication exists. NSAIDs are effective in reducing the amount of opioid needed to control more severe pain and have been found to reduce side effects of opioid agents when used together (Table 3-5).

The primary physiologic process of pain control involves inhibition of prostaglandin production and release. For the NSAID to be effective, the agent must inhibit the cyclooxygenase enzyme that is responsible for the production of prostaglandins. Some agents are competitive inhibitors, but many have effects that disappear slowly. Other agents, such as acetaminophen, are effective only in a low-peroxide environment (e.g., the hypothalamus). Inflammation sites are usually high in peroxides generated by leukocytes; this may account for acetaminophen's poor anti-inflammatory activity in such environments.[3]

Opioid analgesics are commonly used for pain control in a number of situations. When used for acute short-term post-operative pain control, tolerance and physiologic or psychologic dependence are unlikely to develop in patients with no prior history of substance abuse. Patients should be instructed in the analgesic effects and side effects and given control over their dosing. Dosing frequency should be adjusted to prevent "breakthrough" recurrent pain and minimize side effects. Other pain-reducing modalities, such as physical therapy and relaxation techniques, help reduce the need for opioid analgesia.

Opioids relieve pain by binding to opioid receptors outside as well as inside the CNS. Opioid analgesics are classified as full agonists, partial agonists, or mixed agonist-antagonists, according to their means of interacting with opioid receptors. Full agonists produce a maximal response within the cells with which they bind. Partial agonists produce a lesser response. Mixed agonist-antagonists activate one type of opioid receptor and block another type at the same time.[1] The mu receptor type is so named because of its response to morphine. The mu opioid agonists are codeine, hydromorphone, oxycodone, hydrocodone, fentanyl, meperidine, methadone, and levorphanol. Potential side effects of the mu agonists include nausea, constipation, urinary retention, sedation, respiratory depression, or confusion.

Meperidine is a relatively short-acting opioid that may be used for brief courses in healthy patients who are allergic to more effective opioids such as morphine, hydromorphone, or one of the synthetic opioid agents. The dose needed to achieve analgesia equivalent to morphine 10 mg administered every 4 hours is meperidine 100 to 150 mg every 2½ to 3 hours. Meperidine is contraindicated in patients with impaired renal function and those taking MAO inhibitors. Toxic effects of the metabolite normeperidine include cerebral irritation and seizures. In patients

**Table 3-4.** Dosing data for opioid analgesics

| Drug | Approximate equianalgesic oral dose | Approximate equianalgesic parenteral dose | Recommended starting dose > 50 kg body wt (oral) | Recommended starting dose > 50 kg body wt (parenteral) | Recommended starting dose < 50 kg (oral)* | Recommended starting dose < 50 kg (parenteral)* |
|---|---|---|---|---|---|---|
| **Opioid Agonist** | | | | | | |
| Morphine[†] | 30 mg q 3-4 h (around-the-clock dosing) 60 mg q 3-4 h (single dose or intermittent dosing) | 10 mg q 3-4 h | 30 mg q 3-4 h | 10 mg q 3-4 h | 0.3 mg/kg q 3-4 h | 0.1 mg/kg q 3-4 h |
| Codeine[‡] | 130 mg q 3-4 h | 75 mg q 3-4 h | 60 mg q 3-4 h | 60 mg q 2 h (IM/SQ) | 1 mg/kg q 3-4 h[§] | Not recommended |
| Hydromorphone[†] (Dilaudid) | 7.5 mg q 3-4 h | 1.5 mg q 3-4 h | 6 mg q 3-4 h | 1.5 mg q 3-4 h | 0.06 mg/kg q 3-4 h | 0.015 mg/kg q 3-4 h |
| Hydrocodone (in Lorcet, Lortab, Vicodin, others) | 30 mg q 3-4 h | Not available | 10 mg q 3-4 h | Not available | 0.2 mg/kg q 3-4 h[§] | Not available |
| Levorphanol (Levo-Dromoran) | 4 mg q 6-8 h | 2 mg q 6-8 h | 4 mg q 6-8 h | 2 mg q 6-8 h | 0.04 mg/kg q 6-8 h | 0.02 mg/kg q 6-8 h |
| Meperidine (Demerol) | 300 mg q 2-3 h | 100 mg q 3 h | Not recommended | 100 mg q 3 h | Not recommended | 0.75 mg/kg q 2-3 h |
| Methadone (Dolophine, others) | 20 mg q 6-8 h | 10 mg q 6-8 h | 20 mg q 6-8 h | 10 mg q 6-8 h | 0.2 mg/kg q 6-8 h | 0.1 mg/kg q 6-8 h |
| Oxycodone (Roxicodone, also in Percocet, Percodan, Tylox, others) | 30 mg q 3-4 h | Not available | 10 mg q 3-4 h | Not available | 0.2 mg/kg q 3-4 h[§] | Not available |
| Oxymorphone[†] (Numorphan) | Not available | 1 mg q 3-4 h | Not available | 1 mg q 3-4 h | Not recommended | Not recommended |
| **Opioid Agonist Antagonist and Partial Agonist** | | | | | | |
| Buprenorphine (Buprenex) | Not available | 0.3-0.4 mg q 6-8 h | Not available | 0.4 mg q 6-8 h | Not available | 0.004 mg/kg q 6-8 h |
| Butorphanol (Stadol) | Not available | 2 mg q 3-4 h | Not available | 2 mg q 3-4 h | Not available | Not recommended |
| Nalbuphine (Nubain) | Not available | 10 mg q 3-4 h | Not available | 10 mg q 3-4 h | Not available | 0.1 mg/kg q 3-4 h |
| Pentazocine (Talwin, others) | 150 mg q 3-4 h | 60 mg q 3-4 h | 50 mg q 4-6 h | Not recommended | Not recommended | Not recommended |

Key: h = hour; kg = kilogram; mg = milligram; q = every; wt = weight

Note: Published tables vary in the suggested doses that are equianalgesic to morphine. Clinical response is the criterion that must be applied for each patient; titration to clinical response is necessary. Because there is not complete cross-tolerance among these drugs, it is usually necessary to use a lower than equianalgesic dose when changing drugs and to retitrate to response.

Caution: Recommended doses do not apply to patients with renal or hepatic insufficiency or other conditions affecting drug metabolism and kinetics.

*Caution: Doses listed for patients with body weight of less than 50 kg cannot be used as initial starting doses in infants under 6 months. Consult the *Clinical Practice Guideline for Acute Pain Management: Operative or Medical Procedures and Trauma* section on management of pain in neonates for recommendations.

[†]For morphine, hydromorphone, and oxymorphone, rectal administration is an alternate route for patients unable to take oral medications, but equianalgesic doses may differ from oral and parenteral doses because of pharmacokinetic differences.

[‡]Caution: Codeine doses above 65 mg usually are not appropriate due to diminishing incremental analgesia with increasing constipation and other side effects.

[§]Caution: Doses of aspirin and acetaminophen in combination with opioid/NSAID preparations must also be adjusted to the patient's body weight.

From Acute Pain Management Guideline Panel: Acute pain management: operative or medical procedures and trauma. Rockville: Agency for Health Care Policy and Research. AHCPR publication no 92-0032, 1992, pp 112-113.

**Table 3-5.** Dosing data for NSAIDs

| Drug* | Usual adult dose | Usual pediatric dose[†] | Comments |
|---|---|---|---|
| **Oral NSAID** | | | |
| Acetaminophen | 650-975 mg q 4 h | 10-15 mg/kg q 4 h | Acetaminophen lacks the peripheral anti-inflammatory activity of other NSAIDs |
| Aspirin | 650-975 mg q 4 h | 10-15 mg/kg q 4 h[‡] | Standard against which other NSAIDs are compared. Inhibits platelet aggregation; may cause postoperative bleeding |
| Choline magnesium trisalicylate (Trilisate) | 1000-1500 mg b.i.d. | 25 mg/kg b.i.d. | May have minimal antiplatelet activity; also available as oral liquid |
| Diflunisal (Dolobid) | 1000 mg initial dose followed by 500 mg q 12 h | | |
| Etodolac (Lodine) | 200-400 mg q 6-8 h | | |
| Fenoprofen calcium (Nalfon) | 200 mg q 4-6 h | | |
| Ibuprofen (Motrin, others) | 400 mg q 4-6 h | 10 mg/kg q 6-8 h | Available as several brand names and as generic; also available as oral suspension |
| Ketoprofen (Orudis) | 25-75 mg q 6-8 h | | |
| Magnesium salicylate | 650 mg q 4 hr | | Many brands and generic forms available |
| Meclofenamate sodium (Meclomen) | 50 mg q 4-6 h | | |
| Mefenamic acid (Ponstel) | 250 mg q 6 h | | |
| Naproxen (Naprosyn) | 500-mg initial dose followed by 250 mg q 6-8 h | 5 mg/kg q 12 h | Also available as oral liquid |
| Naproxen sodium (Anaprox) | 550-mg initial dose followed by 275 mg q 6-8 h | | |
| Salsalate (Disalcid, others) | 500 mg q 4 h | | May have minimal antiplatelet activity |
| Sodium salicylate | 325-650 mg q 3-4 h | | Available in generic form from several distributors |
| **Parenteral NSAID** | | | |
| Ketorolac (Toradol) | 30- or 60-mg initial dose IM followed by 15 or 30 mg q 6 h. Oral dose following IM dosage: 10 mg q 6-8 h | | IM dose not to exceed 5 days |

*Note: Only the above NSAIDs have FDA approval for use as simple analgesics, but clinical experience has been gained with other drugs as well.

[†]Drug recommendations are limited to NSAIDs when pediatric dosing experience is available.

[‡]Contraindicated in presence of fever or other evidence of viral illness.

From Acute Pain Management Guideline Panel: Acute pain management: operative or medical procedures and trauma. Rockville: Agency for Health Care Policy and Research. AHCPR publication no. 92-0032, 1992, p 110-111.

Key: b.i.d. = twice daily

h = hour

IM = intramuscular

kg = kilogram

mg = milligram

NSAID = nonsteroidal anti-inflammatory drug

with normal renal function, normeperidine is excreted through the kidney with a half-life of 15 to 20 hours.

Opioids in the mixed agonist-antagonist class include pentazocine, butorphanol tartrate, and malbuphone hydrochloride. Symptoms and signs of opioid withdrawal may be seen when a mixed agonist-antagonist is given to a patient already taking any of the mu opioid agonists.

Patient-controlled analgesia is becoming more popular for pain management in both the inpatient and outpatient setting. A dosing schedule of 3 to 5 mg of morphine every five minutes until the acute pain is diminished followed by on-demand doses of 1 mg per minute, up to 10 mg per hour, may be useful in the patient who is waiting for an operating suite or an inpatient bed.

---

**Nonpharmacologic treatment for acute pain**

Physical therapy
   Ultrasonography
   Thermal modalities
   Exercise
Manipulation
Transcutaneous electrical nerve stimulation (TENS)
Acupuncture
Accupressure/massage
Relaxation techniques
Biofeedback
Hypnosis
Visual imagery
Behavior modification

---

## Nonpharmacologic management

The contribution of adjunctive modalities from many cultures is beginning to be appreciated as more data are processed at multidisciplinary pain-management centers of excellence around the world.

Whether the patient's pain is treated at a "pain clinic" or supervised by the patient's primary care physician, a multidisciplinary approach is advisable. Despite limited studies in the past, the following general conclusions have been reached: 1) patients treated at multidisciplinary pain centers fare better than those receiving no treatment or single-modality treatment, 2) improvement can be seen in diminished patient complaints of pain as well as fewer patient visits and increased productivity (e.g., return to work), and 3) the benefits of treatment from pain clinics are sustained over time. This section describes some of the various treatment modalities available to the pain-management team (see box above).

Nonpharmacologic interventions are used in conjunction with pain medications to help return the patient to a full, active life. Patients who respond best to these methods are willing to try new or different concepts and tend to express their emotions. When patients experience persistent or breakthrough pain despite appropriate pharmacologic interventions, nonpharmacologic therapies can provide relief without oversedation.

Cognitive-behavioral modalities help patients better understand their pain, give them a sense of control over their pain, and help them change behaviors that exacerbate their pain. Cognitive-behavioral therapies include education, relaxation techniques, hypnosis, visual imagery, distraction, music distraction, and biofeedback. These strategies may be initiated by the patient prior to the operative procedure and are especially helpful in the patient who is expected to have long-term discomfort.

Physical therapy incorporates several strategies to improve or correct physical dysfunction, change physiologic responses, reduce fears associated with immobility or restricted activity, and provide pain relief. Cold is applied to reduce tissue damage in the initial post-injury phase. Heat can assist the clearance of tissue breakdown. Used alternately, hot and cold applications can reduce muscle spasm, decrease inflammation, and change the pain threshold in the area of injury. Immobilization provides stability to the injured area and reduces the chance of further injury. In extremity injury, immobilization maintains structural alignment and promotes healing. Musculoskeletal exercise helps the patient regain strength and agility when activity has been restricted due to pain. Massage and acupressure can help relieve muscle spasm and increase muscle stretch and tendon length. Acupuncture is a form of physical therapy that has been used in eastern cultures for thousands of years. Although clinical studies of acupuncture by traditional Western medicine methods are limited, this mode of therapy should be considered to supplement more traditional pain management treatments.

### Effective pain management as a process

Coordinating chronic pain management with other caregivers requires a multidisciplinary approach (Figs. 3-3, 3-4). The overall goal is to relieve discomfort and increase activity of patients suffering from acute and chronic pain. Communication between the patient and the pain-management team as well as among the team members is essential to realize any benefits. It is also important to include family members and significant others in the treatment plan.

Educational materials, including printed and audiovisual materials, about various pain-reducing therapies should be available to patients, their families, and members of the pain-management team. Information should include when to use certain therapies, why they work, how to learn self-management techniques, and where to obtain professional consultations. Clinicians should be aware of the available modalities and the indications for their use. Rapid recovery to a more comfortable life is realistic when combined pain-treatment strategies are used with well-informed patients.

### Procedures

Useful medications for painful procedures in the emergency department include intravenous fentanyl and midazolam, or methohexital sodium. Patients must be monitored for respiratory depression, which is usually brief. If oxygen saturation drops below 90%, use a bag-valve mask and oxygen to assist ventilation. Fentanyl can be reversed rapidly with naloxone, and midazolam can be reversed with flumazenil if deep sedation persists.

IV or IM administration of ketamine produces a dissociative state with minimal respiratory depression within five minutes. The recommended dosage is 1 to 4 mg/kg for a 20-minute procedure. A short-acting benzodiazepine should be administered with the ketamine to reduce the side effect of hallucinations or bizarre behavior after the procedure.

Nitrous oxide in combination with oxygen in a 50:50 to 80:20 mixture is useful for painful procedures (see the above section on pediatrics).

## Pain Treatment Flow Chart: Pre- and Intraoperative Phases

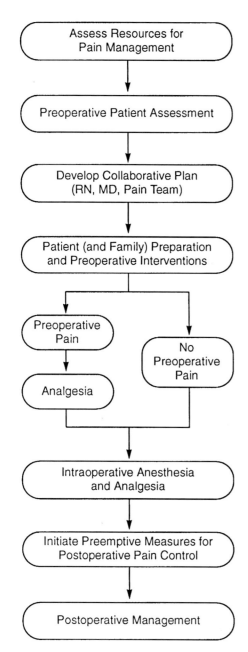

**Fig. 3-3.** Pain treatment flow chart: Preoperative and intraoperative phases.

Local anesthesia is commonly achieved with lidocaine or bupivacaine. The maximum dose for local infiltration of lidocaine is 3 to 5 mg/kg and 5 mg/kg for a peripheral nerve block. To minimize the local irritation, lidocaine can be buffered with sodium bicarbonate at a ratio of 10:1. Lidocaine with epinephrine is sometimes used to reduce local bleeding. There is a greater risk of tissue necrosis when epinephrine is used, and it should never be adminis-

tered in the fingers, nose, penis, toes, or ear. Bupivacaine is available for local infusion in 0.25%, 0.5%, and 0.75%, with or without epinephrine, and has a longer duration of action than lidocaine. The 0.75% solution should not be given to pregnant patients.

Other options for anesthesia include: a) Bier block and mini-Bier block for anesthesia to the hand, wrist, and forearm; b) regional blocks for anesthesia to the hand, wrist, forearm, elbow, and foot; and c) hematoma blocks for anesthesia of fractures of the hand and wrist. Lidocaine is used most commonly for regional and hematoma blocks. It is important to remember that the dose injected is quickly absorbed and can cause toxic reactions if care is not taken to avoid an overdose.

The mini-Bier block is very useful and easily performed.[15] The first step is to establish a small bore IV on the hand of the injured arm. Apply a blood pressure cuff to the upper arm, then raise the arm to drain venous blood. Inflate the blood pressure cuff quickly to exceed arterial pulse pressure using a clamp to ensure that air will not leak back through the tubing. Lower the arm to heart level and inject a 0.5% solution of lidocaine to a total of 1.5 mg/kg IV. Remove the IV and massage the hand to ensure wide distribution of the solution. Within 15 minutes, the arm will become anesthetized. The cuff should remain inflated for at least about 15 minutes. A 1.5 mg/kg dose of lidocaine should not be toxic.

Hematoma blocks are performed by injecting 1% lidocaine into the hematoma at the site of fracture. Complete anesthesia is not always obtained, but significant pain relief is afforded.

Median nerve block at the wrist is useful for fractures of the hand within the distribution of the median nerve. The median nerve is located between the palmaris longus tendon and the flexor carpi radialis tendon on the Volar aspect of the wrist. Use a small bore needle to inject around this nerve.

A block of the posterior tibial nerve at the ankle is sometimes useful. To perform this block, inject 1% lidocaine just posterior to the pulse of the posterior tibial artery, which can be felt posterior to the medial malleolus.

A brachial nerve block is most useful when elbow manipulations are necessary. It is performed by injecting 0.5% lidocaine around the pulse of the brachial artery in the axilla. The patient will feel tingling when the needle is in the correct position.

### Obtaining consent after pain medication

The patient who is experiencing acute pain and may require an operative procedure presents a dilemma to the emergency physician. When should pain control take precedence? Who should give consent? These questions are often asked in this setting. The role of the physician is to reduce pain and suffering without inflicting harm or injury to the patient. If an individual is extremely uncomfortable because

# Pain Treatment Flow Chart:
# Postoperative Phase

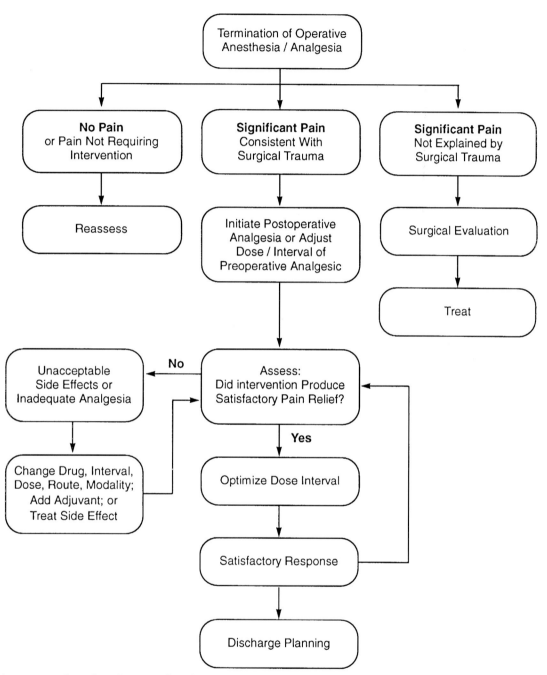

**Fig. 3-4.** Pain treatment flow chart: Postoperative phase.

of acute pain, an analgesic can be safely administered with appropriate monitoring of mental status and vital signs. It is difficult to obtain "informed consent" when a patient is experiencing pain. Some people think that the presence of significant pain unduly influences a patient to give consent.

Family members may be included when informing the patient who has been given analgesic medication. If the procedure is emergent and cannot be delayed, two physicians who are not going to perform the procedure may be included in the consent process.

**Discharge medications**

After the procedure, a limited supply of analgesic medication can be prescribed for the patient to provide pain relief until the follow-up visit. Oral opioids in conjunction with an NSAID or acetaminophen are common discharge medications (e.g., acetaminophen with codeine or hydrocodone, ibuprofen or ketoprofen).

## DISCUSSION

To relieve suffering is one of the primary roles of physicians and nurses. Recent studies have demonstrated the success of organized, multidisciplinary pain-management programs. Treatment of pain incorporates multiple modalities, including nonpharmacologic therapies. The patient's complaint of pain is the best indicator of the level of discomfort. Understanding the patient's perception of pain and overcoming patient fears regarding the pain are essential to the long-term alleviation of suffering. Preventive measures in pain management include telling patients what to expect with an acute injury or with a surgical procedure. When complaints of pain seem to escalate beyond the clinician's expectations, a thorough search for the cause of the pain should be done. Infection, other injury, or exacerbation of the original pain source must be ruled out before dismissing the complaints as undertreatment or patient manipulation. Satisfying outcomes can be realized when patients and clinicians work together toward the common goal—a return to an active, pain-free life.

## REFERENCES

1. Acute Pain Management Guideline Panel: *Acute pain management: operative or medical procedures and trauma. Clinical practice guideline.* Rockville, MD, Agency for Health Care Policy and Research, Public Health Service, U.S. Department of Health and Human Services. AHCPR publication no. 92-0032, 1992.

2. Hill CS: Pain. In Rakel RE, editor: *Conn's current therapy.* Philadelphia, WB Saunders, 1992.

3. Insel PA: Analgesic-antipyretics and antiinflammatory agents: drugs employed in the treatment of rheumatoid arthritis and gout. In: Goodman Gilman A, et al (eds): *The pharmacological basis of therapeutics,* ed 8, New York, Pergamon Press, 1990.

4. Mooney NE: Pain management in the orthopedic patient. *Nursing Clin North Am* 26:73-87, 1991.

5. Osterweis M, et al (eds): *Pain and disability: clinical, behavioral and public policy perspectives.* Washington, DC, National Academy Press, 1987.

6. Deathe A, Helmes E: Evaluation of a chronic pain programme by referring physicians. *Pain* 52:113-121, 1993.

7. Crook J, Weir F, Tunks E: An epidemiological follow-up survey of persistent pain sufferers in a group family practice and specialty pain clinic. *Pain* 36:49-61, 1989.

8. Max MB: Improving outcomes of analgesic treatment: is education enough? *Ann Intern Med* 113:885-889, 1990.

9. Srivatanakul K, et al: Studies with different types of visual analog scales for measurement of pain. *Clin Pharmacol Ther* 34:234-239, 1983.

10. Oden RV: Acute postoperative pain: incidence, severity, and the etiology of inadequate treatment. *Anesth Clin North Am* 7: 4-5, 1989.

11. McGrath PJ, Craig KD: Developmental and psychological factors in children's pain. *Pediatr Clin North Am* 36:825-835, 1989.

12. Max MB: U.S. Government disseminates acute pain treatment guidelines: will they make a difference? *Pain* 50:3-4, 1992.

13. Max MB: American Pain Society quality assurance standards for relief of acute pain and cancer pain. In: Bond MR, et al (eds): *Proceedings of the sixth world congress on pain,* Amsterdam, Elsevier, 1991.

14. Grossman SA, Sheidler VR: *The Johns Hopkins Oncology Center's Narcotic Conversion Program* [on disk]. Philadelphia, Lea & Febiger, 1989.

15. Farrell RG, Swanson SL, Walter JR: Safe and effective IV regional anesthesia for use in the emergency department. *Ann Emerg Med* 14(4): 288-292, 1985.

# Immobilization in the Emergency Department

*Wayne F. Hass*

Today's emergency physician must deal with many problems, not the least of which is the appropriate diagnosis and treatment of orthopedic injuries. Even though some of these injuries are relatively easy to diagnose, each case presents a wide variety of management options. The emergency physician must be able to diagnose and then provide such initial treatments as stabilization until an orthopedic surgeon arrives, temporary immobilization by casting or splinting with follow-up referral to a family practice or orthopedic specialist, or the definitive care of the patient's orthopedic needs, including instructions to follow up with the emergency department. The vast majority of emergency physicians never anticipate acting as the ongoing orthopedic specialist for a patient, but some patients fail to keep their follow-up appointments at an orthopedic clinic. They frequently damage or remove their casts and arrive at the emergency department in various states of disarray, requiring additional care for their fracture. Thus, on occasion, the emergency physician is the de facto orthopedist. This chapter discusses both the pearls of initial management (i.e., immobilization) and the pitfalls of ongoing care.

## HISTORICAL BACKGROUND

Approaches to the treatment of fractures have evolved over time. Certainly the fundamental tenet of fracture management is to reduce pain. Immobilization with some sort of external device wrapped about the fracture undoubtedly did so, even in prehistoric times. The next logical step to take would be to realign the broken limb. One of the earliest accounts, dating to approximately 1000 A.D., is from Albucasis, an Arabian surgeon and medical encyclopedist living in Spain who used bandages or cloth applied to the affected area and stiffened by the application of egg albumin.[1] Elsewhere, in the Arabian world, plaster was being used to immobilize fractures. Initial attempts involved making a box or container around the affected limb and pouring plaster into the box, immobilizing the affected area. Later, they used plaster that had partially set and applied it in its semiformed state to the affected area, again creating a rigid cast. Antonius Mathijson (Flemish army surgeon) is credited with developing plaster of paris bandages in approximately 1852. He prepared a plaster or gypsum material to apply to gauze bandages that were subsequently wetted and applied in multiple layers to the affected area. These would then dry and form a rigid cast. The Montmartre district in Paris held extensive deposits of gypsum (hence the name plaster of paris). The gypsum was found in its natural state and pulverized. Subsequent heating of the pulverized gypsum drove off water molecules. The addition of water at later stages reversed this reaction, allowing for crystal formation and the setting up of a plaster of paris cast.[2] Plaster of paris materials have been refined in the last 140 years; now, we have slow-setting, medium-setting and fast-setting plaster materials. Also, the recent introduction of new synthetic materials has contributed to our ability to immobilize fractures.[1]

## ADVANTAGES

The advantages of immobilization are fairly obvious. They include the following: 1) pain reduction; 2) proper alignment to facilitate healing (such healing should have both cosmesis and function as appropriate end points of therapy); 3) prevention of further injury, especially to neurovascular structures in close proximity to the fracture site or affecting the limb distal from the fracture site; and 4) easier movement of the patient in the prehospital setting, during diagnostic evaluation and x-ray and in the outpatient setting.[1]

## DISADVANTAGES

The disadvantages of immobilization are more difficult to appreciate at first glance. These are discussed under the headings below.

### Fracture disease

The term *fracture disease* applies to a number of changes that are considered secondary to the immobilization and healing of fractures. These changes primarily include 1) chronic edema, 2) the development of joint stiffness, 3) ischemic contractures, and 4) tissue atrophy, involving muscle, tendon, ligament, or bone.[3]

### Effects on calcium metabolism

Calcium is an element that is both stored within our bones and circulated throughout our body. Calcium adds considerably to the bone strength and also takes part in electrophysiologic chemical reactions within the body. Short-term immobilization rarely causes true problems with calcium metabolism. However, long-term immobilization, especially if combined with total body resting (as in patients with multiple trauma, head injury, or fractures requiring external traction) results in the loss of both bone and total body calcium. Newly mobilized calcium is excreted via the kidneys and may lead to renal impairment. This impairment is usually reversible but may persist. Problems associated with hypercalcemia are also encountered during these times. Abnormalities in calcium metabolism seem to be worse in adolescent males treated for fractures that require traction and bed rest.[4] This certainly does not preclude development of the same problems in women or older age groups; the emergency physician must therefore keep this problem in mind when treating patients from nursing homes or other facilities who may be restricted from their full activities while a fracture heals.

### Cast problems

A cast or splint must be neither too tight nor too loose. A cast that is too tight, or one that becomes tight through swelling of the tissue under it, may quickly result in neurovascular compromise and permanent disability for the patient if it is not promptly recognized and corrected. If the cast is tight only in certain places and not in a completely circumferential manner, pressure ulcers may develop, brought on through a process of ischemic necrosis. Such ulcers can develop in as little as two hours. Loose casts, on the other hand, fail to immobilize the fracture site adequately. This results in increased pain and improper healing, which may affect both cosmesis and function and certainly opens the door for additional injuries to neurovascular structures. A loose cast is associated with movement of the cast against the skin in an area of bony prominence; thus, a friction sore may develop. Another problem is that of thermal burns. Just as plaster of paris was formed by an endothermic reaction or baking of the original gypsum, the addition of water to plaster of paris creates an exothermic reaction. Depending on the patient's underlying skin and general condition, as well as on the mass of plaster involved, the heat released from such a reaction can be significant. Second-degree burns are not unheard of due to this problem. Occasional patients may also exhibit an allergic reaction to plaster of paris or other materials within the cast.[1] These must be dealt with as they arise. It is best, however, to prevent such problems from occurring in the first place.

### Other problems

Deep venous thrombosis (DVT) is a relatively common accompaniment of immobilization. While this problem is more frequently encountered with bed immobilization and the use of traction, it can also be found in the patient who is simply casted. The best treatment for this is prevention, which includes recognition of which patients are at higher risk (patients with a previous history of thrombophlebitis or DVT, elderly patients, patients with long leg casts, etc.) and subsequent efforts to minimize the time period of immobilization necessary for proper treatment of the fracture. Elevation of the affected extremity when at rest will facilitate venous return from that leg and will also reduce the risk of DVT, while it also minimizes edema.[1]

The last and perhaps one of the most important aspects of fracture management is the need to match the method of immobilization to the type of patient and fracture. It would be inappropriate to put a firm, full long leg cast on an elderly patient in a nursing home who does not and did not walk before the current injury. It is much more appropriate to treat this patient when possible with a Robert Jones dressing with or without plaster reinforcement. Conversely, the treatment of a young active, athletic individual with an ankle sprain might stress mobilization rather than immobilization; thus, treatment may consist of a simple elastic bandage or perhaps an air or gel cast ankle splint, to allow dorsal and plantar flexion at the ankle but to restrict medial and lateral movement of the ankle joint.

## MOBILIZATION

To allow appropriate fracture healing and return of full function, some injuries require no (or little) immobilization, while others require early immobilization.

### No or little immobilization

If immobilized too long (or even mobilized at all in certain cases) some fractures are complicated by the rapid development of stiffness and loss of function. Other fractures do not require restrictive immobilization, and the patient can be treated in a more liberal fashion, thus regaining full use and function sooner. Examples of these types of fractures and treatment might include simple fractures of the radius head, which are best placed in a sling for limited immobilization; the patient is encouraged to use the injured elbow as soon as possible to prevent subsequent stiffness during pronation, supination, extension, and flexion. Clavicle fractures represent another area where the philosophy regarding proper management has been changing. For many years, immobilization was considered desirable and best achieved with a figure-of-eight or McCleod splint applied so that the shoulders were pulled back and the patient assumed a military "at-attention" posture. Now studies are showing that simple slings to relieve pain and allow rest of the extremity provide very similar results although they certainly do not immobilize as well.[5] Likewise, soft-tissue injuries around joints are frequently splinted for comfort and mobilized as soon as possible. This might include minor sprains and ligament injuries as well as crushing injuries to the fingers. A large number of devices provide some degree of stabilization but not complete immobilization, and thereby facilitate pain reduction and healing. These include neck or cervical (C) collars, back braces,

buddy-taping of the fingers and toes, knee immobilizers, elastic bandages or wraps used in wrist, ankle, and knee areas, and ankle splints that allow motion in the anterior-posterior direction.

Continuous passive motion (CPM) devices also allow early mobilization of joint and soft tissue after surgery, even for injuries that do not involve fractures. These recently developed devices provide a continuous and gentle range of motion (ROM) throughout the day, 24 hours a day, for one to three weeks. The patient then progresses to active ROM. Again, early mobilization is used to stimulate soft-tissue healing around joints and fracture sites, resulting in both earlier and fuller recovery.[6]

### Early immobilization (rapid progression to mobilization)

The practice of immobilizing or keeping a fracture stable is based on the premise that such stabilization enhances the healing process so that the bone will become inherently stable. Through trial and error, various time increments have been recognized as necessary to immobilize a fracture site. Ideally, a fracture would be immobilized until the bone has healed enough to support itself and to perform its role within the body. As an example, one might consider the treatment of middle and distal humerus fractures. Current treatment of these fractures seems to center around the application of a sugar tong or U-type splint starting in the axilla, going down to and around the elbow, and continuing up the lateral humerus and over the top of the shoulder. Continued for four to six weeks, such treatment may be the definitive care of the fracture; however, some authors replace the splint after one week or so with a humerus brace and a cuff and collar support for the forearm to allow early mobility. Patients so treated enjoyed not only increased and earlier mobility but also increased range of motion, decreasing stiffness and apparently more satisfaction. The use of a device such as a brace around the humeral fracture allows the patient to remove it and wash as necessary and also to occasionally tighten up the brace to ensure a snug fit. While this specific study[7] supports one specific fracture and a goal for early mobilization, the concept can and should be applied to all fracture situations.

### Mobilization and rehabilitation

Once a fracture has healed, it is time to loosen up the muscles and begin to use them again. This should be done gradually at first, employing both active and passive ROM, perhaps facilitated with warm soaks and periods of splinting as necessary. This is an extremely important aspect of fracture care and management and, if not properly handled, will result in stiffness and permanent loss of mobility and function. The realities of care within an emergency department dictate that patients be given not only initial instruction on the appropriate management of their fracture, but also a long-term plan, including physical therapy and rehabilitation. If patients fail in their follow-up treatment, the importance

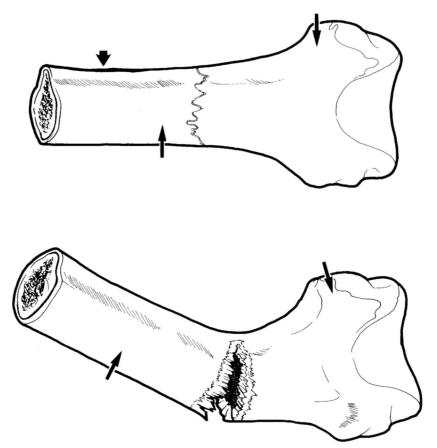

**Fig. 4-1.** A soft-tissue/periosteal hinge allows the cast to stabilize the fracture site via three points of force.

of rehabilitation must be emphasized, and, in some patients, referred to physical medicine and rehabilitation.

### TENETS OF FRACTURE REDUCTION AND CASTING

For a fracture to heal, it must be properly reduced, or realigned. This commonly requires the application of longitudinal traction to the fracture site and a reversal of the forces that caused the fracture. Reduction is more easily accomplished and maintained when there is a strong soft-tissue hinge on one side of the fracture site upon which to pivot the reducing forces and attain proper alignment. The cast or splint that is subsequently applied must stabilize the newly reduced fracture site. This is commonly referred to as a three-point system, or three points of force to maintain the reduction as originally described by Charnley and reemphasized in Rockwood and Green[1] (Fig. 4-1).

See other chapters for information regarding specific fractures, for example, which fractures require reduction and what degree of angulation is acceptable for each. Remember that some fractures are difficult to reduce and to maintain reduction and others are not. While many fractures can be temporarily splinted and others can be definitively casted, one should understand when to call the orthopedic consultant for assistance.

### MATERIALS

Plaster of paris for casting is available in various lengths and widths. It is available as a strip for application of splints or in rolls to facilitate the application of a circular cast. In the last few years, fiberglass and other synthetic materials have become increasingly popular in emergency departments. Some of the original fiberglass casts required an acetone cure, which often resulted in skin rashes; these have since been discontinued.[8] Subsequent efforts involved the light curing of fiberglass, which worked well but was time-consuming to apply. Current synthetics are water-activated polymers that are easy to use but are somewhat more expensive than plaster of paris.[9] Perhaps the most useful new products are the plaster or water-activated polymers (available as rolls in various widths) that can be cut to the desired length. These splinting materials have their own built-in padding and can be simply cut to length and applied as is with an elastic bandage. They can also be modified for special applications such as a thumb spica. They are quick, easy to use, and effective.

Thermolabile plastic materials have been available for a number of years and can be used to make casts but are more commonly used for splints. They are particularly helpful in the physical medicine and rehabilitation departments when specific splints are needed for extended periods.[8] Their use in the emergency department is limited to nonexistent.

Two other materials bear mentioning; these are stockinette and Webril-Curity®. Stockinette is made of cotton and can be applied over the full cast or on the ends only to provide a neat, finished edge. Stockinette by itself is not adequate padding for a cast or a splint and must be used with additional material. Such padding material comes in the form of sheet wadding, which is a multi-layered pad to apply over the stockinette. Another padding product is Webril-Curity®, which can also be applied over the stockinette to provide the additional cushion or padding necessary to allow proper cast fit. Different types of thicker padding may be used for high pressure points under the cast, and large rolls of cotton batting are used to form Robert Jones dressings over fracture sites when a large bulky compression dressing is desired.

## APPLICATION OF THE CAST OR SPLINT

Once the fracture has been diagnosed and the type of cast or splint needed has been identified, assemble the appropriate materials in sufficient size and quantity, perhaps cut to length, and apply the cast or splint as efficiently as possible. The patient should be informed of the type of cast or splint being applied so that he or she can understand and facilitate the proper application of the device. Certain patients and fractures require more than one set of hands to apply a splint or cast; obtaining additional help required before application will speed the application of the cast or splint and reduce the patient's pain and discomfort.

### Application techniques

**Casting.** Stockinette should be applied first, for either the full length of the cast or only at the top and bottom, to facilitate a clean, neat, finished edge on the cast. If the stockinette crosses a joint that has significant angulation (e.g., the ankle joint), care must be taken to avoid a crease in the stockinette, which could create a pressure point and perhaps lead to a pressure ulcer or wound. A crease in such areas can be avoided by making a horizontal cut on the concave side of the bend in the stockinette, and overlapping the stockinette material smoothly (Fig. 4-2). The stockinette chosen should be small enough to fit smoothly around the injured area, but not so loose that it looks sloppy (resulting in creases and pressure points) or so tight that it constricts the injured area.

If additional padding materials such as sheet wadding are needed, it should be rolled from top to bottom of the casted area with an overlap of approximately half of its width on each turn. This will result in a uniform double-thickness layer of Webril-Curity® for the cast. The structure of Webril-Curity® is such that it can be stretched to facilitate a smooth application down the length of the cast. Again, avoid creating any lumps or irregularities and, if it is impossible to continue with one roll, the material should be

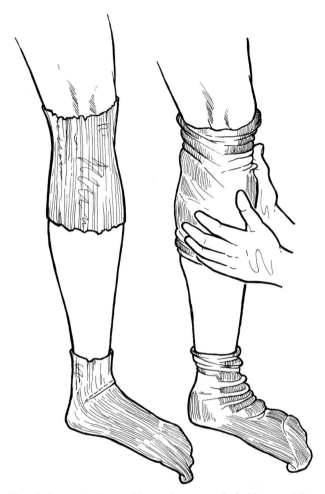

**Fig. 4-2.** Apply the stockinette in a smooth fashion, avoiding creases which could create a pressure point.

torn off cleanly and the application begun anew. Webril-Curity® clings to itself, so it is easy to insert small patches or start and stop the roll as necessary to obtain proper thickness and flow of the padding (Fig. 4-3).

The next step in applying the cast is to wet the cast or splint material to activate either the plaster of paris or the synthetic polymer. While there is some variation in these products, it is generally true that the cooler the water, the longer it takes to set the casting material. Cool-to-tepid water will decrease the time it takes the material to set, allowing more time to work with the cast and properly mold it. It will also retard exothermic reaction, minimizing the pain and discomfort that may be associated with the heat release. When wetting a roll of plaster, it is best to unroll approximately six inches off the end of the roll. This free end is more easily found and facilitates the application. The roll should be held vertically in the water for three to five seconds. Bubbles will escape through the top of the vertical core of plaster material during this time. Slab or splint material should be grasped firmly by the two ends and dipped in the bucket briefly to wet thoroughly. Both materials should be squeezed slightly to remove excess

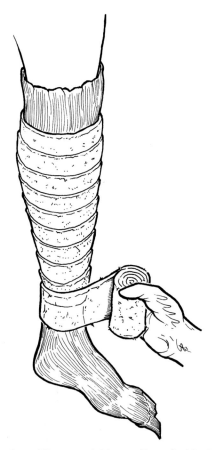

**Fig. 4-3.** Apply padding material in a uniform double thickness. Avoid creating any lumps or irregularities.

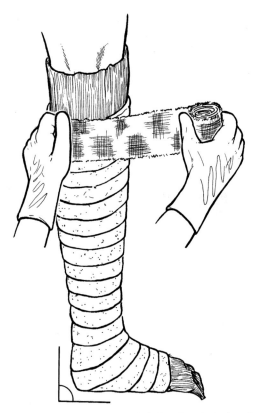

**Fig. 4-4.** Holding the roll in the right hand and placing the free end of the roll at the top of the cast, apply the cast material.

water but not so firmly that all of the plaster is extruded from the material. Dipping plaster of paris cast or splint material for too long or squeezing too tightly will compromise the ultimate strength of the cast or splint. Synthetic materials have an advantage here in that none of the material is compromised by prolonged dipping. However, they must be properly squeezed or rolled out and partially dried before application. Specific instructions regarding this will accompany the type of material chosen for use.

The cast is applied by holding the roll in the right hand (assuming the physician is right-handed) and placing the tail or free end of the roll to the top of the cast (Fig. 4-4). The cast material is then unrolled around the cast length in a continually advancing fashion down or back up the involved area. As the diameter of the area being casted changes, excess material will be noted; this material should be tucked in with the left hand and smoothed down as the rolls comes over it a second time (Fig. 4-5). The plaster material should be applied as rapidly and neatly as possible, again avoiding irregularities and creases that could cause pressure points. The full thickness of the cast should be approximately one quarter of an inch, which represents between 8 and 10 layers of casting material. One should always select the largest-width material that can be comfortably used on the area to be casted. The cast should be made longer than necessary so that the edges can be trimmed back and will, therefore, be firm and solid. Once

the full cast has been applied, it is necessary to form or mold the cast to the body area involved (Fig. 4-6). This should be done with the palms and thenar eminences and not with the fingers, which have a tendency to dent the cast and create pressure points. Firm molding of the cast around the muscles as well as the bony prominences ensures proper and comfortable fit, and minimizes any subsequent motion of the cast. Once the cast has been applied and molded, it is time to finish the ends. This should be done promptly while the cast is still green and requires a scalpel or cast knife to make a strong edge on the cast (Fig. 4-7). Then, the stockinette or padding material can be rolled back over the top and bottom edge of the cast and a final layer of plaster applied to hold that rolled back material in place (Fig. 4-8). This last plaster application is not intended to give any additional structural support to the cast but rather to create a neat, finished look to the cast and an edge that will not injure the patient.

Drying a cast or splint should be a simple matter. However, this step's importance is frequently overlooked, and drying problems can and do occur. After all the time spent on diagnosing, reducing, and treating the fracture, it is also necessary to hold that reduction while the cast material sets. While a plaster of paris cast develops some stability in 20 or 30 minutes, it will not fully set for 24 to 48 hours. Water-activated synthetic materials dry more quickly but still require attention so that the proper reduction is maintained during the early setup or curing time. After the

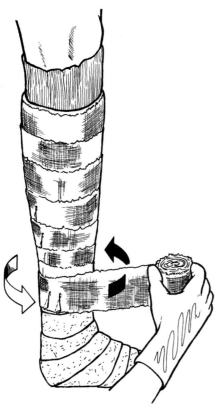

**Fig. 4-5.** Apply the cast material as rapidly and neatly as possible, tucking excess material down and going over the tuck on the next roll.

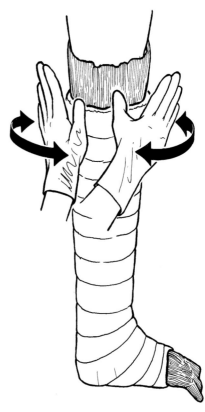

**Fig. 4-6.** Mold the cast firmly with palms and thenar prominence, not with the fingertips, which will dent and create a pressure point.

fracture is reduced and the injury casted, the patient must understand the importance of staying in that position until the initial cast setup is complete. One easy technique is to use pillows, regardless of whether the patient is sitting or lying on a cart. A pillow provides support for the casted extremity while it cures and protects against dents that may occur if a leg is, for instance, left to hang over the end of litter or cart. Once again, instruct the patient to maintain the reduction and if necessary, have an assistant stay with him or her while the casting material cures.

**Splinting.** Splints require much the same preparation and considerations as casts, especially with respect to proper fit and padding. By its nature, a splint will not be as rigid as a circumferential cast, but it may be a very appropriate immobilization device for minor fractures. This type of device should be considered when the risk of swelling is particularly marked. Splints may be applied easily by using premade splinting material, choosing the appropriate width of material, and cutting it to the appropriate length. Manufacturers of premade splint material often supply patterns that can be used to devise particular types of splints. As an alternative to premade splint materials, one can make one's own by laying down on a table a double thickness and proper length piece of Webril-Curity®. The appropriate length and width of plaster is then chosen and cut, dipped in water and gently squeezed, and laid out over the doubled Webril-Curity®. A single length of

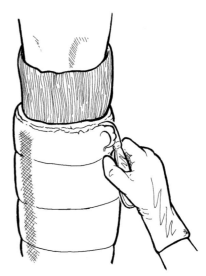

**Fig. 4-7.** Cut the ends of cast with a scalpel or cast knife to ensure uniformly thick and, therefore, a firm edge to the cast.

Webril-Curity® is placed on top, creating a padded, enclosed plaster splint (Fig. 4-9). This splint can be quickly applied to the affected area with an elastic bandage and molded to obtain the proper fit. A variation would be to use stockinette and choose the appropriate width and length of plaster material. Eight to 10 sheets of thickness of plaster material are used and inserted within the stockinette (Fig. 4-10). Additional padding is applied to the area to be

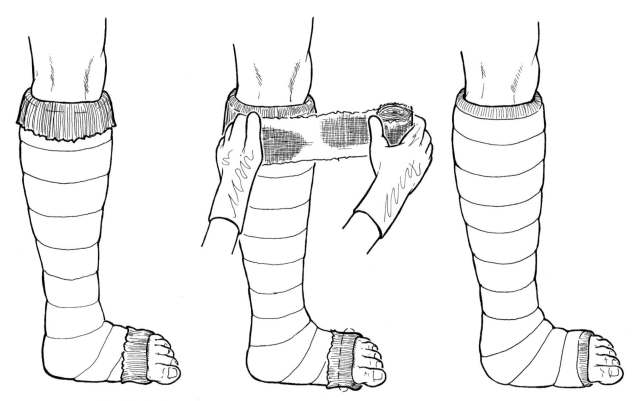

**Fig. 4-8.** Roll stockinette and padding over the edge of cast to create a smooth edge and finish with a plaster overlay.

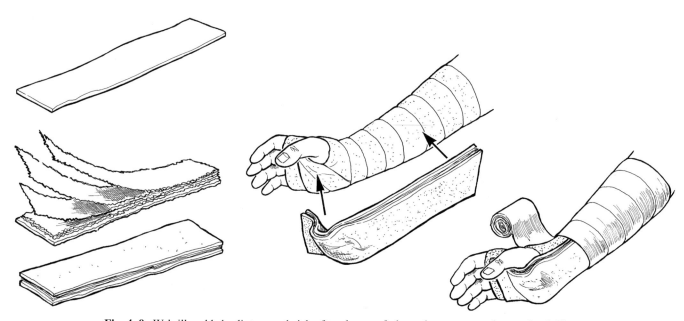

**Fig. 4-9.** Webrill-padded splint, a sandwich of ten layers of plaster between two sheets of webrill padding.

splinted, and the stockinette-encased plaster is then dipped in water, squeezed, applied, wrapped with elastic bandages, and molded. Both of these two homemade splints are effective and inexpensive. However, one should remember that 1) additional padding may be necessary, and 2) the plaster must be covered with some sort of material before the ace or elastic bandage is applied. A bandage that is applied directly to plaster will be impregnated with the plaster and lose its elastic characteristics. It therefore has less ability to stretch with swelling of the affected part.

**Post-casting and splinting.** After a cast has been applied, it is appropriate to ensure not only that it fits properly, but also that the reduction has been maintained. For this reason, a post-reduction and post-casting x-ray film should be obtained. Before the patient is discharged from the emergency department, a circulation, motion, and sensation

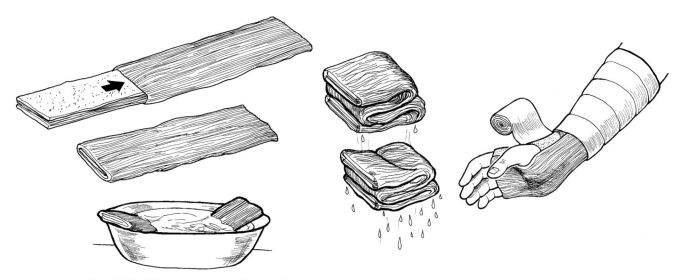

**Fig. 4-10.** Splint made in a stockinette sheath.

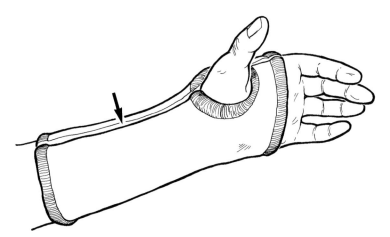

**Fig. 4-11.** Split cast.

(CMS) check should be performed on the body part distal to the cast. The patient should be instructed about cast care, which should include elevation of the area to facilitate venous blood return and minimize swelling as well as the signs and symptoms of a tight cast that will require a return to the emergency department for appropriate modification. If, due to the type of injury involved, there is a strong concern about excessive swelling before the patient even leaves the emergency department, the cast should be split or bivalved. Splitting a cast refers to performing a full length cut upon one aspect or side of the cast with a cast saw (Fig. 4-11). Then, a cast splitter is used to open up the cut. This will allow minimal release of tension from the cast compartment. A further modification of splitting a cast may involve making a second cut approximately 1 cm from the first cut and removal of that 1-cm strip of material (Fig. 4-12). This along with cutting through the Webril-Curity® and stockinette material under the cut, will further release the compression of the casting cylinder. Some fractures require bivalving. This is the process of placing a cut on two sides of the cast, 180° degrees from each other, so that

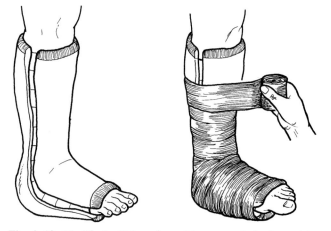

**Fig. 4-12.** Modified splitting of a cast by removal of a 1-cm strip of material.

the cast can be lifted off having both a top and bottom portion. The cast is subsequently kept in place by elastic bandages firmly applied over the newly bivalved halves of the cast (Fig. 4-13).

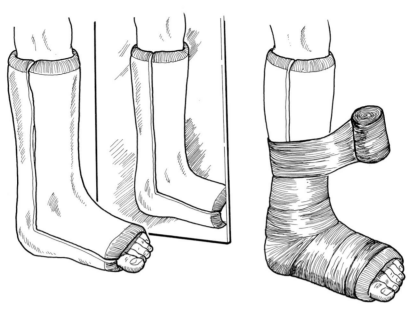

**Fig. 4-13.** Bivalved cast.

**Complications.** Complications secondary to swelling under a cast are of major concern. Be liberal in the decision to 1) admit patients for observation after casting so that elevation can be ensured and the fingers or toes beyond the end of the cast can be assessed to verify that CMS are adequate; 2) use Robert Jones dressings with or without plaster for the grossly swollen fracture. This heavily padded compression dressing provides good support and pain reduction and facilitates the interim phase before casting. Once again, consider hospitalization in such cases, or a return to the emergency department in 12 to 24 hours for a cast change.

### Various casts and splints

**Short arm cast (SAC).** A short arm cast (SAC) extends from the proximal forearm to the palm and dorsal hand. It allows full motion at the metacarpophalangeal (MCP) joints. Therefore, it ends dorsally just short of the MCP joints and extends on the palm side to the distal palmar crease. In a standard short arm cast, the thumb is free to facilitate functional use of the hand (i.e., opposition of the thumb with the fingers). The SAC can be modified with aluminum finger splints as necessary for phalangeal and metacarpal injuries. The aluminum splint is applied to the volar surface of the SAC and held in place with additional layers of plaster of paris. The "outrigger" or distal portion of the splint is appropriately bent to obtain the desired fixation and attached to the fingers with tape. The extended aluminum splint may be applied to one or two fingers, especially when buddy taping to a stable finger is desired. When injuries occur to the thumb, first metacarpal, or navicular bone, it is necessary to incorporate the thumb into the SAC. This is termed a thumb spica and should completely immobilize the thumb, MCP joints and interpha-

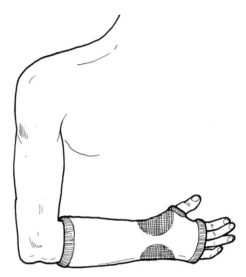

**Fig. 4-14.** Padding about the thumb and ulnar styloid areas should be given special care in the short arm cast.

langeal joints. *Note:* Take special care when padding around the thumb in the standard SAC and when carving the cast in this area. Additional padding should be applied to the ulnar styloid area (Fig. 4-14).

**Long arm cast.** The long arm cast (LAC) extends from the proximal portion of the upper arm or humerus through the elbow area flexed at 90° and onto and over the wrist and palm area. The hand is held in pronation, and the cast allows full motion at the thumb and finger levels. Additional padding should be applied over the bony prominences, olecranon process, medial and lateral epicondyles, and ulnar styloid (Fig. 4-15).

**Short leg cast.** The short leg cast may either be a weight-bearing or a non–weight-bearing type. Both casts

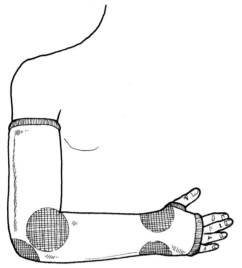

**Fig. 4-15.** Additional padding over the bony prominences should be applied in the long arm cast.

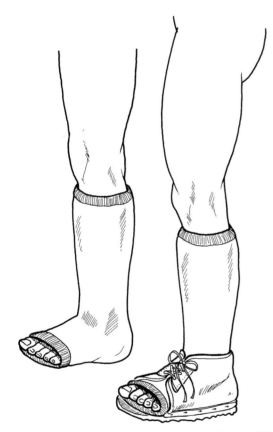

**Fig. 4-16.** Short leg cast with the ankle immobilized at 90°, and placed in a cast boot/shoe.

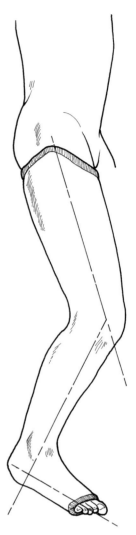

**Fig. 4-17.** Long leg cast with the knee immobilized at 15° to 20° of flexion.

proximal fibular head as well as to the medial and lateral malleoli. Weight-bearing casts were once fitted with walking heels or iron, but currently these have been replaced by cast boots or cast shoes (Fig. 4-16).

**Long leg cast.** The long leg cast is an extension of the short leg cast up and over the knee and to the high thigh area. The knee is immobilized at 15° to 20° of flexion (Fig. 4-17).

**Long leg cylinder cast.** The long leg cylinder cast extends from the high or proximal thigh area to just above the malleoli. It requires additional padding over the fibular head. It must be firmly molded to maintain its position on the leg. There is a natural tendency of this cast to slip down, especially with subsequent atrophy of the muscle. For this reason, various adhesive foams are used to pad this cast and keep it in place. Additional care should be directed to the cutting and padding at the distal end of the cast (Fig. 4-18).

**Splints**

Splints are undeniably the forte of the emergency physician. While a splint does not immobilize as well as a cast, it

extend from just below the knee to the toes. It is customary to incorporate a plantar or volar plate on the cast that will restrict flexion of the toes. The top, or dorsum, of the toes is often exposed, and the ankle is usually in its neutral position at 90°. Additional padding should be applied to the

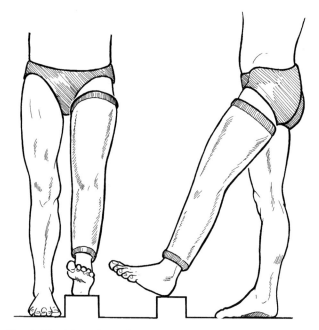

**Fig. 4-18.** A long-leg cylinder cast.

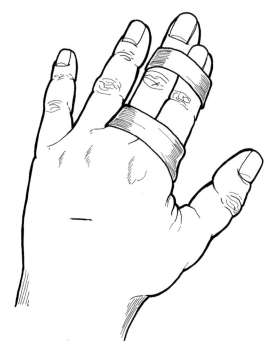

**Fig. 4-19.** Buddy taping of the fingers.

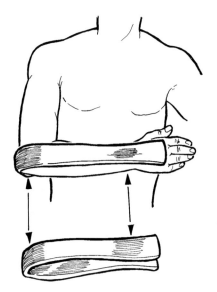

**Fig. 4-20.** A sugar tong splint limiting pronation and supination of the forearm.

still provides good immobilization as well as room for swelling and expansion to a minimal degree. Splints therefore are frequently used to get the patient from the emergency department to a follow-up appointment with the patient's orthopedic physician. The newer synthetic materials, with their incorporated padding, are an attractive, quick, easy, and effective alternative to making a homemade splint.

**Buddy taping.** Fingers and toes can often be treated for minor injuries by buddy taping. Buddy taping is the practice of taping an injured digit to an adjacent, uninjured digit. If necessary, this can done in conjunction with simple aluminum splints or even short arm casts (Fig. 4-19).

**Sugar tong splint.** Sugar tong splints can be applied in

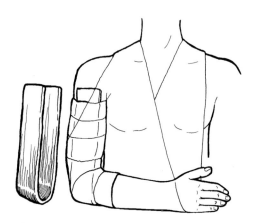

**Fig. 4-21.** A sugar tong splint of the humerus.

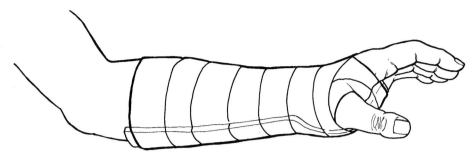

**Fig. 4-22.** Volar forearm splint provides partial immobilization of the wrist.

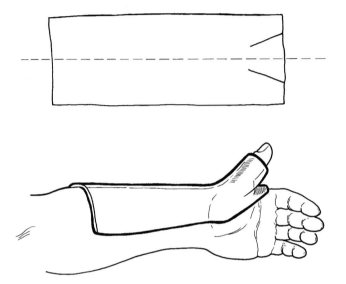

**Fig. 4-23.** Radial thumb spica splint incorporates splinting material over the web space between the thumb and index finger as well as around the thumb.

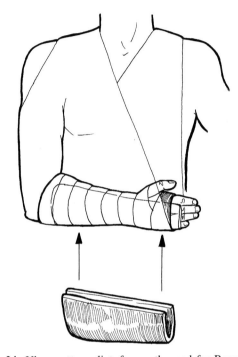

**Fig. 4-24.** Ulnar gutter splint, frequently used for Boxer's fracture.

two directions on the upper extremity. The first mimics a SAC in that it extends from the dorsal hand just proximal to the MCP joints, up the dorsal forearm, around the elbow, and back down the volar forearm to the distal palmar crease. The sugar tong splint in this direction is more effective in limitation of pronation and supination of the forearm than is the SAC. Additional padding is required over the ulnar styloid as well as around the medial and lateral epicondyles (Fig. 4-20).

A sugar tong splint for the humerus is applied from the axilla down the medial aspect of the upper arm, around the elbow, and back up the outside portion of the upper arm, with extension over the shoulder area. Extra padding is required around the elbow over the medial and lateral epicondyle as well as around the olecranon process (Fig. 4-21).

**Volar forearm splint.** This simple splint provides partial immobilization for the wrist and extends from the proximal forearm down the volar aspect of the forearm and to the distal palmar crease (Fig. 4-22).

**Radial thumb spica splint.** The radial thumb spica splint extends from the radial aspect of the proximal forearm, down the forearm in a radial gutter fashion, and onto the thumb. It wraps over the thumb and also incorpo-

rates a small portion of splinting material over the web space between the thumb and index finger (Fig. 4-23).

**Ulnar gutter splint.** The ulnar gutter splint is designed to go in a gutter or U-shaped fashion from the proximal ulnar aspect of the forearm down across the wrist and extending out onto the hand as far as necessary. Because this splint is frequently used to treat metacarpal fractures (boxer's fractures), it should in those applications be extended out to approximately the distal interphalangeal (DIP) joint level. Otherwise, it may be terminated at a more proximal level (Fig. 4-24).

**Sandwich splint.** A sandwich splint is a splint that covers the affected area from both above and below. The sandwich splint is most commonly used on the forearm, extending from the proximal forearm down across the wrist and out onto the hand. Like all previously mentioned devices in this area, it should be appropriately padded with additional padding over the ulnar styloid. This is an excellent splint for metacarpal fractures (Fig. 4-25).

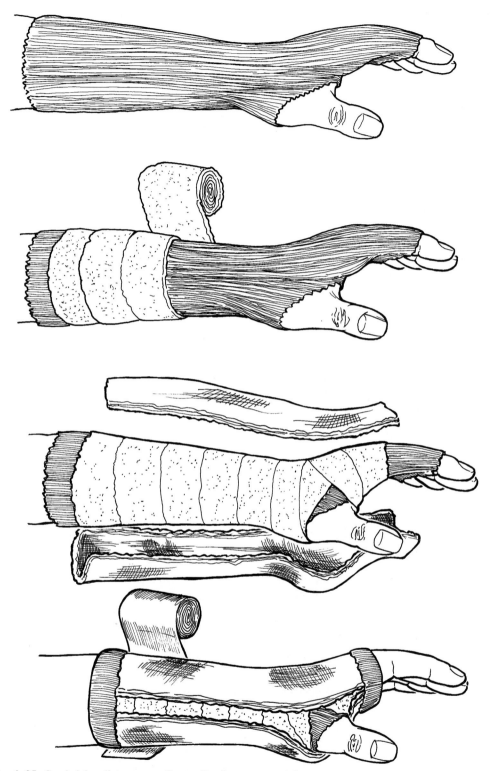

**Fig. 4-25.** Sandwich splint—an excellent splint for metacarpal fractures.

**Ankle splints.** Splints of the lower extremity are confined usually to either a posterior ankle splint, a sugar tong splint, or a U-shaped splint around the ankle. Once again, special padding should be provided for the medial and lateral malleoli as needed (Fig. 4-26).

**Robert Jones dressing.** The Robert Jones or Jones dressing is a heavily padded dressing applied to any fracture site in which compression and immobilization are required but swelling from the injury is considerable. It can be applied as a simple cotton-batting wrapping with large

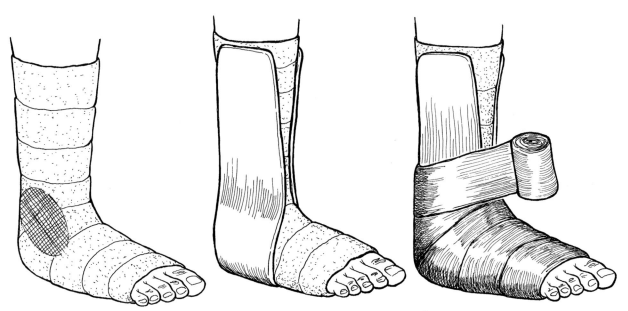

**Fig. 4-26.** Ankle splint should provide special padding around the malleoli.

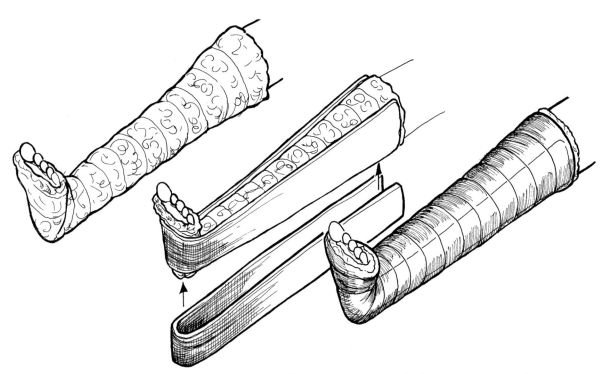

**Fig. 4-27.** A reinforced Robert Jones dressing is commonly used when compression and immobilization are required but swelling is considerable. Plaster reinforcement may be posterior or medial/lateral.

elastic bandages over it, or a plaster slab can be incorporated into the splint to add stability. Once again, if plaster splints are added to this type of dressing or if it is to be used with elastic bandages, it is important to cover the plaster with Webril-Curity® or other feltlike material to preserve the elasticity of the bandages (Fig. 4-27).

## PREMADE DEVICES

A large number of premade immobilization devices are available for use in the emergency department and can be used with very good results. Certainly, if strict attention is needed to exact reduction of an area, a premade device will not suffice in holding the reduction. However, if the fracture or injury is such that limited motion is acceptable, premade devices can be extremely helpful as well as fast and easy to use.

### Aluminum finger splints

These devices come in various lengths and are usually in a position of function, with slight flexion of the digit. They can be quickly and easily taped in place for minor injuries to the digits. Longer finger splints might be incorporated into a SAC with finger extension. Also available is aluminum splinting material of various widths that can be cut to length and formed or angulated as necessary. Again, this material is easily manipulated and can be shaped and used quickly. It works extremely well as a dorsal splint in mallet finger injuries to hold the finger at the DIP in straight extension or slight hyperextension. Distal finger gauntlet-type extension splints are also available for mallet finger injuries, and come in various sizes (Fig. 4-28).

### Forearm splints

Preformed or premade forearm splints are of limited application in the emergency department. Some splints for this area are made of a malleable material that can be quickly affixed to help stabilize the fracture and send the patient safely to x-ray. Most, however, do not lend themselves to definitive treatment or even interim treatment, after which the patient can be discharged from the emergency department. Carpal tunnel and overuse syndromes of the forearms can, however, be successfully treated with some preformed forehand or forearm splints. These splints usually have a contoured volar surface across the wrist area and on the hand and are held in place with Velcro® or similar fastening straps. These devices are usually not prescribed from the emergency department but originate from the departments of occupational medicine or physical medicine and rehabilitation.

### Shoulder immobilizer

The shoulder immobilizer is basically the old sling and swath. A sling supports the forearm from the elbow down through the wrist and onto the hand. The swath holds the arm close to the body by passing over the outside of the humerus and being tied around the thorax. The shoulder immobilizer, as manufactured by various medical device companies, consists of a sling type device as well as Velcro® straps around the distal humerus which attach to matching Velcro® straps on a thorax piece. Shoulder immobilizers are used for upper arm injuries, especially for initial immobilization of first-time shoulder dislocations (Fig. 4-29).

### Sling

As previously mentioned, a sling is a forearm support and should extend from the elbow across the wrist and under the hand. Care should be taken to make sure that the fit of the sling is appropriate for the patient and that the patient understands that the hand is to be supported within the sling. Failure to do this will result in the patient having the wrist drop at the edge of the sling and resultant nerve compression in the wrist area.

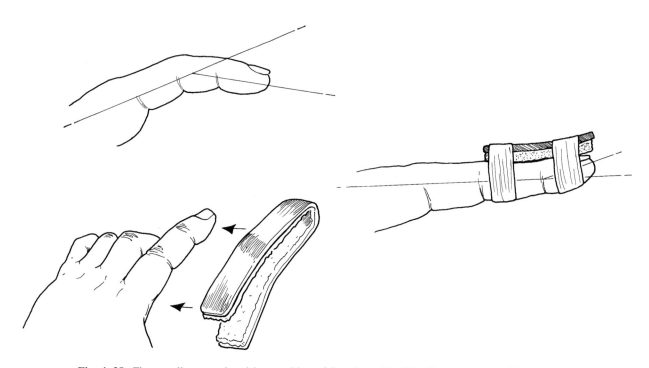

**Fig. 4-28.** Finger splints are placed in a position of function with slight flexion or in straight to mild hyperextension depending on the fracture being treated.

## AC joint splints

The acromioclavicular (AC) joint splint is an attempt to pull down the distal clavicle and hold it in proper alignment for healing of second- and even third-degree AC joint separations. This device resembles a shoulder immobilizer, but instead of a Velcro® strap around the distal humerus, it has a Velcro® strap that attaches to the front of the thorax band, goes up and over the distal clavicle, and attaches posteriorly to the thorax band. This strap can be adjusted to pull down on the distal end of the clavicle. This treatment is in question; many orthopedists prefer to use a simple sling for first- and second-degree AC joint injuries and surgery, when necessary, for third-degree injuries (Fig. 4-30).

## Clavical splints

Simple clavical fractures can be treated with a figure-eight clavical splint made in the emergency department or a premade device such as a McCleod splint. These devices pull the shoulders back, place the patient in a position of military "at-attention" and thus immobilize the fracture and enhance patient comfort (Fig. 4-31).

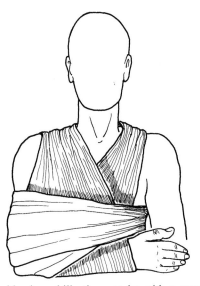

**Fig. 4-29.** Shoulder immobilization can be with a special premade immobilizer or with sling and swath.

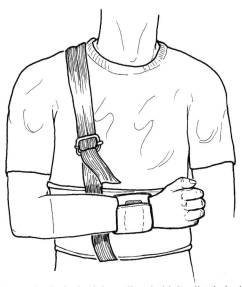

**Fig. 4-30.** Acromioclavicular joint splints hold the distal clavicle down in place.

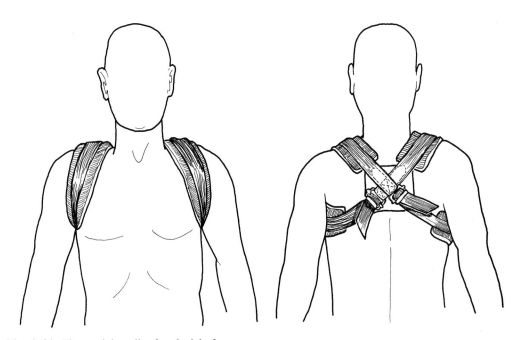

**Fig. 4-31.** Figure eight splint for clavicle fractures.

### Cervical collars

Soft cervical collars are good treatment for simple whiplash injuries. They provide the necessary rest and restriction of neck motion. Philadelphia collars, on the other hand, provide better immobilization. They may be used in the prehospital as well as the hospital setting and as outpatient treatment for minor injuries to the neck. These devices do not provide complete immobilization of the cervical spine but can be very helpful when only limited immobilization is necessary, as in minor ligamentous injuries or stable fractures of the cervical spine (see Chapter 5).

### Back braces

Back braces are rarely used in the emergency department and are more frequently prescribed in the departments of occupational medicine or physical medicine and rehabilitation.

### Knee immobilizer

The knee immobilizer is commonly used and provides very good partial immobilization of the knee, assuming that is all that is necessary. The knee immobilizer is a foam cylinder applied with Velcro® straps from the high thigh to the low tibia-fibula area. It has medial and lateral aluminum stays attached to the immobilizer. There is a potential for pressure by the lateral stay against the peroneal nerve as it crosses near the proximal fibular head. For this reason, many physicians prefer to remove the lateral stay from the knee immobilizer (Fig. 4-32).

### Ankle splints

The elastic bandage is the most convenient and frequently used type of ankle splint. Properly applied in a figure-of-eight configuration about the ankle, it provides compression and minimal stabilization of the ankle joint. More complete immobilization of the ankle, at least in respect to the medial and lateral ligaments, can be provided by various air and gel splints. These splints usually come with good padding on the medial and lateral aspects of the splint and Velcro® straps to hold them firmly in place. They permit plantar and dorsiflexion at the ankle but limit medial and lateral motion.

They are especially good for getting people back on their feet who want to be up and active. These might include people returning to work or those with a strong interest in competitive sports such as basketball (Fig. 4-33).

### Bunion boots

A bunion boot is a wood or synthetic hard-soled material with leather uppers and laces. The bunion boot provides an excellent firm walking surface for the treatment of Jones fractures of the proximal fifth metatarsal. It also can be used for the treatment of other soft-tissue injuries of the foot where a firm, nonbending sole or walking surface is required and, obviously, is designed for the use of the post–operative bunion patient.

### SUPPORT DEVICES

These devices are designed to offer support of the body's weight upon a device carried by the upper extremities so that healing and rest of the lower extremity injury can occur. Crutches, canes, and walkers are used to provide support when necessary for injuries to the lower extremity. Crutches are the most frequently used of these devices. They should be properly measured for the patient in respect to the total height as well as the hand distance from the axilla. The patient should be instructed to bear weight on the hands and not in the axilla, where nerve compression and secondary complications can take place. Crutches are excellent devices and can be used by many patients, but they have limitations as patients become older, overweight, or have other disabilities that preclude their use. In such cases, a walker may be appropriate. Walkers were originally designed to help people get about as they become older and unsteady on their feet, perhaps while recovering from a stroke. However, they are also useful to patients with lower extremity injuries who cannot tolerate crutches. They provide moderate support but can be an acceptable device in the later stages of healing. Canes, on the other hand, provide minimal, if any, support to the lower extremity. This limitation precludes wide acceptance in their use. They are, however, useful for a small number of patients who need only a slight amount of assistance. The cane

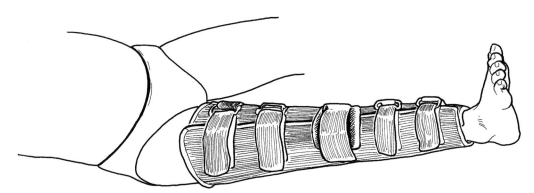

**Fig. 4-32.** Knee immobilizer provides good, but not rigid, immobilization of the knee.

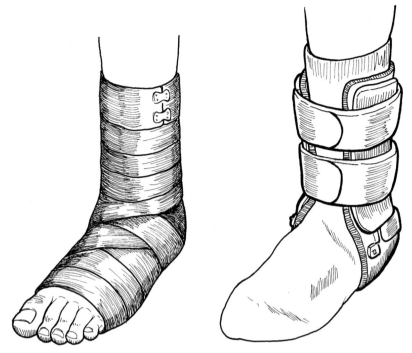

**Fig. 4-33.** Ankle splints can vary from elastic bandages to reinforced air or gel splints.

should be held in the hand on the side of the injured leg to bear weight when the uninjured leg is swung forward.

## IMPROVISATION

First aid courses have often taught how to immobilize fractures in the field with whatever devices were available. This is certainly true for first aiders, first responders, prehospital personnel members of a more advanced organization like the National Ski Patrol, and wilderness or outdoor enthusiasts. Members of many large organizations still wear cravats with which to fashion slings or apply splints. Numerous materials can be used to apply as splints to a broken extremity; these include—but are not limited to—wooden boards, skis, ski poles, wire mesh, newspaper, magazines, and small trees or saplings. These may be held in place with tape, belts, cravats or other bandages or items of clothing, as appropriate.

## DISCUSSION

An important point to remember in treating orthopedic injuries is to choose the right treatment for the right patient. The injury should be treated appropriately, but one should also consider the patient's specific medical condition and limitations, job, sports activities, and routine activities of daily living. Treating the injuries of the handicapped or nursing home patient is far different than treating the same injury in a young, athletic individual. The quadriplegic patient and the patient with a condition resulting in loss of sensation, which limits awareness of constriction or pain, also merits careful attention. Dementia is another condition where the patient will frequently not report complications

with a cast or immobilizing device to the emergency physician or other appropriate person. Also, such patients may not continue to wear devices that facilitate the healing of the injury. Patients with diabetes or other conditions that predispose to infection or skin breakdown may need extra padding and additional or early follow-up care.

The emergency physician should know the follow-up consultant and discuss the patient with him while the patient is in the emergency department receiving initial care and treatment. The consultant may prefer, for example, a figure-of-eight or McCleod splint for a clavicle fracture. Knowing who the consultant is and discussing the case at the time of patient presentation will minimize aftercare problems for the patient. Likewise, the emergency physician should know what kind of cases the orthopedic consultant wants to see and treat personally, Some consultants prefer to see their patients from the time of their initial presentation, while others prefer that the emergency physician provide initial stabilization and treatment, with a follow-up visit in a few days in the consultant's clinic. Knowing when to call the orthopedic or hand specialist is vital to the proper management of complex cases. When in doubt, it is best to call the specialist and discuss the case.

The emergency physician should be especially aware of cast and splint problems. Patients should be made to understand that they must return to the emergency department if any pain, sensory loss, or other problems develop after a splint or cast has been applied. Giving a patient the telephone number of an orthopedic specialist who will conduct a follow-up examination does not close the case for the emergency physician. Finally, one must be sure that patients understand that, if complications arise, they must return to the emergency department or see a specialist as soon as possible for further evaluation and management.

## REFERENCES

1. Harkess JW, Ramsey WC, Harkess JW: Principles of fractures and dislocations. In: Rockwood CA, Green DP, Bucholz RW, (eds): *Rockwood and Green's fractures in adults,* ed 3, Philadelphia, JB Lippincott, 1991.
2. Schneider FR: *Handbook for the orthopedic assistant,* St. Louis, CV Mosby, 1972.
3. Anderson GI: Fracture disease and related contractures, *Vet Clin North Am Small Anim Pract* 21:845, 1991.
4. Andrews PI, Rosenberg AR: Renal consequences of immobilization in children with fractured femurs, *Acta Paediatr Scand* 79:311, 1990.
5. Andersen K, et al: Treatment of clavicle fractures: figure of eight bandage versus a simple sling, *Acta Orthop Scand* 57:71, 1987.
6. Continuous passive motion, an innovative concept enhancing the healing process of bone fractures, *Can Oper Room Nurs J* 7:14, 1989.
7. Camden P, Nade S: Fracture bracing the humerus, *Injury* 23: 245, 1992.
8. Lewis RC: *Handbook for traction, casting and splinting techniques,* Philadelphia, JB Lippincott, 1972.
9. Bowker P, Powell ES: A clinical evaluation of plaster of paris and eight synthetic fracture splinting materials, *Injury* 23:13, 1992.

# CHAPTER 5

# Cervical Spine Injuries

*Brian Mahoney*

Because there is no national injury registry, no none knows the true incidence of significant spinal cord injury in the United States. However, data from the National Spinal Cord Injury Center study of 1975 give us an approximation.[1] This regional study covered a large part of Northern California, and reported the incidence of spinal cord injury was 53.4 per million people, and death occurred in 48 percent. Applying these data to the population of the United States in 1994 yields approximately 14,000 spinal cord injuries and 6700 deaths each year. Many of those deaths could be caused by multiple injuries in addition to cord injury. In slightly more than half of these injuries, the cord damage would be the immediate cause of death, but approximately 7300 patients will survive each year with significant neurologic disability. This is truly a national epidemic, aside from being a personal and family tragedy.

## EMERGENCY MANAGEMENT

When confronted with a patient having possible spinal column or cord injury, the emergency physician has four priorities. The first is to ensure patient survival. The physician should follow the same approach used in the resuscitation of any critically injured patient. A primary survey including airway, breathing, circulation, disability, and exposure (ABCDE) should be done, followed by resuscitation, a secondary survey, and disposition for definitive care. The second priority is to preserve residual spinal cord function. The physician should be cautioned to avoid causing a second injury to the already damaged tissue by not allowing unnecessary motion, hypoxia, poor perfusion, or infection. The third priority is to begin treatment that will allow optimum recovery of the cord-injured patient. Very high-dose methylprednisolone, cord rest by immobilization, skin care, respiratory care, and genitourinary care should be used. The fourth priority is to restore spinal column stability. This, of course, cannot be accomplished in the Emergency Department; however, even the patient who will remain permanently quadraplegic eventually must have spinal column stability.

What are causes of second injury to an already damaged cord? Central nervous system tissue, which includes the brain and spinal cord, does not tolerate hypoxia, poor perfusion, infection, or mechanical irritation from motion of unstable segments. Emergency physicians must attend to all of these, but it is especially important that they not permit any unnecessary motion. The word "unnecessary" is used deliberately here. There are times when it is necessary to move the head of a cord- or column-injured patient to preserve life—for example, a patient in a hazardous environment, such as a vehicle on fire—where careful extrication is impossible. Another example is the patient in the Emergency Department who has an obstructed airway and cannot be ventilated. The emergency physician has many skills and tools available to attain a patent airway without neck manipulation. If despite these, it is still impossible to open the airway and to preserve life, it will be necessary to manipulate the neck to open the airway.

**Primary survey**

The patient with potential cervical spinal column instability or cord injury should be managed in the same fashion as any other seriously injured patient—that is, following the ABCDE approach. The description here is limited to those aspects of this approach that are particular to the cervical spinal cord- or column-injured patient.

**Airway.** The first goal is to obtain and then maintain an open airway without subjecting the patient to unnecessary motion. There are five possible airway approaches, each with its own advantages and disadvantages.

The first is blind nasotracheal intubation. This approach has the advantage of not directly requiring cervical manipulation for tube placement, but also has the disadvantage of possible bucking and gagging that would cause neck motion. To help control this motion, the head and neck should be stabilized using the technique of in-line immobilization. During blind nasotracheal intubation, the patient may suffer a nosebleed that will complicate airway management until intubation is successful. Before intubation, the nose should be prepared with a local anesthetic and neosynephrine, and inspected by placing a gloved, lubricated fifth finger into each nostril to determine which will best accept the nasotracheal tube. The well-lubricated tube can be gently passed medial and along the floor of the nose to limit nosebleeds. The patient's breath sounds coming through the tube can help guide it toward the vocal cords.

The second approach involves use of a fiberoptic bronchoscope as a guide for a nasotracheal intubation. This method can be used in the circumstance where the patient is breathing adequately but requires the airway remain open because of a decreased level of consciousness. The endotracheal tube can be advanced through the nose into the posterior pharynx, and the fiberoptic tube placed through the endotracheal tube and advanced under direct vision through the vocal cords. The scope then serves as a flexible guide for advancing the endotracheal tube over it into the trachea. This approach is relatively slow, and the view through the fiberoptic scope can be blocked by even small amounts of mucus or blood, making intubation very difficult.

A third and somewhat controversial approach is the use of in-line immobilization.[2,3] It is important to understand the difference between in-line immobilization and axial traction. The goal of the person providing immobilization is to do just that, and not to apply axial traction. The patient should be immobilized without rotating, shortening, or stretching the cervical spine, spinal cord, or roots. One study investigated complications from this technique in patients going to the operating room for surgery.[4] These patients had known cervical column and cord injuries. There was no measurable loss of cord function in any of the patients after using in-line immobilization to intubate the patients prior to surgery. The head and neck can be immobilized by hands on either side of the head and a semirigid collar. The intubating physician uses a laryngoscope to intubate under direct vision without placing the neck into the typical sniffing position. In some cases, the vocal cords cannot be seen with the patient in a neutral position. Application of cricoid cartilage pressure (Sellick's maneuver) usually pushes the larynx back into view and allows the physician to pass the tube through the cords under direct vision. Cricoid cartilage pressure should be maintained until the intubation is complete to prevent regurgitation.

A fourth approach to opening an airway is transtracheal catheter ventilation (TTCV). TTCV has the advantage of very rapid and effective ventilation and oxygenation of the patient by using a tidal inflation of 1 second with 35 to 50 lb per square inch wall oxygen source and 4 seconds for the patient to exhale through the vocal cords. A similar approach using a continuous liter flow oxygen source attached to the catheter will oxygenate, but will also have a progressive accumulation of carbon dioxide. The disadvantage of TTCV is that it is a temporary maneuver that does not provide definitive control of the airway.

Cricothyrotomy is the fifth approach. It is a rapid approach that involves no manipulation of the possibly injured cervical column. The disadvantage is a 40% incidence of complications when cricothyrotomy is performed under emergent conditions.[5]

**Breathing.** In any seriously injured patient, it must be determined whether or not breathing is adequate, and then the source of the impairment must be corrected. There is one aspect of breathing that is particular to the spinal cord-injured patient: if the lesion manifests above the C-3 or C-4 level, which innervates the diaphragm via the phrenic nerves, then the patient will require positive pressure ventilation. Patients can live long term with adequate spontaneous ventilation if their phrenic nerves and diaphragm continue to function normally. The emergency physician must be aware that, in a few cases, the level of a cord lesion will ascend over time.[6] The patient who was not initially ventilator-dependent may become so if the lesion ascends to the level of C-3 or C-4.

**Circulation.** In managing circulation, the goal is to find and rapidly correct any respiratory, hemorrhagic, infectious, or cardiac source of shock. For the cord-injured patient, there is an additional cause of shock: spinal shock. Unfortunately, there are two important parts to the term *spinal shock* that can cause confusion. I use the phrase *spinal neurogenic shock* for one commonly used meaning and *spinal shock* for another.

*Spinal neurogenic shock.* Spinal neurogenic shock involves the sudden loss of sympathetic function below the level of the cord lesion. This sudden loss of sympathetic function leads to hypotension, often in the range of 80 to 100 systolic. In addition, it leads to a paradoxic bradycardia. The patient would be expected to have a tachycardia in response to the systolic hypotension, but instead the patient has a relative bradycardia, with the pulse ranging between 60 and 80. In addition, the skin is warm, dry, and well perfused. These are all in contrast to the patient with hemorrhagic shock, who is hypotensive and tachycardic, with cool, moist skin and delayed capillary refill.

*Spinal shock.* Spinal shock here refers to the sudden complete removal of ascending and descending cerebral impulses. This leads to a temporary flaccid paralysis below the level of the lesion and a temporary loss of segmental reflexes such as bulbocavernosus and deep-tendon reflexes below the level of the cord lesion. This temporary effect of spinal shock may last hours to days (typically, about 24 hours). It has significant implications for the emergency physician, because a patient with spinal shock may seem to have a physiologically complete neurologic deficit on physical examination during the time of spinal shock. However, when this phase has passed, the patient may recover a surprising amount of function. This potential for recovery of function after spinal shock has passed makes it impossible for the emergency physician to predict a patient's long-term outcome despite the patient's appearance on presentation. To make such a prediction requires a very thorough second examination after spinal shock subsides. When spinal shock is over (usually within a day), signalled by the return of some segmental reflexes (such as the bulbocavernosus in the male) and the patient is still physiologically complete, the prognosis for recovery becomes grim (Fig. 5-1).

*Occult hemorrhage.* Another aspect of managing patient circulation particular to spinal cord–injured patients is completing the search for areas of occult hemorrhage— areas where a patient can bleed to death without showing blood on the outside. These include the thoracic cavity, the area around the pericardium (causing pericardial tamponade), the peritoneal cavity, the retroperitoneal space, and the pelvis. The usual patient history and physical findings are of very limited value in identifying injuries in the patient who is anesthetic below the level of the cord lesion. On initial presentation, the injured patient with evidence of hypotension should be treated as having possible hemorrhagic shock until the search for occult hemorrhage is complete. The emergency physician must evaluate these hidden anatomic spaces if the mechanism of injury or findings suggest any possibility of injury to these body parts. The typical evaluation involves a chest radiograph with possible echocardiogram, peritoneal lavage or abdominal CT, and pelvic radiograph with either cystopyelogram or abdominal CT scan if there is a pelvic fracture or evidence of hematuria. The emergency physician must exercise caution with volume resuscitation of the potential cord-injured patient. Such patients can develop pulmonary edema if they receive excessive hydration in a futile attempt to correct their hypotension with volume if the hypotension is really the result of loss of sympathetic tone. Occult hemorrhage should be ruled out and then maintenance fluids and dopamine administered to maintain appropriate cord and brain perfusion.

**Disability.** There is very little that is different about the possible cord-injured patient in terms of the disability examination of the primary survey. The patient's level of consciousness and pupillary reactivity will be based on head injury or other global causes such as hypoglycemia, hypoxia, or intoxication. Cord injury plays no role in level of consciousness. The disability examination can be completed by measuring response to voice or pain above the lesion and pupillary reactivity. In an unconscious cord-injured patient, it is impossible to use the response to painful stimuli in the extremities to localize intracranial injury.

**Exposure.** In managing the issue of exposure, the emergency physician must remember that the patient cannot feel anything below the level of the lesion. It is therefore crucial that the physician see and examine everything in much greater detail than in the patient who can describe pain or tenderness. The examining physician should perform a careful examination and order a radiograph of any areas of the body that show bruising or other evidence of injury. These multiple radiographs may need to be delayed when evaluating and managing the patient with evidence of unstable vital signs or life-threatening injuries. However, careful examination and radiographs must be performed when patient stability allows.

### Resuscitation

During the resuscitation phase, two large-bore intravenous tubes should be inserted and blood tests initiated. A nasal or

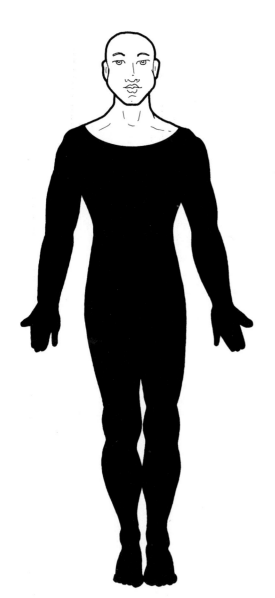

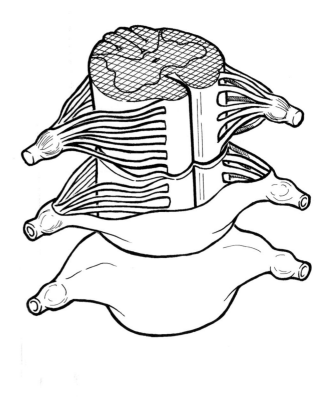

**Fig. 5-1.** A complete spinal cord lesion is physiologically complete far more often than anatomically transected.

orogastric tube can be placed if the patient is unconscious, nauseated, or requires oral contrast for abdominal CT examination. After rectal and meatal examination, a Foley catheter can be placed. Later, this catheter will likely be replaced by intermittent catheterization to decrease the risk of urinary infection.

**High-dose steroids.** Based on a national multicenter study, it has become standard practice to administer very high-dose methylprednisolone to the cord-injured patient.[7] This controlled, prospective, randomized, double-blind study included patients who had suffered blunt injury of the spinal cord within 8 hours of presentation to the study center. The patients received a 30 mg/kg bolus over 15 minutes of methylprednisolone followed by a 45-minute waiting period. Next, patients received a 23-hour, continuous 5.4 mg/kg/hr methylprednisolone drip. Overall, the treatment group showed significantly improved motor and

sensory outcome. In addition, there was no significant difference between the study group and the control group in complications or mortality.

## SECONDARY SURVEY

The survey involves a careful, complete physical examination of every organ system. This detailed examination may need to be delayed when managing a hemodynamically unstable or deteriorating patient. The neurologic component of this survey is discussed elsewhere in this chapter.

### Immobilization

Patients with post-traumatic neck pain or tenderness should be immobilized, as well as patients who present with an unknown reason or a traumatic mechanism for unconsciousness. The latter patients cannot provide a good history and cannot answer whether or not they have neck pain or post-traumatic neck tenderness. Patients who have evidence of a neurologic deficit should also be immobilized. This patient group includes not only the quadriplegic or quadraparetic, but also those who have suffered paresthesias at the time of injury or any time following. The paresthesia indicates pinching of the cord or a nerve root and is associated with cervical stenosis and unstable ligamentous injuries.[8] This patient should be protected until adequate examination and radiograph studies can rule out the possibility of an unstable column that could cause a second injury. Patients involved in a very high-energy mechanism of injury should also be immobilized. In the emergency department, it may be possible to remove a patient's immobilization without radiograph examination if there are no positive findings on careful history and physical examination. Patients who have multiple painful injuries and a mechanism for cervical injury should be immobilized as well. These distracting painful injuries make it difficult for the patient to report any post-traumatic neck pain or tenderness. These patients may or may not require cervical radiographs, depending on their ability to focus on the post-traumatic neck pain or tenderness and the likelihood of cervical injury based on their mechanism.

Occasionally, an injured person may be found walking around an accident scene. This patient can sometimes be mistaken as having a stable spinal column. The argument against cervical spine films would then be that the patient has already stood the test of time. However, it can take approximately 6 weeks for spinal ligaments and bone to heal sufficiently enough that a sudden loss of function would no longer be expected. After the 6-week period, the patient may gradually develop angulation and with it progressive cord disability, but a sudden deterioration may not be expected. Until that time, the emergency physician should not accept the argument that the patient has stood the test of time. Unfortunately, there have been tragic cases in which such an ambulatory patient has presented neurologically intact and suffered an acute subluxation and neurologic disability.

There are also well-documented cases of patients who have presented with subacute instability.[9] Typically, these are patients with ligamentous injury who on initial presentation had enough muscular tone in their neck to hold their neck stiffly so that bony instability was not visible on radiographs. On a second visit at the 2- to 3-week period, the muscular spasm in these patients had eased and evidence of ligamentous instability was elicited on flexion and extension views.

The key tool for immobilizing the patient and consequently preventing second injury caused by unnecessary motion is the long spine board. If the patient is securely attached to this board, it can be used to log-roll the patient if they regurgitate. A radiograph study has shown that a log-rolled patient does not maintain a straight spinal column, but airway protection and preservation of life require log rolling.[10] Semirigid collars, such as the Philadelphia®,

the Nec-Lok®, or the Stiff-Neck® collars, are an important adjunct to be used with a spinal immobilization board. However, radiograph studies have shown that no collar can totally immobilize a patient's neck.[11] Hence, these collars cannot totally replace the spinal immobilization board, but they do serve as an important adjunct. The Philadelphia® collar is more comfortable for the patient, but it provides less immobilization. The Stiff-Neck® collar can be applied in the prehospital setting with less manipulation of the patient's neck and provide immobilization, at the price of more patient discomfort. The semirigid collar should be left in place until complete cervical spine films have been completed and carefully reviewed. The semirigid collar may need to be temporarily opened to examine the neck. At our hospital, we typically leave these collars on overnight for any patient admitted with possible cervical spine injury.

A sponge-type cervical collar may be used for patient comfort after radiographs have shown that the spinal column is stable. Sponge collars provide very little immobilization and work mostly as a reminder to limit the patient's motion. These are not effective immobilizing devices and should not be used until after radiographic studies have proven cervical stability.

When presented with a potential cord- or column-injured patient, the prehospital crew should advise the patient to stay still, and the semirigid collar should then be applied. The patient should either be lifted with the spinal column moving as a straight unit, or log-rolled slowly onto their side. When the patient is lateral, an examination of the back should be completed prior to returning the patient to the spinal immobilization board. There is some controversy regarding which crew member should direct the procedure in such situations. One suggestion is the crew member at the head of the patient should give the orders, because they control the most mobile part of the spinal column and the area most at risk for injury. The converse argument is that the person controlling the trunk has the heaviest area to manage and it is easier for other crew members to assist them, therefore he or she should give the orders. At our hospital, the crew member managing the patient's head is the one assigned to give the orders for moving the possibly injured patient.

**Neurologic examination.** The sensory examination for perception of pain will rapidly help to localize the level of the patient's injury. The emergency physician must know the arrangement of the dermatomes or have a dermatome map (Fig. 5-2) available for reference. Sensory and reflex function around the anus should be examined. Sacral sparing of neurologic function may be the only indication of a partial cord syndrome versus physiologic completeness. If a point of transition from anesthetic to intact is identified, it is helpful to draw an ink line on the skin to show this transition. This will help to identify the patient whose level is ascending.

A change in the patient's neurologic function is a key

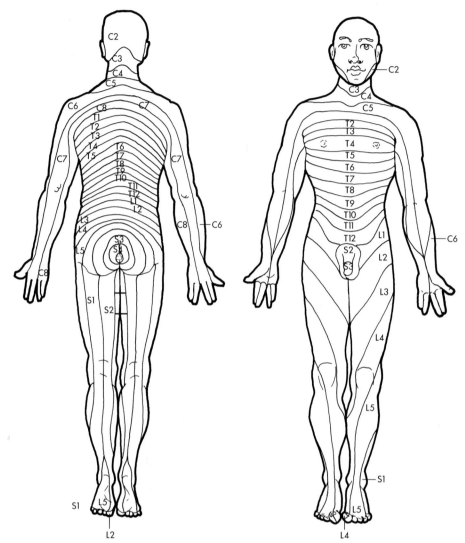

**Fig. 5-2.** The dermatome map varies somewhat from patient to patient.

parameter that strongly influences how the cord-injured patient will be managed. A patient's change for the worse, plateauing, or improvement in neurologic function significantly influences whether the patient will require a myelogram and possible surgery for decompression. To be able to identify this change, the emergency physician must perform a careful baseline neurologic examination again within the context of how hemodynamically stable the patient is. An adequate baseline examination would at a minimum include motor examination of all four extremities and sensory examination involving at least pinching of all four extremities, assessing deep tendon reflexes, and assessing anogenital reflexes (Table 5-1). Motor function is conducted along the lateral corticospinal tract and pain sensation along the spinothalamic tract (Fig. 5-3). In addition, an often-overlooked area of examination is the assessment of posterior column function. This can be performed by checking vibratory sensation in the

extremities, but checking for gross proprioception is readily available and does not require any tools. The patient who presents with priapism should be assumed to have a cord injury and should be treated as such. Alert the crew members who might potentially manipulate the patient's cervical spine (such as the respiratory therapist) to this finding and its implications.

## PARTIAL CORD SYNDROMES
### Anterior cord syndrome

In the acute anterior cord syndrome (Fig. 5-4), a lesion either causes direct injury or ischemic injury to the anterior aspect of the cord. This damage is caused by direct crushing injury to the cord or ischemic injury resulting from compression of the anterior spinal artery. Causes of this syndrome include bony instability, disc herniation, hematoma formation, or other mass-occupying lesions. This syndrome can be identified by finding loss of function below the level

**Table 5-1.** Motor, sensory, and reflex tests by nerve root levels

| Nerve Root Level | Motor | Sensory | Reflex |
|---|---|---|---|
| C-3 | | lower neck | |
| C-4 | diaphragm | clavicular area | |
| C-5 | deltoid, biceps | lateral upper arm | biceps |
| C-6 | extensor carpi radialis | thumb and lateral forearm | brachioradialis |
| C-7 | triceps, wrist flexors, finger extensors | middle finger | triceps |
| C-8 | finger flexors | little finger | |
| T-1 | hand intrinsics | medial forearm | |
| T-4 | intercostals | nipples | |
| T-10 | abdominals | umbilicus | |
| T-12 | | supra pubic area inguinal ligament | |
| L-1 } L-2 } | iliopsoas | upper thigh | |
| L-3 } | | lower anterior thigh | |
| L-4 } | quadriceps | medial calf | quadriceps |
| L-5 | extensor hallucis longus | dorsal foot | |
| S-1 | gastrosoleus, flexor hallucis longus | little toe | Achilles tendon |
| S-2 } S-3 } S-4 } | anal sphincter bladder | perineum | bulbocavernosus anal wink |

From Trafton PG. Spinal Cord Injuries. Surg Clin N Am 62:64, 1982.

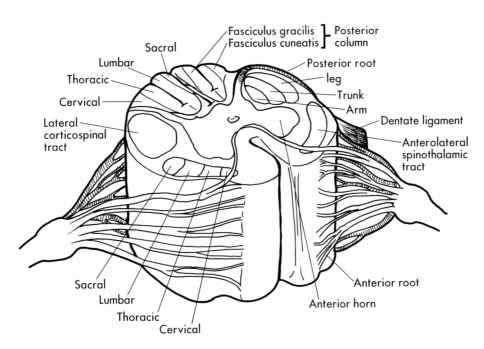

**Fig. 5-3.** Cross section of spinal cord.

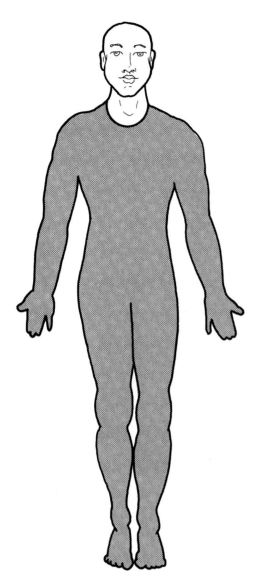

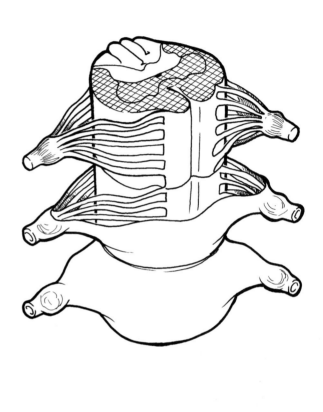

**Fig. 5-4.** Anterior cord syndrome.

of lesion in those neurologic functions served by the anterior cord, including motor, pain, light touch, and temperature sensation. In addition, there is preservation of the functions of the posterior columns including vibration, pressure, and gross proprioception. Unfortunately for these patients, the prognosis is relatively grim. After primary survey and resuscitation, these patients should be placed in axial traction to achieve complete bony alignment. If this is impossible, then the bony displacement must be at least reduced to achieve a medullary canal two thirds of its normal anteroposterior diameter. After bony reduction, the patient usually undergoes a rapid CT or myelogram to determine if there is an extrinsic mass pressing arteriorly on the spinal cord. If such an extrinsic mass is discovered, the patient is sent for an emergency laminectomy to decompress the cord.

### Brown-Séquard syndrome

Another partial-cord syndrome is Brown-Séquard (Fig. 5-5). This syndrome can be caused by disc, bone, hematoma, or tumor. If caused by injury, a penetrating wound is the most common cause. The classic findings are those of a crossed lesion. The motor loss is on the same side of the lesion distal to the level of injury because the motor fibers cross in the medulla. There is a simultaneous loss of sensory function on the opposite side of the body approximately two segmental levels lower than the motor loss. This is caused by the sensory fibers that enter the cord at the dorsal root, and then travel in the cord on the ipsilateral side for two levels prior to crossing to the contralateral side. The patient presents with the peculiar findings of paralysis or paresis in one leg that has preservation of sensory function, and the other leg has retained motor function but is

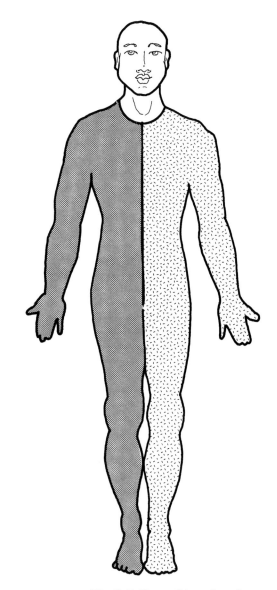

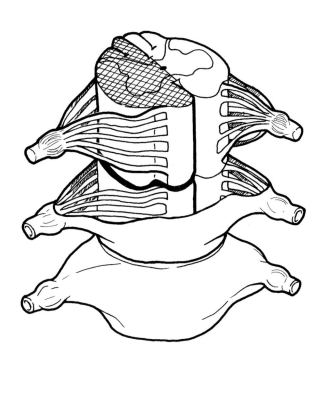

**Fig. 5-5.** Brown-Séquard syndrome.

anesthetic or hypoesthetic. Prognosis is poor for patients with penetrating injuries.[12]

### Central cord syndrome

The acute central cord syndrome (Figs. 5-6 and 5-7) is one that typically afflicts patients with narrowing of the spinal medullary canal. It occurs most commonly in older patients with cervical degenerative spine disease. It is typically a lesion caused by a hyperextension injury and is thought to arise from buckling of the ligamentum flavum during hyperextension. Although the exact mechanism is unknown, physical findings on autopsy studies show evidence of damage to the central portion of the spinal cord. The sensory losses are patchy in this syndrome. The key physical finding is more motor loss in the upper extremities than in the lower extremities. A typical patient is pro-

foundly paralyzed in the upper extremities from the level of the cervical cord lesion but has at least some preserved function in the lower extremities. This evidence of preserved function can be as simple as the ability to wiggle a toe. These patients have a relatively good prognosis, and typical treatment is nonoperative.[13]

### ANATOMY

The first seven vertebrae compose the cervical spine. C-1 or the atlas has a small vertebral body. Much of a person's flexion and nodding motion occurs at the atlanto-occipital junction. The odontoid or dens of C-2, the axis, fills the space that would typically form the body of C-1. Much of a person's neck rotation occurs about the C-1–C-2 junction. The spinal medullary canal is surrounded and protected by the vertebral body anteriorly, the two pedicles and lateral

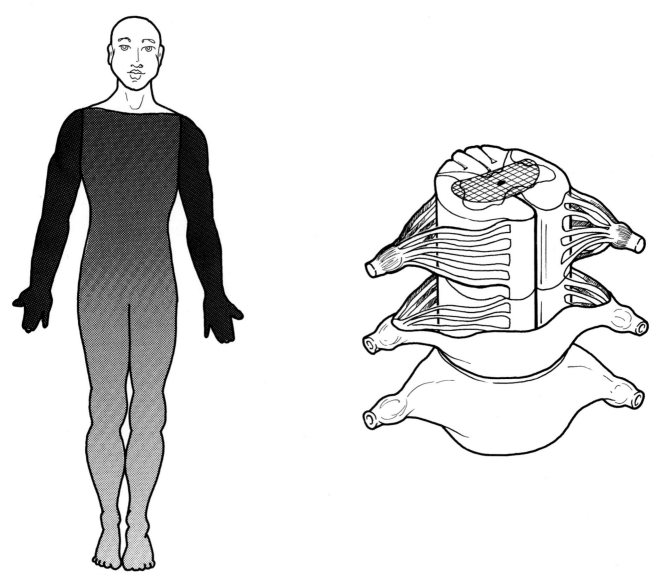

**Fig. 5-6.** Central cord syndrome.

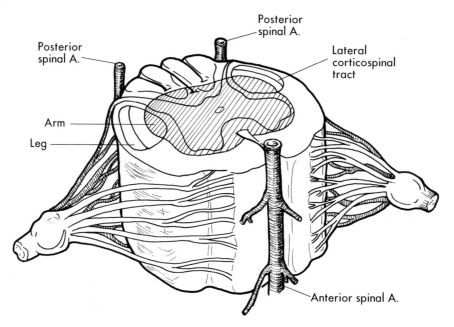

**Fig. 5-7.** Detail of central cord syndrome showing medial motor fibers at greater risk of injury in the lateral corticospinal tract.

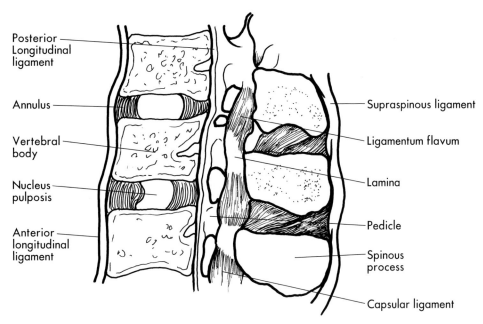

**Fig. 5-8.** Ligaments of the spinal column.

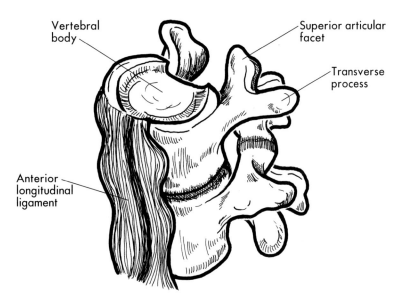

**Fig. 5-9.** Oblique view of the spinal column.

masses, and the two laminae that join and give rise to the spinous processes (Fig. 5-8). The lateral masses give rise to the transverse processes, and the superior and inferior articulating facets (Fig. 5-9).

The anterior longitudinal ligament (Fig. 5-10) arises from the base of the skull and travels anterior to the vertebral bodies. It is a relatively narrow but thick and tough ligament. The posterior longitudinal ligament (Fig. 5-11) arises from the anterior aspect of the foramen magnum starting as the tectorial membrane and continuing as the posterior longitudinal ligament. This ligament is very broad yet thin. Removing this ligament at the level of C-1,

C-2 exposes the transverse ligament and the alar check ligaments of the odontoid (Fig. 5-11). The spinal cord lies next to this posterior longitudinal ligament, separated only by the epidural space. The ligamentous structures involved from anterior to posterior are the anterior longitudinal ligament, disc, posterior longitudinal ligament, facet capsular ligament, intertransverse ligament, ligamentum flavum, interspinous ligament, ligamentum nuchae, and a thickening of this ligament called the supraspinous ligament.

In the neck, the numbered root exits the spinal canal above the pedicle of its associated vertebral body until the root of C-8 exits inferior to the pedicle of C-7. From

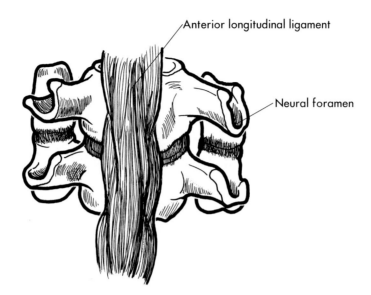

**Fig. 5-10.** Anterior view of the spinal column.

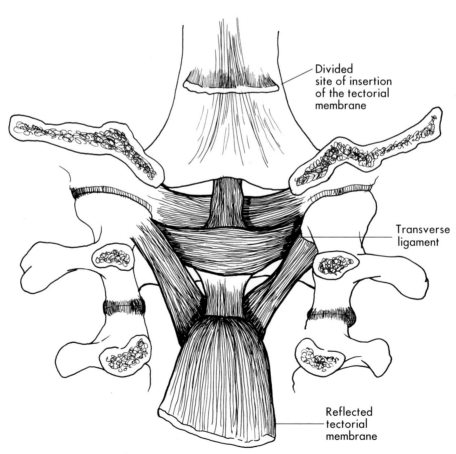

**Fig. 5-11.** Coronal section posterior view after removing posterior elements and spinal cord, dividing, and reflecting the tectorial membrane which is a continuation of the posterior longitudinal ligament.

T-1, the root exits inferior to the pedicle of the similarly numbered vertebral body.

Cervical spine injuries in children up to 7 years of age are almost completely limited to the three upper cervical segments.[14] After 8 years of age, the pattern of injury gradually shifts to an adult pattern, with the greatest number of injuries occuring at C-4, C-5, C-6.[14] The susceptibility to injury of the upper cervical segments in young children is related to their relatively larger heads, ligamentous laxity, and nearly horizontal facet joints. Most fractures in the child less than 8 years of age occur through the odontoid epiphyseal plate (Fig. 5-12).

## PLAIN RADIOGRAPHS
### Indications

The patient history and physical examination should be used as the main tools to determine if a patient has sustained a cervical injury. Cervical radiographs should be performed on patients with post-traumatic neck pain or tenderness, patients with impaired consciousness who cannot accurately report any cervical pain or tenderness, patients with high-energy mechanisms of injury or with other painful injuries that distract them from accurately reporting cervical pain or tenderness, and patients with neurologic deficits, including paresthesias at the time of injury or any time following.

### Lateral view

The lateral view of the neck (Fig. 5-13) is the principal screening tool used to determine if the injured cervical spine is stable. In 90% of patients, the single true lateral view will either answer this question or lead to further studies. The open-mouth odontoid view will determine this most of the time in the remaining 10%. In reading the study results of the lateral view of the spine, it is acceptable for the emergency physician to first scan for obvious injuries. However, it is important that the physician have a more systematic approach so that less-obvious injuries are not missed.

Each bone of the cervical spine should be carefully examined for evidence of injury. In addition, the adjacent structures of the jaw and lower skull should be examined to ensure there is no significant pathology there. Common findings that may be overlooked include a skull fracture or enlargement of the sella turcica. A normal lateral view gives only a fair degree of certainty that the spinal column is stable. The patient should remain in the semirigid collar until time or the patient's condition allows completion of further cervical radiograph studies.

**Seven and one third vertebrae.** The first step is to ensure that all seven cervical vertebrae are visible on the film, and at least the upper portion of the first thoracic vertebra. The emergency physician should count from the body of C-1 through the upper portion of T-1. If these vertebrae are not visible, the film can be used for as much as it shows. However, the patient must remain immobilized until an adequate view showing the first seven and one third vertebrae can be obtained. It is vital that the top of T-1 be seen in that injuries of the C-7–T-1 interspace are neither rare nor common.[15] Often, the superimposed den-

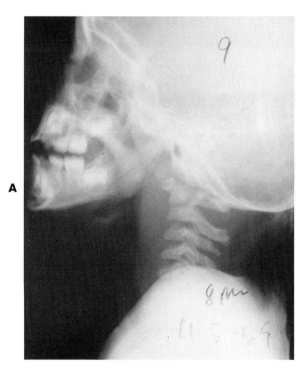
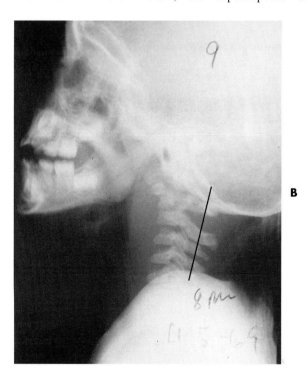

**Fig. 5-12. A,** Pediatric odontoid fracture through the epiphyseal plate. Note retropharyngeal soft-tissue swelling, and angulation of odontoid. **B,** Note posterior displacement of the spinolaminal line of C-2 in relation to C-1 and C-3.

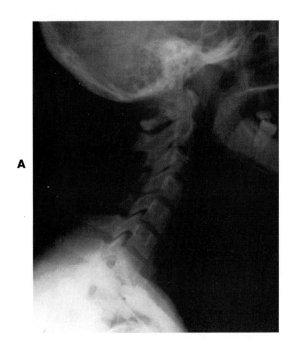

A

**Fig. 5-13. A,** Normal lateral radiograph. **B,** Schematic of normal lateral radiograph.

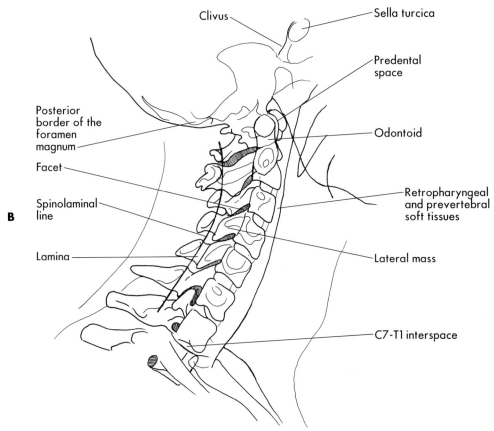

B

Clivus — Sella turcica

Predental space

Posterior border of the foramen magnum

Odontoid

Facet

Spinolaminal line

Retropharyngeal and prevertebral soft tissues

Lamina

Lateral mass

C7-T1 interspace

sity of the patient's shoulders will make it difficult, if not impossible, to clearly see the lower cervical segment, especially the C-7–T-1 interspace.

***Supplemental techniques.*** There are several techniques that the emergency physician can use to view the C-7–T-1 interspace more clearly. Traction should first be applied to

both arms to help move the shoulders out of the way, clearly showing the lower cervical segments. Wearing a lead apron, the physician should place the patient's feet against their thighs, ask the supine patient to relax the shoulders, and apply traction to both arms. This technique is limited by serious injury to the patient's arms. Force such that the patient's shoulders lift off the table should not be used. The second technique is the swimmer's view (Fig. 5-14). In this technique, the patient is positioned as doing the freestyle crawl, typically with the right arm abducted above the head when lying supine. The left arm is then pulled down toward the foot. Neither of these motions should be done with such force that the patient's body moves on the table. If the patient is awake, they should be asked to relax the shoulders and allow the lower shoulder to be displaced. The effect of this view is to place one shoulder totally in the way, but move the other totally out of the way. Using the hot light, the lower cervical segments show well enough to indicate gross alignment. Of course, the upper cervical segments were previously viewed on the earlier, inadequate lateral view. It may require multiple attempts using this technique to achieve a successful diagnostic view. When managing a critically injured patient, time may be saved in airway management decision-making by shooting a swimmer's view immediately after the lateral view. The swimmer's-view radiograph should be ordered before obtaining results from the lateral-view radiograph. If the lower cervical segment cannot be seen despite these maneuvers, then tomograms or CT examination will be required to clear the patient's lateral cervical spine.

**Facet superimposition.** It should be specifically decided if the lateral view is a true lateral. This can be determined by close examination of the facets. On a true lateral, the facets are superimposed behind each other such that only one facet is visible at each vertebral level. On a slightly obliqued projection, the facets are displaced one from the other and create additional shadows. This slightly obliqued projection can be very difficult to read when trying to assess vertebral alignment. A second view in a true lateral projection should be performed if there is any question about cervical pathology. When the slightly obliqued view is caused by a patient's head rotation, the facets will be gradually displaced from C-7 to C-3. This is in contrast to unilateral facet dislocation, where the spine changes from a true lateral projection to a markedly obliqued view at a single interspace.

**Detecting instability.** In addition to deciding whether the cervical spine is injured, the physician must also decide

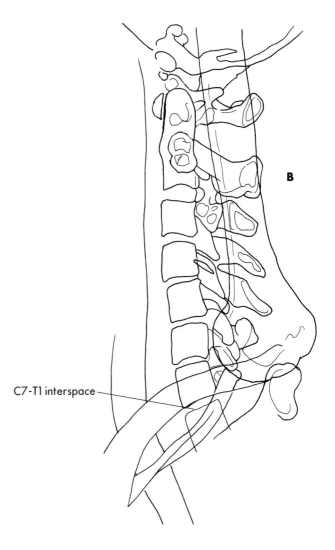

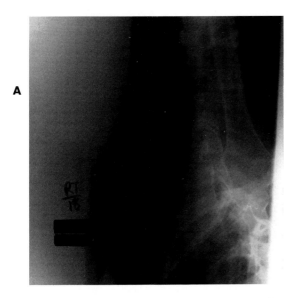

C7-T1 interspace

**Fig. 5-14. A,** Normal swimmer's view. **B,** Schematic of normal swimmer's view.

whether or not the injury is stable (see the box on this page). Panjabi defines clinical instability as "the loss of the ability of the spine under physiological loads to maintain relationships between the vertebrae in such a way that there is neither damage nor subsequent irritation to the spinal cord or nerve roots and, in addition, there is no development of incapacitating deformity or pain due to structural changes."[16] The emergency physician should "consider as potentially unstable any motion segment in which all of the anterior elements or all of the posterior elements are either destroyed or unable to function."[16] The anterior elements begin with the anterior longitudinal ligament and end at the posterior longitudinal ligament. The posterior elements begin with the posterior longitudinal ligament and end with the supraspinous ligament of the ligamentum nuchae.

*Soft tissue clues.* To assess ligamentous stability on the lateral view, the physician should specifically look for the size of the predental space (Fig. 5-13B). This is the distance between the back of the body of C-1 and the anterior aspect of the surface of the odontoid. In the average adult, on a lateral film, this distance should be no greater than 3 mm.[17] About 10% of normal adults will have a predental space up to 5 mm in length. If the predental space exceeds 3 mm in length, then the possibility of injury to the transverse and alar ligaments must be evaluated (Fig. 5-15). The physician must specifically measure the size of the retropharyngeal soft tissue. The tissue should be less than 5 mm thick on a

---

**The spectrum of acute instability in cervical spine injuries**

*Most unstable*

1. Rupture of transverse atlantal ligament
2. Fracture of dens
3. Burst fracture with posterior ligamentous disruption ("flexion teardrop")
4. Bilateral facet dislocation (or equivalent posterior disruption)
5. Burst fracture of vertebral body without posterior ligamentous disruption
6. Hyperextension fracture dislocation
7. Hangman's fracture
8. Extension teardrop fracture (stable in flexion)
9. Jefferson fracture (burst of C1)
10. Unilateral facet dislocation (or equivalent posterior disruption)
11. Anterior subluxation
12. Simple wedge compression fracture without posterior disruption
13. Pillar fracture
14. Fracture of posterior arch of C1
15. Spinous process fracture ("clay shovelers")

*Least unstable*

From Trafton PG. Spinal Cord Injuries. Surg Clin N Am 62:65, 1982.

---

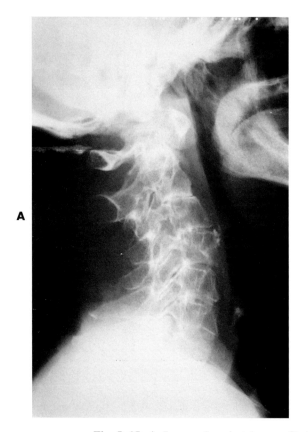
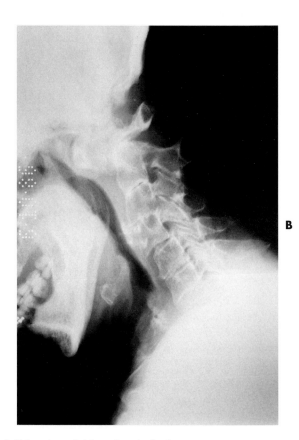

**Fig. 5-15. A,** Increased predental space. **B,** Atlantoaxial dislocation of this patient in flexion.

lateral film through the level of C-4.[18] If the tissue exceeds 5 mm, it implies possible swelling due to hematoma or abscess. At the C-4 level, the glottis and esophagus create a much more variable size to the prevertebral soft tissue. Beginning at C-4, the normal range of size is so broad (14–22 mm) that it is rarely a diagnostic measurement.

*Anterior and posterior longitudinal ligament lines.* In assessing the lateral cervical view for ligamentous stability, there are several lines to follow. The first passes along the anterior aspect of the vertebral body and corresponds to the location of the anterior longitudinal ligament. This line should have a smooth, sweeping curve consistent with normal cervical lordosis. Unfortunately, this line can be distorted by lipping and spurring caused by cervical degenerative spine disease. The second line is one that follows along the posterior aspect of the cervical vertebral bodies. This line corresponds to the location of the posterior longitudinal ligament, and should be smooth in that the spinal cord lies immediately next to it. This line should also have a smooth sweep consistent with normal cervical lordosis. This line can have a step-off of up to 3.5 mm on a lateral film and still be within normal limits.[16] However, in the presence of acute trauma, the patient should have further evaluation before this is dismissed as a normal variant. This evaluation may involve CT, magnetic resonance imaging (MRI), or carefully performed flexion-extension views to prove stability. This is done by showing no further displacement of the vertebral bodies, one on the next during flexion and extension. These dynamic studies determine if the measured displacement (up to 3.5 mm) is a fixed one and therefore a normal variant, or if it increases and is therefore a sign of instability. If this line changes by 11° or greater at a single interspace, the patient must be protected from possible ligamentous instability.[16] Further investigation to prove or disprove the possibility of acute instability should be carefully conducted.

*Spinolaminal line.* The next line that should have a smooth lordotic sweeping curve to it is the spinolaminal line. This line is formed by the junction of the lamina and the spinous processes at each vertebra. This junction shows up as a bright white line on the lateral view. The spinolaminal line is particularly useful in evaluating for subtle injuries of the upper cervical segment. Subtle injuries of the odontoid may be discovered by connecting the spinolaminal line of the middle of C-1 with the middle of the spinolaminal line of C-3 (Fig. 5-12). The spinolaminal line of C-2 should lie within 1 mm of a line drawn connecting these two spots. Displacement greater than 1 mm suggests the possibility of injury of the odontoid with either anterior or posterior displacement, or the possibility of bilateral fracture of the C-2 pedicles (also known as a hangman's fracture) (see Fig. 5-20).

Until approximately 8 years of age, there can be a remarkable degree of subluxation of C-2 on C-3 and, to a lesser extent, C-3 on C-4.[19] This is known as *physiologic*

*subluxation* or *pseudosubluxation.* To differentiate pseudosubluxation from a true injury, the spinolaminal line can again be used. A line should be drawn, connecting the center of the spinolaminal line of C-1 with that of C-3. The center of the C-2 spinolaminal line should be either on this line or within 1 mm. If it is off by greater than 1 mm, an unstable injury should be assumed. The most likely injury will be a fracture dislocation through the epiphyseal plate of the odontoid.

*Tips of the spinous processes.* The fourth line to examine is one that is much more variable, and that is connecting the tips of the spinous processes. The variable size of spinous processes makes this line of limited value.

**Degenerative disease and spinal stenosis.** Cervical degenerative spine disease can distort the lines corresponding to the anterior and posterior longitudinal ligaments. Distortion of the line of the anterior longitudinal ligament often lacks clinical significance. In contrast, lipping and spurring of the posterior aspect of the vertebral body narrows the anteroposterior diameter of the spinal canal, placing the patient at risk for injury due to stenosis. Patients with stenotic canals often present with acute central cord injuries after relatively minor hyperextension injury (Figs. 5-6 and 5-7). Physicians should specifically look for the anteroposterior (AP) diameter of the spinal medullary canal. This diameter can be dangerously narrowed as a cause of congenital stenosis or degenerative changes. The usual adult spinal cord is 9.3 mm in AP diameter, and the spinal canal should appear at least 10 mm deep on CT.[20] Considering the magnification of a standard 72-inch lateral view of the cervical spine, the measurement on the plain film should allow for at least 13 mm of AP diameter to fit the average adult spinal cord. The emergency physician should measure the distance from the back of any degenerative spur or the back of the vertebral body to the spinolaminal line. This spinolaminal line is the bright line created by the junction of the spinous process and the two laminae. If this distance is less than 13 mm, even minor trauma will place the patient at risk for significant spinal cord injury.

## Odontoid view

In most of the remaining 10% of patients with instability not seen or suspected on the lateral view, the open-mouth odontoid view will reveal if the patient's cervical spine is stable. This view is difficult to achieve in the unconscious or uncooperative patient. A good view clearly shows the body of C-2 extending up to the odontoid, the lateral masses of C-1, and the symmetric relationship of these lateral masses to the body of C-2 (Fig. 5-16).

## Anteroposterior view

The anteroposterior view provides less than 1% of the information yielded by plain cervical radiography (Fig. 5-17). On occasion, it shows a vertical fracture through the vertebral body with fracture line in an anteroposterior

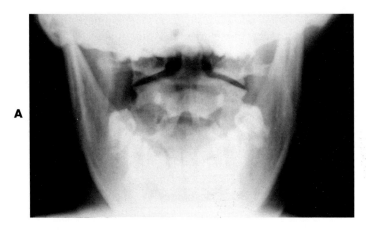

**A**

**Fig. 5-16. A,** Normal open-mouth odontoid view. Displacement of central incisors indicates slightly rotated view. **B,** Schematic of normal open-mouth odontoid view.

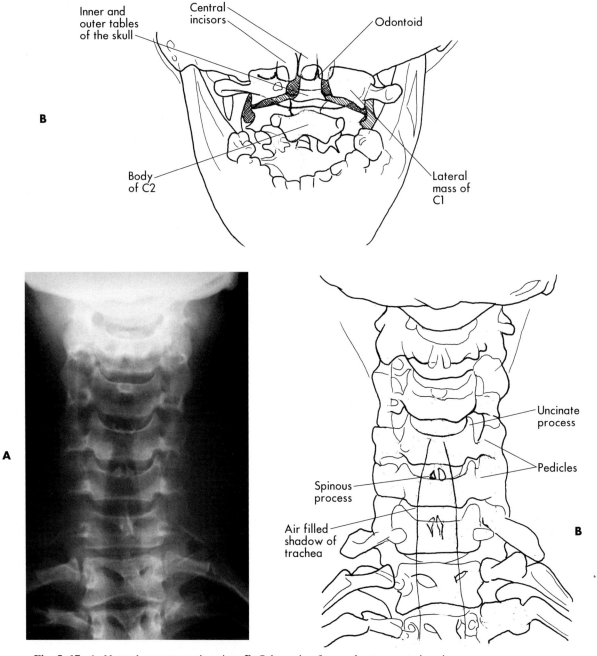

**Fig. 5-17. A,** Normal anteroposterior view. **B,** Schematic of normal anteroposterior view.

direction. This orientation makes it difficult to see on the lateral view. The AP view can also be helpful in locating fractures of the spinous processes with the fractured process displaced laterally. The physician should not be confused by bifid spinous processes that are common through C-4. In the presence of a burst fracture, the pedicles may be moved laterally and not form the usual string of pearls. This finding is more helpful in interpreting thoracic spine injury in that the cervical burst fracture would be clearly visible on the lateral. Sometimes the AP view shows an uncinate process fracture that is not visible on the lateral view.

### Indications for additional views

Patients whose lateral, open-mouth odontoid, or AP views are diagnostic of an unstable spinal column should have further evaluation by the neurosurgeon or orthopedic surgeon, as dictated by local practice. There are other patients whose film results suggest a low possibility of instability, but they are much more likely to have a stable cervical spine. In these patients, the emergency physician should conduct careful flexion-extension views, CT, or MRI to assess the stability of the spine. Examples of patients that may be stable or unstable are those with avulsion fractures of the anterior-inferior lip of the vertebral body, or those with up to 3.5 mm of displacement of one vertebra on the next without additional signs of ligamentous instability.

**Flexion and extension views.** When doing careful flexion-extension views, the physician should instruct the patient to remain supine and to slowly and carefully flex their neck. The patient should stop if he or she suffers pain or paresthesias. If the patient cannot cooperate with these instructions, CT examination should be done in place of flexion-extension views. In the awake, cooperative patient who is able to flex their neck without pain or paresthesias, a wedge pillow can be placed behind their head and the radiograph performed. A similar process of slowly extending the neck should be used, stopping for pain or paresthesias, when performing a careful extension view. The most important signs of instability on flexion are subluxation of the posterior aspects of the vertebral bodies along the line associated with the posterior longitudinal ligament, or evidence of abnormal fanning out between the spinous processes of one vertebra on the next. The extension view should be assessed for similar evidence of subluxation of one vertebral body on the next, as evidenced by displacement along this posterior longitudinal ligament line.

**Oblique views.** Posterior oblique and anterior oblique views are particularly helpful in revealing any restriction in the size of the nerve root canals (Fig. 5-18). On the posterior oblique view, the foramina visible refer to the roots of the opposite arm. On an anterior oblique view, these apply to the arm of the same side. Oblique views are helpful in determining the size of the foraminal canal, the integrity of the pedicle, the integrity of the lamina, and the alignment of the facets at each level. The lamina and associated facets should align similar to shingles on a roof.

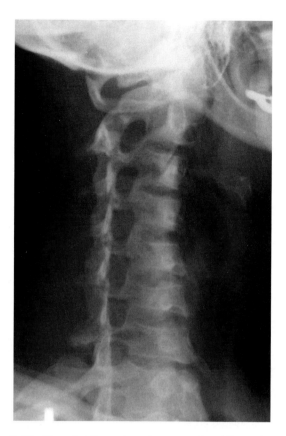

**Fig. 5-18.** Normal oblique view. On an anterior oblique view, the visible foramen are on the same side as the labelled side. On a posterior oblique view, the visible foramen are on the side opposite the labelled side.

## ADDITIONAL STUDIES

Additional studies such as CT or MRI may be necessary in the patient whose degree of pain seems out of proportion to the visible evidence of injury on plain films. There are patients who present with apparent acutely stable cervical spines who will develop subacute instability. This may be caused by initial muscle spasm that holds the spine relatively secure. As this spasm gradually decreases, the spine relies on ligamentous integrity to hold its position, which may allow a subacute instability to emerge. A follow-up appointment at the 2- to 3-week period will help to identify those patients with subacute instability.[9] A CT scan will add substantial detail to that shown on plain films (see Fig. 5-21A). Often, additional unsuspected fractures are found. A CT scan is generally more effective in defining bony detail, and MRI is better for soft-tissue evaluation. Early MRI is often impossible to perform because the patient cannot safely tolerate the prolonged time needed.

After the best reduction of an unstable injury, a patient would require myelography (see Fig. 5-21B), CT myelography, or MRI for two reasons. The first is continued loss of function; this deteriorating condition suggests the possibility of continued pressure on the cord, leading to further damage resulting from direct pressure or ischemia.

Myelography will identify an extrinsic mass pressing on the cord that may be reduced by laminectomy. The second reason for emergent evaluation for pressure by an extrinsic mass is the anterior cord syndrome (Fig. 5-4). This lesion may be caused by continued pressure on the anterior aspect of the cord or pressure on the anterior spinal artery (Fig. 5-7). Although the prognosis is poor, myelography is performed to determine if a soft-tissue mass not visible on plain films is present. If one is found, decompression by laminectomy is done to eliminate the mass as a cause of possible continuing damage.

## CERVICAL TRACTION

In the prehospital and initial hospital phase, the patient is immobilized using a semirigid collar and a rigid spinal board. The application of such devices should not involve the use of traction, because distraction of an unstable column can cause cord or root injury. Plain films should be taken after initial history, physical examination, and stabilization. Emergency traction can be initiated if the film results show bony dislocation that narrows the spinal medullary canal. This condition is often managed by the neurosurgeon or orthopedic surgeon, according to local hospital practice. Initial traction and relocation may be undertaken by any skilled physician. Serial radiographs and physical examinations guide this process. Weight in 5- to 10-lb increments should be added up to specified limits, with an additional radiograph and physical examination after each increase to ensure there is no evidence of distraction of an interspace greater than 5 mm on the lateral radiograph or evidence of neurologic deterioration.[21] The treating physician must know that distraction of nervous tissue can equal permanent destruction of the spinal cord or roots. If the patient survives, atlanto-occipital injuries are able to be managed with just 2 lbs of traction.

Traction is applied by one of several devices, such as the Gardner-Wells tongs. The patient should lie on a circle bed, turning frame, or serial auto-inflating device to protect their skin. The Gardner-Wells tongs should be applied above the bony auditory canal after aseptic preparation and local anesthesia. No incision should be made, as the points are self-seating. The points can be placed anterior or posterior to the bony auditory canal depending on patient stability in extension or in flexion. As the two prongs are screwed into the skull, a pressure-sensitive indicator protrudes from inside the tong. When the indicator protrudes 1 mm from its port, the tong can be rocked gently to seat it, and the prongs screwed in again, stopping when the pressure indicator again protrudes 1 mm. The prongs are secured in place by tightening the locking nuts. These tongs are also available in graphite for patients who will be undergoing CT or MRI examination.

The goals of traction are to achieve and maintain early realignment. The goal is complete anatomic position, but if this cannot be achieved, reduction should accomplish at least a two-thirds width of the normal spinal canal. Reduction should not be hasty, but it should be expeditious.

Remarkable degrees of neurologic recovery have been reported after closed reduction[22] and open reduction with surgical decompression.[23]

## FRACTURES
### Jefferson fracture

In the Jefferson fracture, the patient suffers an axial loading mechanism of injury. This causes the ring of C-1 to burst, with the base of the skull serving as a wedge. Sometimes fractures of the ring of C-1 show on the lateral view because of visible cortical discontinuity in the lateral mass or lamina of C-1. On the open-mouth odontoid view, the lateral masses will typically be displaced laterally to the body of C-2. There can be some degree of lateral displacement and disc space asymmetry created by rotation of the patient's head. In such a case, the presence of rotation can be seen by locating the space between the upper central incisors that should be in the midline in an unrotated view. In addition, the lateral mass of C-1 should be laterally displaced on the side of rotation and medially displaced on the opposite side.

### Odontoid fracture

Usually the patient with an odontoid fracture (Fig. 5-19) will present either neurologically intact[24] or dead on arrival. This is because injury here permits motion with damage to the medulla and subsequent cardiorespiratory arrest. The front and back of the body of C-2 should clearly lead to the odontoid. Prognosis for neurologic recovery of those who survive is good.[24] Closed versus open treatment is controversial, with nonunion being a frequent complication.

### Hangman's fracture

The hangman's fracture (Fig. 5-20) is an injury of the pedicles of C-2, suffered during hyperextension. This appears paradoxical in that the body of C-2 displaces anteriorly on C-3 despite the extension mechanism. This can be a devastating, fatal fracture; however, considering the degree of displacement often seen, it can be surprisingly associated with minimal or no cord injury,[25] due to the anterior displacement and the relatively large size of the medullary canal at the C-2 level. The emergency physician will encounter this injury typically when treating a motor-vehicle accident with hyperextension mechanism. Judicial execution by hanging also creates this injury, with marked distraction and immediate cardiorespiratory arrest. However, this is a very unusual injury to see in suicide hangings because almost all such hangings are strangulation injuries with no associated column injury. Suicide hangings do not cause the extreme hyperextension and distraction forces intentionally created during judicial hangings.

### Burst fracture

The burst fracture occurs when there are flexion and compressive forces that explode the vertebral body with fragments moving both anteriorly and posteriorly into the spinal medullary canal. This injury is often associated with

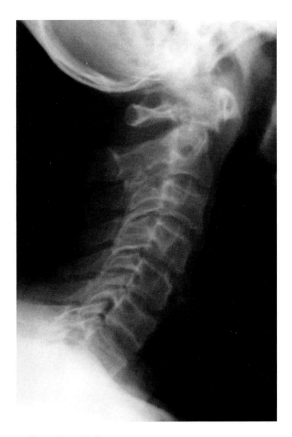

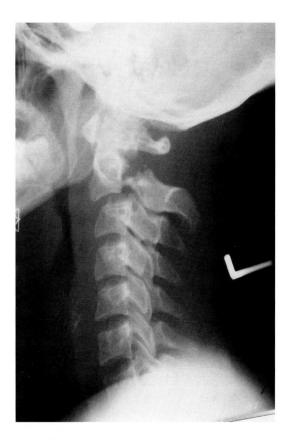

**Fig. 5-19.** Odontoid fracture.

**Fig. 5-20.** Hangman's fracture.

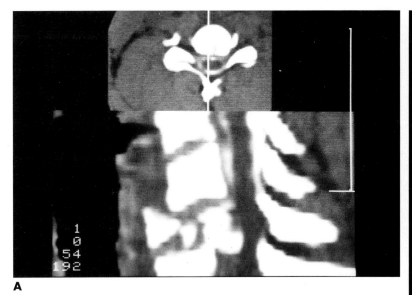

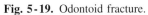

**A**

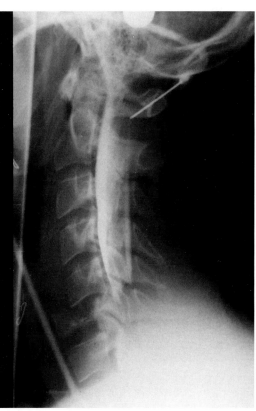

**B**

**Fig. 5-21. A,** Detail from computed tomography (CT) of C-6 burst fracture. Note fragments retropulsed into spinal canal. **B,** Myelogram of C-6 burst fracture. The contrast material cannot pass the level of injury due to retropulsed fragments compressing the spinal cord.

devastating degrees of spinal cord injury. CT (Fig. 5-21A) should be used to define the bony details of this injury, as there are often small fragments in the canal that are difficult or impossible to identify on plain films. Myelogram (Fig. 5-21B) or CT myelography will show if the cord is compressed to the point of preventing flow of contrast material past the level of injury.

### Spinous process fracture

The clay shoveler's injury (Fig. 5-22) is one historically described as an avulsion of the tip of the spinous process because of traction created by the shoulder muscles during heavy physical labor. It is an unusual injury to see from this mechanism and is much more commonly associated with a direct blow to the back of the neck. Typically, this occurs during a motor-vehicle accident or an assault. In the classic clay shoveler's injury, only the tip of the spinous process is avulsed. Although this may be painful, it does not have any effect on stability of the spinal column and as such presents no risk to the spinal cord. However, it is vital that the emergency physician recognize the difference between such a relatively benign clay shoveler's fracture of the tip of the spinous process and fractures associated with strong flexion injury, causing fracture through the base of the spinous process or laminae with associated ligamentous injury (Fig. 5-23). The first injury presents no risk to the spinal cord; the second may present critical risk to the spinal cord, depending on the extent of associated ligamentous disruption.

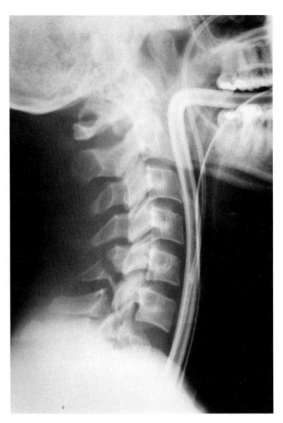

**Fig. 5-23.** Fracture of the base of the spinous process and lamina of C-5, fracture of the lamina of C-6, and anterior subluxation of C-6 on C-7.

## CERVICAL SPRAINS

The emergency physician must not only determine if there is bony injury, but also if there is ligamentous injury. The patient may have no fracture, and yet have a severe sprain of cervical ligaments, allowing an unstable spinal column to move (Fig. 5-24), rendering the patient quadriplegic. A sprained neck can range in severity from a minor, temporary source of discomfort to gross instability, risking permanent quadriplegia. Ligamentous integrity should be assessed by attention to the alignment and relationship between the cervical vertebrae. A patient may have a sprained neck and no fractures but have an unstable column and devastating cord injury.

### Atlanto-occipital dislocation

An uncommon but extremely dangerous sprain injury that the emergency physician must specifically watch for is the atlanto-occipital (AO) dislocation (Fig. 5-25). In this injury, the skull disconnects from the cervical spine as a result of ligamentous injury. Immediate death occurs if the head displaces from the neck during or following injury. There have been a few survivors of this injury who are neurologically intact.[26] Several systems are used to attempt to identify this injury by establishing ratios and various measured distances.[27] These include the X-line, Wholey Dens-

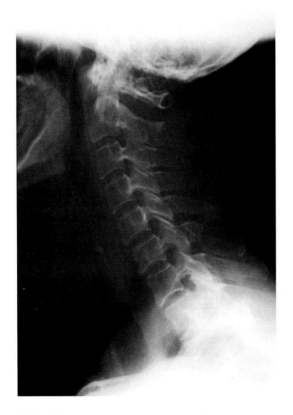

**Fig. 5-22.** Spinous process or clay shoveler's fracture.

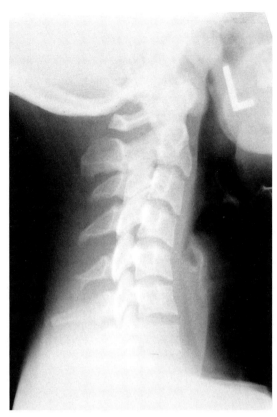

**Fig. 5-24.** Third-degree sprained neck. Note angulation greater than 11° at C-4 on C-5. There is likely a rupture of the supraspinous, interspinous, ligamentum flavum, facet capsular, and posterior longitudinal ligaments. This is an unstable injury.

Basion line, Powers ratio, and Dublin method. Unfortunately, none of these systems are reliably diagnostic for anterior, posterior, and translational AO dislocations in adults and children. In the obvious case, the posterior aspect of the foramen magnum is not in relationship to the spinolaminal line of the ring of C-1. In addition, the bony canal of the ear is not above the body of C-1, and a line drawn through the clivus at the base of the skull does not continue through the tip of the odontoid process. It should be noted that even minimal degrees of traction can drastically displace the skull from the cervical spine, causing distraction injury to the medulla.

**Facet dislocation**

Unilateral facet dislocation involves a flexion and rotation mechanism.[28] These forces cause one facet to slide up and over the facet inferior to it, creating an injury that skips and locks in terms of returning to the normal position. This is most often a stable injury. The degree of additional ligamentous injury determines stability. This injury can be identified on the lateral cervical view by the sudden transition from a true lateral view to a markedly obliqued view at a single disc interspace. In addition, the superior vertebral body subluxes approximately 30% or less of the width of the inferior body. Reduction is often accomplished by

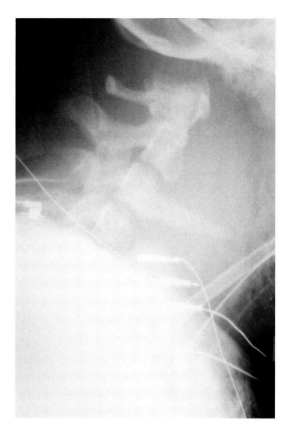

**Fig. 5-25.** Atlanto-occipital dislocation.

traction, but may require operative intervention to remove part of the facet if traction is unsuccessful. Some neurosurgeons leave the patient in the unilaterally dislocated position if traction is unsuccessful in achieving reduction. On the AP view, this lesion can sometimes be spotted by the spinous process suddenly angulating to the right or left at a single interspace.

A bilateral facet dislocation occurs as a result of a flexion mechanism.[29] With this injury, the facets of the superior vertebra on both sides slide up and over the immediately inferior facets. In some of these patients, the tips of the facets perch on each other; in others, a complete skipped and locked position occurs. This lesion is markedly unstable in that it involves massive injury to ligamentous structures. It is locked in terms of returning to the normal position, but not locked in terms of falling off into further flexion, causing catastrophic cord damage. This lesion can be identified by subluxation of approximately 50% or more of the width of the inferior vertebral body and by no transition from true lateral to suddenly obliqued view, as described for unilateral facet dislocation. This lesion is often reduced by traction; if this is not possible, surgery is used to partially remove the blocking facets to allow relocation. This injury is unstable and requires fusion.

**KEY POINTS**

Key points for emergency personnel to remember are as follows:

1. Immobilize and do not apply traction until more is known about the stability or instability of a patient's lesion.

2. When moving a patient, attempt to keep the spinal column in an anatomic line.

3. When evaluating the patient, manage the patient as any other: first ensuring that the patient survives by attention to the ABCDE method of resuscitation.

4. In those patients who are anesthetic, the usual history and physical examination cannot be relied upon to discover sources of occult bleeding or injury. The emergency physician should complete the search for occult bleeding and injuries whenever the mechanism or vital signs suggest their possibility.

5. Because change is a key parameter, it is vital that an adequate neurologic examination be performed. The emergency physician must remember to test not only motor and sensory examination but also for posterior column function, such as gross proprioception or vibration.

6. Early in the management of a patient with a cord injury, the patient should receive very-high-dose methylprednisolone.

7. The lateral view provides 90% of the information needed to determine the stability of the patient's cervical spine. The open-mouth odontoid view will provide most but not all of the remaining 10%.

## REFERENCES

1. Kraus JF, Franti CE, Riggins RS et al: Incidence of traumatic spinal cord lesions, *J Chron Dis* 28:471-492, 1975.
2. Bivins HG, Ford S, Bezmalinovic Z et al: The effect of axial traction during orotracheal intubation of the trauma victim with an unstable cervical spine, *Ann Emerg Med* 17:1, 25-29, 1988.
3. Majernick TG, Bieniek R, and Houston HG: Cervical spine movement during orotracheal intubation, *Ann Emerg Med* 15:4, 417-420, 1986.
4. Holley J, Jorden R: Airway management in patients with unstable cervical spine fractures, *Ann Emerg Med* 18:11, 1237-1239, 1989.
5. McGill J, Clinton JE, and Ruiz E: Cricothyrotomy in the emergency department, *Ann Emerg Med* 11:7, 361-364, 1982.
6. Yablon IG, Ordia J, Mortara R et al: Acute ascending myelopathy of the spine, *Spine* 14:10, 1084-1089, 1989.
7. Bracken MB, Shepard MJ, Collins WF et al: A randomized, controlled trial of methylprednisolone or naloxone in the treatment of acute spinal-cord injury, *New Engl J Med* 322:20, 1405-1411, 1990.
8. Torg JS, Pavlov H, Genuario SE et al: Neuropraxia of the cervical spinal cord with transient quadriplegia, *J Bone Joint Surg* 68:9, 1354-1370, 1986.
9. Herkowitz HN, Rothman RH: Subacute instability of the cervical spine, *Spine* 9:4, 348-357, 1984.
10. McGuire MA, Neville S, Green BA, Watts C: Spinal instability and the log-rolling maneuver, *J Trauma* 27:5, 525-531, 1987.
11. Kaufman WA, Lunsford TR, Lunsford BR, Lance LL: Comparison of three prefabricated cervical collars, *Ortho Prosthet* 39:4, 21-28, 1986.
12. Oller DW, Boone S: Blunt cervical spine Brown-Séquard injury: a report of three cases, *Am Surg* 57:6, 361-365, 1991.
13. Merriam WF, Taylor TK, Ruff SJ, McPhail MJ: A reappraisal of acute traumatic central cord syndrome, *J Bone Joint Surg* 68:5, 708-713, 1986.
14. Hill SA, Miller CA, Kosnik EJ, Hunt WE: Pediatric neck injuries, *J Neurosurg* 60:4, 700-706, 1984.
15. Nichols CG, Young DH, and Schiller WR: Evaluation of cervicothoracic junction injury, *Ann Emerg Med* 16:6, 640-642, 1987.
16. Panjabi MM, White AA: Basic biomechanics of the spine, *Neurosurgery,* 7:1, 76-93, 1980.
17. Williams CF, Bernstein TW, and Jelenko C: Essentiality of the lateral cervical spine radiograph, *Ann Emerg Med* 10:4, 198-204, 1981.
18. Weir DC: Roentgenographic signs of cervical injury, *Clin Ortho Rel Res* 109:9-17, 1975.
19. Cattell HS, Filtzer DL: Pseudosubluxation and other normal variations in the cervical spine in children, *J Bone Joint Surg* 47A:7, 1295-1309, 1965.
20. Stanley JH, Schabel SI, Frey GD, Hungerford GD: Quantitative analysis of the cervical spinal canal by computed tomography, *Neuroradiology* 28:139-143, 1986.
21. Fried LC: Cervical spinal cord injury during skeletal traction, *JAMA* 229:2, 181-183, 1974.
22. Brunette DD, Rockswold GL: Neurologic recovery following rapid spinal realignment for complete cervical spinal cord injury, *J Trauma* 27:4, 445-447, 1987.
23. Ljunggren B, al Refai M, Sharma S et al: Functional recovery after near complete traumatic deficit of the cervical cord lasting more than 24 hours, *Br J Neurosurg* 6:4, 375-380, 1992.
24. Apuzzo MLJ, Heiden, JS, Weiss, MH et al: Acute fractures of the odontoid process, *J Neurosurg* 48:1, 85-91, 1978.
25. Seljeskog EL, Chou SN: Spectrum of the hangman's fracture, *J Neurosurg* 45:7, 3-8, 1976.
26. Bools JC, Rose BS: Traumatic atlantooccipital dislocation: two cases with survival, *Am J Neuroradiol* 7:5, 901-904, 1986.
27. Lee C, Woodring JH, Goldstein SJ et al: Evaluation of traumatic atlantooccipital dislocations, *Am J Neuroradiol* 8:1, 19-26, 1975.
28. Rorabeck CH, Rock MG, Hawkins RJ, Bourne RB: Unilateral facet dislocation of the cervical spine, *Spine* 12:1, 23-27, 1987.
29. Maiman DJ, Barolat GB, and Larson SJ: Management of bilateral locked facets of the cervical spine, *Neurosurgery* 18:5, 542-547, 1986.

# CHAPTER 6

# Thoracolumbar Spine

*Paul R. Haller*
*Ross M. Huelster*

## ANATOMY

The spinal column provides support to the musculoskeletal system and houses and protects the spinal cord. The column itself consists of bony vertebrae, intervertebral discs, and connecting ligaments.

Each vertebra is composed in an upright, cylindrical body. Projecting posteriorly from this cylinder are a pair of pedicles (Fig. 6-1). Paired laminae sweep medially and posteriorly from these pedicles to make up the ring of the vertebral foramen. The laminae form a posterior spinous process in the midline and extend lateral to the pedicles to become the transverse process. The pedicles, laminae, and spinous processes form the neural arch, protecting the spinal cord in its descent from the brain. Each vertebra articulates with the body above and below it by means of a set of superior and inferior articular facets. Demifacets exist in the thoracic vertebrae for rib articulation.

The vertebral bodies are stacked one upon another, with discs intervening. Posteriorly, they articulate with their facets. A series of ligaments that course the length of the spinal column provide stability. The anterior and posterior longitudinal ligaments run along the front and back of the discs and connect the vertebral bodies (Fig. 6-2). The ligamentum flavum attaches to subsequent laminae, providing the dorsal border of the spinal canal. Posteriorly, the interspinous ligaments connect the spinous processes. The

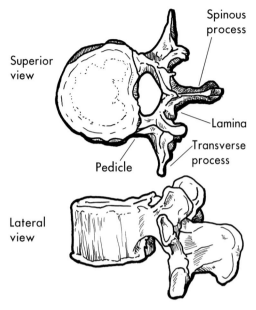

**Fig. 6-1.** Superior and lateral vertebral body.

supraspinous ligament is adjacent to the spinous processes and runs the length of the column. Intercapsular ligaments connect the facets.

The portion of the spinal column responsible for weight-bearing is the vertebral bodies and the intervertebral discs. The discs have a thick outer capsule, the anulus fibrosis, which surrounds the gelatinous nucleus pulposus. The anulus fibrosis attaches to the inferior and superior margin of the adjacent vertebral bodies. The anulus is reinforced by the broad anterior longitudinal ligament, and less so by the posterior longitudinal ligament.

Each of the twelve vertebral bodies of the thoracic spine is buttressed by a rib. The head of the rib attaches to the intervertebral disc and to the demifacets of the adjacent vertebral bodies. As the rib arches posteriorly and laterally, it again articulates with the spine at the anterior wall of the transverse process. Thus, the ribs provide considerable support to the thoracic spine. Although the parallel arrangement of the ribs allows rotation, there is minimal flexion, extension, or lateral bending in the thoracic spine. This support helps to explain the paucity of fractures or dislocations occuring in the upper thoracic region. When they do occur, displaced fractures of the thoracic spine may also involve injury to the sternum or rib cage. Most thoracic spine injuries occur in the lower T-10 to T-12 region, where the ribs are less developed.

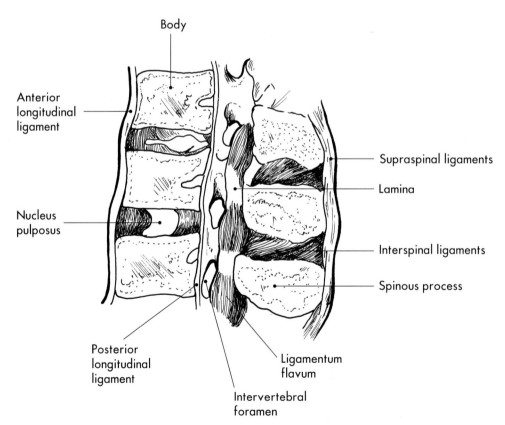

**Fig. 6-2.** Sagittal section of the mid-lumbar vertebral column showing the vertebral bodies, intervertebral disks, and associated ligaments.

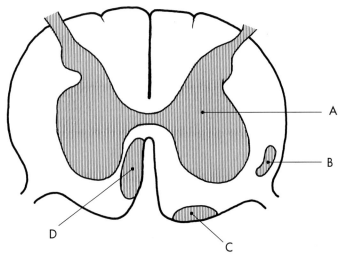

**Fig. 6-3.** Cross-section of the spine demonstrating the (A) posterior column, (B) lateral spinothalamic tract, (C) anterior spinothalamic tract, and (D) corticospinal tract.

The bodies of the five lumbar vertebrae are the largest in the spine. Their spinous processes are heavier and the transverse processes more developed than in the thoracic spine. The lumbar spine allows significant mobility and carries most of the body's weight.

## NEUROANATOMY

The spinal cord extends from the brainstem (exiting at the foramen magnum) to the L-1–L-2 level. It is broader in the cervical and lumbar regions, where more nerve roots are needed to innervate the upper and lower extremities, respectively. The conus medularis is the conical termination of the spinal cord. Extending from the conus is the filum terminale, a fibrous extension of the pia mater that attaches to the coccyx.

A cross-section of the spinal cord shows the centrally located, butterfly-shaped gray matter that is made up of cell bodies and their processes. On the periphery run white bundles or tracts of myelinated fibers (Fig. 6-3). Although there are a number of tracts in the white matter, for present purposes these can be simplified into: 1) the posterior tract that contains sensory modalities to detect vibration and two-point discrimination; 2) a lateral tract that transmits pain and thermal sensation; and 3) an anterior lateral tract that carries the motor and sensory pathways. Ascending tracts are sensory in function; descending tracts are motor in function.

Each of these pathways crosses from one side of the body to the other in its route from the peripheral nerve to the opposite side of the brain. The tracts for vibration, pain, and temperature cross the midline at the level at which they enter the spinal cord. The anterior lateral tracts, carrying motor and sensation, do not cross until they reach the midbrain. The fact that nerves decussate at different levels in their path to the brain is evident in findings from examination of patients with partial spinal cord injuries.

In the anterior cord syndrome, vibration and light-touch modalities remain intact below the level of the lesion, but there is a loss of pain and temperature sensation, along with autonomic dysfunction and motor paralysis below the injury. Lateral hemisection of the cord, known as Brown-Séquard syndrome, results in loss of motor function and light touch on the side of the injury to the spinal cord. Pain and temperature, along with vibratory sensation, are lost on the contralateral side to the injury.

Thirty-one pairs of nerve roots exit the spinal cord in its descent through the column: eight cervical, 12 thoracic, five lumbar, five sacral, and one coccygeal. Each nerve root in the thoracic and lumbar spine exits the vertebral canal just below the vertebra of the same number. After exiting the spinal cord, the nerve roots descend within the spinal canal until they pass through their vertebral foramen. Because the cord is shorter than the vertebral column, this route within the spinal canal is longer for each successive nerve root moving caudally (Fig. 6-4). Below the level of L-1–L-2, the spinal canal no longer contains a spinal cord, but rather is filled with a group of descending nerve roots called the *cauda equina.*

The paired nerves exiting the spinal canal consist of a sensory root and a motor root. Motor roots are axons from the anterior horn cells, which are located within the spinal cord; thus, damage to a motor root after it has exited the spinal cord is a postganglion process similar to insult to a peripheral nerve, and carries a good prognosis for recovery. In contrast, sensory roots leave the spinal canal but do not synapse with the sensory ganglia until they near the intervertebral foramen (Fig. 6-5). Thus, injury to sensory roots within the spinal canal is a preganglion process and carries a poor prognosis for recovery.

Each of the 31 pairs of nerves has specific dermatomal sensory and motor distribution. Dermatomal distribution of these fibers is shown in Fig. 6-6. Clinically pertinent motor function of these roots is listed in Table 6-1.

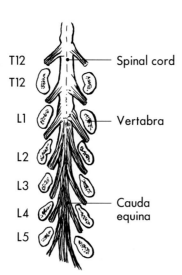

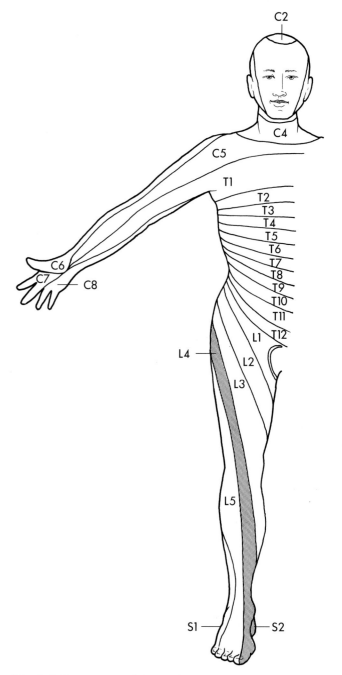

**Fig. 6-4.** Cross-section of the spinal column demonstrating successive elongation of the vertebral roots in their pathway from the spinal cord to the intervertebral foramen. Also note distal to the L-1–L-2 vertebral bodies, the nerve roots constitute the cauda equina.

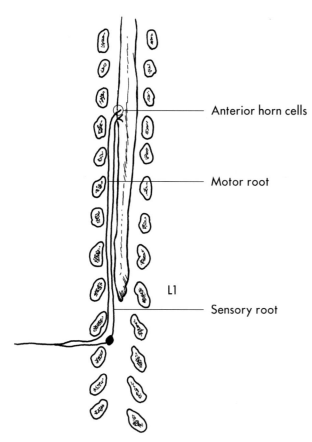

**Fig. 6-5.** Cross-section of the spinal column. The sensory ganglia of the nerve is located near the intervertebral foramen as the nerve exits the spinal column. The anterior horn cell of the motor root is located within the spinal cord itself.

**Fig. 6-6.** Dermatomes of the anterior and posterior aspects of the body.

**Table 6-1.** Clinically pertinent motor function of nerve roots

| Nerve root | Motor |
| --- | --- |
| C-5–C-6 | Biceps, deltoid |
| C-7 | Triceps |
| | Wrist extensors |
| C-8 | Intrinsic hand muscles |
| L-4 | Quadriceps |
| L-5 | Anterior tibial (foot dorsiflexors) |
| S-1 | Gastrocnemius (foot plantar flexors) |

## SPINAL CORD INJURIES

Trauma to the spinal cord proper may result in complete cord injury or an incomplete cord syndrome. Complete cord injury is characterized by immediate motor paralysis (a flaccid paralysis) and areflexia involving all caudal muscle groups. Loss of all sensory modalities also occurs below the same level. Dysfunction of the automatic nervous system is characterized by anhidrosis and piloerection. Initially, urinary and fecal incontinence also occur. After the spinal cord recovers from the initial injury, the subsequent paralysis is usually that of spasticity and hyperreflexia caused by loss of inhibitory input to the anterior horn cells from higher centers in the brain. With time, the bladder and bowels regain spontaneous contractility.

Neurogenic shock often results from complete spinal cord injury. It is caused by a lack of vasomotor tone and is characterized by hypotension and bradycardia. The patient appears quite well and has evidence of adequate perfusion of the brain, kidneys, and periphery, with normal mental status, good urine output, strong pulses, and warm skin. The term *shock* is a misnomer, as this state does not involve inadequate tissue perfusion. Cardiac output is normal or increased, with increased vascular reserve due to dilated arterioles and veins. Hypotension may be treated with volume expansion and, if necessary, vasopressors. In trauma patients, hemorrhagic shock should be ruled out before attributing hypotension to neurogenic shock.

Respiratory function is controlled by both the diaphragm (innervated by C-3 through C-5) and the intercostal muscles of the thorax (served by the thoracic vertebrae as low as T-5). Thus, injuries to the spinal cord above the level of C-4 typically result in complete loss of spontaneous respirations and death. When the level of injury is found caudally to this, more of the respiratory musculature (i.e., chest wall and intercostal muscles) remains intact, thereby enabling a patient to increase respiratory volume, cough, and clear secretions. Injuries below T-5 level are not associated with respiratory embarrassment.

### Incomplete cord syndromes

Several incomplete cord syndromes may result from either blunt or penetrating trauma to the spinal cord.

**Anterior cord syndrome.** This syndrome is usually the result of a flexion injury with a herniated disc or bony fragments pushing into the anterior aspect of the spinal cord. Motor function is lost below the level of the lesion, as is pain and temperature sensation. Light touch, deep pain, and vibratory sensation remain intact.

**Central cord syndrome.** This syndrome involves motor loss that is more severe in the upper extremities than in the lower extremities. Most often, it is seen in cervical spine injuries. Sensory loss is symmetric, with loss of deep pain sensation and intact superficial pain sensation. It is typically seen in older patients who have fallen and disrupted the anterior longitudinal ligament. Patients fre-

quently experience spontaneous improvement in their neurologic function.

**Hemisection of the cord (Brown-Séquard syndrome).** This syndrome is usually secondary to a posterior wound, such as a stab wound, and results in loss of light touch, vibration, and position sensation and motor function on the side of the injury. Contralateral loss of pain and temperature sensation is experienced below the same level.

**Spinal cord concussion.** Spinal cord concussion is similar to concussion of the brain. There is transient neural dysfunction without pathologic abnormality. Spontaneous recovery of neural function occurs shortly after the trauma. This is usually seen in athletes involved in contact sports and may be characterized by a burning sensation in or dysesthesias of the extremities.

### Treatment

Acute treatment of spinal cord injury includes stabilization of fracture and dislocations and supportive care for the patient. Associated injuries must be cared for. The early use of steroids has been shown to improve long-term motor and sensory function in spinal cord–injury patients.[1] To be effective, steroids must be administered within 8 hours of the injury. The regimen calls for a 30 mg/kg bolus of methylprednisolone, followed by a constant infusion at 5.4 mg/kg/h for the next 23 hours. Because of the need for early initiation of steroids, it is the emergency department physician's responsibility to begin this treatment. Complications such as gastritis and infection are minimized by the short duration of steroid use.

## MECHANISM OF INJURY

The spinal column consists of a stack of 24 vertebrae, connected together by joint capsules, ligaments, and discs. A force acting on one area of the spinal column may be strong enough to tear these ligaments, fracture the bone, or both. With this destruction, a shift in position of one vertebral body on another can occur. If the shift is large enough to impinge on the spinal cord, neurologic damage results.

The direction of the force acting on the spinal column determines the pattern of the resulting injury. Knowing how the injury actually occurred can predict radiologic findings, and vice versa. Mechanical forces on the spine may be a result of flexion, extension, lateral bending, distraction, compression, or shear.

Flexion injuries (Fig. 6-7A) are the most common type of spinal trauma. They commonly occur at the thoracic-lumbar junction, an area where the spine changes from the stiffness of the thoracic spine imparted by the rib cage to the more mobile lumbar spine. Flexion injuries occur to a lesser extent in the lower lumbar spine. The resulting injury to the spine is usually in the anterior compression fracture or a wedge fracture.

Although hyperextension is a common cause of cervical spine injury, it is rarely the etiology for thoracolumbar

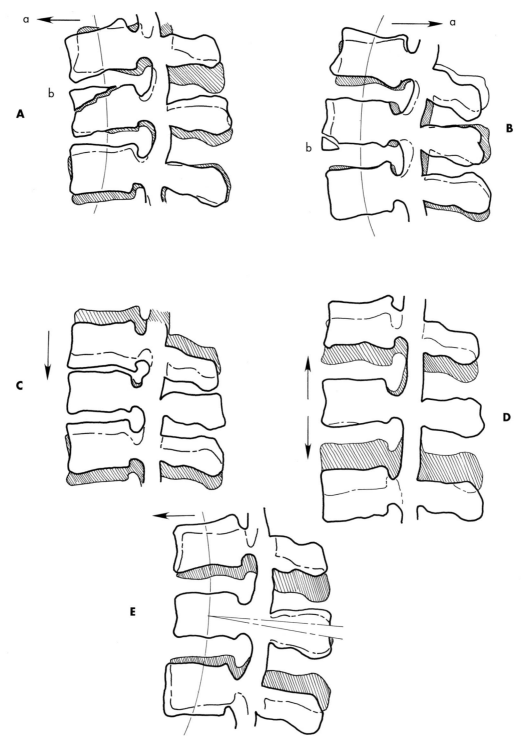

**Fig. 6-7. A,** Flexion injury. The lower aspect of the vertebral column remains stationary and forces push the upper aspect anteriorly (a), resulting in a compression fracture anteriorly (b). **B,** Hyperextension injury. With the force applied to the upper spinal column directed posteriorly (a), an avulsion fracture of the lower anterior vertebral body is demonstrated (b). **C,** Axial load. Compressive forces oriented directly downward. **D,** Distraction forces acting to pull the vertebrae directly away from each other. **E,** Chance fracture. This injury is caused by simultaneous distraction and flexion forces causing an injury to the spinal column, which starts at the posterior aspect of the spinal column and propogates anteriorly.            *Continued.*

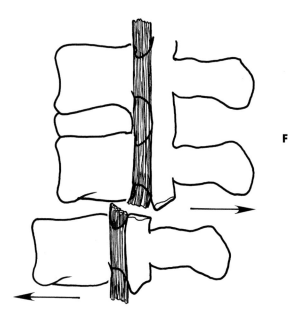

F

**Fig. 6-7, cont'd. F,** Minimal horizontal movement of one vertebral body on the other causes a marked reduction of the spinal canal diameter.

spine damage (Fig. 6-7B). Hyperextension injury may occur in athletes who have repeated, forced extension of the spine, such as football linemen or gymnasts. Distracting forces act on the anterior part of the spine, resulting in an avulsion fracture of the vertebral body or fracture of the pars interarticularis.

Compression forces are the result of a direct downward (axial) load on the spinal column (Fig. 6-7C). The weight-bearing portion of the spinal column consists of the discs and the vertebral bodies. The discs are primarily composed of fluid, which because of its incompressible nature, transmits the force to the vertebral bodies. Thus, large compression forces typically result in damage to the vertebral body when the disc remains intact. With a small axial load on the spinal column, the disc transmits the force to the vertebral body, resulting in a bending-type deformity of the end plate. If the force is large enough, a burst fracture of the body with displacement of fracture fragments occurs. Fracture fragments may be projected laterally; however, displacement more commonly occurs in an anterior-posterior direction.

Distraction forces act in the opposite direction of compression. Here, the vertebral column is pulled apart in its longitudinal direction (Fig. 6-7D), as occurs in hanging from inversion boots, for example. In the emergency setting, this mechanism is most commonly found in a victim of a motor vehicle accident who was restrained by a lap belt but not by a shoulder harness. The belt holds the pelvis stable, and the weight of the upper torso distracts the spine. Because the patient is bent at the waist at the time of injury, the fracture or ligamentous injury begins in the posterior part of the spinal column and propogates anteriorly (Fig. 6-7E).

A shear force acts to move one vertebral body horizontally in relation to its adjacent vertebrae. This may be in either the anterior, posterior, or lateral directions. Because a small horizontal movement in any direction markedly decreases the lumina of the spinal canal (Fig. 6-7F), this injury frequently results in spinal cord damage. The ligamentous destruction that accompanies a horizontal shift of one body on another causes a grossly unstable spine. This type of injury most often occurs in the upper two thirds of the lumbar spine.

Lateral bending forces are similar to flexion-extension. These are uncommon injuries and result in wedge fractures of the lateral aspect of the vertebral bodies. Similar to anterior compression fractures, they are stable and are not associated with neurologic injury.

## SPINAL STABILITY

Injuries to the spinal column are classified as stable or unstable. In an unstable fracture, the fracture fragments may move, causing new damage to the spinal cord. An unstable fracture is frequently viewed as needing internal fixation. In a stable injury, by contrast, there is enough ligamentous or bony continuity to prevent further movement of the column.

To classify stability, the spine is divided into three columns.[2] The anterior column is made up of the anterior longitudinal ligament, the anterior aspect of the anulus fibrosis, and the anterior portion of the vertebral body (Fig. 6-8). The middle column consists of the posterior longitudinal ligament, the posterior portion of the anulus fibrosis, and the posterior part of the vertebral body. The posterior column is made up of the neural arch, along with the interspinous and supraspinous ligaments, ligamentum flavum, and the intercapsular ligaments.

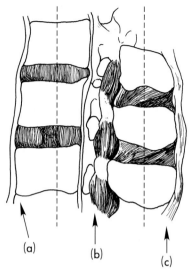

**Fig. 6-8.** Columns of the spinal cord. The anterior column (a) consists of the anterior aspect of the vertebral body, the anterior portion of the disk, and the anterior longitudinal ligament. The middle column (b) consists of the posterior aspect of the vertebral body, the posterior portion of the intervertebral disk, and the posterior longitudinal ligament. The posterior column (c) is made up of the spinous processes, the interspinous ligaments, and the supraspinous ligament, along with the intervertebral facets.

Fracture stability is determined on the basis of these three columns. An injury to two of the columns is mechanically unstable; if it is not immobilized, it has the potential for further displacement and neurologic injury caused by bony fragments. The anterior compression fracture, which involves only the anterior column with intact middle and posterior columns, is a stable fracture. Burst, chance, and shear fractures are unstable fractures. Burst fractures in-

volve both the anterior and middle columns. Subsequent axial load (as in weight-bearing) could further displace fracture fragments into the spinal canal, injuring the cord. Chance fractures are often seat belt–induced. There is disruption of the posterior and middle columns, and they are unstable when the spine is flexed. For a shear fracture or fracture dislocation to occur, all three columns must be disrupted.

## COMPRESSION FRACTURES
### Mechanism of injury

Anterior compression fractures of the thoracolumbar spine typically occur after a flexion type of injury, such as a fall onto the buttocks with axial load. Important in understanding this type of fracture is attention to the direction of forces applied. Weight is carried by the spine on an axis that runs close to the center of the intervertebral disc. In flexion injuries, this axis becomes the point of a fulcrum, with compression forces acting anterior to this axis and distraction forces, posteriorly (Fig. 6-9). Because the distance from the fulcrum to the posterior spinous ligament is four times the distance from the axis to the anterior longitudinal ligament, the anterior compression force during flexion injury is four times greater than the distraction force that occurs posteriorly. It is for this reason that these flexion forces leave the posterior portion of the spine intact when causing a compression fracture of the anterior vertebral body.

### Signs and symptoms

The patient's primary complaint is pain that is better when recumbent, and worse with motion, cough, or sitting upright. The physical examination is often unimpressive. The

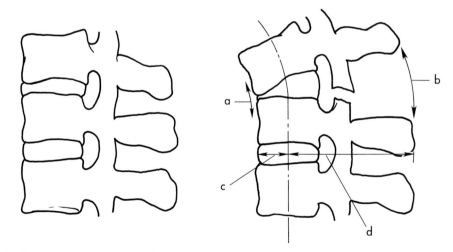

**Fig. 6-9.** Anterior compression fracture. Because the compressive forces are much greater, fracture of the interior border of the vertebral body occurs when posterior ligaments remain intact. In this figure, compressive forces are acting anteriorly (a) when distraction forces are acting posteriorly (b). The distance from the axis to the anterior border of the vertebral bodies (c) is four times the distance from the axis to the posterior spinous process (d). Because distance "d" is four times that of "c," the compressive forces are four times greater than the extension forces acting posteriorly.

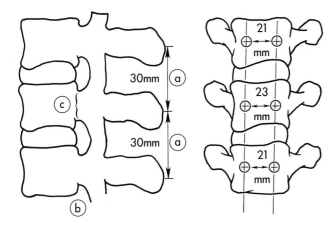

**Fig. 6-10.** Characteristics of compression fracture. Lateral view: the posterior aspect of the spinal column remains intact as demonstrated by identical distances between adjacent spinous processes (a). Posterior spinous line shows no posterior displacement of the vertebral bodies (b). Height of the posterior pole of the vertebral bodies is identical (c). Anteroposterior view: the interpedicular distance varying by less than 3 mm characteristic of anterior compression fracture without posterior involvement.

findings may include tenderness over the involved area or spasm of the paravertebral muscles. Clues to the need for radiographs are gleaned more from the patient history than the physical exam.

### Radiographic findings

The lateral film is critical in making an accurate diagnosis. The findings consist of a wedge-type deformity at the anterior aspect of the vertebral bodies. The height of the anterior face of the vertebra should be compared with adjacent vertebrae. Anterior compression should be limited to less than 50% of the original height of the body to avoid instability. The lateral film should be scrutinized for findings suggestive of a more serious fracture. Particular attention should be paid to: 1) the distance between the posterior spinous processes; 2) the height of the posterior portion of the vertebral body (a collapsed posterior margin signifies a burst fracture and the possibility of fragments extruding into the spinal canal); 3) the posterior spinous line; and 4) the interpedicular distance of the involved vertebrae, in comparison with adjacent vertebrae (Fig. 6-10).

### Diagnosis

The proper diagnosis of an anterior compression fracture is made with a history of mechanism of injury, examination, and evaluation of the anteroposterior (AP) and lateral radiographs. Because this is a stable fracture managed by conservative treatment, it is critical to differentiate it from more serious injuries. The two injuries most easily confused with the anterior compression fracture are burst and chance fractures.

The chance fracture is more commonly seen after a seat belt injury. Its associated findings may include widening of

the posterior spinous processes and fracture through the spinous process or parsinterarticularis, or even through the posterior pole of the vertebral body.

Burst fractures occur after an axial load on the spine, such as landing flat-footed after a fall. In an unstable burst fracture, the posterior spinous line appears displaced on the lateral film. The AP film may show widening of the intrapedicular distance of the involved vertebrae in comparison with adjacent vertebrae.

Differentiating recent compression fractures from old ones may be difficult. A new fracture tends to be painful, and often the patient recalls a specific traumatic event. Old films of the spine may help to distinguish new from old.

### Management

Trauma significant enough to fracture a vertebral body can also cause related soft-tissue injuries. Retroperitoneal hematoma associated with the fracture can result in ileus or gastric dilitation. These usually occur within 24 hours and can be treated conservatively with nasogastric suction and nothing-by-mouth orders.

Pain management for anterior compression fractures is achieved by bedrest and appropriate analgesics. Typically, the patient is kept flat in bed for at least a few days, although the length of time depends on degree of wedging and pain tolerance. This is followed by upright sitting and ambulation as tolerated.

External spine supports are of questionable value in compression fractures with minimal loss of vertebral height. With more severe compressions, these molded plastic braces become more useful. Long-term management is best directed by a specialist, as 20% of the patients have significant persistent disabilities, and another 45% have persistent and mild discomfort without disability.[3]

### BURST FRACTURES

A downward (axial) load on the spine transmits its force to both the intervertebral discs and vertebral bodies. Because these discs are primarily made up of noncompressible water, it is the vertebral bodies that become disrupted when the axial load becomes too great. This load causes a bending of the superior and/or inferior vertebral body endplates, and, with sufficient force, a fracture or burst of the vertebral body occurs. The fragmentation of vertebrae often results in a loss of height of the body. This shattering also produces a disruption of the neural arch: the pedicles shift laterally, and to accommodate this, an associated fracture occurs in the posterior lamina, most commonly at its junction with the posterior spinous process (Fig. 6-11).

Burst fractures are unstable. Movement of the posterior fracture fragments may impinge on the spinal cord, causing permanent neurologic damage.

### Mechanism of injury

Burst fractures result from axial compression of the vertebral column. Typically, this is the result of a fall. The injury

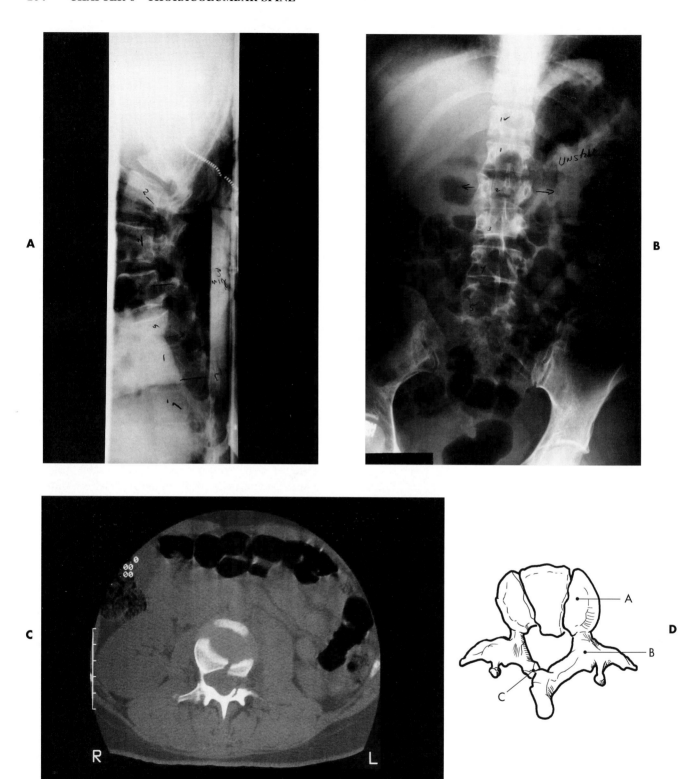

**Fig. 6-11. A, B, C,** Burst fracture. **D,** Characteristic burst fracture with comminution of the vertebral body (A). Part of the vertebral body has shifted laterally, taking the pedicle with it (B). A disruption of the neural arch must occur to accommodate this shift. This typically occurs near the posterior spinous process (C).

usually occurs in the T-10–L-2 region, where the spinal column is in transition from the kyphosis of the thoracic spine to the lordotic curvature of the lumbar spine. It is this neutral position of the vertebrae that predisposes this location to burst fractures.

### Signs and symptoms

The patient presents with pain at the level of the injury. There may be associated spasm and tenderness on examination. A thorough neurologic examination is essential, as these fractures may be accompanied by a neurologic injury.

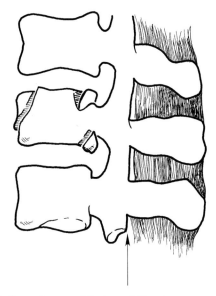

**Fig. 6-12.** Burst fracture. The lateral film demonstrates posterior displacement of a chip of the superior pole of the vertebral body into the vertebral canal itself.

When the injury involves the upper lumbar spine, most of the motor and sensory nerves have already exited the spinal canal above the injury; thus, this fracture may result in an incomplete or partial cord syndrome. Survey of the patient is carried out with attention to spinal immobilization.

### Radiologic findings

Critical in the evaluation of this injury is the involvement of the middle column (the posterior third of the vertebral body, the posterior longitudinal ligament, and the posterior aspect of the anulus fibrosis). The lateral spine radiograph is viewed with attention to the posterior vertebral body line. Clues to the presence of a burst fracture include: 1) posterior displacement of the posterior vertebral line with respect to the adjacent vertebrae; 2) posterior displacement of a chip of the superior or inferior aspect of the vertebral body; and 3) obliteration of all or part of the posterior vertebral line (Fig. 6-12).

The AP film is evaluated for a widening of the space between pedicles. The interpedicular space should vary by no more than 3 mm when compared with the interpedicular spaces of adjacent vertebrae. An AP film may also be the only clue to a burst fracture where the fragments have moved laterally rather than posteriorly. Here, the radiograph shows loss or displacement of the lateral margin of the vertebral body.

### Diagnosis

After patient history review and physical, the review of the AP and lateral radiograph leads to the diagnosis. Further evaluation with a CT scan is indicated. The CT scan demonstrates the amount of intrusion (if any) of the fracture fragments into the spinal canal. The amount of encroachment on the spinal canal by the fragments is not necessarily a predictor of neurologic injury. Significant narrowing may

be associated with injury, but the opposite is also true. The CT scan may show the final resting place of the fragment but does not demonstrate the maximal displacement that occurred during the injury. CT scanning also delineates fractures involving the neural arch (pedicles, posterior lamina, and spinous process). The posterior lamina is frequently fractured near the spinous process (Fig. 6-11).

### Treatment

The amount of trauma necessary to shatter a vertebral body is obviously capable of producing injury to other organs. As this fracture is frequently unstable, it is capable of further subluxation or movement resulting in neurologic disability. The emergency department evaluation must be carried out with spinal immobilization. Definitive treatment of this injury requires patient admission and the involvement of a spine specialist. Thorough evaluation of the neurologic status and any changes in the exam are documented and discussed with the spine specialist. Decisions on timing of surgery (immediate vs. semielective) are influenced by the presence of a change in the neurologic examination; progressing neurologic deficits are operated on promptly.[4] The early use of steroids in spinal cord–injured patients has been shown to decrease long-term neurologic dysfunction.[1]

## FRACTURE-DISLOCATION

The least stable spinal injuries are dislocations or fracture-dislocations. These involve the disruption of the alignment of the spinal column, with a shift of one vertebral body on another. This movement disrupts all three columns of the spine. Fracture-dislocations have a high incidence of spinal cord injury (up to 50% of cases). When the thoracic spine is involved, cord injury is usually complete. In the lumbar region, complete or incomplete syndromes may be seen.

### Mechanism

The thoracic spine is stabilized in part by the rib cage, which prevents lateral bending and anterior and posterior flexion. However, the parallel arrangement of the ribs does allow shear or translational injuries to occur in the thoracic spine. Forces causing fracture-dislocations may be either shear, rotation, or flexion-extension associated with shear or rotation.

### Signs and symptoms

The forces that cause the fracture-dislocation are capable of causing injury outside the vertebral column. Such injuries may be obvious or subtle. Evaluation of the back may demonstrate tenderness over the involved site. Widening or malalignment of the posterior spinous process may also be detected on examination. A soft spot may be palpable between spinous processes, indicating a complete tear of the posterior longitudinal ligament. Physical examination and subsequent radiographs should be performed with attention to immobilization of the potentially unstable spine.

Findings of the neurologic examination may be normal or may reveal complete or partial cord syndrome. Detailed serial neurologic examinations are crucial, as treatment plans are determined in part on the basis of whether a neurologic deficit is progressing or remaining stable.

### Radiologic findings

Pathognomonic of this injury is a malalignment of the spinal column. This dislocation may be obvious on the lateral or AP films. Rotational deformity may be less obvious, and recognition may be enhanced by attention to alignment of the pedicles and posterior spinous process on the AP film. Translational injuries can be identified by the shift of one vertebral body on another. These are frequently accompanied by fractures of the posterior spinous process or the neural arch. Fractures or dislocations of the facets are not well seen with plain radiography. CT scanning of the spine may better visualize the facet fracture-dislocation that accompanies these injuries. The scan may also reveal an injury to the posterior ligaments. Tomography also demonstrates injury to the anterior and middle columns, such as disruption of the disc or vertebral body.

### Diagnosis

Careful physical examination distinguishes the degree of neurologic impairment and bony involvement. The diagnosis is often obvious on AP and lateral-spine films. Because the supine position may reduce the dislocation, it is possible though rare, to have nearly normal supine radiographs. CT scanning often further defines the injury, the position and integrity of the facets, and possible injury to the soft tissues, such as discs and ligaments, and resulting destruction of the spinal canal.

### Treatment

Disruption of the spinal column can also create life-threatening injuries. Priority is given to the treatment of such injuries, though the spine is immobilized during this time. Additional neurologic examinations document spinal cord injury and any developing progression. Care of these injuries is best directed by a spine specialist, with subsequent reduction and stabilization of the dislocation. Timing of surgery is affected by stability as documented by neurologic examination. High-dose steroids reduce subsequent neurologic morbidity when administered within 8 hours of injury.[1]

### SEAT BELT INJURIES

These injuries occur most commonly when seat belt lap restraints are worn without shoulder restraints. The passenger is thrown forward and distraction forces are applied to the spine. Injuries involving the thoracolumbar spine rarely occur above the T-11 region, and complete spinal cord injury is infrequent. There is a high incidence (up to 90% in children) of associated abdominal injuries.[5]

One subtype of this group of injuries was originally described by Chance in the 1940s, prior to the advent of seat belts; hence, the same mechanism may occur in other types of trauma.

### Mechanism of injury

The mechanism involves flexion of the spine with the fulcrum located anterior to the spinal column (i.e., the anterior abdominal wall). A classic example is deceleration injury in a person restrained by a lap belt (Fig. 6-13). When this happens, the belt applies forces anterior to the spinal column. The posterior aspect of the spinal column is subject to distraction forces. Fractures or ligamentous injuries originate posteriorly and then propogate anteriorly.

There are three types of distraction injuries: 1) purely ligamentous injuries, in which the posterior innerspinous ligament is disrupted with subluxation of facets (Fig. 6-14A); 2) purely bony involvement injuries, with fracture through the posterior spinous process, pedicles, and vertebral body (the classic Chance fracture, Fig. 6-14B); and 3) a combination of ligamentous and bony fracture (Fig. 6-14C).

### Signs and symptoms

Findings on examination frequently include contusions and abrasions over the lower abdominal wall from the lap belt. Pain occurs over the site of the spinal cord injury. The examination may show tenderness over the injured area along with gibbous deformity. Increased distance between the spinous process may be detectable. Neurologic examination may reveal a complete cord injury; more commonly, however, no spinal cord injury is found.

### Radiologic findings

This injury is essentially a tearing of the spinal column. The tear progresses from the posterior aspect of the column anteriorly. In its route though the spinal column, it may disrupt ligaments or bone, and it may involve adjacent vertebrae. The lateral spine film may show the pathognomonic horizontal split of the transverse process and pedicles, with or without spinous process involvement. Distraction at the fracture site may be seen, as well as increased height at the posterior aspect of the vertebral body.

Injuries of ligaments can only be quite subtle radiographically. Findings would include widening of the interspinous space and opening up of the facets.

CT scanning does not significantly aid in the diagnosis. A CT scan without sagittal or vertical reconstruction may be entirely normal.

### Diagnosis

Mechanism of injury, physical examination, and lateral spine films should combine to make the diagnosis straightforward. The evaluation of abdominal injuries is crucial to these patients. Surgical consultation with diagnostic peritoneal lavage or abdominal CT are used liberally.

### Treatment

Although this fracture affects both the posterior and middle columns, it is a relatively stable fracture when it is not

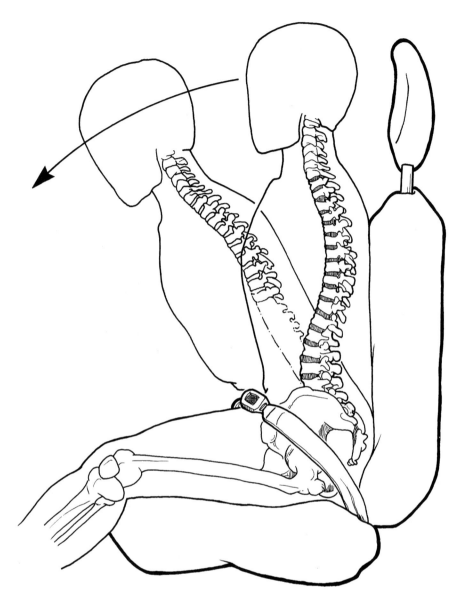

**Fig. 6-13.** In seat belt injuries when the lap belt is worn without a shoulder harness, the upper torso is thrown forward in a deceleration accident and the pelvis and lower lumbar spine remain stationary. This results in simultaneous flexion and distraction forces.

subjected to further flexion forces. This is caused by the intact anterior longitudinal ligament acting as a hinge to stabilize the spine. Therefore, although immobilization is necessary, any urgent injuries, especially those to the abdomen, can be cared for first. High-dose steroids are used for neurologic injuries. Partial cord deficits resulting from this injury have a relatively good prognosis.

## FRACTURE OF THE TRANSVERSE PROCESS AND SPINOUS PROCESS

Fractures isolated to either the posterior spinous process or the transverse process are benign in that they do not affect the structural integrity of the spinal column itself. Fractures of the transverse process typically occur after lateral bending; the process on the convex side of the spine is avulsed from the neural ring. Injury to the spinous process may be

caused by either a direct blow or by hyperflexion of the back. This is the lumbar equivalent of the clay shoveler's fracture.

### Signs and symptoms

The patient frequently has associated injuries that cause the emergency department visit. Examination of the back shows tenderness over the fracture site. Transverse process fractures typically occur at the L-2, L-3 or L-4 regions. It is common to involve more than one of these sites. As the hematoma accompanying the transverse process fracture may cause an ileus, the patient may have complaints of nausea, vomiting, and abdominal distension. Examination of the abdomen could reveal absent bowel sounds. Examination of the urine is also appropriate, as these injuries may be accompanied by renal contusion or damage to the vascular pedicle of the kidney.

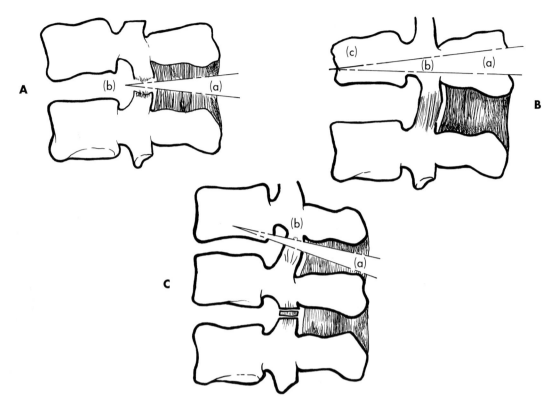

**Fig. 6-14.** Seat belt injury. **A,** Ligamentous injury only. Ligamentous distraction injury involving (a) interspinous ligament and (b) dislocation at the facets. **B,** Chance fracture (bony injury only). Fracture involving the spinous process (a), pedicles (b), and the vertebral body (c) as it moves anteriorly. **C,** Ligamentous and bony injury. As the fracture moves from posterior to anterior, it involves the infraspinous ligament (a) and the vertebral body (b).

### Radiographic findings

Unless the physician is specifically looking for a fractured transverse process, the diagnosis will frequently be missed. Avulsion of the transverse process detected on the AP film can involve multiple contiguous sites. It is important to scrutinize the AP film for evidence of a lateral compression fracture on the side of the spine opposite the broken process. The lateral film will best define the spinous process. In the lumbar area, these are large structures requiring significant force to affect their integrity.

### Treatment

Transverse spinous fractures can be treated with local care such as application of ice for the first 48 hours, then heat application. Bedrest for 3 to 5 days is appropriate as are oral analgesics. As these may be accompanied by paralytic ileus, some recommend an initial 24 hours of inhospital observation. Significant hematuria should be evaluated with an intravenous pyelogram and treated accordingly.

Fractures of the posterior spinous process are treated in a similar fashion with local care, bedrest, and appropriate analgesia.

Both spinous process and transverse process fractures may at times result in nonunion. If this is a cause of residual pain, the avulsed fragments may be surgically excised.

### PENETRATING INJURIES TO THE SPINE

Gunshot and knife wounds lag behind blunt trauma as a cause of spinal cord injury to our society. However, penetrating trauma is gaining rapidly. In 1991 in Texas, fatalities secondary to gunshot surpassed those due to motor vehicle accidents.

Penetrating trauma to the spine differs from bony trauma in several aspects: 1) knife and gunshot injuries seldom affect structural stability of the spinal column; 2) penetrating injuries introduce the complication of infection; 3) bullets and blades traverse other areas in the process of injuring the spinal column; and 4) partial cord syndromes are more likely to result from penetrating trauma.

### Management

Management of patients with sustained penetrating spinal trauma begins with the ABCs of resuscitation. Most penetrating injuries to the spine also enter the thorax or abdomen, and these injuries must be surveyed. A neurologic exam demonstrates the extent of damage to the spinal cord. Radiographs may show fractures or a lodged bullet. Subcutaneous air and bullet fragments may mark the path of the bullet. Cord damage caused by a bullet may be secondary to direct penetration of the spinal canal or may occur without violation of the canal; these spinal contusions are more likely to be seen after entry from high-velocity projectiles (eg, hunting rifles).

Standard management of penetrating spinal injuries was initially based on aggressive treatment developed during wartime. During World War II and the Korean conflict, the common treatment of ballistic injuries was laminectomy with tissue debridement and shrapnel removal. However, conservative management may be more appropriate if the offending weapons are nonmilitary, as their lower velocity and smaller diameter result in less tissue destruction.

Because bullet and knife wounds tend to leave the spinal canal structurally stable, the primary focus in management is conservative versus operative treatment of the wound. The goal of treatment is to prevent local infections, meningitis, and leak of cerebrospinal fluid (CSF), and to optimize the long-term outcome in terms of neurologic disability and pain.

Several studies have evaluated the incidence of infection in patients with spinal cord injury from penetrating trauma. Romanick et al[6] found that infections were more likely to occur if the missile perforated the colon prior to its entry into the spinal canal. Subsequently, a study by Roffi[7] found that bowel perforations treated with a prolonged course of antibiotics was effective in preventing infections, and that operative intervention did little to decrease the incidence of infection. Roffi[7] also retrospectively examined the incidence of CSF leak and meningitis in operative versus conservatively treated patients and found the operative group to have a higher incidence of leaks and infections.

Investigations of neurologic outcome with and without bullet removal consistently found that: 1) complete cord injuries do not improve under either circumstance; and 2) partial cord injuries improve equally well with either conservative or aggressive treatment.[8-11] There has been some suggestion that when the lesion is low in the spine, greater recovery is seen with bullet removal.[11]

Neither surgery nor conservative management reduces the chronic pain associated with penetrating spinal injury.[12,13]

## LOW BACK PAIN

Few emergency physicians entered the specialty specifically for the purpose of treating patients with low-back pain. For a number of reasons, it is difficult to deal with this problem. First, patients presenting with complaints of low-back pain may have other motivations aside from the relief of pain. They may be seeking drugs or attempting to build a case for litigation or workman's compensation. These patients often present with the same symptoms as patients who truly have pathology. Second, the ability to make a specific pathophysiologic diagnosis is limited. History and physical examination can rule out serious causes of low-back pain but can only infrequently point to the exact etiology. Radiology is rarely helpful.[12] Third, the mainstays

of treatment, bedrest, and pain medication such as acetaminophen or ibuprofen are easily available to the patient; hence, the physician can prescribe no magic bullet. Although acute low-back pain is common—up to 90% lifetime prevalence and 5% annual incidence[14]—it is at times a manifestation of a serious disease, such as a ruptured abdominal aortic aneurysm or osteomyelitis.

Low-back pain is defined as involving the regions from the rib cage to the buttocks. At times, the pain may radiate into the upper legs. *Sciatica* is defined as a pain in the distribution of a specific nerve root, usually with sensory and motor deficits in the same nerve root.

Low-back pain can occur as a result of a number of benign causes. Inflammation of facet joints, capsules, spinous ligaments, and intervertebral discs can all cause pain. Often there is spasm in the paraspinal muscles exacerbating the pain. It is difficult to distinguish these etiologies clinically. Fortunately, conservative therapy is usually sufficient for each of these, making such a distinction not critical.

Although the differential diagnosis of back pain is broad, several diseases must be ruled out before the patient leaves the emergency department. Intense pain in a patient who is writhing is suggestive of renal stone or, in the elderly, a vascular catastrophe such as ischemic bowel or ruptured abdominal aneurysm. Pain that is not relieved by rest is characteristic of an infectious process such as osteomyelitis, discitis, or epidural abscess. Metastatic or primary malignancy of the spinal column can cause intense pain at rest. An epidural tumor can cause pain with local neurologic symptoms. Disc herniation, which compresses a nerve root, can also inflict pain that is typically of a sciatic nature. On rare occasions, a disc herniates centrally (posteriorly); this central disc herniation can compress the center of the spinal cord or cauda equina, causing a progressive neurologic deficit with urinary and fecal incontinence or retention and caudal anesthesia. In this case, diagnostic testing and treatment should begin immediately.

Ancillary tests in previously healthy young patients with acute low-back pain are frequently of limited value. Standard AP and lateral radiographs have proven unnecessary for patients with no prior trauma or for patients who have no other underlying medical conditions such as cancer, diabetes, immunosupression, or drug abuse.[12] In the evaluation of sciatic type of pain, radiography is often insensitive to the presence of disc disease.[13,14] Elevated erythrocyte sedimentation rate can be used as a marker for infectious causes of low-back pain, such as osteomyelitis, or malignant involvement of the spinal column.

Despite the high incidence of low-back pain and its causes, controlled studies to evaluate what is effective treatment are not plentiful.[15] Bedrest is the mainstay of treatment. Wiesel[16] demonstrated that with military recruits randomized to either treatment with bedrest or continuing ambulation, the former group was able to return to full activity in 6.6 days, versus 11.8 days for the ambulatory group. Subsequently, Wiesel showed that 2 days of bedrest were as effective as 7 days for patients with low-back pain in the ambulatory care setting.

In the treatment of acute low-back pain, analgesic medication with a short half-life (e.g., ibuprofen, acetaminophen, or indomethacin) may be superior in that steady-state plasma levels may be reached more quickly. No specific nonsteroidal medication has been shown clinically to be more effective than others, although particular patients may respond better to one agent than another. The use of muscle relaxants may be productive if spasm seems to be playing a large role in the pain. Steroid injection for the treatment of acute low-back pain is generally not recommended.

Initial treatment of sciatica is also conservative, with bedrest and acetaminophen, phenylbutazone, or indomethacin, all of which have been shown in prospective trials to decrease pain. Sciatica symptoms that do not resolve with such conservative measures warrant evaluation by a back specialist.

## HERNIATED DISC DISEASE

Herniation of a portion of the nucleus pulposis into the spinal canal may cause compression or irritation of the adjacent nerve root, resulting in sciatic-type pain. The vertebral disc is made up of an anulus fibrosis, a thick connective tissue that surrounds the disc like a tire. The anulus fibrosis attaches to the superior and inferior vertebral bodies, each of which has a cartilaginous covering providing the upper and lower borders of the disc. The front part of the anulus fibrosis is reinforced by the anterior longitudinal ligament running the length of the vertebral column. Similarly, the posterior longitudinal ligament provides support to the back of the anulus fibrosis. Most disc herniations are not oriented posteriorly; rather, they occur just lateral to the posterior longitudinal ligament.

In addition to the typical lateral herniation of a disc, the nucleus pulposis can at times bulge into the superior or inferior cartilaginous end plates, producing a Schmorl's nodule in the adjacent vertebral body, an incidental radiographic finding.

A disc can also herniate posteriorly on rare occasion. When midline posterior herniation occurs, a cauda equina syndrome may develop. Because the vertebral canal below the L-2 level contains only the cauda equina (basically peripheral nerves), compression in this area produces unilateral or bilateral motor and sensory patterns consistent with peripheral nerve lesion (e.g., decreased reflexes, weakness, and sensory loss, often in a saddle-type distribution). Along with this, the cauda equina syndrome causes autonomic dysfunction with loss of bowel and bladder control, manifested by either fecal incontinence with lax anal tone, or urinary changes (e.g., retention or incontinence).

**Table 6-2.** Changes in reflexes as defined by level of herniated disc

| Disc | Root | Sensory | Motor | Reflex |
|------|------|---------|-------|--------|
| L-3–L-4 | L-4 | Anterior thigh; anterior-medial calf | Quadriceps | Knee jerk |
| L-4–L-5 | L-5 | Anterior calf; medial dorsum of foot | Foot; dorsiflexors | — |
| L-5–S-1 | S-1 | Lateral calf; lateral dorsum of foot | Foot; plantar flexors | Ankle jerk |

Nerve roots are named for the vertebral bodies at which they exit. Because the nerve roots exit rather high in relation to the disc space, a protrusion of the disc usually affects the nerve exiting below that area (Table 6-1). For example, herniation of the L-4–L-5 disc compresses the L-5 nerve root, producing motor and sensory changes in this distribution.

### Mechanism

The vertebral discs are able to withstand considerable loads (1000 lbs) before failure occurs. When injuries from axial load do occur, they tend to involve the vertebral cartilaginous end plates. However, with age, fissures may develop in the anulus fibrosis. Axial loads can then produce herniation of the nucleus pulposis, either through these fissures or through an attenuated area of anulus fibrosis. At times, the pulposis may herniate completely through the anulus fibrosis and lie free in the spinal canal. Herniated discs are most likely to occur in the 3rd to 5th decade of life. The injury is usually one of a flexion, although herniation can occur without a known traumatic event. Over 95% of thoracolumbar disc herniations occur at the L-4–L-5 or L-5–S-1 disc spaces, with the L-3–L-4 disc comprising most other herniations. Herniation of other areas of the thoracolumbar spine is rare. Herniations are typically unilateral.

### Signs and symptoms

Herniated discs can cause either acute, recurrent, or chronic symptoms. Patients with sciatica from herniated discs tend to have had prior episodes of low-back pain. The components of sciatica resulting from a nerve root compression include pain, sensory changes, and motor findings. The back pain may be a dull ache or severe and lancinating with radiation into the buttocks or hips in a dermatomal distribution (Table 6-2). Pain is worse with Valsalva (i.e., coughing, sneezing, or straining) and when standing or sitting. If the pain is not relieved by lying flat, other etiologies should be considered. Sensory changes may be hypesthesia or pins-and-needles, prickly sensations in the leg. The patient may be able to localize the pain to the nerve root involved.

Inspection of the patient in a position of comfort shows an attempt to flatten the lumbar spine: forward tilting of the trunk with flexion of the hip and knee of the affected side. If the patient is supine, the hips will be slightly flexed. Palpation may reveal spasm of the paraspinous muscles and spinous process tenderness.

The straight-leg–raise test is performed with the patient supine. With the knees extended and the foot plantar flexed, the examiner lifts the patient's leg by gradually flexing at the hip until the patient develops pain. Patients without nerve root compression may flex to 90° before the onset of discomfort, whereas patients with herniated discs begin to develop pain at 30° to 40° of flexion. If flexion of the opposite side (well-leg–raise test) elicits pain, this suggests either a large herniated disc or one herniated in the midline.

Changes in reflexes are defined by the level of the herniated disc (Table 6-2). Longstanding disc herniation may cause not only weakness in the affected muscle but also atrophy. If the herniation is at the L-4–L-5 disc space, the muscles involved are the peroneals, anterior tibial, and extensor hallicus longus. Pain and sensory changes may involve the great toe, particularly the web space between the great and second toes, and dorsum of the foot, although reflexes may be normal. A foot drop is a common finding. Herniation at the L-5–S-1 level causes a diminished ankle reflex, decreased sensation over the lateral foot or ankle, and weakness of plantar flexion of the foot.

### Radiologic findings

Plain radiographs of the lumbosacral spine are frequently negative when the cause of pain is herniated disc. Occasionally, the radiographs show loss of the normal lordotic curvature of the spine. The films may be used to rule out osteoarthritis, fracture or involvement of the spine by tumor, or infection when clinically indicated.

Acute radiographic diagnosis of herniated disc incorporates the use of a CT scan or magnetic resonance imaging (MRI). Because most herniated discs may be treated conservatively (eg, pain medications and bedrest), with referral to a back specialist, it is at times wise to allow the surgeon to select the radiographic modality best suited to the particular patient when seen in follow-up.

### Diagnosis

In the emergency department, the diagnosis of herniated disc is a clinical one. Laboratory and radiographic data available in the emergency setting may rule out other etiologies for the pain, but do not confirm the herniation. WBC and erythrocyte sedimentation rate (ESR) may be useful to distinguish from metastatic or infectious involvement of the spine. Intravenous pyelography (IVP) may be used if renal stone is considered as a potential cause of the back pain. In the elderly, abdominal aneurysm and mesenteric ischemia must be considered.

The diagnosis of disc herniation is made from the following: 1) patient history of injury and pain; 2) pain worse with Valsalva in the upright position and better with recumbency; 3) pain involving an appropriate dermatome; 4) physical examination showing a positive straight-leg–raise test; and possibly 5) motor or sensory changes in the affected region of the disc.

When the disc is herniated posteriorly, a cauda equina syndrome may develop. The patient may have bilateral sensory changes, possibly with pain or hypesthesia in a saddle distribution. The patient also has bowel or bladder symptoms, typically involving urinary retention but possibly incontinence of urine or stool. On examination, patients with cauda equina syndrome have decreased rectal tone in addition to other findings seen with lateral disc herniation.

### Treatment

The initial treatment for herniated disc is nonoperative unless cauda equina is suspected. Patients are placed at bedrest, analgesics are used, and muscle relaxants are prescribed if spasm plays a significant role in the patient's illness. Steroid administration has not been shown to be beneficial. Physical therapy with traction or heat application may be added to the conservative regimen. Patients with sciatica secondary to disc herniation should be referred to a specialist for follow-up. Those who fail to respond to conservative treatment would then be candidates for discectomy. If the patient has developed cauda equina syndrome, aggressive management is indicated with the immediate involvement of the spine specialist.

## CANCER AND SPINAL CORD DISEASE

Despite advances in the field, cancer still is the second leading cause of death in America. However, new therapeutic modalities have increased the lifespan of the patient with cancer. Given this, it is not surprising that the emergency department physician frequently evaluates patients with cancer for acute related or unrelated medical problems. One of the devastating complications of cancer is its spread to the spinal column with associated neurologic impairment.[17] This is not an infrequent occurrence, as up to 40% of patients who die of cancer have vertebral column involvement at the time of their death.

### Pathophysiology

Cancerous involvement of the spine may be primary or metastatic. Primary spinal tumors are rare; thus, the vast majority (>95%) of spinal tumors are caused by metastasis. There are three ways tumors can involve the spinal column: 1) bony involvement of the spinal column, particularly common when the primary tumor is prostate, breast, or lung; 2) spread between the bony paravertebral spaces from a tumor lying adjacent to the spinal cord, such as a lymphoma or a renal cell tumor; and 3) metastasis directly to the spinal cord itself, which is a rare occurrence. The relatively impermeable dura mater protects the spinal cord from direct spread of adjacent tumors. Therefore, neurologic signs and symptoms of spinal metastasis result from cord compression rather than invasion. Cord compression may be caused by collapse of an eroded vertebral body or by direct pressure from a tumor mass. A tumor can compress the cord's blood supply, causing vasogenic cord damage.

Metastasis to the spine may be either single or multiple. Multiple noncontiguous sites are found in 10% to 38% of patients. Metastasis favors thoracic spine 70% of the time, lumbar 20%, and the cervical spine 10%.

## Diagnosis

Because the outcome of cord involvement is affected most by the extent of symptoms at the time of diagnosis, evaluation must be prompt. Historical questions include a previous diagnosis of cancer (although one-third of patients with metastases carry no prior diagnosis), social history (tobacco use, diet, and alcohol use), work history, family history, quality of pain, radicular signs and symptoms, weight loss, trauma-overuse, and history of arthritis.

Differentiation from the discomfort of degenerative joint disease of the spine includes a more severe pain with cancer that worsens when recumbent, a prior history of backache with degenerative joint disease (DJD), and a predilection of DJD for the lumbar spine. Also, progression to radicular signs and symptoms is not commonly seen with DJD.

On physical exam, the cancer patient may have difficulty finding a comfortable position. There will be pain with percussion over the tumor site (also found in trauma and discitis). The neurologic exam will confirm deficits.

Plain radiographs will show bone loss or collapse of vertebral bodies when 25% to 30% of the bone has eroded. These film results are almost always positive by the time neurologic signs and symptoms arise. Plain film results will miss excursion of tumors through foramina (as seen with lymphoma). Here, a CT or MRI scan is required.

Bone scans are more sensitive for detecting bony metastases from solid tumors but not from myelomas.

Evaluation of compression of the spinal cord is accomplished with MRI or CT scans, although myelography is sometimes used. As multiple sites are involved in up to one-third of the patients, study of the entire spine is prudent.

Cerebral spinal fluid examination is nonproductive and lumbar puncture is probably contraindicated, as it may cause conization of the cord due to a decrease in column pressure distal to the obstruction. This can worsen neurologic symptoms.

## Treatment

The most important prognostic indicator is the degree of neurologic disease at onset of radiation therapy. Patients who are ambulatory at initiation of treatment are likely to retain their ability to walk; those with paraplegia are unlikely to do so.

The three forms of treatment available include radiation therapy, steroid therapy, and surgery. Radiation therapy is the standard modality; fractionated doses are directed at the tumor with ports to minimize damage to surrounding tissue. Patients with progressing neurologic deficits are an emergency, and radiation should begin immediately. Steroid therapy should be initiated promptly in the emergency department. Although there are a wide range of dosages available, 10 mg of intravenous dexamethasone every 6 hours would be considered acceptable. Steroid therapy decreases edema of surrounding tissue, but is only a temporary measure until radiation therapy begins to affect the tumor mass.

Surgical intervention is less commonly used than other modalities. Surgery may be considered when neurologic symptoms continue in spite of radiation therapy. Surgery may also be used in patients who have received radiation therapy in the past, making subsequent dosing toxic to the surrounding tissue. Patients with tumors known to be resistant to radiation therapy may also benefit from surgery. Often, these patients are high-risk surgical candidates because of their underlying disease.

## REFERENCES

1. Bracken MB, Shepard MJ, Collins WF et al: A randomized controlled trial of methylprednisolone or naloxone in the treatment of acute spinal cord injury, *N Engl J Med* 322:1405-1411, 1990.
2. Denis F: The three column spine and its significance in the classification of acute thoracolumbar spinal injuries, *Spine* 8:817-831, 1983.
3. Young MH: Long term consequences of stable fractures of the thoracic and lumbar vertebral bodies, *J Bone Joint Surg* 55B:295-300, 1973.
4. Yashon D, Jane JA, and White RJ: Prognosis and management of spinal cord and cauda equina injuries in sixty-five civilians, *J Neurosurg* 32:163-170, 1970.
5. Sivit CJ, Taylor GA, Newman KD et al: Safety belt injuries in children with lap–belt ecchymosis: CT findings in 61 patients, *AJR* 157:111-114, 1991.
6. Romanick PC, Smith TK, Kopaniky DR et al: Infection about the spine associated with low–velocity–missile injury to the abdomen, *J Bone Joint Surg* 67A;8:1195-1201.
7. Roffi RP, Waters RL, and Adkins RH: Gunshot wounds to the spine associated with a perforated viscus, *Spine* 14:808-811, 1989.
8. Richards JS, Storer SL, and Jaworski T: Effect of bullet removal on subsequent pain in persons with spinal cord injury secondary to gunshot wound, *J Neurosurg* 73:401-404, 1990.
9. Simpson RK, Venger BH, and Narayan RK: Treatment of acute penetrating injuries of the spine: A retrospective analysis, *J Trauma* 29:42-46, 1989.
10. Stauffer ES, Wood RW, and Kelly EG: Gunshot wounds of the spine: The effects of laminectomy, *J Bone Joint Surg* 61A:389-392, 1979.
11. Waters RL, Adkins RH: The effect of removal of bullet fragments retained in the spinal cord, *Spine* 16:934-939, 1991.
12. Liang M, Komaroff AL: Roentgenograms in primary care patients with acute low back pain: A cost-effective analysis, *Arch Intern Med* 142:1108-1112, 1982.
13. Frymoyer JW: Back pain and sciatica, *N Engl J Med* 318:291-300, 1988.

14. Deyo RA, Diehl AK: Lumbar spine films in primary care: Current use and effects of selective ordering criteria, *J Gen Intern Med* 1:20-25, 1986.

15. Deyo RA, Diehl AK, and Rosenthal M: How many days of bed rest for acute low back pain? A randomized clinical trial, *N Engl J Med* 315:1064-1070, 1986.

16. Wiesel SW, Cuckleo JM, DeLuca F et al: Acute low back pain: An objective analysis of conservative therapy, *Spine* 5:324-330, 1980.

17. Byrne TN: Spinal cord compression from epidural metastasis, *N Engl J Med* 327:614-620, 1992.

# Pelvic, Sacral, and Acetabular Fractures

*Ernest Ruiz*

Pelvic fractures constitute an enormous cause of traumatic mortality and morbidity throughout the world. In the United States, these fractures directly and indirectly cause the deaths of thousands of people each year. Recent reports of trauma center experience using multifaceted and multispeciality approaches to the pelvic fracture patient have indicated that the mortality and morbidity of this injury can be reduced. Whether in a trauma center or a small rural hospital, prompt, studied, and effective resuscitation by the emergency physician who initiates care is a key element.

## EPIDEMIOLOGY

In an autopsy study of 127 patients dying of injuries received in traffic accidents, Perry and McCellan[1] found that pelvic fractures were the third leading cause of death, accounting for 12% of all traffic deaths. With traffic accidents causing 47,713 deaths in 1982, one can extrapolate to a figure of more than 5000 fatal pelvic fracture cases yearly in the United States alone.[2] Another estimate that may help put this injury in perspective is that about 5% of patients admitted to hospitals because of trauma have pelvic fractures.[3] As reported in the recent literature,[4-8] the overall mortality of patients surviving to reach the hospital is 5% to 15%. A review of pelvic ring fractures in children revealed an 11% mortality. However, this mortality was usually due to an accompanying head injury.[9]

Three trauma centers with a rural and urban catchment area reported the following mechanisms of injury for 538 patients admitted with acute pelvic fractures: motor vehicular trauma, 40%; falls, 28%; pedestrians struck by automobiles, 17%; motorcycle accidents, 9%; crush injuries, 5%; assaults and ski injuries, 1%.[7]

In addition to mortality, the morbidity suffered by victims of pelvic fracture is substantial. Of 30 pelvic fracture patients (Malgaigne fractures) who were contacted 2 to 12 years after injury, Semba et al.[10] found 11 patients with paresthesias of the legs, nine with gait disturbances, eight with severe low back pain, four with groin pain, and two with fecal incontinence. Impotence and urinary incontinence are also long-term complications of pelvic fractures.

The initial management and evaluation of pelvic fracture is a complex process because of the many possible injuries these patients can suffer. The severity of injury varies from minor to catastrophic. At the same time, the combinations of injuries vary from simple fractures to multiple-organ system involvement. Mucha and Farnell[3] found that of 34 fatal cases involving pelvic fractures, 23 had head injuries, 22 had thoracic injuries, and 15 had abdominal injuries. The pelvic fracture was the major cause of death in four patients, a contributing factor in 18, and a minor factor in 12. In addition, a pelvic fracture is a significant marker for thoracic aorta rupture, with a two- to fivefold increase in incidence among pelvic fracture patients.[11,12] Unfortunately, the type of fracture seen on radiography cannot rule out bleeding or other injury with enough reliability to allow the resuscitating physician to proceed complacently.[5,7,13] The resuscitation of these patients is truly a multispecialty challenge.[7]

## OBJECTIVES

Hemorrhage is estimated to be the cause of death in about 50% of fatal pelvic fracture cases.[5,7] Some pelvic fracture victims are dead on arrival at the emergency department. Some exsanguinate in a matter of minutes or hours,[3] while others do not bleed at all. Because the worst-case scenario must be anticipated for each case, evaluation and priority-setting must proceed rapidly.

The emergency physician and his or her colleagues must have a prepared plan of action if the patient is to be managed safely. The major objectives of this chapter are to provide information on the pathophysiology of pelvic fracture injuries and to outline a logical and efficient emergency department algorithm for resuscitation of the pelvic fracture patient.

## ANATOMY AND PATHOPHYSIOLOGY
### The bones and ligaments

**The pelvic ring.** The pelvis is comprised of two innominate bones and the sacrum. This structure is spatially complex and exquisitely formed to provide strength for weight-bearing, a stable fulcrum for powerful muscle function, a conduit for childbirth in women, a site for hemopoiesis, and protection of the pelvic organs. Each innominate bone is formed by an ilium, a pubic bone, and the ischium. In children, the ossification centers of these three components meet at the triradiate cartilage of the acetabulum. This cartilage persists until age 16 to 18 years when the bones fuse together.

The ilium and pubic bone on each side and the alar and proximal vertebral portion of the sacrum form a distinct ring that is the weight-bearing ring of the pelvis. This ring is also called the *iliopectineal line* or the *arcuate line.* The pelvis above this ring is the false pelvis and is a part of the abdomen. The pelvis below this ring is the true pelvis. The pubic bone portion of the ring functions as a strut, keeping the ring from opening or closing. When sitting, weight is borne by the ischium, transmitting force up posterior to the acetabulum to the weight-bearing ring. This portion of the innominate bone is called the *posterior column* of the acetabulum. When standing upright, the force imparted by the head of the femur to the acetabulum is carried by an anterior column to the weight-bearing ring. The ring forms the entrance to the true pelvis from the abdomen.

Figures 7-1 and 7-2 offer three-dimensional views of the bony and ligamentous pelvis. The primary ossification centers of the pubis and sacrum fuse at the pubic rami at age 6 or 7 years.[14] The ages for fusion of the secondary ossification centers of the pelvis are listed in Table 7-1.[16]

**The sacrum and coccyx.** The sacrum starts out looking like a lumbar vertebral body, then abruptly flattens out and curves backward to become a concave dish. Because it is really a series of five vertebral bodies fused together, the sacrum has four anterior and posterior foramina that communicate with each other and the spinal canal of the sacrum. The spinous processes of the vertebral bodies that

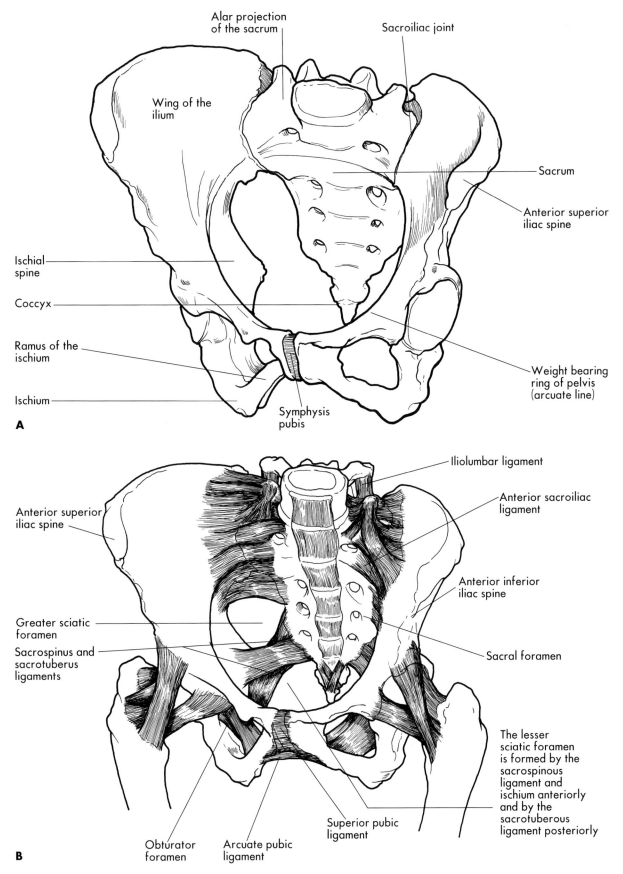

Alar projection of the sacrum

Sacroiliac joint

Wing of the ilium

Sacrum

Anterior superior iliac spine

Ischial spine

Coccyx

Ramus of the ischium

Ischium

Symphysis pubis

Weight bearing ring of pelvis (arcuate line)

**A**

Iliolumbar ligament

Anterior superior iliac spine

Anterior sacroiliac ligament

Anterior inferior iliac spine

Greater sciatic foramen

Sacrospinus and sacrotuberus ligaments

Sacral foramen

The lesser sciatic foramen is formed by the sacrospinous ligament and ischium anteriorly and by the sacrotuberous ligament posteriorly

Obturator foramen

Arcuate pubic ligament

Superior pubic ligament

**B**

**Fig. 7-1. A** and **B**, Anterior oblique views of the bony pelvis and ligaments. Note the iliolumbar ligaments connecting the transverse processes of L-5 to the ligaments of the sacroiliac joints. Transverse process fractures of L-5 often accompany sacroiliac disruption. The pelvic ring separates the false pelvis from the true pelvis. The inguinal ligaments connect the anterior superior iliac spines with the pubic tubercles. The muscles and fascia of the anterior abdominal wall attach to the inguinal ligaments and the pubis.

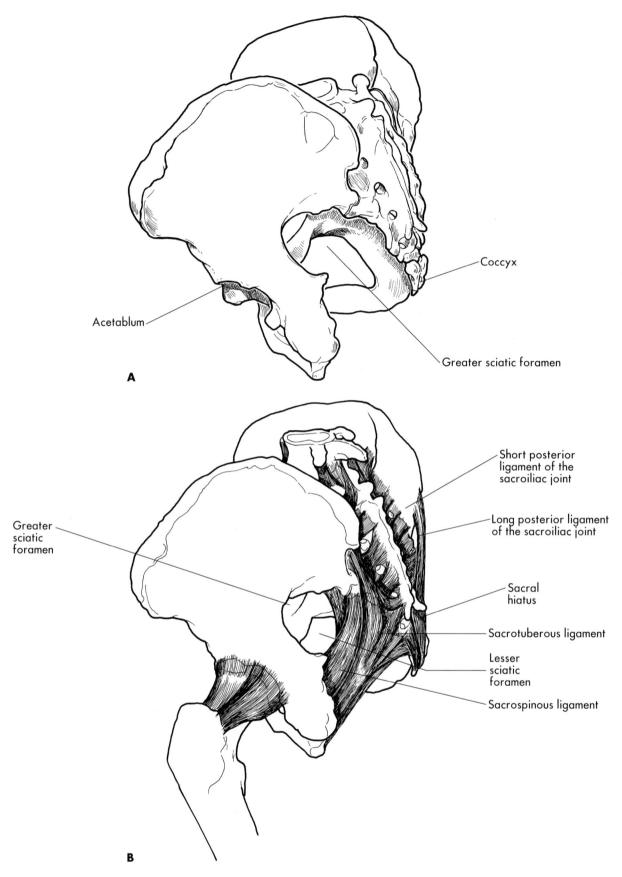

Coccyx

Acetablum

Greater sciatic foramen

**A**

Short posterior ligament of the sacroiliac joint

Long posterior ligament of the sacroiliac joint

Sacral hiatus

Sacrotuberous ligament

Lesser sciatic foramen

Sacrospinous ligament

Greater sciatic foramen

**B**

**Fig. 7-2. A** and **B**, Posterior oblique views of the bony pelvis and ligaments. Note how the sacrospinous and sacrotuberous ligaments form the greater and lesser sciatic foramina. The sacral articulation with the innominate bones is wider anteriorly than posteriorly, so it is not a keystonelike wedge in the ring. The strength of this articulation is due to the sacroiliac ligaments, especially the posterior ligaments.

**Table 7-1.** Age when human fusion of the secondary ossification centers of the pelvis occurs

| Ossification center | Approximate age of fusion |
| --- | --- |
| Iliac crest | 20–25 |
| Ischial apophysis | 20–25 |
| Anteroinferior iliac spine | 16 |
| Pubic tubercle | 20–25 |
| Lateral wing of the sacrum | 25–30 |

Adapted from Goss CM: *Gray's anatomy,* ed 29, Philadelphia, 1973, Lea & Febiger.

comprise the sacrum are fused together so that the spinal canal is closed posteriorly except at its distal end, where the canal is open. This opening is called the *sacral hiatus.* The dural sheath of the spinal cord ends at the third sacral vertebral level, but the filum terminale continues on to attach to the proximal coccyx. The ventral and dorsal roots of the sacral nerves exit the anterior and posterior foramina, respectively. Fortunately, the foramina are large relative to the size of the nerves. Two alar projections of the proximal portion of the sacrum form the sacral articulations of the sacroiliac joints. Because these joints slant inward posteriorly toward the midline, the sacrum is not a true keystone in the weight-bearing ring.

The sacroiliac joints themselves do not offer much resistance to a shearing or opening force. Rather, the stability of the ring is due to strong ligaments located anteriorly and posteriorly that firmly hold the sacroiliac joints together.[17] The posterior ligament has three components consisting of short fibers directly crossing the joint (the interosseous sacroiliac ligament), longer fibers obliquely crossing the sacroiliac joint (the short posterior sacroiliac ligament), and fibers fanning out from the posterior iliac spine to connect to the sacrum and the sacrotuberous ligament (the long posterior sacroiliac ligament). The sacrum and the sacroiliac joints are also joined to the lumbar vertebrae by strong ligaments. The ligaments between the sacroiliac joints and the transverse processes of the fifth lumbar vertebra are called the *iliolumbar ligaments.*

The coccyx is formed by three to five rudimentary vertebral bodies. In women, the sacrum and coccyx are more exposed to direct trauma from behind because of the greater diameter of the true pelvis in women.[18]

**The innominate bones and the acetabula.** The innominate bones articulate with the femora through the cup-shaped acetabula. The acetabulum is formed at the junction of the ischium, pubis, and ilium (Fig. 7-3). Each of these bones contributes to its articular surface. The triradiate cartilage is subject to traumatic changes, as are

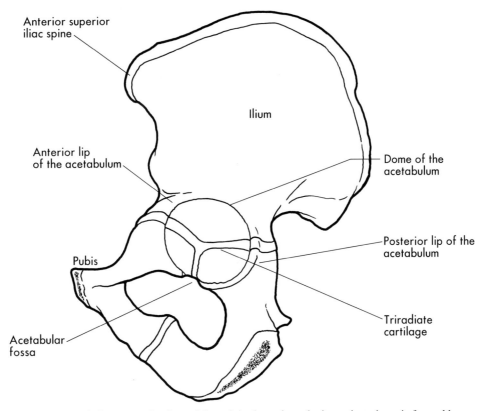

**Fig. 7-3.** This semi-diagrammatic view of the pelvis shows how the innominate bone is formed by the pubis, ischium, and ilium, which come together at the center of the acetabulum. This junction remains cartilaginous (the triradiate cartilage) for approximately 17 years.

growth plates in other areas. Premature or irregular fusion of this cartilage leads to significant morbidity.[14] The center of the cup is occupied by the acetabular fossa, which accommodates the ligament of the head of the femur and a fat pad. The anterior (iliopubic) and posterior (ilioishial) columns of thickened bone that transmit force from and around the acetabulum are difficult to visualize on a single view but are depicted in Fig. 7-4. The acetabular cup is deepened by a lip of bone for most of its circumference. For descriptive purposes, this lip is divided into the anterior and posterior lips. The lip of the acetabulum does not cross the acetabular fossa inferiorly. The superior and inferior pubic rami and the ischium form the obturator foramen on either side. The pubic bones meet medially at the symphysis pubis. A fibrocartilagenous disk, the interpubic disk, is interposed between the pubic bones. Strong superior and arcuate pubic ligaments hold the pubic bones firmly together.

The strong anterior and posterior sacroiliac and pubic symphysis ligaments have already been described. Two other pairs of ligaments help shape and hold the floor of the true pelvis: the sacrospinous and sacrotuberous ligaments.

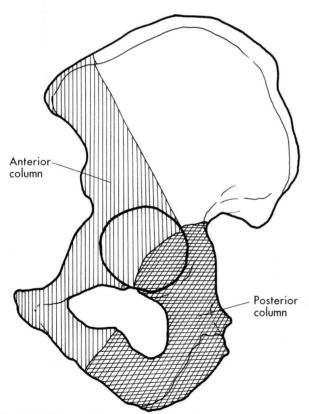

**Fig. 7-4.** This semi-diagrammatic view of the pelvis depicts the anterior and posterior columns of thick, dense bone that transmit force through and posterior to the acetabulum. The posterior column transmits force from the ischium to the weight-bearing ring, and the anterior column transmits force from the dome of the acetabulum to the weight-bearing ring.

The sacrospinous ligament is attached to the spine of the ischium and fans out to attach to the ventral surface of the ischium and coccyx. The sacrotuberous ligament is located posterior to the sacrospinous ligament and extends out from the lateral border of the sacrum and coccyx to attach to the ischial tuberosity. These ligaments define the greater and lesser sciatic foramina (Figs. 7-1 and 7-2).

**Fracture patterns**

**The pelvic ring.** Single breaks of the weight-bearing pelvic ring occur rarely, presumably due to ligamentous stretching; two or more breaks in the ring is the general rule when this rigid ring is disrupted.[4] In children, single breaks may be more common because of greater elasticity of bones and ligaments.[14] Because the ring is rigid, with areas of relative weakness and strength, a force causing it to fracture produces predictable combinations of fractures, depending on the direction and magnitude of the force. The segments of the ring that are most likely to fracture or separate are the symphysis pubis, the pubic rami, and the ilium at or just lateral to the sacroiliac joint. Pennal et al.[20] at the Shock Trauma Center of the Maryland Institute for Emergency Medical Services Systems have evolved the Young classification system, which classifies pelvic ring disruptions; this system takes advantage of this predictability.[4,19-21]

Lateral compression (LC) fractures are caused by a transverse compression fracture of the pubic bone or its rami, combined with a compression fracture of the sacrum on the side of impact (Fig. 7-5).[22] This fracture is usually impacted and runs through the ala of the sacrum and through the foramina on the same side. With more force, the iliac wing is also fractured; with still more force, the opposite side of the pelvis opens up due to an anteroposterior compression (APC) force imparted to it as the other side caves in. These are termed LC-I, LC-II, and LC-III fractures, respectively. Note that in these fractures the sacrospinous and sacrotuberous ligaments are compressed rather than torn apart on the side of impact. Fractures of the LC type constitute about 40% of all pelvic ring fractures. LC-I injuries constitute 33.5%, LC-II injuries, 6.4%, and LC-III injuries, 1.5%.[6] Patients with LC-type fractures suffer an overall mortality of about 13%.[6]

Anteroposterior compression opens the ring like a book and causes symphyseal diastasis or vertical fracture of the pubic bone or its rami, combined with a degree of sacroiliac joint disruption (Fig. 7-6). Again, these fractures are termed APC-I, APC-II, and APC-III according to the magnitude of force required to produce them. In APC-I injuries, the symphysis is separated by less than 2 cm. Note that the sacrospinous and sacrotuberous ligaments are torn apart in APC-II and APC-III injuries. The iliolumbar ligament sometimes avulses the transverse process of L-5 when the sacroiliac joint is disrupted.[23] Fractures of the APC type constitute about 26% of all pelvic ring fractures. APC-I injuries constitute 9%; APC-II injuries, 9%; and APC-III

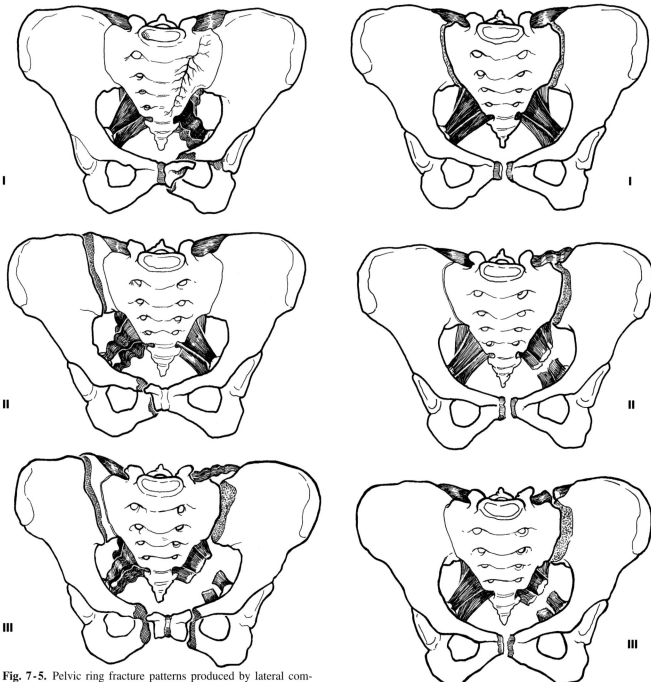

**Fig. 7-5.** Pelvic ring fracture patterns produced by lateral compression (LC). The sacral compression fracture seen in LC-I fractures may or may not be impacted. Note that the sacrospinous and sacrotuberous ligaments are intact on the side of impact, and that the anterior fractures have a transverse configuration.

**Fig. 7-6.** Pelvic ring fracture patterns produced by anteroposterior compression (APC). These fractures are sometimes called "open-book fractures" for obvious reasons. In APC-II fractures, the posterior sacroiliac ligaments remain intact. Note that the anterior fractures have a vertical configuration.

injuries, 8%.[6] Patients with APC-type fractures suffer an overall mortality of about 26%.[6]

A vertical shear (VS) force fracture can be imparted by falling on an outstretched leg or by the knee striking the dashboard in an automobile accident. In these cases, as in APC fractures, there is an anterior fracture, but with cephalad displacement. Likewise, the posterior sacroiliac

joint or iliac wing fracture is displaced cephalad (Fig. 7-7). Note that the ligaments are disrupted. VS-type fractures constitute about 5% of all pelvic ring fractures.[6] Patients with this type of fracture suffer an overall mortality of 25%.[6]

Combined injuries, such as those that occur when a victim is rolled on the pavement by a vehicle or is crushed

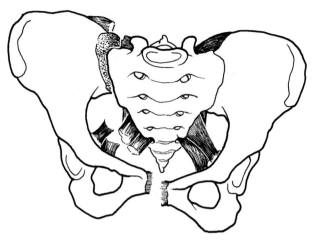

**Fig. 7-7.** Pelvic ring fracture pattern produced by a vertical shear force. The anterior and posterior fractures are displaced cephalad.

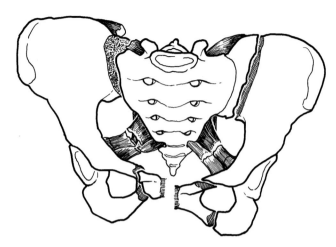

**Fig. 7-8.** Pelvic ring fractures produced by a combined mechanism. A lateral compression and vertical shear force injury is a common combination.

**Table 7-2.** The Young classification system for pelvic ring fractures

| Category | Pattern description |
|---|---|
| **Lateral compression (LC) injury** | |
| LC-I | Transverse fracture of pubis or pubic rami; sacral compression fracture on side of impact |
| LC-II | Transverse fracture of pubis or pubic rami; iliac wing fracture on side of impact |
| LC-III | LC-I or LC-II injury on side of impact with contralateral anteroposterior injury |
| **Anteroposterior compression (APC) injury** | |
| APC-I | Slight widening of the symphysis with stretched but intact sacroiliac ligaments; sacrospinous and sacrotuberous ligaments intact |
| APC-II | Symphyseal diastasis or vertical rami fractures; widened sacroiliac joint anteriorly; anterior sacroiliac, sacrospinous, and sacrotuberous ligaments disrupted; posterior sacroiliac ligaments intact |
| APC-III | Symphyseal diastasis or vertical rami fractures; complete sacroiliac joint and ligament disruption; sacrospinous and sacrotuberous ligaments disrupted |
| **Vertical shear (VS) force injury** | |
| | Symphyseal or pubic rami vertically disrupted with displacement anteriorly or posteriorly; fracture through the sacroiliac joint, iliac wing, or sacrum with vertical displacement |
| **Combined mechanism (CM) of injury** | |
| | Combination of other injury patterns |

Adapted from Burgess AR: The pelvic ring. In Rockwood CA Jr, Green DP, and Bucholz RW, eds: *Fractures in adults,* ed 3, Philadelphia, 1991, JB Lippincott.

by an immense weight, are termed combined mechanical (CM) injuries. Figure 7-8 shows a combined VS and LC injury. CM injuries constitute about 10% of all pelvic ring fractures.[6] Patients with these injuries suffer an overall mortality of 18%.

The Young classification system is outlined in Table 7-2. The Kane modification of the Key and Conwell classification system is also widely used and is shown in the box on the next page. The term "Malgaigne fracture" is generally applied to fractures of the VS type with displacement.[24]

---

**The Kane modification of the Key and Conwell pelvic fracture classification system**

*Fractures without a break in the continuity of the pelvic ring*

Avulsion fractures
Anterosuperior iliac spine
Anteroinferior iliac spine
Ischial tuberosity
Fractures of the pubis or ischium
Fractures of the wing of the ilium (Duverney)
Fractures of the sacrum or coccyx

*Single break in the pelvic ring*

Fracture of two ipsilateral rami
Fracture near or subluxation of the symphysis pubis
Fracture near or subluxation of the sacroiliac joint

*Double break in the pelvic ring*

Double vertical fractures or dislocation of the pubis (straddle fractures)
Double vertical fractures or dislocation (Malgaigne)
Severe multiple fractures

*Fractures of the acetabulum*

Small fragment associated with dislocation of the hip
Linear fracture associated with nondisplaced pelvic fracture
Linear fracture associated with hip joint instability
Fracture secondary to central dislocation of the acetabulum

(Adapted from Kane WJ: Fractures of the pelvis. In Rockwood CA Jr, Green DP, eds: *Fractures in adults,* ed 2, Philadelphia, 1984, JB Lippincott.)

---

Joseph Malgaigne was a French surgeon who described this fracture based on clinical findings in 1859.[25]

**The acetabulum.** When the head of the femur is driven into the acetabulum, either the anterior or posterior column can be fractured, depending on the direction of the force and the position of the femoral head. When the femoral head is internally rotated, the posterior column is usually fractured; when the rotation is external, the anterior column is usually fractured. When the femur is adducted, the superior aspect of the acetabulum is commonly fractured; when the femur is abducted, the inferior aspect may be fractured.[26] When the weight-bearing ring of the pelvis is involved, there is severe pelvic fracture. A transverse fracture through the acetabulum can also result (Fig. 7-9). When the head of the femur is forcibly dislocated anteriorly or posteriorly, a chunk of the lip of the acetabulum, with or without a piece of the dome of articulation, is often broken off (Fig. 7-10). Combinations of these fractures also occur, as Tile[26] has summarized. Acetabular fractures frequently involve the weight-bearing ring of the pelvis, accounting for about 18% of all pelvic ring fractures.[6]

**The sacrum alone.** Isolated sacral fractures are uncommon and comprise about 4.5% of all pelvic fractures.[27] Sacral fractures resulting from direct trauma, such as that suffered in a fall backward, are transverse through the foramina usually at the S-4 level (Fig. 7-11A).[18] Another mechanism of isolated sacral fracture occurs when the pelvis is fixed and a strong extending force is applied to the lumbar spine. Falls from a great height and motor-vehicle accidents generally produce this injury, which is characterized as a transverse fracture across the foramina at the S1-2 level (Fig. 7-11B).[18,28]

**The coccyx.** The coccyx is frequently fractured in backward falls on the buttocks, especially in women, in whom the coccyx lies in a vulnerable position. The true incidence is unknown because these injuries are not usually included in pelvic fracture compilations. They are transverse fractures and are usually displaced anteriorly by the pull of the levator ani, coccygeus, and anal sphincter muscles.[14]

**Avulsion fractures.** Avulsion fractures of the pelvis, which generally occur in young athletes, are located at the growth cartilage of the apophyseal plates.[29] The muscles of the abdominal wall attach to the apophysis of the iliac crest, the sartorius muscle to the anterior superior iliac spine, the rectus femoris muscle to the inferior iliac spine, and the hamstring muscles to the ischial apophysis. Excessive muscle strain can avulse these apophyses. The apophyseal plates at these locations close in the late teenage years or early twenties.

**Iliac wing fractures.** Isolated fractures of the iliac wing without involvement of the weight-bearing ring are not uncommon, comprising 6% to 18% of pelvic fractures.[14] These fractures were first described by Duverney in 1751 and are known by his name. They occur as a result of direct trauma but can also be associated with intra-abdominal injuries. Abdominal muscle spasm and pain can hide these injuries.[14]

**Fracture of a single pelvic ramus.** Isolated fractures of a pelvic ramus were formerly thought to be common injuries, particularly in elderly patients injured in falls. However, some trauma surgeons feel that these injuries are rare and that additional radiographic views of the pelvis often detect occult associated fractures.[22]

**The nerves**

The nerves exiting the lumbar spine and sacrum are peripheral nerves, as compared with the spinal cord, and so are more resistant to permanent injury. Likewise, there is much communication among visceral fibers. Muscle weakness and paresthesias of the lower extremities, fecal and urinary incontinence, and impotence are all complications of pelvic and sacral fractures.[10,30-32] However, improvement in function over time has been the general experience in patients with these fractures, and return of strength and sensation has been noted over 12 to 18 months in some cases.[18,33]

The pelvis contains several complex networks of ventral, dorsal, and autonomic nerves, which are interdigitated with

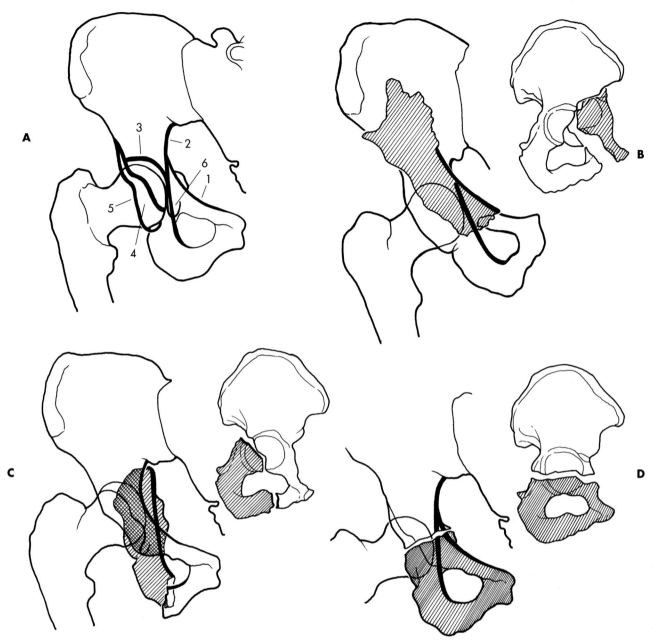

**Fig. 7-9.** Common patterns of acetabular fractures shown diagrammatically, as seen on an anteroposterior radiographs. **A,** Lines to follow when attempting to identify acetabular fractures on an anteroposterior radiograph: 1) the arcuate line; 2) the ilioischial line, which is an imaginary line connecting the arch of the sciatic notch to the arch of the inferior ring of the obturator foramen in a smooth manner; 3) the roof of the acetabulum; 4) the margin of the anterior lip of the acetabulum; 5) the margin of the posterior lip of the acetabulum; and 6) the "teardrop," or "U" formed by the acetabular fossa. **B,** Anterior column fracture. Note that the arcuate line is disrupted, signifying a pelvic ring fracture. **C,** Posterior column fracture. Note that the ilioischial line is disrupted. Although the pelvic ring is intact, fracture through the greater sciatic foramen can put major blood vessels at risk. **D,** Transverse acetabular fracture. This type of fracture disrupts both columns and the pelvic ring.

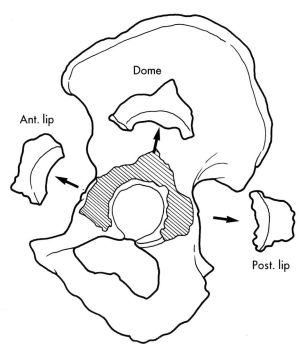

**Fig. 7-10.** Lip and dome fractures of the acetabulum, which are commonly associated with hip dislocation.

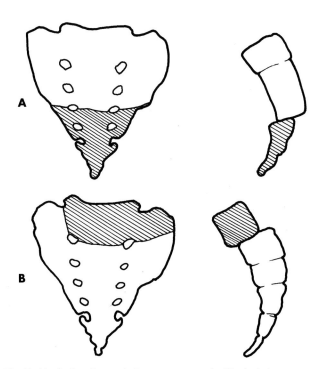

**Fig 7-11.** Isolated sacral fracture types. **A,** Typical transverse fracture of the sacrum at the S-4 level secondary to direct trauma. **B,** Uncommon transverse fracture of the sacrum at the S1-2 level secondary to hyperextension of the spine. Sacral nerve injuries are common with these fractures.

muscles, ligaments, and blood vessels in the pelvis (Fig. 7-12). Almost any pelvic fracture can involve nerve injury.

**The femoral nerve.** The lumbosacral plexus gives rise to the motor and sensory femoral nerve, which lies on the iliacus muscle on the inner surface of the ilium above the true pelvis and exits under the inguinal ligament lateral to the femoral artery. It sends motor branches to the quadriceps femoris. Ventral motor branches of the L-2, L-3, and L-4 roots are contained in the femoral nerve.

**The sciatic nerve.** The lumbosacral plexus also gives rise to the motor and sensory sciatic nerve, the largest nerve in the body, which courses over the brim of the true pelvis at the sacroiliac joint and out through the greater sciatic notch formed by the ilium, the sacrum, and the sacrospinous ligament. It contains motor branches of the L-4, L-5, S-1, S-2, and S-3 roots and innervates the hamstring group of muscles in the thigh and all of the muscles of the leg. The sciatic nerve courses anterior to the ischium and posterior to the hip joint, where it can be trapped easily and damaged by posterior hip dislocation. Figure 7-13 describes this relationship.

**The obturator nerve.** The motor and sensory obturator nerve also rises from the lumbosacral plexus. It travels around the true pelvis just under the brim to exit through the obturator foramen. It contains motor fibers from the L-2, L-3, and L-4 roots innervating the adductors of the thigh.

**The pudendal nerve and pelvic plexus.** The pelvic plexus, which lies in the deepest portion of the pelvis, is made up of fibers from S-2, S-3, S-4, and S-5, the coccygeal nerve, and sympathetic and parasympathetic fibers. This plexus and the pudendal nerve, arising from the ventral roots of S-2, S-3, and S-4, innervate the pelvic and genital organs, namely the rectum, urinary bladder, prostate, seminal vesicles, uterus, vagina, vulva, scrotum, and penis. A branch of the pudendal nerve, the inferior rectal nerve, innervates the sphincter ani externus and provides fecal continence and sensation around the anus. Another branch of the pudendal nerve, the perineal nerve, provides motor and sensory innervation of the labia, clitoris, scrotum, and penis. Parasympathetic nerve fibers arising from S-2, S-3, and S-4, sympathetic fibers arising from the sympathetic trunk, and motor and sensory fibers from the pudendal nerves all play a role in urinary continence and penile erection. Interruption of the blood supply to the penis is another possible cause of impotence after pelvic fracture.[20]

**Cauda equina syndrome.** Injury to the branches of the cauda equina with sacral fracture produces cauda equina syndrome, which consists of a loss of pain and tactile sense in the saddle region, sometimes extending down the back of one or both legs. This area of anesthesia corresponds to the S-2, S-3, S-4, and S-5 sensory distribution seen in Fig. 7-14. Motor function of these nerves is also affected. Anal sphincter function tends to be incompletely disturbed.[34]

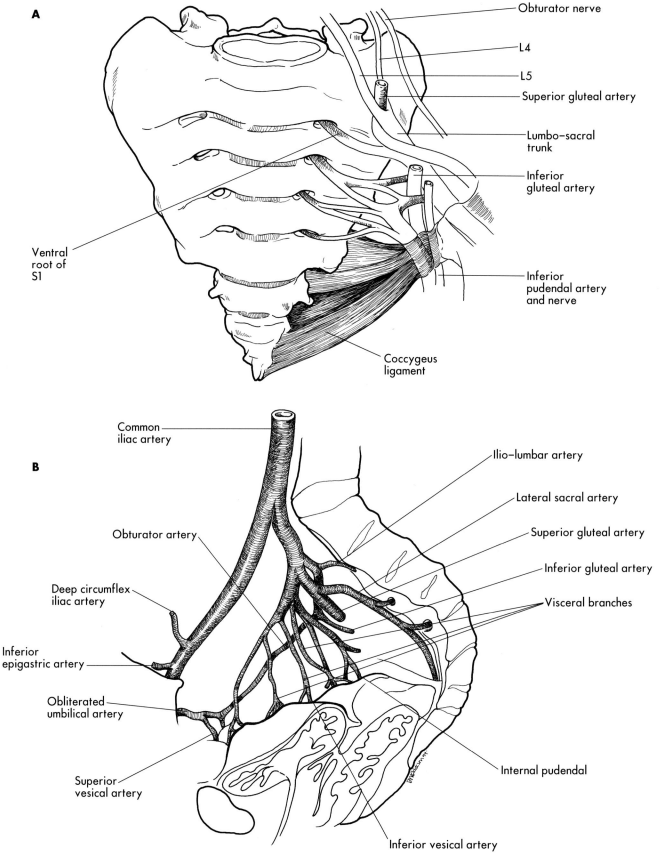

**Fig. 7-12. A**, Diagram of the lumbosacral and pelvic plexuses. Note how the nerves interdigitate with blood vessels and muscles. **B**, Diagram of the arteries in the pelvis.

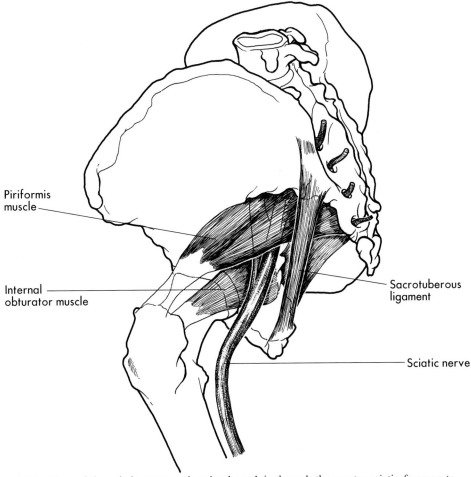

**Fig. 7-13.** View of the sciatic nerve as it exits the pelvis through the greater sciatic foramen to course behind the hip joint. The sciatic nerve can be trapped against the ischium when the hip is dislocated posteriorly. Note the piriformis and internal obturator muscles exiting the pelvis through the greater sciatic foramen and the lesser sciatic foramen, respectively.

Patients may also experience radiating pain over this distribution.[22]

**The muscles of the pelvis**

**Muscles within the false pelvis.** Two muscles occupy the false pelvis formed by the wings of the innominate bones. The psoas muscle descends from the posterior abdomen over the posterior iliac crest then, staying lateral to the brim of the true pelvis, exits under the inguinal ligament to insert on the lesser trochanter of the femur. The iliacus muscle arises from and fills the fossa of the inner surface of the iliac wing then courses under the inguinal ligament lateral to the psoas muscle to also attach to the lesser trochanter.

**Muscles of the floor of the true pelvis.** Two muscles arise within the true pelvis to help form the pelvic floor and wall then exit to attach to the femur. The piriformis muscle arises from the anterior surface of the sacrum and exits the pelvis through the greater sciatic foramen to attach to the greater trochanter. The obturator internus muscle is a broad muscle that arises from the bones that outline the obturator foramen and the obturator membrane. It exits the pelvis through the lesser sciatic foramen to insert on the greater trochanter. These two muscles can be seen in Fig. 7-13.

Two muscles lie entirely within the pelvis and form the remainder of the pelvic floor. The coccygeus muscle arises from the spine of the ischium and the sacrospinous ligament and inserts on the sacrum distal to the origin of the piriformis muscle. It also inserts on the margin of the coccyx. The remainder of the pelvic floor is comprised of the levator ani, which arises from the superior pubic ramus, the obturator membrane, and the spine of the ischium. It inserts on the ligmentous anococcygeal body that extends from the coccyx to the anal sphincter mechanism and to the central tendon of the perineum, the perineal body, which lies anterior to the anus (Figs. 7-15 and 7-16). The levator ani blends into the anal sphincter mechanism. Ventral to the perineal body, the levator ani separates and allows passage of the urethra in males and the urethra and vagina in females. The urogenital diaphragm, containing fascial lay-

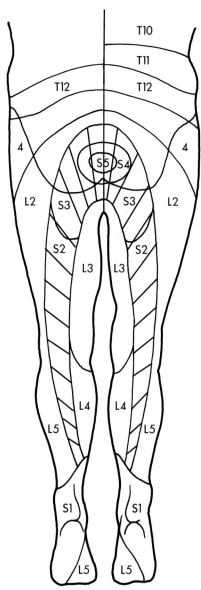

**Fig. 7-14.** Sensory changes of the cauda equina syndrome. The sensory distributions of the S-2, S-3, S-4, and S-5 nerve roots are affected. The distribution may be asymmetrical.

ers, the urethral sphincter, and the transversus perinei profundus muscle, reinforces this opening.

**Muscles attached to the external surfaces of the pelvis.** The muscles of the abdominal wall are attached to the iliac crests, the inguinal ligaments, and the pubis. These muscles are not depicted here.

The muscles of the hip and thigh are attached to the external surface of the pelvis and can be divided into five groups:

1) The glutei consist of the gluteus maximus, the gluteus medius, and the gluteus minimus. They originate on the external surface of the ilium (Fig. 7-17).

2) The hamstring group consists of the long head of the biceps femoris, the semitendinosus, and the semi-

membranosus. These muscles originate on the posterior surface of the ischium (Fig. 7-17).

3) The rotators of the hip consist of the piriformis, the gemelli, the obturator internus, the obturator externus, and the quadratis femoris. The piriformis and obturator internus arise inside the pelvis and attach to the greater trochanter. The gemelli arise on the posterior surface of the ischium, on either side of the obturator externus as it exits through the lesser sciatic foramen (Fig. 7-18). The obturator externus and the quadratis femoris originate on the anterior surfaces of the inferior pubic ramus and the ischium (Fig. 7-19).

4) Two muscles arise on the anterosuperior iliac spine and the anteroinferior iliac spine. They are the sartorius and the rectus femoris, respectively (Fig. 7-19).

5) The muscles of the adductor group, consisting of the pectineus, adductor brevis, adductor longus, gracilis, and adductor magnus, arise from the anterior surface of the pubis, the inferior pubic ramus, and the anterior surface of the ischium (Fig. 7-20).

### The blood vessels

**Arteries.** The abdominal aorta bifurcates at or just above the pelvic brim into the common iliac arteries, which follow the brim of the pelvis around to the sacroiliac joints. There they bifurcate into the internal and external iliac arteries. The external iliacs continue along the pelvic brim to exit under the inguinal ligaments as the femoral arteries. The internal iliacs dive steeply into the pelvis and quickly divide into iliolumbar, lateral sacral, superior gluteal, inferior gluteal, pudendal, and obturator arteries, as well as visceral branches to the pelvic organs (Fig. 7-12B). The superior gluteal artery curves under the sciatic notch to reach the buttocks.

Ben-Menachem et al.[35] have described several mechanisms of injury to pelvic blood vessels. The piriformis muscle, which originates from the ventral surface of the sacrum and exits the pelvis through the greater sciatic foramen on its way to the greater trochanter, has a sharp fascia that can sever the superior gluteal artery. The inferior gluteal and internal pudendal arteries traverse the lesser sciatic foramen, where they are in close proximity to the sacrospinous and sacrotuberous ligaments and are at risk of injury when these ligaments are damaged. The obturator artery is at risk as it passes through the obturator foramen when the pubic rami are fractured. Figure 7-21 depicts these structures. Holting et al.[36] found that fractures of the pubic ramii and the acetabulum were associated with obturator artery lesions, and fractures of the symphysis and sacroiliac joints were associated with pudendal artery lesions.

The external iliac arteries may be subject to stretching forces in APC injuries, with resulting intimal tears, contusion, and occlusion.[38,39] In one such case, peripheral pulses were present initially then disappeared during resuscita-

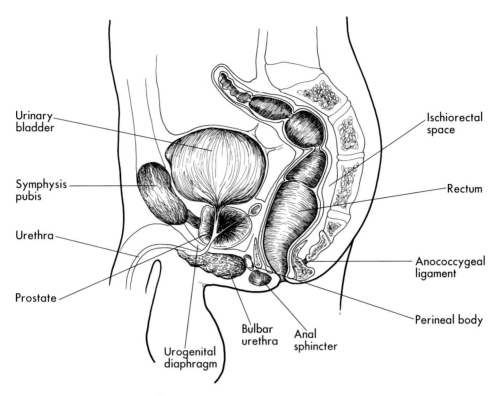

**Fig. 7-15.** Median section of the male pelvis. The urogenital diaphragm lies anterior to the central tendon of the perineum, the perineal body, and consists of sphincter muscle and the transversus perinei profundus muscle between layers of fascia. It is penetrated by the membranous urethra.

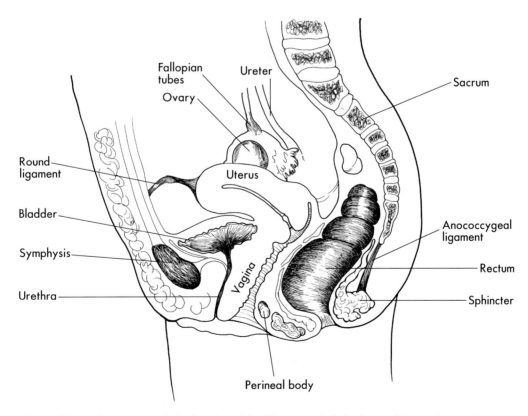

**Fig. 7-16.** Median section of the female pelvis. The urogenital diaphragm lies anterior to the perineal body and is penetrated by the urethra and vagina.

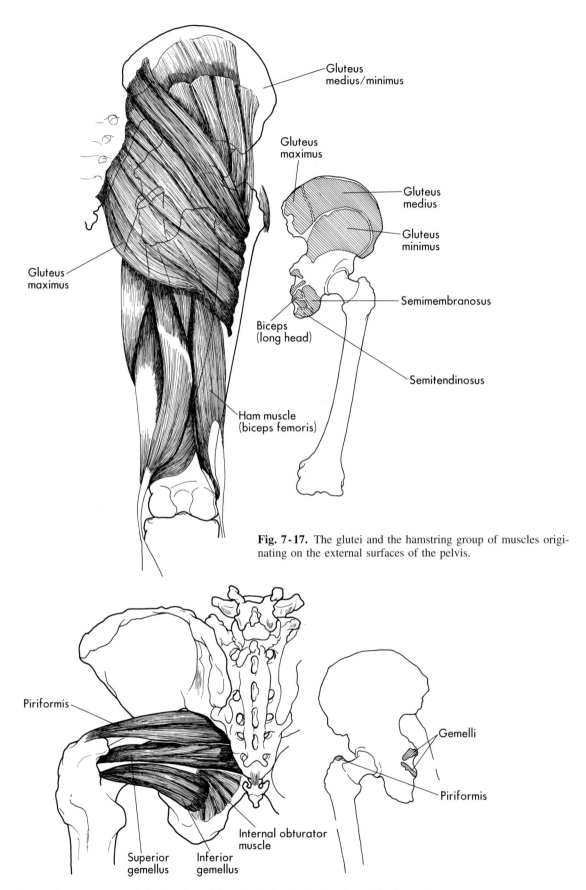

**Fig. 7-17.** The glutei and the hamstring group of muscles originating on the external surfaces of the pelvis.

**Fig. 7-18.** The rotators of the hip viewed from behind. The piriformis and the internal obturator muscles arise from inside the pelvis. The gemellus superior and the gemellus inferior flank the internal obturator muscle as it exits the pelvis.

Fat embolism and tissue fat embolism can result from venous lacerations as well as from disruption of marrow by fractures. One patient suffered a fatal large-tissue embolus of fat when she was positioned for an upright chest radiograph to rule out a widened mediastinum seen on a supine film.[111] The author has also seen a fatal case of the usual microscopic variety of fat embolism that occurred within 4 hours of injury. This patient exhibited tachypnea, tachycardia, cyanosis, and confusion. Petechiae, pyrexia, and thrombocytopenia are also seen with fat embolism, with the syndrome usually appearing 3 to 4 days after injury.[41] Early fixation and immobilization of fractures are important in the prevention of this complication.[41,42] In patients with a pelvic fracture plus a long bone fracture, the incidence of fat embolism is about 11%.[43]

### The pelvic viscera at risk

Figures 7-15 and 7-16 show median sections of the male and female pelvis.

**The rectum and anus.** Rectal and anal injury in association with pelvic fracture is not uncommon. Two trauma centers reported eight cases in 5 years and six cases in 10 years, respectively.[44,45] The distal colon becomes a retroperitoneal structure at the S-3 level. As such, it does not have a serosal surface, and is subject to rupture secondary to bony fragment penetration and from a tearing force extending from the perineum.[46] The superior rectal artery is a continuation of the inferior mesenteric artery. The middle and inferior rectal arteries are visceral branches of the pudendal artery branches of the internal iliac arteries. Severe crushing injury can devascularize the rectum.[46,47] Rectal injuries resulting from blunt trauma are accompanied by frank blood in the rectum that can be detected by performing a digital rectal examination; however, a high index of suspicion is necessary, and proctoscopy should be performed if there is any question about the integrity of the rectum.[46]

**The male urethra.** In males, the urethra is long and vulnerable to injury. The incidence of urethral injuries in males range from 1.4% to 11%.[48] The anterior urethra extends from the meatus to the urogenital diaphragm. The posterior urethra consists of the membranous urethra and the prostatic urethra. The membranous urethra is about 2 cm long and traverses the urogenital diaphragm, where it is firmly fixed.[49] There are two expansions of the anterior urethra, one near the tip of the penis and one at the proximal end; these are called the navicular fossa and the intrabulbar fossa, respectively, and are shown in Fig. 7-15. The male urethra is most at risk for disruption as it enters the urogenital diaphragm.[48,50] In a series of 74 urethral injuries, Cass[51] found 50 pelvic fracture cases associated with 46 posterior urethral and four anterior urethral injuries. In his series of 48 cases of posterior urethral injuries, there were 25 complete ruptures (52%) and 23 (48%) partial ruptures. Blood at the meatus was seen in 28 (58%) of these patients. Cass also reported 26 cases of anterior urethral injury in his

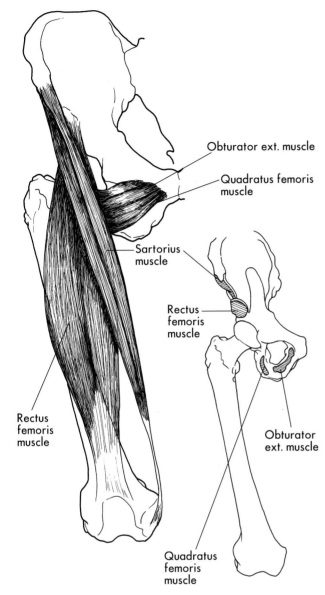

**Fig. 7-19.** The rotators of the hip viewed from the front. The quadratus femoris and the obturator externus muscles arise from the anterior surfaces of the bones forming the obturator foramen. Two thigh muscles arise on the anterosuperior spine and the anteroinferior spine of the ilium. They are the sartorius and rectus femoris muscles, respectively.

tion.[39] This case was also remarkable for the absence of a significant pelvic hematoma. Major vascular injuries of this magnitude are estimated to occur in about 1% of pelvic fracture cases.[38]

**Veins and marrow channels.** External, internal, and common iliac veins accompany the arteries. A rich plexus of veins surrounds the pelvic organs and the walls of the pelvis itself. Many experienced surgeons ascribe most pelvic hemorrhage resulting from pelvic fracture to venous and bone marrow bleeding.[23] Movement of patients with pelvic fractures can stimulate venous and arterial bleeding.[7,13]

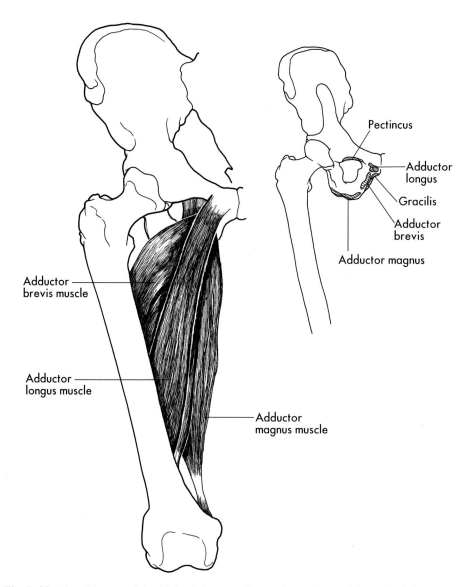

**Fig. 7-20.** The adductors of the thigh originate on the anterior surfaces of the pubis, inferior pubic ramus, and ischium.

series, with two complete ruptures (8%). Blood at the meatus was present in 24 cases (92%).

**The prostate.** The prostate gland is attached firmly to the urogenital diaphragm and connected to the pubis by the puboprostatic ligament.[52] It receives the seminal vesicle and ductus deferens ducts (Fig. 7-22). In the adult man, the prostate is a firm structure that is not commonly disrupted in pelvic fracture cases. In children, the immature prostate and the prostatic urethra are more commonly disrupted.[52] With complete rupture of the membranous urethra, the prostate gland rises in the pelvis and is frequently surrounded by blood or urine, giving it a boggy feeling on rectal examination. This finding alone is enough to make the diagnosis of complete urethral disruption.

**The female urethra.** In females, the urethra is shorter but injury can occur. In a recent report, Perry and Husmann[31] found six urethral injuries in 130 female patients with pelvic fractures, for an incidence of 4.6%. Orkin[53] also reported a review of 2000 pelvic fracture cases in females, with a urethral injury rate of 6%. This injury is generally underestimated in its significance and incidence.[54] Urethral transection appears to be less common in females, but partial disruption with or without bladder neck injury appears to be more common. Figure 7-23 shows a typical configuration of urethral injury in women. Unfortunately, this involvement of the bladder neck was associated with long-term urinary incontinence in Perry and Husmann's experience. It is recommended that a careful vaginal examination precede placement of a Foley catheter because there may be a communicating vaginal laceration or hematoma. These findings provide valuable clues as to the presence of a urethral injury that can lead to fatal sepsis if not appreciated.[31]

**The vagina and uterus.** Vaginal laceration with pelvic

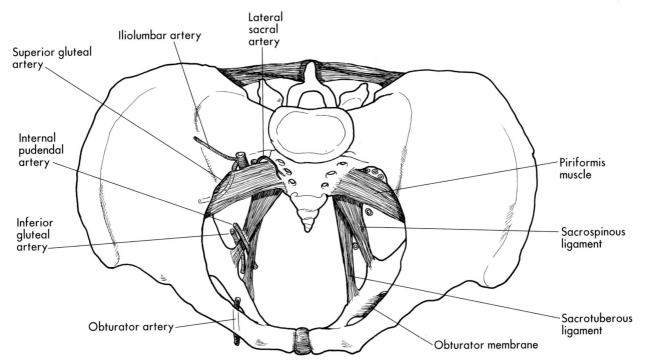

**Fig. 7-21.** Diagrammatic portrayal of the points of exit of blood vessels of the pelvis with adjacent bony, ligamentous, and fascial structures, as described by Ben-Menachem et al.[35]

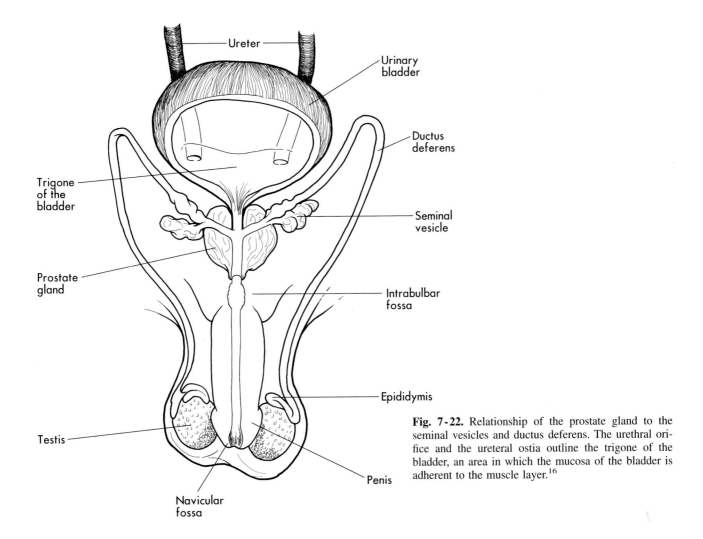

**Fig. 7-22.** Relationship of the prostate gland to the seminal vesicles and ductus deferens. The urethral orifice and the ureteral ostia outline the trigone of the bladder, an area in which the mucosa of the bladder is adherent to the muscle layer.[16]

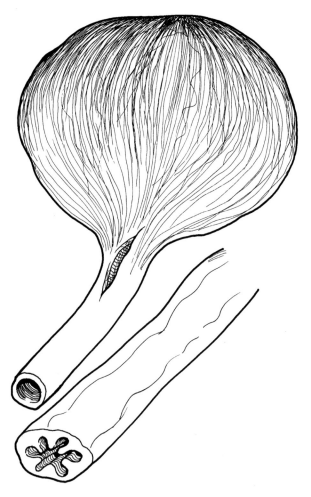

**Fig. 7-23.** Diagrammatic portrayal of a bladder neck laceration in a female, as described by Perry and Husmann.[31]

fractures is uncommon but not rare. Sinnott et al.[45] found two cases in a 10-year series of 27 open pelvic fracture cases. Vaginal bleeding is present in all or most reported cases. Perry and Husmann[31] advise that vaginal lacerations be explored carefully so that a communicating urethral injury is not missed. Perineal lacerations may extend into the vagina.[55] The uterus can be involved in severe open pelvic disarticulating cases.[55] A case of uterine and ovarian injury by bony spicules has been reported.[56]

**The urinary bladder.** The urinary bladder is a muscular extraperitoneal sac that is situated in the pelvis in older children and adults. In children younger than about 6 years, it is predominantly an abdominal organ.[49] Bladder rupture occurs in about 5% to 10% of pelvic fracture cases. About 15% to 45% of these ruptures are into the peritoneal cavity, and about 50% to 85% rupture extraperitoneally.[57] In the case of intraperitoneal rupture, the bladder ruptures at its weakest point when it is full and intravesical pressure rises abruptly. The weakest area of the bladder is its intraperitoneal portion, where it is unsupported by adjacent structures and its muscle is thinnest.[49] In the case of extraperitoneal rupture, one postulated mechanism of injury is that the partially or nearly empty bladder is abruptly compressed from increased intra-abdominal pressure, forcing it to rupture within the confines of the pelvis.[49] It was formerly believed that extraperitoneal ruptures were the result of direct penetration of bony spicules. However, it has been shown that most of these ruptures occur at sites away from the fracture.[58] The capacity of the bladder is about 500 ml in adults and 5 ml/kg in children. The presence of prostatic hypertrophy can result in bladder distention and bladder diverticula that can confuse the

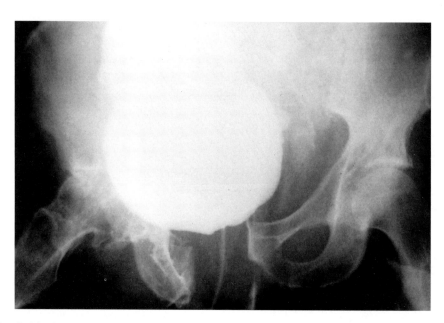

**Fig. 7-24.** Cystogram in an elderly man with prostatic hypertrophy. Bladder diverticula can confuse the unwary. This radiograph shows a large and a small diverticulum that could be confused with bladder rupture.

uninitiated. Figure 7-24 shows a cystogram revealing diverticula. Figure 7-25 shows the effect of pelvic lipomatosis, a normal variant, on the shape of the bladder.[110] The fat, however, is relatively radiolucent, so it should not be confused with pelvic hematoma. Figure 7-26 shows a cystogram with an intravesical blood clot.

Bladder distention can stimulate voluntary or involuntary contraction. If the patient has suffered a urethral injury precluding the placement of a Foley catheter, urine is extravasated into the surrounding tissues and, possibly, the pelvic hematoma, increasing the risk of infection and sepsis. Perry and Husmann[31] found that when urine extravasation occurred in a series of women with urethral injuries, life-threatening sepsis ensued. In non–trauma center hospitals, when a urologist is not immediately available to perform a suprapubic cystostomy, the resuscitating

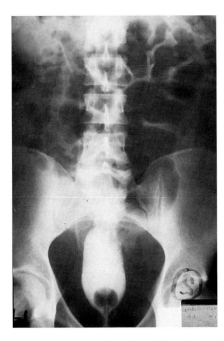

**Fig. 7-25.** Cystogram revealing deformity of the bladder by pelvic lipomatosis, a normal variant. The fat outlining the bladder is less dense than hematoma.

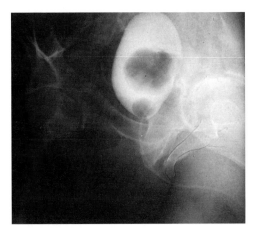

**Fig. 7-26.** Cystogram revealing an intravesical blood clot.

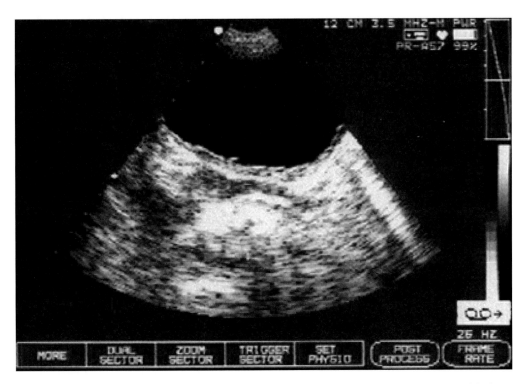

**Fig. 7-27.** Ultrasound image of a distended urinary bladder. The clear, homogeneous black appearance of the urine-filled bladder is different than that of a hematoma, which has a stippled appearance.

physician should do so if the bladder is distended on clinical or ultrasound examination. Figure 7-27 shows the appearance of the distended urinary bladder on ultrasound. Urine has a clear homogenous black appearance as compared with clot, which has a stipled appearance. If the bladder is distended, placement of a suprapubic catheter is easily performed using a 14F Percutaneous Cavity Drainage Catheter (Arrow International Inc.; Reading, PA) or similar Seldinger technique catheter. The bladder is located with an exploring needle and a guidewire inserted. The skin opening is enlarged with a scalpel, and a dilator is passed over the guidewire to enlarge the path into the bladder. The drainage cannula is then passed over the guidewire into the bladder and attached to drainage tubing. Figure 7-28 shows the catheter coiled up in position in the bladder. The 10-in catheter is long enough to be retained in the emptied bladder. If the returns are bloody, a small amount of contrast should be injected through the catheter and an X-ray obtained to confirm correct placement.

The intraluminal pressure generated by the ureters can exceed 50 cm of water (36.78 torr).[60] Obstruction of ureters

by pelvic hematoma is only a theoretic consideration. However, bladder neck obstruction has been reported secondary to the deformity produced by a pelvic hematoma, and this possibility should be considered when urine output falls inexplicably during resuscitation.[61] Operative hematoma decompression may be necessary if this occurs.

### Pelvic hemorrhage

**Continuous bleeding.** Serious pelvic hemorrhage following pelvic fracture injury is a form of continuous hemorrhage. The continuous hemorrhage shock model has produced very pertinent findings that ring true to trauma surgeons. In 1966, Milles et al.[62] studied uncontrolled peripheral arterial hemorrhage in dogs and found that dogs that received no blood or fluids had a better mortality than those that received saline while bleeding continued. This and similar studies were inconclusive but were affirmed in 1991 when Bickell et al.[37] reported the results of a study designed to test the recommendation that hemorrhagic shock of an estimated volume be reversed by three times that volume of electrolyte solution (the three-for-one

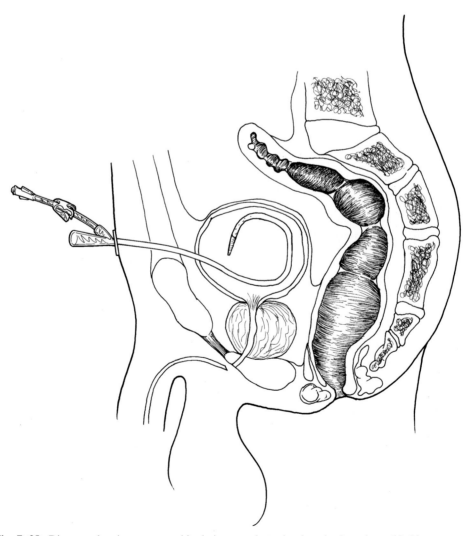

**Fig. 7-28.** Diagram showing a suprapubic drainage catheter in place in the urinary bladder.

rule).[63] In Bickell et al.'s porcine model,[37] animals receiving lactated Ringer's solution fared poorly after aortotomy. All of the untreated control animals survived the 2-hour experimental period, while all of the treated animals died. Kowalenko et al.[64] found that survival (87.5%) was improved with fluid resuscitation in a porcine model of continuous aortic hemorrhage when a *mean* aortic pressure of 40 torr was used as an endpoint versus 80 *torr* (37.5%). Hemodilution with decreased blood viscosity, hypothermia, and coagulopathy have been implicated in the increased bleeding in this model.[65] This experimental work supports the experience of trauma surgeons during World War II.[66]

With this evidence, how should the resuscitating physician respond to shock in a bleeding pelvic fracture patient? The goal should probably be to achieve and maintain a systolic blood pressure of about 100 torr with an infusion of units of packed red cells reconstituted with saline (250 ml/unit) and administered through a blood warmer until measures have been taken to control the bleeding. If blood is not available or delayed, the blood should be supplemented with warm saline solution, but an attempt should be made to avoid hemodiluting the patient. Type O Rh-negative or type O Rh-positive blood (in males and postmenopausal women) should be given until type-specific blood becomes available.

**Hypothermia.** Hypothermia is often a severe problem in trauma and can develop quickly and insidiously during resuscitation. The administration of cold fluids and blood, the undressing of the trauma victim in an air-conditioned resuscitation room, and the presence of shock itself produce hypothermia. Several studies have documented the problem.[67,68] Bleeding and the administration of cold blood are clearly implicated. Control of ambient temperature with heating lamps; warming of infused blood, blood products, and electrolyte fluids with fast and effective blood-warming devices; monitoring of core temperature; and, of course, control of hemorrhage are extremely important responsibilities of the resuscitating team. The author recommends mounting a commercial quartz-type 3200-W infrared heating lamp on the ceiling over the resuscitation cart to keep the patient warm.

**Coagulopathy.** The effect of hypothermia and hemodilution on coagulation is complex and not well understood. Standard clotting tests (prothrombin time and partial thromboplastin time) performed at 37° C may be normal in the face of a disseminated intravascular coagulation defect–like clinical picture in a hypothermic trauma patient. Some authors[69] recommend not giving any "shotgun" treatments, but recommend simply rewarming the patient. Nevertheless, the prudent resuscitating physician will alert the blood bank about the probable need for fresh-frozen plasma units and platelet packs as soon as it becomes evident that the patient is bleeding significantly. Administering warmed blood instead of electrolyte solution as replacement therapy may help avert this coagulopathy. "Massive" or class IV bleeding generally means loss of about 40% to 50% of a patient's blood volume.[63] Since the adult blood volume is 65 to 75 ml/kg, a 70-kg patient would have to bleed about 2000 ml to qualify. Flint et al.[70] defined severe pelvic bleeding as that requiring more than 1000 ml of blood in the first 2 hours after initial resuscitation or more than 2000 ml of blood in the first 8 hours following admission.

**Tamponade with external pressure.** Venous, small arterial, and bone marrow bleeding are thought to result from movement of the pelvic fracture patient. The only effective splint available for such a patient is the pneumatic antishock garment (PASG). McSwain[71] has thoroughly reviewed the use of the PASG. Flint et al.[70] used retrospective controls in a study of its use in bleeding pelvic fracture cases, and found that mortality and blood requirements were reduced in 10 patients in whom the PASG was used. These authors used pressures of 50 torr in the leg compartments and 40 torr in the abdominal compartment. No significant complications were seen with the PASG. Others,[7,72] however, have noted an incidence of compartment syndromes in the legs and thighs with prolonged use of the PASG. Christensen[73] studied trancutaneous oxygen pressure ($TcPO_2$) in healthy volunteers who had air splints applied to their legs, and found that at inflation pressures over 20 torr, $TcPO_2$ fell to anoxic levels. He recommended that the PASG be used at a pressure of 20 torr whenever it is used for more than 1.5 hours.

Several trauma center teams use the PASG on a selective basis for the management of pelvic hemorrhage in conjunction with algorithms for overall management, usually at a pressure of 40 torr.[5,7,13,70,74,75] In addition to acting as a splint, the PASG undoubtedly provides some tamponade for bleeding. Pearse et al.[76] reported a case of uncontrollable venous pelvic bleeding in a patient undergoing radical hysterectomy. The pelvis was packed with packing extending through the vagina. Postoperatively, bleeding continued until the patient was placed in a PASG at 40 torr pressure. No further bleeding occurred. Figure 7-29 shows a commercially available PASG with manometer attached.

**Tamponade with external fracture fixation.** Pelvic bleeding is felt by many surgeons to be due, at least in part, to the expanded volume of the pelvis that is created when the weight-bearing ring is opened by fractures, with subsequent loss of the tamponade effect provided by space limitation. It has been estimated that the retroperitoneal space will accommodate 4000 ml of blood before venous tamponade occurs.[77] Using geometric principles, it has been estimated that if the symphysis pubis is separated by 3 cm, the volume of the pelvis doubles.[78] The PASG has been shown to reduce pelvic fractures; however, several trauma centers have found external skeletal fixation to be more effective and practical for overall management.[7,79] Flint et al.[13] obtained excellent overall results (three deaths in 60 severe hemorrhage cases) using an algorithm that included use of the PASG as a primary method of controlling hemorrhage. The PASG was inflated for 24 hours to an extremity compartment pressure of 40 torr and an abdomi-

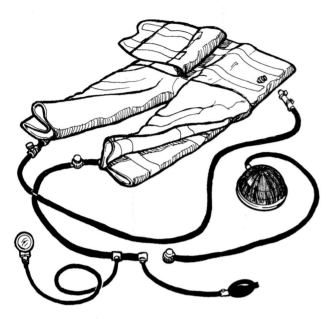

**Fig. 7-29.** Drawing of a commercially available pneumatic anti-shock garment (MAST; Armstrong Medical Industries, Lincolnshire, IL), with gauge and pump enabling control and adjustment of compartment pressure.

nal compartment pressure of 30 torr. It was then deflated at 2- to 3-hour intervals to check for compartment syndromes. Two patients developed compartment syndromes necessitating fasciotomy. Use of the PASG alone was successful in controlling bleeding 11 out of 12 times. Emergency application of external fixation was also used successfully with primary bleeding control in three of four cases.[13]

External fixation as a primary means of controlling hemorrhage has the advantage of allowing accurate fracture reduction, when the fracture geography is favorable, and early mobilization of the patient without the increased risk of compartment syndrome. The "external fixator" method of tamponade and splinting, sometimes combined with traction or internal fixation, is growing in favor.[7] The 5-mm, self-tapping external fixation pins are inserted percutaneously into the iliac crest by the orthopedist, then twisted and advanced so that they seek their own position between the inner and outer tables of bone of the ilium. They should lodge in the strong bone above the acetabulum,[59] which can be accomplished in 15 to 20 minutes.[80] A frame of rods is then applied to the pins to aid in fracture reduction and stabilization. Alternatively, if the patient is undergoing laparotomy anyway, plates can be attached to the reduced symphysis to obtain stability.[59] Ward et al.[81] estimate that a simple external fixation frame restores about 10% of the pelvis' rigidity, and a more complex frame can restore up to 25% of this rigidity. Figure 7-30 shows a fixator in place.

**Transarterial embolization.** Transarterial embolization of bleeding pelvic arteries has been used successfully for bleeding from vessels as large as the superior gluteal artery as well as from smaller arteries and veins. Mucha and

Welch[75] describe the technique in detail, citing a success rate of 85% to 95% when the bleeding site can be visualized. Figure 7-31 shows angiographic examples of bleeding from the superior gluteal artery as well as pudendal and obturator artery bleeding. The embolization should be as selective as possible using absorbable materials such as Gelfoam (Upjohn; Kalamazoo, MI).[75] Ben-Menachem et al.[35] recommend an aggressive use of embolization, including "scatter embolization" of the larger branches of the internal iliac artery. In their experience, 20% of patients with APC-, VS-, or CM-type injuries benefit from embolization if primary control of bleeding is not obtained quickly. In their opinion, an invasive radiologist should be on-call to the trauma center at all times for these cases. When the trauma surgeon is forced to operate because of patient instability or grossly positive diagnostic peritoneal lavage (DPL), he or she can embolize the hypogastric arteries under direct vision or, alternatively, pack the pelvis and take the patient to angiography.[7,40] Holting et al.[36] emphasized the need for angiographic embolization within 6 hours of injury to achieve the best results. Klein et al.[82] recommend that the angiographer be alerted when the patient has received four units of blood and that the patient be moved to angiography when the sixth unit is given.

**Diagnostic peritoneal lavage in pelvic bleeding.** The pelvic hematoma is commonly conceptualized as lying posterior as it dissects out of the pelvis. However, it usually encircles the lower abdomen, including the properitoneal fat layer of the anterior abdominal wall. For this reason, DPL must be performed using an open technique to visualize the peritoneum for puncture.[7] The supraumbilical approach is recommended for the same reason.[79] The presence of a pelvic hematoma can result in the diapedesis, or more likely, leakage of red blood cells through small defects or lacerations through the peritoneum into the abdomen.[75] Probably for this reason, DPL as usually interpreted results in an excessive false-positive rate.[7,79,83] Moreno et al.[7] determined that only the return of frank blood on initial aspiration indicates the need for immediate surgery. Flint et al.[13] defined frank blood returns as 8 ml of blood on initial aspiration. If the results of the DPL were positive based on cell count alone, laparotomy could be safely deferred while other studies, such as computed tomography (CT) or angiography, took place. When the aspirate was positive for frank blood, 87% of cases justified emergency laparotomy on review.[7]

**The open pelvic fracture**

In a review of blunt open pelvic fractures, Snyder[84] found the incidence to be 2% to 13% of all pelvic fractures. The mechanism of injury was usually high-energy motorcycle or pedestrian vehicular accidents. In a review of the literature, Sinnott et al.[45] found a range of mortality of 5.5% to 60% of open pelvic fracture cases, with an average of 41%. He found a mortality of 15% in his own series. An open pelvic fracture is defined as one that communicates with the skin or mucous membrane.

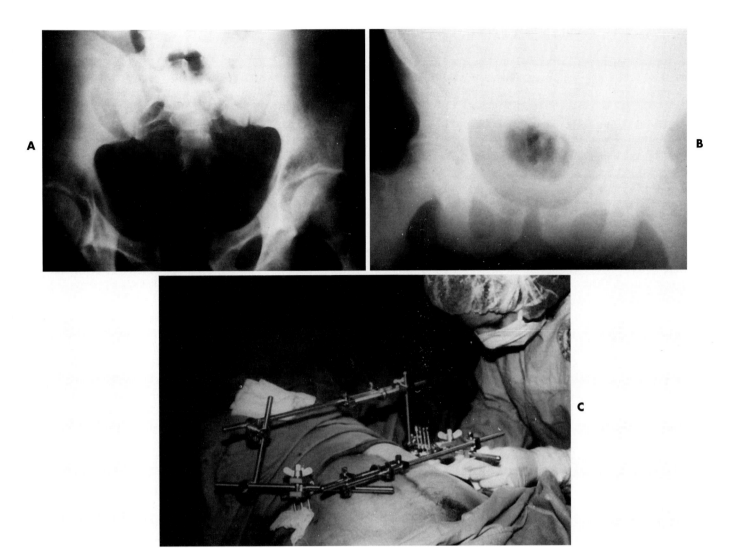

**Fig. 7-30. A**, Diastasis of the symphysis is present in an anteroposterior compression fracture. **B**, Reduction of the diastasis using an external fixator. **C**, Photograph of the external fixator in place on the same patient. (From Russell TA: Fractures of hip and pelvis. In Crenshaw AH, ed: *Campbell's operative orthopaedics,* ed 8, St. Louis, 1992, Mosby-Year Book, p. 969. Used by permission.)

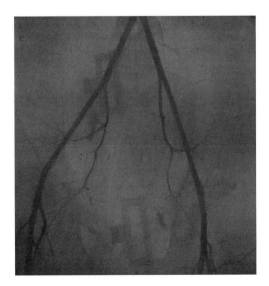

**Fig. 7-31.** Exsanguinating hemorrhage occurring from a branch of the right superior gluteal artery and the left pudendal artery in a fatal case.

The mortality and morbidity of this injury relates to hemorrhage and infection.[84]

**Hemorrhage.** When the pelvic fracture communicates with the skin, the tamponade effect of tissue containing the hematoma is lost. Exsanguinating hemorrhage sometimes occurs through the open wound. Collecting data over 4 years in a series of seven patients with open pelvic fractures, Evers et al.[79] reported three that bled massively, requiring packing with use of the PASG or embolization for control. One patient died of sepsis. Sterile vaginal packing gauze is a recommended packing material.[45] When there is massive devitalizing injury, hemipelvectomy may be necessary.[7,45]

**Infection.** Three recent open pelvic fracture series cite a very low mortality secondary to sepsis.[45,55,85] Of the 69 patients in these three series, only two deaths were attributed to sepsis. Broad-spectrum antibiotics, irrigation and débridement of the open wound, diverting colostomy, distal colon washout, and primary repair of rectal tears (when feasible) along with presacral space drainage, were measures that were employed successfully. Failure to accomplish these procedures led to wound infection, sepsis, and multisystem organ failure.[85] Obviously, the first step is discovery; therefore, a thorough examination of the patient is critically important.

Intravenous antibiotics should be started as soon as an open pelvic fracture is identified. This therapy is not prophylactic, since contamination has already occurred. The common microbial flora of the gut should be covered—*Escherichia coli, Pseudomonas, Klebsiella, Enterococcus, Bacteroides fragilis, Peptostreptcoccus,* and *Clostridium.*[86] The second-generation cephalosporin, cefoxitin, covers most of these potential pathogens adequately and has gained favor because it replaces the need for triple-drug therapy (penicillin or ampicillin with an aminoglycoside and clindamycin) when simplicity is needed.[86] Typically, a loading dose of 2 g of cefoxitin, or 30 to 40 mg/kg in children, is given during resuscitation of the open pelvic fracture patient. Cefmetazole and cefotetan are two other second-generation cepholosporins with similar coverage. Ampicillin/sulbactam is a β-lactamase–resistant ampicillin that has also been recommended recently because of improved enterococcus and anaerobe coverage.[87] For the penicillin-allergic patient, a combination of gentamicin and clindamycin can be used.[88]

Irrigation and débridement of open wounds should be conducted in the operating room. Uncommonly, wounds such as an isolated vaginal tear can be closed primarily after urethral involvement has been ruled out.[31] However, most wounds should be left open and strong consideration given to performing a diverting colostomy to divert the fecal stream from the perineum.[44,45,55,85] Shannon et al.[44] described the performance of a loop colostomy over a penrose drain using a stapler to isolate the proximal and distal portions of the loop. A Foley catheter is placed in the distal portion for distal rectosigmoid washout using a 1% povidone antiseptic solution followed by an antibiotic-containing saline solution.[44] When it can be accomplished, the authors recommend repair of rectal lacerations combined with presacral space drainage to further protect against continued soilage.[46,85] The trauma surgeon should consult his or her orthopedic colleagues regarding placement of the colostomy, so that the orthopedist is not prevented from selecting an anterior approach for fixation of fractures.[7,13,80]

Pelvic fracture splinting or fixation is also felt to be important in the prevention of sepsis as well as hemorrhage.[89] Leenen et al.[90] recommend internal fixation of grossly unstable pelvic fractures, even in the presence of fecal contamination, as a means of preventing sepsis.

### Pelvic fracture in pregnancy

The pregnant uterus and its contained fetus may be at considerable risk in pelvic trauma. It is estimated that trauma occurs in 7% of pregnancies.[91] A study conducted in Cook County, Illinois, covering 1986 to 1990, found that trauma accounted for 46% of maternal deaths and was the leading cause of maternal death.[92] Fetal demise is a well-known complication of pelvic fracture in pregnant women. In a recent study of pelvic fracture cases,[93] the incidence of fetal demise was 56%. Other recent studies[94] have indicated that the mother's death is not the most common cause of fetal death, as previously believed, but rather the severity of the mother's injuries correlates with fetal mortality.

**Maternal vital signs.** During the second trimester, there is a 5- to 15-torr fall in maternal blood pressure, which returns to near-normal levels at term. Maternal heart rate increases by 15 to 20 beats per minute beyond normal. Minute ventilation increases during pregnancy with a resulting hypocapnea, with an arterial $PaCO_2$ of about 30 torr.[95]

**Maternal blood volume changes and fetal distress.** Maternal blood volume increases by 40% to 55% from the 6th to the 34th week of gestation. During this time, the mother is able to maintain normal vital signs with significant blood volume loss. The placental circulation is very sensitive to circulating catecholamines, however, and the fetus will be deprived of oxygen before the mother decompensates. To detect fetal distress as a guide to fluid resuscitation,[96] fetal heart rate should be monitored closely via ultrasound or external fetal monitoring.

**Supine hypotensive syndrome.** Maternal hematocrit is only about 35% at term. The resulting lowered blood viscosity combined with the expanded blood volume helps explain the increased cardiac output in pregnancy. However, the weight of the uterus on the inferior vena cava can decrease venous return, with a drop in cardiac output by about 35% when the mother is supine and beyond about 20 weeks' gestation. This is sometimes called the *supine hypotensive syndrome.*[95] Inflation of the abdominal compartment of the PASG is contraindicated in the pregnant patient because of the potential for exacerbating this effect.[97] It is recommended that during resuscitation the patient be turned toward her left side, with due precautions regarding possible spinal injury, to take the weight of the uterus off the vena cava.[63]

**Abruption of the placenta.** The placenta contains no elastic tissue, so shear forces in trauma can easily separate the placenta from the elastic and contractile myometrium. Abruption of the placenta is probably the most common cause of fetal demise in blunt pelvic injury to the pregnant woman.[98] This separation cannot be seen reliably on ultrasound examination.[99] In a large series of pregnant women who experienced major trauma, the "classic" findings of uterine tenderness, vaginal bleeding, and amniotic vaginal discharge were not seen.[15] Bleeding from the fetal circulation into the maternal circulation, consumption of fibrinogen, and amniotic fluid leak into the maternal circulation are uncommon but serious results of abruption.

Fetomaternal hemorrhage can be detected by the Kleihauer-Betke smear of maternal blood. However, this test is very institution-dependent in quantitative terms, so trends rather than absolute values are probably more important.[93] Amniotic fluid embolization is manifested by respiratory failure and coagulopathy. Baseline clotting studies, as well as fibrinogen levels when indicated, should be obtained and followed during resuscitation.[100]

**Maternal isoimmunization.** Isoimmunization of an Rh-negative pregnant mother who suffers trauma is probable. All such women should receive Rh-immune globulin, 50 μg if injured during the first trimester and 300 μg if injured later in pregnancy.[96] The results of blood typing should, of course, be made known to the resuscitating physician.

**Uterine rupture.** During the second and third trimesters, the uterus is an abdominal organ and is subject to direct trauma. Uterine rupture with expulsion of the fetus into the abdomen can occur with or without direct fetal injury.[100] DPL is not contraindicated by pregnancy.[94] An open supraumbilical approach would be advisable.

**Radiation of the fetus.** The radiation dose to the gravid uterus can be significant during resuscitation of the pregnant patient with blunt trauma.[15] It behooves the resuscitating physician to obtain a urine pregnancy test immediately for all trauma victims of child-bearing age unless clearly unneeded. Essential radiographic studies should be obtained, but other radiographic or CT scans may be deferred.

**Postmortem cesarean section.** Pre- or postmortem cesarean section should be considered when the mother is fatally injured and the estimated gestational age is greater than about 20 weeks (uterus palpable above the umbilicus). Ideally, an emergency ultrasound examination is performed to determine whether the fetus is viable and has a beating heart. Otherwise, clinical judgment alone will have to suffice.

## RADIOGRAPHY OF PELVIC FRACTURES
### The routine anteroposterior view of the pelvis

A routine anteroposterior (AP) radiographic view of the pelvis is recommended in all multiple trauma cases.[63] However, in alert, competent trauma patients without signs or symptoms of pelvic injury and without other serious injuries such radiographs need not necessarily be taken.[101] The AP pelvic view should be carefully reviewed in order to get as much information as possible. Depending on the weight and height of the patient, a large or small portion of the abdomen will also be seen.

**Flank stripes and dog ears.** The properitoneal fat stripes seen in each flank of the abdomen are normally separated from the lumen of the large bowel only by the peritoneum and the wall of the colon. When fluid collects in the abdominal cavity, the colon is displaced medially by a water density "stripe." Lesser quantities of fluid collect first in the pelvic recesses beside the sacrum and the rectum. Because the urinary bladder is usually faintly outlined by a layer of fat, it has the appearance of a dog's head, and the recesses appear as "dog ears" when they are filled with fluid. Normally, these recesses are filled with

loops of bowel variably containing fluid, feces, and air, so that the homogeneous appearance of free fluid is lacking (Fig. 7-32).[102,103]

**Reading the anteroposterior radiograph for fractures.** Pelvic fractures are often difficult to distinguish on a single AP view; however, almost all of them can be picked up or inferred from the fracture pattern. The box on page 143 lists the areas that should be inspected closely for evidence of fracture. If the mechanism of injury is known, the examiner can expect to find certain combinations of fractures.

Figure 7-33 is a radiograph of an LC-I pelvic fracture. The pubic rami on the side of injury are fractured transversally. The sacrum has suffered an impacting fracture through the foramina and ala on the side of the injury. Figure 7-34 is a radiograph of an LC-II pelvic fracture. In this case, the ilium was fractured by the force of the trauma. Figure 7-35 is a radiograph of an LC-III fracture that resulted in an opening of the contralateral half of the pelvis. Figure 7-36 shows an APC-III fracture with gross widening of both sacroiliac joints and wide displacement of the symphysis—the typical "open book fracture." In this in-

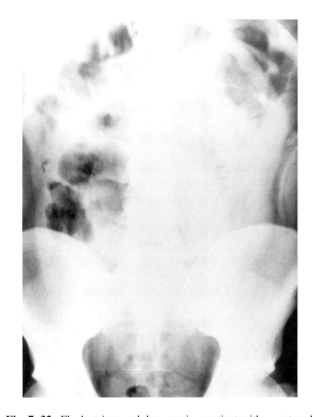

**Fig. 7-32.** Flank stripes and dog ears in a patient with a ruptured urinary bladder. Note how the angle of the liver is blurred at the right flank. The wall of the colon is separated from the radiolucent properitoneal fat layer on both flanks by a water-density stripe, signifying fluid in the peritoneal cavity. Note that the urinary bladder is outlined by a fat layer. The space on either side of the sacrum above the urinary bladder is occupied by a water-density collection of fluid that equals the bladder density, and gives the bladder the appearance of a dog's head. These spaces normally contain air-speckled feces.

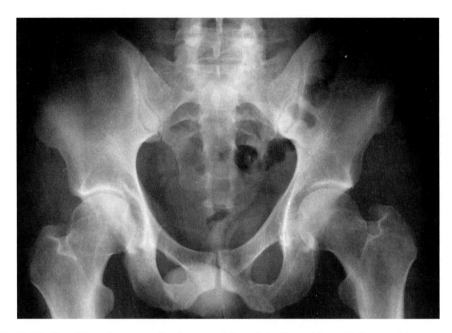

**Fig. 7-33.** Type I lateral compression fracture of the pelvis. The pubis and inferior pubic ramus on the left are fractured with a transverse, overlapping configuration. A vertical fracture line can be seen faintly on the left side of the sacrum. The upper arc of the second sacral foramen also reveals a fracture. The sacral component of this injury is usually difficult to see and may only be visualized by computed tomography.

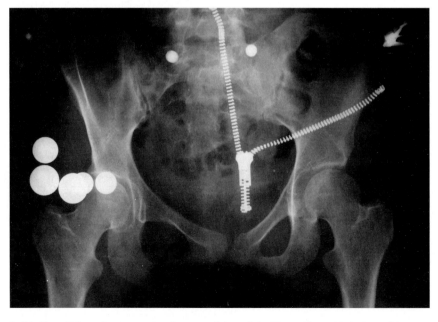

**Fig. 7-34.** Type II lateral compression fracture of the pelvis. The pubis and inferior pubic ramus on the left are fractured with a transverse, overlapping configuration. The sacroiliac joint on the left is opened. Although not well seen on this reproduction, the left L-5 transverse process is fractured.

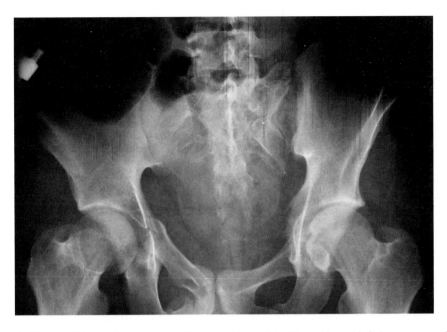

**Fig. 7-35.** Type III lateral compression fracture of the pelvis. The pubis and inferior ramus on the right are fractured transversely. The sacrum is fractured on the right. The left half of the pelvis is opened with a disrupted sacroiliac joint. An anterior column fracture of the left acetabulum is present, with disruption of the arcuate line. A transverse fracture of the acetabulum is seen on the right.

---

**Areas to inspect on review of an anteroposterior radiographic view of the pelvis for signs of fracture**

Arcuate lines
Ilioischial lines
Sacroiliac joints
Transverse processes of L-5
Ala of the sacrum
Lateral borders of the sacrum
Arcs of the sacral foramina
Symphysis pubis
Pubic rami
Dome of the acetabula
Anterior and posterior lips of the acetabula
Wings of the ilia
Head and neck of the femura

---

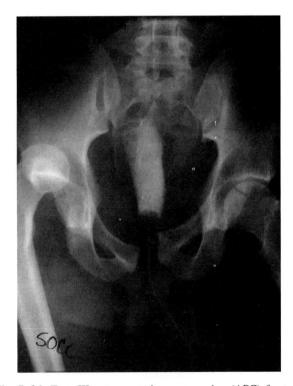

**Fig. 7-36.** Type III anteroposterior compression (APC) fracture of the pelvis. Bilateral APC fractures can be seen, with disruption of both sacroiliac joints and wide separation of the symphysis. There is also a right posterior hip dislocation involving the dome of the acetabulum as a fragment, and an undisplaced posterior column fracture of the left acetabulum. Note the massive distortion of the bladder by a pelvic hematoma. This patient exsanguinated before embolization could be completed.

jury, one would expect all of the ligaments on both sides to be disrupted. Figure 7-37 shows a VS fracture with cephalad displacement of half of the pelvis. Figure 7-37 shows a CM fracture with features of both LC and VS fractures.

Figure 7-38 shows anterior and posterior column fractures of the acetabulum. Figure 7-35 demonstrates a transverse fracture of the acetabulum. Figure 7-36 shows a posterior hip dislocation, including dislocation of the dome of the acetabulum. Figure 7-39 shows an avulsion fracture of the anterosuperior iliac spine in a young athlete.

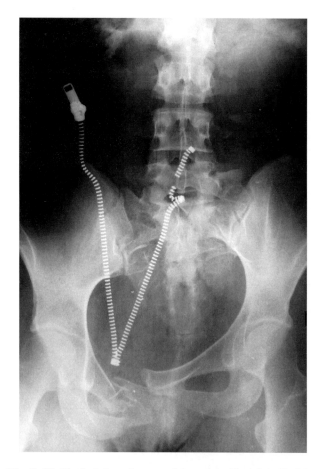

**Other plain films.** The resuscitating physician should be aware of other plain films that may be indicated, if and when there is time to spare. These extra views can help the orthopedist plan possible internal fixation surgery, although CT scans will probably be necessary anyway. These radiographs are shown diagrammatically in Fig. 7-40. They are inlet and outlet views of the pelvis and obturator and iliac 45° oblique (Judet) views of the pelvis when an injured acetabulum is suspected.

### The urethrogram

A urethrogram is indicated when blood is present at the urethral meatus or when there is a high suspicion of urethral injury. In an average-sized adult man, a 14- or 16F Foley catheter is inserted into the urethra so that the balloon is at

**Fig. 7-37.** Vertical shear fracture of the pelvis. The left half of the pelvis is vertically displaced with a fracture of the pubis and sacrum and disruption of the left sacroiliac joint. This example also qualifies as a combined mechanical injury because there is a lateral compression injury on the right, with transverse rami fractures and a compression fracture of the sacrum.

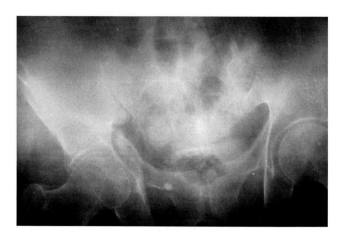

**Fig. 7-38.** Posterior column fracture of the acetabulum. Note the disruption of the ilioischial line. The arcuate line is also disrupted, making this an example of a both-column fracture.

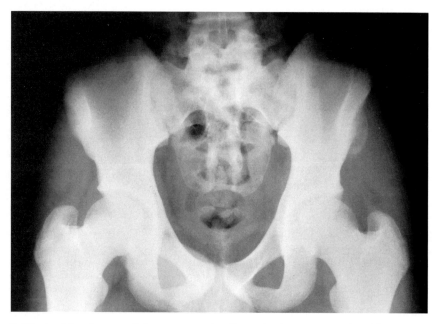

**Fig. 7-39.** Avulsion fracture of the anterosuperior iliac spine in a young male athlete.

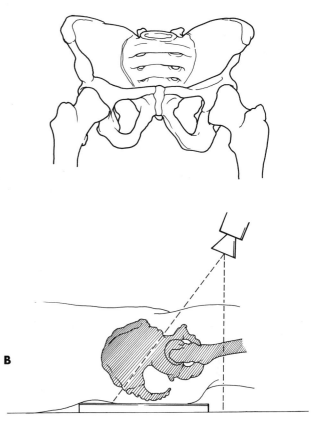

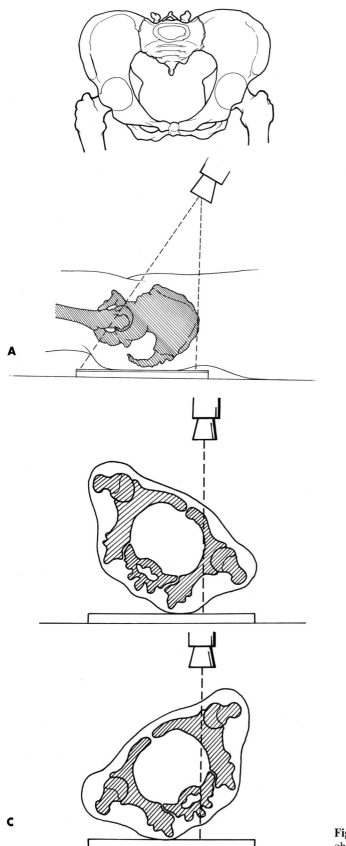

**Fig. 7-40.** Extra plain radiographic views of the pelvis may be obtained in stable patients. **A** and **B**, Inlet and outlet views. **C**, Judet (obturator and iliac) oblique views.

the level of the navicular fossa. The length of the catheter is kept sterile. A 0.5 milliliter of saline (just enough to occlude the urethra) is used to inflate the balloon using a small syringe. Thirty ml of contrast solution is then injected into the urethra using a large catheter-tipped syringe, and an oblique radiograph is obtained while the last 10 ml is injected.[49] If the study is negative or the injury is minor, the catheter can be advanced into the bladder. Figure 7-41 shows a disruption of the posterior urethra at the urogenital diaphragm.

### The cystogram

In the author's opinion, a cystogram is indicated in every instance of pelvic ring fracture. Others[104,105] have condemned such use of the cystogram because, unless there is grossly bloody urine present, the possibility of identifying bladder rupture is negligible. The reason for obtaining the cystogram, however, is to both quantify pelvic hemorrhage and identify bladder rupture. If the bladder is fully distended when the cystogram is obtained, it outlines the extent of the pelvic hematoma. If there is significant bladder displacement, then the patient is bleeding significantly from the pelvis. Knowing this allows the resuscitating team to make better decisions regarding the priorities of management. A shocky patient with little or no bladder displacement is bleeding somewhere else; a shocky patient with gross bladder displacement and no frank blood on DPL should go to angiography for embolization.

The technique is to attach a 500-ml bottle of contrast to the Foley catheter using tubing designed for this purpose, and to run it in by gravity from a height of about 3 feet above the patient. The author uses an 8.5% organically bound iodine solution (Cystograffin; Squibb, New Brunswick, NJ). When the entire bottle has drained into the patient, or when contrast solution leaks around the Foley catheter, the tubing is clamped and an AP radiograph of the pelvis obtained. The Foley catheter is then attached to a drainage bag,

the contrast allowed to drain entirely from the bladder, and the bladder irrigated with saline. Another AP radiograph of the pelvis is obtained so that extravasation from an extraperitoneal rupture is not hidden from view by the full bladder. CT is not as sensitive as the cystogram in detecting bladder rupture.[78]

Figures 7-42 and 7-43 show intraperitoneal and extraperitoneal rupture of the bladder, respectively. Figure 7-44 shows a small pelvic hematoma distortion of the bladder, and Fig. 7-45 shows massive bladder displacement.

### Computed tomography

Computed tomography is a valuable adjunct in the management of pelvic fracture cases. However, CT scans entail time and movement, and other priorities can supervene. Resnik et al.[106] recently reported a series of 50 pelvic fracture cases studied with plain radiography and CT. The plain radiographs included inlet and outlet views in 25 of the patients and oblique views in 12 patients with acetabular injuries. These 50 cases harbored 162 bony injuries, of which only 14 (9%) were not seen on the plain films. Acetabular intra-articular fracture fragments, however, were missed 80% of the time by plain films. The authors concluded that plain films are sufficient to detect virtually all clinically important fractures and dislocations of the pelvis, with the exception of acetabular fractures.[106] Dunn et al.[107] compared CT scans with AP radiographic views of only the pelvis in 20 pelvic fracture patients and found that clinically important new information was garnered in 13 (65%).[107] It would appear that a plain AP radiograph of the pelvis is adequate for the unstable patient. Inlet and outlet views and CT scans should be reserved for the resuscitated patient who remains stable. All patients with acetabular fractures need

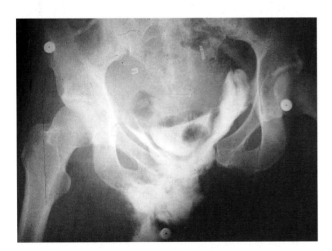

**Fig. 7-41.** Urethrogram showing disruption of the membranous urethra above and below the urogenital diaphragm. Some contrast solution entered the bladder, indicating that this might not be a complete disruption.

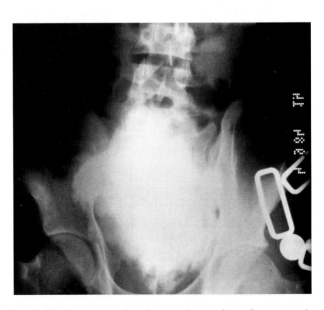

**Fig. 7-42.** Cystogram showing an intraperitoneal rupture. An extraperitoneal rupture with perivesical extravasation of contrast can also be seen. Note that contrast can be seen between loops of bowel, cinching the diagnosis of free intraperitoneal rupture.

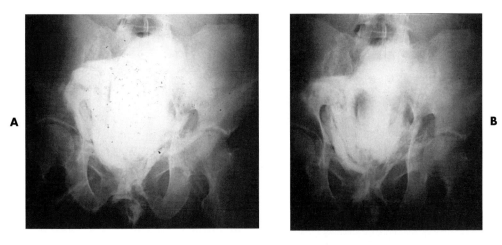

**Fig. 7-43.** Extraperitoneal rupture. **A,** Cystogram with the bladder filled. Note that there is contrast in the perivesical space. **B,** Second view cystogram, with the bladder emptied of contrast. Note that the contrast that is not in the bladder remains.

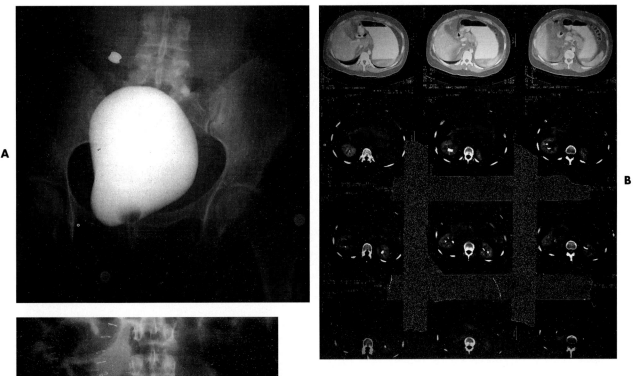

**Fig. 7-44.** Example of how a cystogram can aid in decision making. **A,** Cystogram showing only a small pelvic hematoma in a patient with a pelvic fracture. **B,** Retroperitoneal hematoma seen on computed tomography. **C,** The results of operative reduction and fixation. This patient was in shock and the cystogram led to immediate surgery with repair of an inferior vena cava tear. The CT was obtained postoperatively and the internal fixation of the pelvic fracture performed subsequently.

CT scans prior to internal fixation of this fracture. Figure 7-46 shows examples of sacral, sacroiliac, and acetabular fractures seen on computed tomography.

## INITIAL MANAGEMENT OF PELVIC RING FRACTURE CASES
### Prehospital management

Emergency medical technicians are trained to detect and manage respiratory and hemodynamic instability during a primary survey. This is followed by a second survey that entails a rapid head-to-toe inspection for injury. Part of this survey includes manual compression of the pelvis to detect pain, motion, and crepitance.

**Prehospital use of antishock trousers.** Hypotensive patients with abdominal or pelvic trauma are placed in a PASG. The compartments of the garment should be inflated to a pressure of about 100 torr, at which time the hook and loop fasteners begin to separate, or to a pressure that results in a satisfactory blood pressure. Awake patients are made more comfortable during transport by the PASG, and at least some bleeding is averted by compression and immobilization. If the patient is not hypotensive but has clinical pelvic instability or complains of pelvic pain on transfer, the PASG should be inflated to a pressure of about 40 torr. The abdominal portion of the PASG should not be inflated in pregnant patients with a palpable gravid uterus. Respiratory compromise may occur with inflation of the abdominal portion of the PASG. Ventilation may have to be assisted or the PASG deflated. If prolonged transport time is anticipated, the PASG pressure should be reduced to 40 torr to help avoid the possible occurrence of compartment syndromes.

**Mechanism of injury.** The emergency medical technicians should note the mechanism of injury in detail, and this information should be related to hospital personnel for documentation. If the patient was thrown or fell, how far was the fall? Did he or she land sideways or feet first? Was the patient crushed in an AP direction or from side to side? Was the patient subjected to rolling trauma? Was a seatbelt worn? Did an air bag deploy? Did the patient straddle an object on falling?

### Emergency department evaluation and management

The ABCs of trauma evaluation and management are discussed in Chapter 1. Part of that process is obtaining trauma series x-rays and performing manual compression

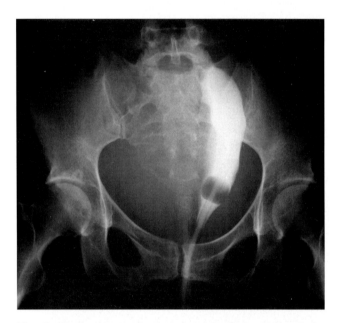

**Fig. 7-45.** Cystogram showing massive displacement of the bladder in a patient with a type I lateral compression (LC) fracture of the pelvis. Many units of blood were needed to resuscitate this patient. Bleeding was controlled subsequently with embolization of bleeding branches of the obturator artery. Although pelvic bleeding is uncommon in LC-I fractures, every pelvic ring fracture must be considered dangerous.

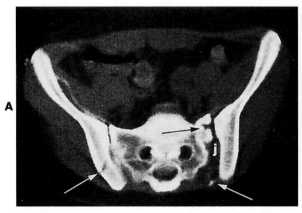
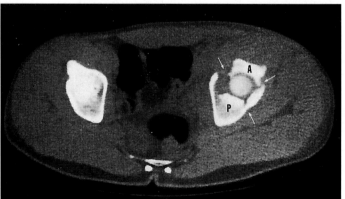

**Fig. 7-46.** Fractures seen on computed tomography. **A,** Fractures of both iliac bones *(white arrows)* and a sacral alar fracture *(black arrow)* with sacroiliac joint (j) disruption. **B,** Left acetabular fracture with involvement of both the anterior *(A)* and posterior *(P)* columns. (From Sartoris DJ, Resnik D: The musculoskeletal system. In Haaga JR, Alfidi RJ, eds: *Computed tomography of the whole body,* ed 2, St. Louis, 1988, CV Mosby, p. 1342. Used by permission.)

of the pelvis in the horizontal and AP planes. If the patient is responsive, it is important to ask about last void and defecation, bladder sensation, and saddle area sensation, in addition to the usual questions.

**Manual compression test.** Manual compression of the pelvis should be gentle. Moving a pelvic fracture can stimulate bleeding. Multiple examiners should not repeat this maneuver. When the patient is log-rolled for examination of the back, the sacrum and posterior aspects of the sacroiliac joints should be palpated for pain, swelling, or crepitance.

**Clues on the routine anteroposterior pelvic radiograph.** The pelvic radiograph, including what is visible of the abdomen should be reviewed carefully to look for flank stripes, dog ears, air in the tissues, and transverse-process fractures of the lumbar spine, as well as for integrity of the pelvic ring, the femura, and the lumbar spine.

**Setting the stage.** When a pelvic ring fracture is discovered, the clinician should expect and prepare for the worst. The patient should be kept warm. All fluids and blood should be warmed. If he or she has not already been notified, the trauma surgeon should be alerted. Packed cells of O-negative or O-positive blood should be kept on hand. The patient should be prepared for transfer to a trauma center if the admitting hospital is not set up to manage the complications of severe pelvic fracture.

**Identifying and treating injuries.** Figure 7-47 is an algorithm for the emergency department management of the patient with a pelvic ring fracture.

First, the clothing should be cut away at the crotch of the PASG without deflating it, and the clothing inspected for blood. The perineum should be palpated and visually inspected, separating any skin folds. The scrotum should also be inspected and palpated, feeling both testicles.

- If the patient is bleeding heavily from an open wound, it should be packed with sterile vaginal packing or laparotomy pads using a ring forcep. Use of the PASG should be continued at 40-torr pressure.
- If there is a perineal wound that is not bleeding, it should not be explored, lest a clot be disturbed and exsanguinating hemorrhage ensue.
- If there is any perineal laceration, intravenous antibiotics covering the fecal flora should be administered. Cefoxitin, 2 g (40 mg/kg in children), or other antibiotic or combination of antibiotics of equivalent coverage can be used.
- If there is a perineal laceration, a diverting colostomy will be needed. The surgeon should be alerted to this finding.
- If a testicle is swollen and tense, testicular rupture should be considered. This requires emergent surgical decompression. A urologist should be involved in setting priority.

Second, the groins should be palpated for femoral pulses. Notation should be made of whether the pulses are decreased or absent.

- An absent pulse in a patient with an APC-II or -III pelvic fracture means that the external iliac artery has probably been stretched and has clotted. Emergency vascular surgery is needed. The involved limb will be at risk for compartment syndromes after revascularization.
- A decreased pulse may mean that the common iliac or external iliac artery has been injured and may be bleeding or clotting. This finding should be monitored closely.

Third, the treating physician should put on clean gloves and perform a rectal examination, noting sphincter tone. The prostate gland should be palpated and its consistency and position noted. Following examination, the physician should check his or her finger for frank blood.

- Decreased sphincter tone may accompany a sacral fracture. A sensory examination should be performed later to detect a cauda equina syndrome.
- A high-riding, boggy prostate indicates that the membranous urethra has been transected, probably above the urogenital diaphragm. A urethrogram is not necessary at this time, and a Foley catheter will not be inserted. If the patient is to be transferred to another hospital, a suprapubic catheter will be needed later. A urologist must be involved at this stage in setting priorities.
- If the prostate findings are equivocal, a urethrogram is needed within a few minutes. Contrast solution, a large catheter-tipped syringe, and a Foley catheter tray should be prepared.
- If there is frank blood in the rectum, there has been rectal penetration or disruption. Intravenous antibiotics should be started and the surgeon informed of this finding. A diverting colostomy, fecal washout, and presacral space drainage are necessary. If findings are equivocal, a proctoscopic examination will be needed later.

Fourth, the penis should be inspected and palpated while looking for blood at the meatus.

- Most urethral injuries are accompanied by blood at the meatus. If blood is seen, a urethrogram is performed. If there is urethral transection, passage with a Foley catheter should not be attempted. If the injury is minor, a Foley catheter can be passed gently into the bladder.
- If there is swelling or other evidence of injury on rectal examination or on palpation of the penis, a urethrogram should be performed. Passage of the Foley catheter into the bladder should be attempted if there is only a minor injury.

Fifth, the vulva should be inspected and palpated, and spread to reveal the urethral meatus and the vagina. Any blood or lacerations should be noted. A bimanual vaginal examination should be performed, feeling for lacerations and swelling. In the presence of menstruation, a speculum examination is necessary.

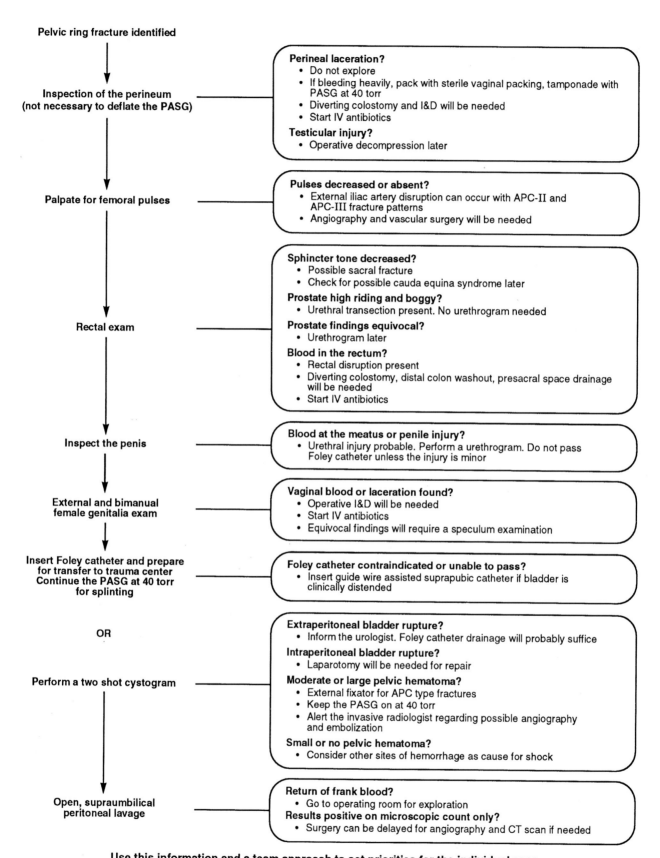

**Fig. 7-47.** An algorithm for management of pelvic ring fractures for use in the emergency department.

- Anterior vaginal injury may indicate a urethral injury. However, unless there is laceration into the urethra from the vagina, a Foley catheter can be passed into the bladder without the need of a urethrogram because urethral transection is rare in females. A urethrogram will eventually be needed if there is suspicion that a urethral injury has been produced.
- Vaginal lacerations must be débrided and explored in the operating room. The surgeon should be informed of this finding and intravenous antibiotics started.

Sixth, a Foley catheter should be inserted in the bladder and, if planned, the patient prepared for transfer. If that is not the plan, go to Step 7. The patient should be left in the PASG at 40 torr during transport.

- The receiving physician should be informed of all physical findings, including the emergency medical technician's reports, radiographs, flow sheets, and lab reports.
- If a Foley catheter is not indicated because of urethral injury, and the bladder is clinically distended, a suprapubic catheter should be inserted into the bladder using the Seldinger technique.

Seventh, a two-shot cystogram should be performed using a volume of about 500 ml, or 5 ml/kg in children.

- If there is no hematoma or a small hematoma deforming the bladder, it is unlikely that pelvic bleeding is present.
- If there is a moderate or a large hematoma deforming the bladder and the patient is hypotensive, significant pelvic bleeding is occurring. The patient should remain in PASG at 40-torr pressure. An immediate open suprapubic peritoneal lavage should be performed. If frank blood is obtained on insertion, the patient should be taken to the operating room for exploratory laparotomy. If there is no blood, the patient should undergo angiography for possible selective embolization of bleeding vessels. If the lavage is positive only on the basis of cell count, laparotomy can be delayed until after angiographic control of pelvic bleeding.
- If there is a moderate or a large hematoma deforming the bladder and the patient is hemodynamically stable, the patient may be a candidate for external fixation, depending on the fracture geography (anterior separation and intact anterior iliac crests). An orthopedic consultant should be present.
- If the fracture is not suitable for external fixation, the patient should remain in the PASG at 30 to 40 torr, with release of pressure every 2 hours to check for compartment syndromes.

### Definitive management of adult pelvic ring fracture cases

The definitive management of each pelvic fracture case entails the treatment of associated injuries as well as management of the fracture itself. In general, the orthope-

dist will elect the following treatments for the various pelvic ring fracture types, if the clinical situation allows.

LC-I injuries are treated with 1 to 5 days of bedrest followed by progressive weight-bearing and ambulation; LC-II injuries are treated with 3 to 6 weeks of bedrest followed by progressive weight-bearing and ambulation; and LC-III, APC-II, APC-III, and CM injuries with undisplaced but unstable sacroiliac joints ideally are treated with open internal fixation within a few days of injury. Otherwise, 6 to 8 weeks of bedrest are required. Traction and external fixation may be used acutely prior to surgery when there is rotatory instability of the sacroiliac joint.

Vertical shearforce and CM injuries with vertically displaced sacroiliac joints ideally are treated with open internal fixation within a few days of injury. Skeletal traction, using a supracondylar femoral or proximal tibial pin, is often used acutely to obtain length prior to surgery. Otherwise, bedrest and traction for 12 weeks are required. External fixation may also be used in combination with traction and internal fixation.[22]

Whether or not the pelvic ring is involved, displaced acetabular fractures almost always require operative repair and fixation. This surgery is usually postponed until the patient has stabilized from associated injuries, but ideally is performed within a few hours of injury.[26]

### Pelvic ring fractures in children

Aside from the obvious differences in size, the ability to communicate, blood volume, and drug dosage, the same steps apply to children as well as adults in the evaluation and management listed in the pelvic ring fracture resuscitation algorithm.

McIntyre et al.[108] reviewed a series of 57 pelvic fractures in children. Although the mortality rate was only 1.7%, blood replacement, external fixation, arterial embolization, bladder repair, and vascular surgical repair were all necessary in some of the children. The definitive management of pelvic ring fractures in small children is more conservative than that in adults, with bedrest and traction being used instead of internal fixation in some cases.[14]

## MANAGEMENT OF FRACTURES NOT INVOLVING THE PELVIC RING
### Isolated sacral fractures

Isolated fractures of the sacrum are relatively uncommon. However, they are difficult to see on radiography and may be underreported for that reason. The sacrum's thin cortex and curving configuration make it difficult to see cortical breaks. Physical examination may identify the fracture: direct pressure on the sacrum may produce pain, and rectal examination may reveal pain on gentle posterior palpation. The physician should be careful not to produce a rectal perforation by palpating a sharp bone fragment. Anal sphincter tone may be decreased, and the patient may not be able to void due to sacral nerve injury. A cauda equina syndrome may be present.

The prognosis for recovery from sacral nerve injury is good.[18] These isolated fractures are caused by considerable direct trauma to the sacrum from behind. Conservative bedrest management is used; however, strong consideration should be given to hospital admission, given the amount of force involved and the potential for other injuries as well as bowel and bladder difficulties.

## Coccygeal fractures

Fractures of the coccyx are common; they occur mostly in women because the wider female pelvis exposes the coccyx to direct trauma in a backward fall. They are not life-threatening, but are very painful and aggravating. Muscles of both the floor of the pelvis and the anal sphincter pull the distal fragment, producing severe pain. Reduction of the fracture is useless because of the muscle pull. Conservative management with bedrest for about 1 week, with Sitz baths to help relieve muscle spasm, is usually successful; hospitalization is not necessary. Stool softeners are helpful. Patients may need to use a donut-ring cushion when sitting. Rarely, surgical excision of the distal fragment is needed for relief of chronic symptoms.

## Iliac wing fractures

Isolated fractures of the iliac wings (Duverney fractures) are not uncommon and are due to direct compression or force. Displacement is usually minimal because muscle pull tends to restore position. This type of fracture is not threatening in terms of blood loss, and conservative management with bedrest is recommended. Hospital admission is not ordinarily necessary unless the fracture is associated with an open wound or there is significant abdominal muscular spasm that makes abdominal examination difficult and painful.[14]

## Avulsion fractures

Avulsion fractures of the pelvis are uncommon, comprising 4% to 13% of all pelvic fractures. However, many if not most patients seek attention in clinics rather than emergency departments.[14,29] Patients with avulsion fractures are likely to come to the emergency department with chronic pain following a remote incident. Radiography will reveal an avulsion fracture in a healing stage, sometimes alarming the emergency physician, who may think that a bone tumor is present. Ewing's sarcoma and osteomyelitis enter into the differential diagnosis.[109] The trabecular pattern of the adjacent bone is intact, however. Excessive callus formation is particularly likely with avulsion fractures of the ischial apophysis; and surgical intervention is sometimes required.[14] Symptomatic management with rest at home in a comfortable position followed by walking with crutches is all that is needed. Follow-up with an orthopedist is obviously necessary.

## Acetabular fractures

Fracture of the acetabulum is caused by severe trauma, usually related to a motor vehicle accident, with force applied relatively directly through the greater trochanter or through the shaft of the femur, as in knee-versus-dashboard injury. Femur fractures, hip fractures, hip dislocation, and knee injuries commonly accompany these fractures. When the ring of the pelvis is disrupted, these fractures should be managed according to the algorithm discussed above. Generally, the acetabular fracture itself takes lower priority than other considerations in such patients.

Acetabular fractures are associated with significant long-term disability. Orthopedic consultation should be obtained as soon as possible because studies must be obtained to delineate the exact extent and displacement of these fractures. This way, early operative intervention to restore anatomic relationships and stability can be undertaken. Aside from the immediate relocation of traumatic hip dislocation, there are few steps for the emergency physician to take during initial resuscitation. All patients, including both adults and children,[14,22] with acetabular fractures should be admitted to the hospital. As with hip dislocation, early reduction and fixation results in a better long-term prognosis.

## DISCUSSION

Rapid and efficient evaluation and emergency management of pelvic fracture victims is a major responsibility for emergency physicians, whether they practice in rural emergency departments or urban trauma centers. Rural practitioners are responsible for rapid stabilization, evaluation, and transfer to a trauma center in pelvic ring fracture cases. In trauma centers, a multispecialty approach results in an institution-wide commitment to the optimum care of such patients. Emergency physicians in trauma centers should seek consensus among their colleagues as to the optimum approach. Trauma surgeons, orthopedists, invasive radiologists, urologists, pediatricians, obstetricians, as well as emergency physicians should help formulate an institutionally accepted algorithm for the evaluation and care of these patients.

## REFERENCES

1. Perry JF Jr, McCellan RJ: Autopsy findings in 127 patients following fatal traffic accidents, *Surg Gynecol Obstet* 119:586-590, 1964.
2. Committee on Trauma Research: *Injury in America: a continuing public health problem,* Washington, DC, 1985, National Academy Press, p. 23.
3. Mucha P Jr, Farnell MB: Analysis of pelvic fracture management, *J Trauma* 24:379-385, 1984.
4. Burgess AR, et al: Pelvic ring disruptions: effective classification system and treatment protocols, *J Trauma* 30:848-856, 1990.
5. Cryer HM, et al: Pelvic fracture classification: correlation with hemorrhage, *J Trauma* 28:973-979, 1988.
6. Dalal SA, et al: Pelvic fracture in multiple trauma: classification by mechanism is key to pattern of organ injury, resuscitative requirements and outcome, *J Trauma* 29:981-1000, 1989.
7. Moreno C, et al: Hemorrhage associated with major pelvic fracture: a multispecialty challenge, *J Trauma* 26:987-993, 1986.

8. Poole GV, et al: Pelvic fracture from major blunt trauma: outcome is determined by associated injuries, *Ann Surg* 213:532-538, 1991.

9. Bond SJ: Gotshall CS, and Eichelberger MR: Predictors of abdominal injury in children with pelvic fracture, *J Trauma* 31:1169-1173, 1991.

10. Semba RT, Yasukawa K, and Gustilo RB: Critical analysis of results of 53 Malgaigne fractures of the pelvis, *J Trauma* 23:535-537, 1983.

11. Ochsner MG Jr, et al: Pelvic fracture as an indicator of increased risk of thoracic aortic rupture, *J Trauma* 29:1376-1379, 1989.

12. Ochsner MG Jr, et al: Associated aortic rupture - pelvic fracture: an alert for orthopedic and general surgeons, *J Trauma* 33:429-434, 1992.

13. Flint L, et al: Definitive control of mortality from severe pelvic fracture, *Ann Surg* 211:703-706, 1990.

14. Canale ST: Part I: fractures of the pelvis. In Rockwood CA Jr, Wilkins KE, and King RE, eds: *Fractures in children,* Philadelphia, 1984, JB Lippincott, pp. 733-781.

15. Drost TF, et al: Major trauma in pregnant women: maternal/fetal outcome, *J Trauma* 30:574-578, 1990.

16. Goss CM: *Gray's anatomy,* ed 29, Philadelphia, 1973, Lea & Febiger, pp. 121, 234.

17. Buckley SL, Burkus JK: Computerized axial tomography of pelvic ring fractures, *J Trauma* 27:496-502, 1987.

18. Sabiston CP, Wing PC: Sacral fractures: classification and neurologic implications, *J Trauma* 26:1113-1115, 1986.

19. Pennal GF, et al: Results of treatment of acetabular fractures, *Clin Orthop* 151:115-123, 1980.

20. Pennal GF, et al: Pelvic disruption: assessment and classification, *Clin Orthop* 151:12-21, 1980.

21. Young JWR, Burgess AR: *Radiologic management of pelvic ring fractures: systematic radiographic diagnosis.* Baltimore, 1987, Urban & Schwarzenberg.

22. Burgess AR: Part I: the pelvic ring. In Rockwood CA Jr, Green DP, Bucholz RW, eds: *Fractures in adults,* ed 3, Philadelphia, 1991, JB Lippincott, pp. 1399-1442.

23. Trafton PG: Pelvic ring injuries, *Surg Clin North Am* 70:655-669, 1990.

24. Griggs S, Kulenovic E, and Seligson D: Malgaigne's fracture: the Larrey variant—a case report, *J Trauma* 31:1553-1554, 1991.

25. Malgaigne JF: *Treatise on fractures,* Philadelphia, 1859, JB Lippincott, p. 523.

26. Tile M: Part II: fractures of the acetabulum. In Rockwood CA Jr, Green DP, and Bucholz RW, eds: *Fractures in adults,* ed 3, Philadelphia, 1991, JB Lippincott, pp. 1442-1479.

27. Dunn AW, Morris HD: Fractures and dislocations of the pelvis, *J Bone Joint Surg* 50-A:1639-1648, 1968.

28. Takahara T, et al: Isolated fracture-dislocation of the sacrum: case report, *J Trauma* 34:600-601, 1993.

29. Lambert MJ, Fligner DJ: Avulsion of the iliac crest apophysis: a rare fracture in adolescent athletes. *Ann Emerg Med* 22:1218-1220, 1993.

30. Ellison M, Timberlake GA, and Kerstein MD: Impotence following pelvic fracture, *J Trauma* 28:695-696, 1988.

31. Perry MO, Husmann DA: Urethral injuries in female subjects following pelvic fractures, *J Urol* 147:139-143, 1992.

32. Van Arsdalen KN, et al: Erectile failure following pelvic trauma: a review of pathophysiology, evaluation, and management, with particular reference to the penile prosthesis, *J Trauma* 24:579-584, 1984.

33. Sidhu JS, Dhillon MK: Lumbosacral plexus avulsion with pelvic fractures, *Injury* 22:156-158, 1991.

34. Rengachary SS: Examination of the motor and sensory systems and reflexes. In Wilkins RH, Rengachary SS, eds: *Neurosurgery,* New York, 1985, McGraw-Hill, pp. 122-147.

35. Ben-Menachem Y, Coldwell DM, and Young JWR: Hemorrhage associated with pelvic fractures: causes, diagnosis and emergent management, *Am J Radiol* 157:1005-1014, 1991.

36. Holting T, et al: Diagnosis and treatment of retroperitoneal hematoma in multiple trauma patients, *Arch Orthop Trauma Surg*111:323-326, 1992.

37. Bickell WH, et al: The detrimental effects of intravenous crystalloid after aortotomy in swine, *Surgery* 110:529-536, 1991.

38. Frank JL, Reimer BL, and Raves JR: Traumatic iliofemoral arterial injury: an association with high anterior acetabular fractures, *J Vasc Surg* 10:198-201, 1989.

39. Birchard JD, Pichora DR, and Brown PM: External iliac artery and lumbosacral plexus injury secondary to an open book fracture of the pelvis: report of a case, *J Trauma* 30:906-908, 1990.

40. Mansour MA, Moore FA, and Moore EE: Hypogastric arterial embolization in pelvic fracture: case report, *J Trauma* 30:1417-1418, 1990.

41. Riska EB, Myllynen P: Fat embolism in patients with multiple injuries, *J Trauma* 22:891-894, 1982.

42. Goesling HR, Donohue TA: The fat embolism sydrome, *JAMA* 241:2740-2742, 1979.

43. Fabian TC, et al: Fat embolism syndrome: prospective evaluation in 92 fracture patients, *Crit Care Med* 18:42-46, 1990.

44. Shannon FL, et al: Value of distal colon washout in civilian rectal trauma: reducing gut bacterial translocation, *J Trauma* 28:989-993, 1988.

45. Sinnott R, Rhodes M, and Brader A: Open pelvic fracture: an injury for trauma centers, *Am J Surg* 163:283-287, 1992.

46. Strate RG, Grieco JG: Blunt injury to the colon and rectum, *J Trauma* 23:384-387, 1983.

47. Froman C, Stein A: Complicated crushing injuries of the pelvis, *J Bone Joint Surg [Br]* 49B:24-32, 1967.

48. Sandler CM, et al: Posterior urethral injuries after pelvic fractures, *Am J Radiol* 137:1233-1237, 1981.

49. Spirnak JP: Pelvic fracture and injury to the lower urinary tract, *Surg Clin North Am* 68:1057-1069, 1988.

50. Colapinto V, McCallum RW: Injury to the male posterior urethra in fractured pelvis: a new classification, *J Urol* 118:575-580, 1977.

51. Cass AS: Urethral injury in the multiple-injured patient, *J Trauma* 24:901-906, 1984.

52. Devine PC, Devine CJ: Posterior urethral injuries associated with pelvic fractures, *Urology* 20:467-470, 1982.

53. Orkin LA: Trauma to the bladder, ureter, and kidney. In Sciarra JJ, ed: *Gynecology and obstetrics,* Philadelphia, 1991, JB Lippincott, pp. 1-8.

54. Carter CT, Schafer N: Incidence of urethral disruption in females with traumatic pelvic fractures, *Am J Emerg Med* 11:218-220, 1993.

55. Govender S, Sham A, and Singh B: Open pelvic fractures, *Injury* 21:373-376, 1990.

56. Doman AN, Hoekstra DV: Pelvic fracture associated with severe intra-abdominal gynecologic injury, *J Trauma* 28:118-120, 1988.

57. Montie J: Bladder injuries, *Urol Clin North Am* 4:59-67, 1977.

58. Corrierre JN Jr, Sandler CM: Mechanisms of injury, patterns of extravasation and management of extraperitoneal bladder rupture due to blunt trauma, *J Urol* 139:43-44, 1988.

59. Kellam JF, et al: The unstable pelvic fracture: operative treatment, *Orthop Clin North Am* 18:25-41, 1987.

60. Kiil F, Setekleiv J: Physiology of ureter and renal pelvis. In Geiger SR, Orloff J, and Berliner RW, eds: *Handbook of physiology; Section 8,* Washington, DC, 1973, American Physiological Society, pp. 1033-1057.

61. Kluger Y, et al: Acute obstructive uropathy seconday to pelvic hematoma compressing the bladder: report of two cases, *J Trauma* 35:477-478, 1993.

62. Milles G, Koucky CJ, and Zacheis HG: Experimental uncontrolled arterial hemorrhage, *Surgery* 60:434-442, 1966.

63. American College of Surgeons Committee on Trauma: *Advanced trauma life support course, instructor manual,* Chicago, 1989, ACS.

64. Kowalenko T, et al: Improved outcome with hypotensive resuscitation of uncontrolled hemorrhagic shock in a swine model, *J Trauma* 33:349-353, 1992.

65. Stern SA, et al: Effect of blood pressure on hemorrhagic volume and survival in a near-fatal hemorrhage model incorporating a vascular injury. *Ann Emerg Med* 22:155-163, 1993.

66. Beecher HK: Resuscitation of men severely wounded in battle. In DeBakey ME, ed: *Surgery in World War II, vol 11: General surgery,* Washington, DC, 1955, Office of the Surgeon General, Department of the Army.

67. Jurkovich GJ, et al: Hypothermia in trauma victims: an ominous predictor of survival, *J Trauma* 27:1019-1022, 1987.

68. Luna GK, et al: Incidence and effects of hypothermia in seriously injured patients, *J Trauma* 27:1014-1018, 1987.

69. Reed RL II, et al: The disparity between hypothermic coagulopathy and clotting studies, *J Trauma* 33:465-470, 1992.

70. Flint LM Jr, et al: Definitive control of bleeding from severe pelvic fractures, *Ann Surg* 189:709-716, 1979.

71. McSwain NE Jr: Pneumatic anti-shock garment: state of the art 1988, *Ann Emerg Med* 17:506-525, 1988.

72. Aprahamian C, et al: MAST-associated compartment syndrome (MACS): a review, *J Trauma* 29:549-555, 1989.

73. Christensen KS: Pneumatic anatishock garments (PASG): do they precipitate lower-extremity compartment syndromes? *J Trauma* 26:1102-1105, 1986.

74. Mears DC, Rubash HE: Acute resuscitation. In Mears DC, Rubash HE, eds: *Pelvic and acetabular fractures,* Thorofare, NJ, 1986, Slack, pp. 429-486.

75. Mucha P Jr, Welch TJ: Hemorrhage in major pelvic fractures, *Surg Clin North Am* 68:757-773, 1988.

76. Pearse CS, Magrina JF, and Finley BE: Use of MAST suit in obstetrics and gynecology, *Obstet Gynecol Survey* 39:416-422, 1984.

77. O'Keefe TJ: Retroperitoneal abscess, *J Bone Joint Surg* 60-A:1117-1121, 1978.

78. Mee SL, McAninch JW, and Federle MP: Computerized tomography in bladder rupture: diagnostic limitations, *J Urol* 137:207-209, 1987.

79. Evers BM, Cryer HM, and Miller FB: Pelvic hemorrhage: priorities in management, *Arch Surg* 124:422-424, 1989.

80. Riemer BL, et al: Acute mortality associated with injuries to the pelvic ring: the role of early patient mobilization and external fixation, *J Trauma* 35:671-675, 1993.

81. Ward EF, Tomasin J, and Vander Griend RA: Open reduction and internal fixation of vertical shear pelvic fractures, *J Trauma* 27:291-295, 1987.

82. Klein SR, et al: Management strategy of vascular injuries associated with pelvic fractures, *Cardiovasc Surg* 33:349-357, 1992.

83. Nallathambi MN, et al: The use of peritoneal lavage and urological studies in major fractures of the pelvis: a reassessment, *Injury* 18:379-383, 1987.

84. Snyder HS: Blunt pelvic trauma, *Am J Emerg Med* 6:618-627, 1988.

85. Davidson BS, et al: Pelvic fractures associated with open perineal wounds: a survivable injury, *J Trauma* 35:36-39, 1993.

86. Hofstetter SR, et al: A prospective comparison of two regimens of prophylactic antibiotics in abdominal trauma: cefoxitin versus triple drug, *J Trauma* 24:307-310, 1984.

87. Weigelt JA, et al: Abdominal surgical wound infection is lowered with improved perioperative enterococcus and bacteroides therapy, *J Trauma* 34:579-584, 1993.

88. Willey SH, et al: Effects of clindamycin and gentamycin and other antimicrobial combinations against enterococci in an experimental model of intra-abdominal abscess, *Surg Gynecol Obstet* 169:199-202, 1989.

89. Latenser BA, et al: Improved outcome with early fixation of skeletally unstable pelvic fractures, *J Trauma* 31:28-31, 1991.

90. Leenen LPH, et al: Internal fixation of open unstable pelvic fractures, *J Trauma* 35:220-225, 1993.

91. Baker DP: Trauma in the pregnant patient, *Surg Clin North Am* 62:275-289, 1982.

92. Fildes J, et al: Trauma: the leading cause of maternal death, *J Trauma* 32:643-645, 1992.

93. Kissinger DP, et al: Trauma in pregnancy: predicting pregnancy outcome, *Arch Surg* 126:1079-1086, 1991.

94. Scorpio RJ, et al: Blunt trauma during pregnancy: factors affecting fetal outcome, *J Trauma* 32:213-216, 1992.

95. Wasserstrum N: Maternal physiology. In Hacker NF, Moore JG, eds: *Essentials of obstetrics and gynecology,* Philadelphia, 1986, WB Saunders, pp. 34-46.

96. Towery R, English TP, and Wisner D: Evaluation of pregnant women after blunt injury, *J Trauma* 35:731-735, 1993.

97. Davis SM: Antishock trousers: a collective review, *J Emerg Med* 4:145-155, 1986.

98. Crosby WM: Automobile injuries and blunt abdominal trauma. In Buchsbaum HF, ed: *Trauma in pregnancy,* Philadelphia, 1979, WB Saunders, pp. 101-127.

99. Jeanty P, Romero R: *Obstetrical ultrasound,* New York, 1984, McGraw-Hill, p. 204.

100. Landers DF, Newland M, and Penny LL: Multiple uterine rupture and crushing injury to the fetal skull after blunt maternal trauma: a case report, *J Reprod Med* 34:988-993, 1989.

101. Koury HI, Peschiera JL, and Welling RE: Selective use of pelvic roentgenograms in blunt trauma patients, *J Trauma* 34:236-237, 1993.

102. Perrin RW: Radiographic demonstrations of small amounts of intra-peritoneal fluid, *Texas Med* 67:80-86, 1971.

103. Swischuk LE: Abdominal fluid collections (ascites, perotinitis, hemoperitoneum). In Swischuk LE, ed: *Emergency radiology of the acutely ill or injured child,* ed 2, Baltimore, 1986, Williams & Wilkins, pp. 175-184.

104. Fuhrman GM, et al: The single indication for cystography in blunt trauma, *Am Surg* 59:335-337, 1993.

105. Hochberg E, Stone NN: Bladder rupture associated with pelvic fractures due to blunt trauma, *Urology* 41:531-533, 1993.

106. Resnik CS, et al: Diagnosis of pelvic fractures in patients with acute pelvic trauma, *Am J Radiol* 158:109-112, 1992.

107. Dunn EL, Berry PH, and Connally JD: Computed tomography of the pelvis in patients with multiple injuries, *J Trauma* 23:378-382, 1983.

108. McIntyre RC, et al: Pelvic fracture geometry predicts risk of life-threatening hemorrhage in children, *J Trauma* 35:423-429, 1993.

109. Kane WJ: Fractures of the pelvis. In Rockwood CA Jr, Green DP, eds: *Fractures in adults,* ed 2, Philadelphia, 1984, JB Lippincott, pp. 1093-1208.

110. Keats TE: *An atlas of normal roentgen variants that may simulate disease,* ed 3, Chicago, 1984, Year Book Medical Publishers, p. 889.

111. Mayron R, et al: Tissue-fat pulmonary embolism occurring in a patient with severe pelvic fracture, *J Emerg Med* 2:251-256, 1985.

# CHAPTER 8

# The Scapula and Clavicle

*David W. Plummer*

The scapula and the clavicle, along with their associated articulations (the glenohumeral, sternoclavicular, acromioclavicular, and thoracoscapular), comprise the shoulder girdle. This complex, taken together, comprises an anatomically complicated and robust kinematic structure. This complex, which displays many degrees of freedom, is required for normal functioning of the upper extremity in humans.[1,2] Failure to detect or treat any component can result in a permanent functional deficit of the upper extremity. These deficits can be severely debilitating for patients whether they occur in the dominant or nondominant extremity and almost irrespective of the patient's expected activity of daily living. As a result, initial assessment, diagnosis, treatment, and appropriate referral are important for a functional and cosmetic outcome. This chapter covers these topics for acromioclavicular, clavicular, sternoclavicular, and scapular injuries.

## ACROMIOCLAVICULAR INJURIES

Acromioclavicular (AC) injuries are among the most common injuries of the upper extremities presenting to the emergency department. This injury, although becoming more common in women, is between five and ten times more common in men.

### Anatomy

The AC joint is formed by the articulation of the distal clavicle with the acromion process of the scapula (Fig. 8-1). This articulation comprises a diarthrodial joint, covered with a thin capsule, with articular surfaces covered with fibrocartilage and cushioned with interarticular disks. The stabilizing ligaments of the distal clavicle are the acromioclavicular and the coracoclavicular ligaments. The coracoclavicular ligament is composed of two components, the conoid and the trapezoid, and acts as the prime suspensory mechanism for the arm. Injury to the AC joint inevitably involves injury to one or both of these ligaments.

### Mechanism of injury

AC injury usually results from a direct force applied from above onto the lateral aspect of the shoulder while the arm is adducted. Rarely, AC injury results from a forward fall onto an outstretched hand. A predictable progression of injury occurs, with increased direct force applied to the lateral shoulder.[3] A small-to-moderate force stretches or ruptures the AC ligament, resulting in a stable injury. A heavier blow disrupts the coracoclavicular ligament and results in complete dislocation.[4] Seldom do AC injuries occur in isolation in children, and when they do, they are usually associated with a good outcome.[5,6]

### Physical examination

Examination of the AC joint is straightforward. The joint can be found subcutaneously and is easily inspected and palpated. When injured, it is painful and tender. The patient's discomfort will be worsened by any motion of the upper extremity. The patient often holds the ipsilateral arm in adduction across the body supported by the contralateral arm. Bringing the involved extremity into extreme adduction by placing the involved hand on a contralateral shoulder will worsen the symptoms. In more severe or higher grade AC injuries, the distal clavicle appears free-floating with superior displacement, whereas the involved ipsilateral shoulder appears depressed. Fig. 8-2 illustrates the types of AC injuries that will be described subsequently.

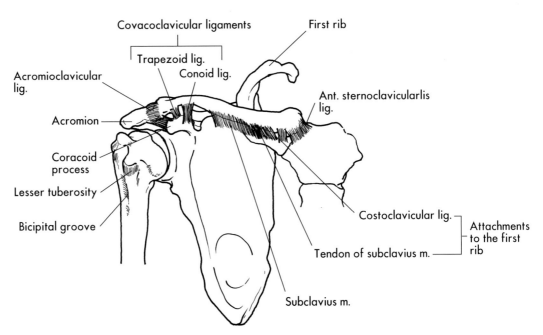

**Fig. 8-1.** Normal anatomic relationships and ligamentous attachments for the acromioclavicular and sternoclavicular joints.

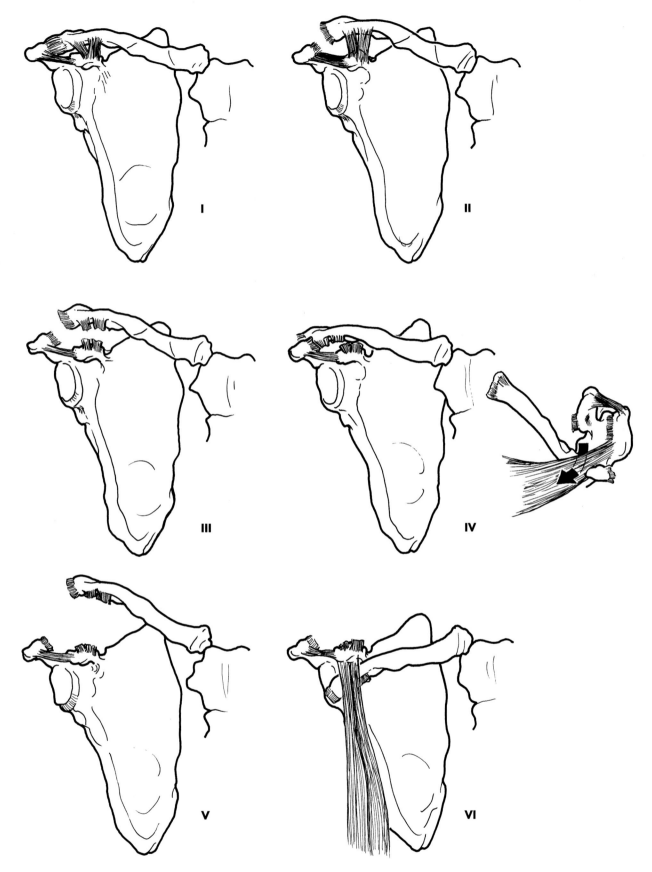

**Fig. 8-2.** Acromioclavicular injuries associated with the six types of acromioclavicular injuries. Refer to the text for complete description.

## Radiographic examination

Physicians may use a variety of radiographic techniques to assess the AC joint.[7] An adequate assessment requires a minimum of two views obtained in orthogonal planes.[8] Most commonly, this includes the standard anteroposterior (AP) and lateral views. However, because the AC joint is superimposed on the spine of the scapula in a standard AP view, the beam should have a slight superior angulation of between 15° and 30°.[9,10] These two views alone are usually sufficient to demonstrate the degree of injury to determine initial treatment. Additional views may be needed, particularly to reveal the amount of posterior displacement in type IV injuries. These additional views include the axillary view and the lateral scapula view. Historically, physicians use stress views of the injured and contralateral joint to distinguish between type II and type III injuries. Perform this by tying a gauze figure-of-eight, attached to a weight of 10 to 15 lb, around the patient's wrist. Allow the patient to stand in an upright position for a time sufficient to fatigue the shoulder girdle musculature. Obtain a simultaneous contralateral view for comparison of the AC space. Recent work suggests that this technique is insensitive and may actually mask some cases of type III injury.[11] As a result, most emergency physicians do not obtain stress radiography during the initial assessment of acromioclavicular injury.

## Radiographic variants

When assessing AC radiographs in children, be particularly careful to distinguish true AC disruption from a pseudodislocation and lateral epiphyseal injury. Pseudodislocation of the AC joint appears as a wide AC space without anatomic disruption of the AC ligament.[12] This occurs in children as a normal variant.[13] Lateral epiphyseal injury with separation may appear clinically identical to a type III AC injury. The distinction between these two are important because lateral epiphyseal fractures with displacement to this degree often require operative repair. In addition to plain radiography, many authors have reported a variety of medical imaging techniques to assess the acromioclavicular joint. These include computed tomography (CT) scan, tomography, magnetic resonance imaging (MRI), and sonography. These advanced techniques are rarely required.[14]

## Classification

Injuries to the AC joint are classified with respect to the amount of injury sustained to the AC and coracoclavicular ligaments. The physical exam and radiologic findings determine the degree of injury.

Type I injuries present with a painful, tender but stable AC joint. This injury involves a stretching but incomplete disruption of the coracoclavicular ligament. Radiographic examination is normal with less than 3-mm difference in the AC joint space when compared with the contralateral side.[11] Restrict the use of the term *acromioclavicular sprain* to this type I injury.

Type II injuries display some degree of subluxation at the AC joint. This requires that some degree of AC disruption has occurred. The coracoclavicular ligament remains intact in type II injuries. The amount of AC subluxation is less than half the diameter of the clavicle and between 3- and 5-mm difference in joint space from the normal side.[15]

Type III injuries display displacement greater than 5 mm or half the diameter of the clavicle (Figs. 8-3 and 8-4). Type III injuries are essentially the same as type II except that they display a larger degree of subluxation on presentation. This injury requires disruption of both the AC and coracoclavicular ligaments. As a result, there may be superior displacement of the distal clavicle on physical examination. The coracoclavicular disruption is usually ligamentous; it can occasionally present as a coracoid avulsion fracture.

Type IV injuries are rare and are essentially type III injuries with extreme posterior displacement of the distal clavicle (Fig. 8-5). This posterior displacement may involve penetration and entrapment of the distal end of the clavicle through the body of the trapezius.

Type V injury, which is also rare, is a type III injury with extreme superior displacement of the distal clavicle. This degree of displacement may lodge the distal clavicle as cephalad as the base of the neck.

Type VI injury is another rare injury. It involves complete disruption of the AC and coracoclavicular ligaments by extreme direct force on the lateral aspect of the clavicle resulting in inferior displacement.[16,17] The degree of inferior displacement may result in locking of the distal clavicle in the subcoracoid or subacromial space.[18,19] An *untyped* AC dislocation has been reported that involved complete AC and coracoclavicular disruption from a posteriorly applied force, resulting in an anterior displacement of the distal end of the clavicle.[20] This may require special radiographic investigation to document if it is not evident on clinical exam.

## Treatment

The optimal treatment for AC injuries is unknown, and authors continue to debate both old and new methods in the literature. The following represents a summary of treatment based on the type of AC injury.

**Type I and type II.** Most authors agree that almost all type I and type II injuries can receive nonoperative therapy. This most often entails *skillful neglect* which uses sling immobilization of the involved extremity. The sling adequately supports the arm and approximates the AC joint. Although this is adequate initial treatment for all type I and type II injuries, it is particularly good for elderly patients, sedentary patients, and injuries to the nondominant arm. Therapy should be maintained for 10 to 14 days after which the patient should be encouraged to resume normal range of motion.

Orthopedic devices include mechanisms for approximating the AC joint. The most commonly used device at this time is the Kenny Howard splint (Fig. 8-6). A disadvantage with this and similar splints is that it requires constant attention by

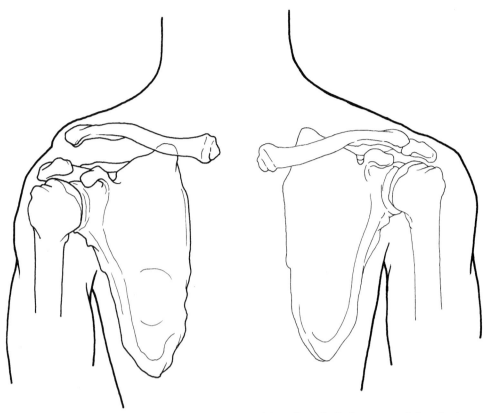

**Fig. 8-3.** Type III acromioclavicular separation with unilateral displacement of the distal clavicle superiorly.

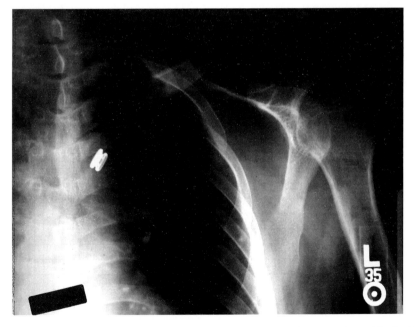

**Fig. 8-4.** This plane radiograph shows a Type III acromioclavicular separation with significant displacement of the distal clavicular head.

a reliable patient to ensure an unyielding approximation of the AC joint for weeks. In addition, overzealous patients have incurred secondary injury by ischemic necrosis of the skin on the superior aspect of the shoulder. However, in competent reliable patients receiving early orthopedic follow-up, this device may be used. Despite which of the above closed techniques is used initially, nearly all patients with type I and over 90% of patients with type II injuries recover fully.

**Types IV, V, and VI.** Most authors currently agree that AC injuries Type IV, V, and VI require immediate operative repair.[21,22,23,24,25]

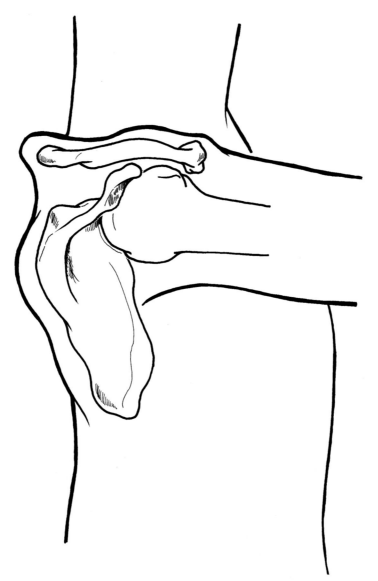

**Fig. 8-5.** Final placement of the distal clavicular head in a Type IV acromioclavicular separation markedly posterior to the normal acromioclavicular articulation.

**Type III.** The gray area that receives significant debate in the orthopedic literature involves the most appropriate treatment for Type III injuries. Some authors prefer surgical treatment of all Type III injuries.[26,27] Others advocate immediate surgical repair only if the patient is athletic or requires heavy physical exertion in their activities of daily living such as heavy laborers.[28] Others prefer to treat all Type III injuries with the conservative mechanisms outlined above and to employ operative repair only after conservative treatment fails. Surgical repair involves a variety of techniques but most commonly includes insertion of a coracoclavicular screw or plating with tension banding.[29,30]

**Special circumstances.** In addition, operative repair should be considered for patients with simultaneous distal clavicular fracture.[31] Late repair should be performed in patients who have continuous pain from the involved joint or the sensation of popping with movement of the upper extremity.

### Disposition

Discharge with appropriate referral those patients receiving closed treatment for type I and II injuries. Patients having an open injury or type IV–VI require hospital admission and surgical repair. Patients with type III benefit from orthopedic consultation.

### Prognosis

Nearly all patients with type I and over 90% of those with type II injuries recover fully. These patients should avoid heavy lifting for 8 to 12 weeks and be referred to an orthopedic surgeon. The late complications associated with AC injuries are uncommon. These include punctate calcification of the AC and coracoclavicular ligaments, resulting in an impingement syndrome of the shoulder.[32,33] In addition, a syndrome of osteolysis, or demineralization of the distal clavicle, is seen after AC injuries. This occurs after both open and closed techniques and may be due to

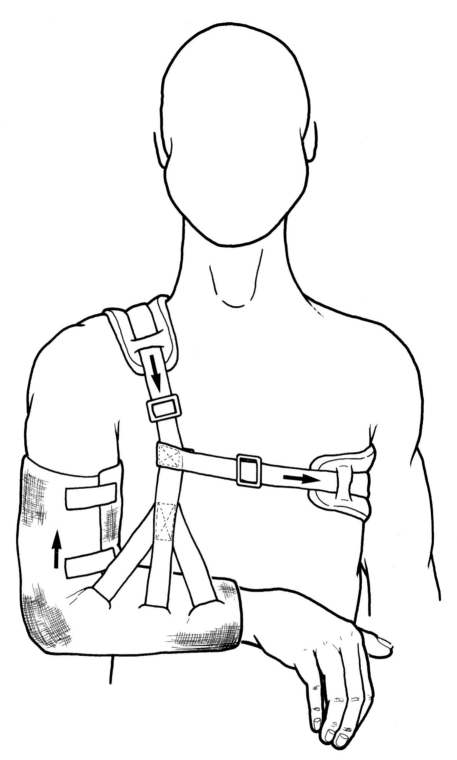

**Fig. 8-6.** Application and final position of a Kenny Howard splint used to treat unstable acromioclavicular separations.

repeated trauma.[34,35] This repeated trauma may be very minor[36] or recurrent,[37] and typically patients recall no traumatic episode.[38] This demineralization of the distal clavicle appears to occur exclusively in men; no cases in women have been reported. Other late complications include degenerative arthritis of the AC joint, which may eventually lead to a posttraumatic frozen shoulder syndrome.[39]

## Associated injuries

The same mechanism of injury most commonly responsible for AC injuries may also cause other simultaneous orthopedic injuries. The most commonly associated injuries are distal clavicular fracture[40,41,42] and acromion fractures.[43] Occasionally, an associated coracoid fracture[44,45,46,47] or even avulsion fracture of a coracoid epiphysis may occur.[48]

Patients can rarely demonstrate simultaneous luxatio erecta,[49] brachial-plexus injury[50,51] or even scapular body fractures.[45] Therefore, examine the entire shoulder girdle carefully in patients presenting with acromioclavicular injuries and supplement this examination with x-rays of any area suspicious of injury.

## CLAVICLE

Injuries to the clavicle are extremely common in emergency medicine and physicians should be well versed in clavicular anatomy, categorization of injury, and initial treatment. Fractures to the clavicle are common in all age groups. In children, clavicular fracture requires very little force and usually heals rapidly and without complication. Unfortunately, many physicians experienced in the treatment of clavicular fractures of children inappropriately apply the same principles and good prognosis to adults. In adults, clavicular fracture usually results from a much greater proportional force, is more often associated with other injuries, and is more likely to heal with complication.

### Anatomy

The clavicle is essentially a tubular strut with flattened ends that supplies anterior support for the breadth of the shoulder. This strut is S-shaped, with a majority of its curvature confined to the middle one third of the clavicle. The clavicle is secured laterally by the coracoclavicular and AC ligaments, as described above, and is secured medially at the sternoclavicular joint by the sternoclavicular ligament and costoclavicular ligaments (Fig. 8-1). Biomechanical analysis of the clavicle reveals its weakest portion is the middle one-third, which is susceptible to forces applied either perpendicular to the axis of the clavicle or an axial load.[52] Because of its function in supporting the breadth of the shoulder, fractures of the clavicle allow the shoulder to slump forward and downward. Muscles inserted into the clavicle include the sternocleidomastoid and the subclavius, which both play roles in the direction and degree of displacement of fragments in clavicular fractures. In addition to these structures, physicians should be aware that the subclavian neurovascular bundle lies immediately posterior to the clavicle.

### Mechanism of injury

The mechanism of injury of clavicular fractures was commonly believed to be a fall on an outstretched hand.[53] However, recent work, supported by both clinical studies and biomechanical models, indicates that the most common mechanism of injury is via a direct blow (94%), a fall on a outstretched hand being much less common.[54] Factors predisposing to clavicular injury include an active lifestyle, particularly participation in contact sports. Competitive weight-lifting and body training predispose to clavicular fracture caused by distal clavicular osteolysis with demineralization.[35] Medical conditions predisposing to clavicular fracture include osteopenia[55] as well as uncontrolled seizure disorder.[56]

### Physical examination

Examination of the clavicle is straightforward. The clavicle runs a subcutaneous course throughout its entire length and is easily inspected and palpated because there are no muscular attachments on its anterior surface. Clavicular injury is usually made apparent by localized swelling, pain, and tenderness. In addition, the shoulder may appear in a downward presentation and the patient often holds the ipsilateral arm in adduction supported by the contralateral arm. Examination of the clavicle is not complete without evaluation of the neurovascular status of the upper extremity.[57]

### Classification

Clavicular fractures are categorized according to which anatomic segment of the clavicle sustains the fracture.[58]

**Middle one-third fractures.** Fractures in the middle one third of the clavicle comprise 80% of all clavicular fractures[59] (Fig. 8-7). These fractures may be subdivided further into fractures that are undisplaced (type I) and those that are displaced (type II). The proximal fragment in type II clavicular injuries displays a superior displacement caused by the pull of the sternocleidomastoid muscle.

**Lateral one-third fractures.** Lateral clavicular fractures comprise 10% of clavicular injuries (Fig. 8-8). These lateral fractures also occur most commonly as a result of direct force[60] and are more likely to require operative repair. They may also be subdivided in the following manner. Type I injuries occur lateral to the coracoclavicular ligament. They present with no instability about the shoulder girdle and can be treated conservatively (Fig. 8-9). Type II fractures occur medial to the coracoclavicular ligament. These are unstable, have a high incidence of nonunion,[61] and may require operative stabilization. The distinction between type I and type II distal clavicular fractures may require weighted radiographic examination. As mentioned previously, however, these stress radiographic studies are not sensitive and may mask more serious injury.[11] Additional radiographic techniques are outlined below.

### Radiographic examination

Radiographic examination for clavicular injury requires at least two views, taken preferably from orthogonal planes. Routine AP and lateral films are generally sufficient to detect most fractures; however, some fractures are easily missed by these views.[62] In addition, it may be difficult to distinguish a fracture from other radiographic findings such as congenital pseudoarthrosis,[63,64,65,66] lateral epiphyseal injury,[67] and the unilateral *wavy clavicle syndrome*.[68] Various other views may be taken to help delineate the nature of the clavicular injury. The scapular plane view should help

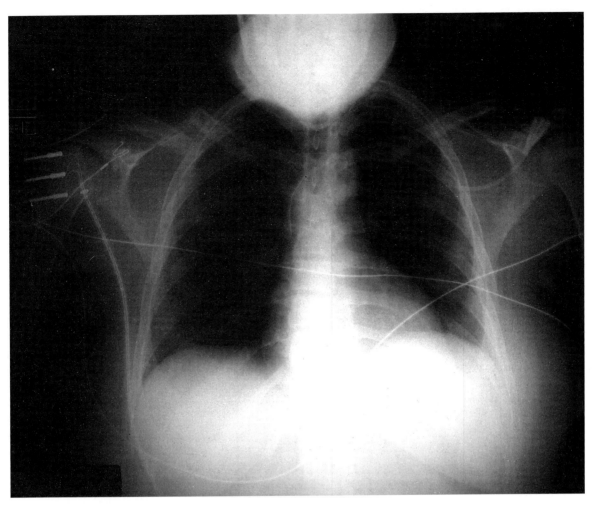

**Fig. 8-7.** This radiograph demonstrates a clavicular fracture in the medial one-third of the shaft. Note the superior displacement of the proximal fragment.

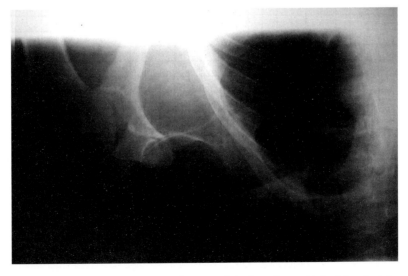

**Fig. 8-8.** Radiography shows a displaced fracture of the lateral one-third of the clavicle.

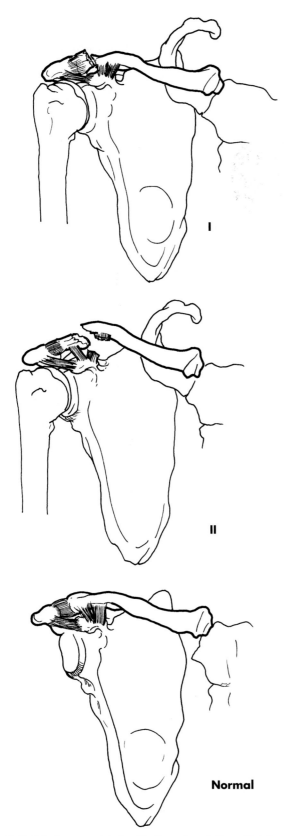

I

II

**Normal**

**Fig. 8-9.** Injuries associated with Type I and Type II lateral clavicular fractures. Note the relationship of the fracture line to the coral clavicular ligament. See the text for a complete description.

assess the degree of displacement in any anterior or posterior displaced fragments. The abduction lordotic view[69] and the apical oblique view[70,71,72] are particularly useful in assessing the medial third of the clavicle. They aid in detecting nondisplaced fractures of a clavicle and, as a single view, may be the most helpful screening test for the detection of clavicular fracture.

### Associated injuries

Many injuries have been associated with clavicular fracture. These result from an extension of the force that initially caused the injury. They are multiple and, occasionally, life-threatening. Because many patients who suffer clavicular fractures have sustained a high-energy impact, the physician must not focus immediately on treatment of the clavicular fracture before considering other injuries. Although many of these injuries are uncommon, failure to recognize them may result in catastrophic outcomes. The physician should seek evidence of pneumothorax, either from blunt trauma or as a result of penetration by the clavicular fracture.[73,74] The close proximity of the neurovascular bundle to the clavicle renders it susceptible to injury during clavicular fracture. Specifically, laceration of the subclavian artery[75] and compression of the subclavian vein,[76] with or without thrombosis,[77,78] have all been reported. Historically, the presence of a clavicular fracture in a patient with altered mental status prompted a search for an occult cervical spine and spinal cord injuries. However, recent work has refuted the association between clavicular injury and cervical spine injury.[79] Medial clavicular fractures presenting with large degrees of displacement have been associated with tracheal disruptions and lacerations[80,81] Clavicular fractures, especially those of the middle third, have reportedly caused both pacemaker malfunction as a result of lead fracture[82,83,84] as well as fracture of ipsilaterally placed infusion catheters.[85] Thus, medical devices implanted on the ipsilateral side require assessment of function prior to patient discharge. Patients sustaining clavicular fracture from seat-belt injuries during high-speed motor vehicle accidents may display one of several immediately life-threatening injuries, including laryngeal fracture, cervical spine or thoracic spine and interthoracic injuries.[86] These patients must be examined fully and carefully before concentrating on the clavicular fracture. Rarely, isolated clavicular fracture causes delayed cardiac arrest, which is currently believed to be secondary to vagal irritation from the developing hematoma.[87] This is an extremely rare complication and has virtually no identifiable risk factors. Finally, the examining physician must be aware that clavicular fractures in children may be the only presenting sign of otherwise occult child abuse.[88] When identified, this abuse may be overt physical abuse to the child but is more commonly a result of unintentional abuse such as repeated exposure to inappropriate rough play or, rarely, inappropriate manipulation by a chiropractor.[89,90]

Many other orthopedic injuries have been associated with clavicular fractures. These injuries, although generally not immediately life-threatening, require recognition for appropriate therapy. Of these, one of the most interesting and least recognized has been called the *costoclavicular outlet syndrome* or the posttraumatic *thoracic outlet syndrome*.[91,92,93,94,95] This syndrome results from compression of the structures immediately posterior to the clavicle, between it and the first rib. This compressive injury can result from either the direct force during clavicular fracture, the impingement caused by a hypertrophic callus formation during healing,[96,97] or during the late contraction of scar tissue around the neurovascular bundles.[98] Ironically, the standard figure-of-eight treatment for clavicular fractures may contribute to the development of this thoracic outlet syndrome.[99,100,101]

This syndrome most commonly presents as the highly variable neuropathy associated with brachial plexus injury.[102,103,104] Clavicular fractures may also be associated with AC dislocation,[40,41,42] sternoclavicular dislocation,[105,106] and luxatio erecta, or inferior dislocation of the shoulder.[49,107] Physicians must specifically seek evidence of this injury since distal clavicular fracture may mask the typical findings in shoulder dislocation. Rarely, when higher degrees of injury are responsible for the clavicular fracture, the fracture may be associated with ipsilateral fracture of the scapula.[108] This associated injury constitutes a double instability of the shoulder and requires open fixation (Figs. 8-10 and 8-11).[109] Also, clavicular injury may be associated occasionally with immediate or late peripheral neuropathy.[110,111]

## Treatment

Treatment of clavicular fractures in children is relatively straightforward and may require nothing more than either a sling or a figure-of-eight dressing. Treatment in the adult is considerably more complicated for two reasons: 1) over two-hundred published different methods exist for the closed treatment of clavicular fractures; and 2) despite this abundance of different closed treatment techniques, there continues to be a relatively high rate of late complication with treatment of adult clavicular fractures.

**Treatment of middle one-third fractures.** Most physicians initially treat fractures involving the middle third with either a figure-of-eight dressing or a simple sling, with or without a swath. Recent work indicates that patients experience fewer complications and less pain wearing a simple sling.[99] In addition, there is no difference between the two techniques in the time required to heal,[112] and most authors now advocate the use of simple sling alone.[113]

**Treatment of lateral one-third fractures.** Treatment strategies are more controversial for adults sustaining fractures of the lateral one-third of the clavicle. Prospective studies indicate that conservative treatment is adequate with the majority of patients remaining asymptomatic after 15

years.[114,115] However, other authors currently advocate the routine open treatment of lateral unstable fractures.[116,117]

**Treatment of medial one-third fractures.** Fractures of the medial one third of the clavicle may also be treated conservatively but must be distinguished from medial epiphyseal fractures which may require open fixation.[118] There are many techniques described for the open treatment of clavicular fractures.[119,120,121]

**Special circumstances.** Consider open treatment for patients sustaining open fracture,[122] irreducible fractures that, due to soft-tissue interposition[60,123] are unstable,[124] or in patients who are for any reason unable to tolerate prolonged conservative therapy.[119] In addition, patients sustaining multiple fractures are much more likely to require open fixation. These include patients presenting with ipsilateral arm fracture, bilateral clavicular fractures, simultaneous proximal and distal fracture,[125] multifragmented clavicular fractures,[126,127] ipsilateral glenoid neck fracture,[128] or ipsilateral scapular fracture (Figs 8-10 and 8-11).[109] Clavicular fracture that presents simultaneously with AC separation,[41,31,117,129] or ipsilateral sternoclavicular dislocation[105] also requires open reduction. Patients sustaining brachial plexopathy[129,130] or nonunion of the shaft[94,131,132] also benefit from open reduction. Many authors report good outcome with open surgical techniques of the clavicle despite the high rate of associated injuries.[133]

## Disposition

Patients sustaining closed injuries and requiring conservative treatment may be discharged with early appropriate follow-up care. Patients with open fractures or associated injury require consultation and hospital admission.

## Prognosis

Complications of clavicular fracture are relatively rare in children and more common in adults.[134] These include malunion and nonunion (most commonly seen in the adult), degenerative arthritis (most commonly seen with lateral fractures) and, rarely, reflex sympathetic dystrophy of the involved extremity.[135]

## STERNOCLAVICULAR JOINT
### Anatomy

The sternoclavicular joint is formed by the articulation of the medial aspect of the clavicle and the manubrial portion of the sternum. This articulation is a diarthrodial joint and is supported by the sternoclavicular, costal clavicular, and capsular ligaments. Although the clavicle is the first bone in the human to ossify (accounting for its relatively high rate of fracture at birth), its medial epiphysis is the last in the body to close. The medial clavicular epiphysis does not close until the third decade of life, and injuries to this medial epiphyseal plate must be distinguished from sternoclavicular injuries. The sternoclavicular joint acts like a ball and socket mechanism and, therefore, moves in virtually all

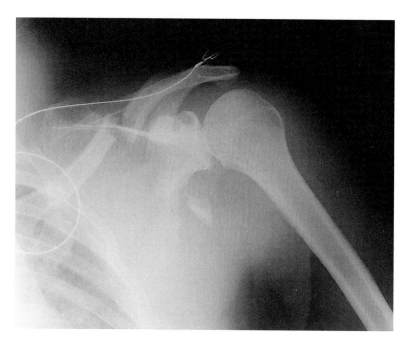

**Fig. 8-10.** This radiograph demonstrates concomitant fracture of the middle one-third of the clavicle and fracture of the neck of the scapula (Type C).

planes, including rotation, around the long axis of the clavicle. It is one of the most frequently used joints in the human body because almost any movement in the upper extremity requires movement at the sternoclavicular joint.

## Mechanism of injury

Injury to the sternoclavicular joint is uncommon, accounting for only 1.5% of all dislocations[136] primarily because of the large force required to cause sternoclavicular dislocation (Fig. 8-12). The most common mechanisms of injury are the high-speed motor vehicle accidents, followed by injuries incurred in contact sports. When this large force is applied directly to the medial clavicle, the dislocated medial end of the clavicle lies posterior to the plane of the sternum. When the force is applied to the lateral aspect of the shoulder, the final position of the medial clavicular head depends on the direction of rotation of the scapula on the thorax. When the scapula rotates anteriorly on the thoracic wall during the application of lateral force, a dislocation at the sternoclavicular joint results in a posterior position of the medial clavicular head (Fig. 8-13). Alternatively, if the scapula rotates posteriorly on the thoracic wall during the application of lateral force, the resulting dislocation will demonstrate an anterior position of the medial clavicular head.

## Classification

Sternoclavicular dislocations can be categorized according to the degree of damage incurred by the supporting ligaments and the final position of the medial clavicular head.

**First-degree sternoclavicular dislocation.** A first-degree sternoclavicular dislocations is incomplete. Ana-

tomically, it demonstrates a stretching without disruption of the supporting ligamentous complex, resulting in a stable injury.

**Second-degree sternoclavicular dislocation.** A second-degree sternoclavicular dislocation demonstrates some subluxation of the medial clavicular head. Anatomically, this injury requires rupture of the sternoclavicular ligament and is unstable.

**Third-degree sternoclavicular dislocation.** A third-degree sternoclavicular dislocation is a complete dislocation. Anatomically, this injury requires a rupture of both the sternoclavicular and costoclavicular ligaments, resulting in gross displacement of the medial clavicular head to either the anterior or posterior plane of the sternum (Fig. 8-12). These are both unstable injuries. The medial clavicular head will lie in the anterior plane in almost 90% of cases and in the posterior plane in approximately 13% of the presentations.[137]

## Physical examination

Examination of the sternoclavicular joint is straightforward. The normal joint can be palpated immediately lateral to the suprasternal notch. The clavicle extends slightly superior to the manubrial component of the sternum. Patients with injuries to this joint frequently present holding the ipsilateral arm across the trunk supported by the contralateral arm. There will be pain at the joint with almost any motion at the glenohumeral joint. The patient will demonstrate direct tenderness over the sternoclavicular joint and this will be exacerbated on the application of a lateral-to-medial force on the humeral head. In addition, the affected shoulder may appear shortened and in a downward displacement.

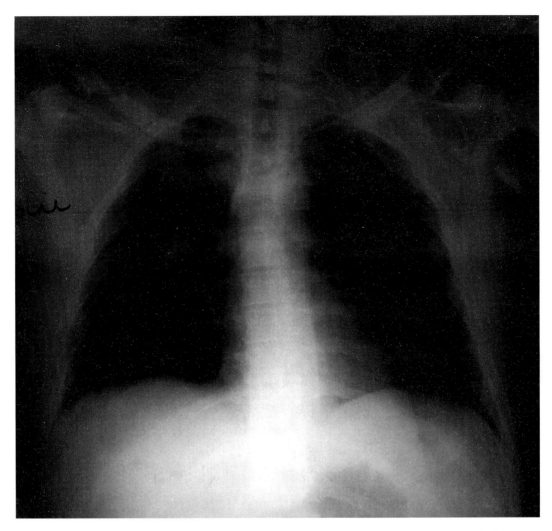

**Fig. 8-11.** This radiograph reveals bilateral closed fractures of the middle one-third of the clavicle associated with concomitant fracture of the neck of the scapula on the left (Type C).

Patients with an anterior sternoclavicular dislocation will have a palpable mass anterior to the plane of the sternum over the sternoclavicular joint caused by the dislocated medial clavicular head. Patients with a posterior dislocation may present with a more confusing physical examination. Because of the swelling that occurs at the joint with this injury, true posterior dislocations may also present with a mass anterior to the plane of the sternum that masquerades as an anterior dislocation. It is critical to avoid making the final diagnosis on physical examination alone because of the high association between posterior sternoclavicular dislocations and mediastinal damage.

### Radiographic examination

The radiographic examination of the sternoclavicular joint is difficult to interpret.[138] This examination includes views taken from two orthogonal planes[8] and begins with the standard AP and lateral techniques described above. However, because of the density of the superimposed mediastinal structures, these standard views are particularly difficult to

interpret. Additional special views have been developed and used by several authors to help rectify this. Each of these views attempts to image the sternoclavicular joint using a beam orientation approaching the coronal plane. This allows for a more accurate determination of the final position of the medial clavicular head. Of these, the views of Hobbs,[139] which includes a modified PA with a cephalocaudal tilt and a serendipitous view that utilizes a modified AP with a 40° cephalic tilt, appear to be adequate for this purpose. Additional views, as suggested by Heinig and Kattan, may also be required.[136] When interpreting plane radiographic studies, it is important to distinguish between dislocation about the sternoclavicular joint from displaced epiphyseal fracture of the medial clavicle.[140,141] Occasionally, accurate diagnosis requires other special medical imaging techniques. These include CT scans, tomography, or MRI of the sternoclavicular joint.

### Associated injuries

Although sternoclavicular dislocations occur in isolation in 41% of patients[137] a number of other associated injuries

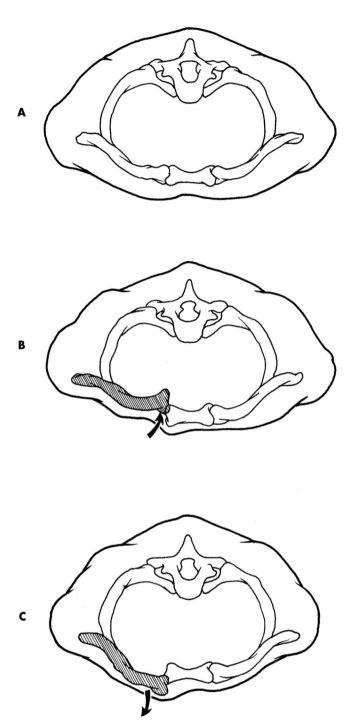

**Fig. 8-12.** The sternoclavicular relationship in a thoracic cross-sectional view: **A,** Normal anatomy; **B,** The relationship with a posterior dislocation of the sternoclavicular joint; and **C,** The final position of the clavicular head and anterior dislocation of the sternoclavicular joint. Please see the text for a complete description.

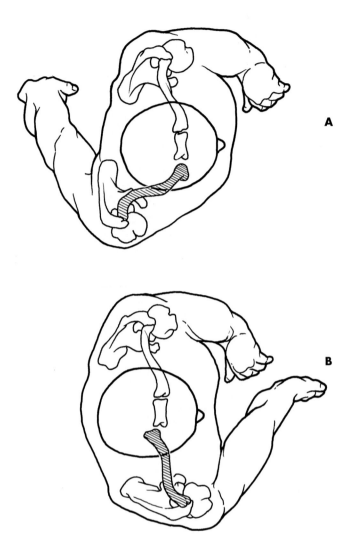

**Fig. 8-13.** The final position of the medial clavicular head and sternoclavicular dislocation depends on the position of the arm at the time of injury. **A,** When the arm is outstretched behind the patient at the time of injury, the dislocation is more likely anterior; **B,** When the arm is outstretched in the forward position at the time of injury, the dislocation is most likely posterior.

have been reported. These injuries generally fall into two categories: those that are immediately life-threatening and due exclusively to posterior dislocation of the sternoclavicular joint, and those that are not immediately life-threatening. Life-threatening injuries from posterior dislocations include major vascular injury,[142] esophageal injury,[143] tracheal injury,[143] and brachial plexus injury.[144] Associated orthopedic injuries include clavicular fracture[105] that requires surgical repair. A variety of scapular fractures are also associated with sternoclavicular dislocations and may be seen in as many as 55% of these patients.[137]

## Treatment

Treatment of the sternoclavicular injuries is dependent on the degree of injury. First-degree injury requires only the application of ice and a sling to the ipsilateral upper extremity. Encourage early mobilization with range-of-motion (ROM), particularly for elderly patients. Refer these patients to an orthopedic surgeon.

Second-degree injuries require treatment similar to first-degree injuries, except that their immobilization includes either a figure-of-eight dressing along with a sling or a sling and swath.

Although some authors advocate treating all third-degree sternoclavicular dislocations surgically,[136] most initially apply closed techniques.[137] The maneuver used for closed reduction is the same for both posterior and anterior dislocations of the sternoclavicular joint. The patient lies supine with the arm abducted while the physician applies lateral traction to the arm. In anterior dislocations, the medial clavicle may require direct force applied in a posterior direction to aid relocation. Occasionally, in patients with posterior dislocations, additional lateral traction must be supplied directly to the clavicle in order to obtain reduction. Accomplish this by using sterile technique to prepare the midshaft of the clavicle and encircle the cortical bone of the midshaft of the clavicle with a sterile towel clip. This provides a rigid handle to achieve additional lateral traction. After reduction, apply a figure-of-eight splint and sling or a sling and swath.

### Disposition

Patients with closed first- or second-degree dislocations or closed, anterior third-degree dislocations may be discharged after treatment with early follow-up. All open dislocation or any posterior one-third dislocation requires consultation.

### Miscellaneous sternoclavicular abnormalities

Miscellaneous sternoclavicular abnormalities may present clinically as sternoclavicular dislocations. However, any condition that results in an inflammation of the sternoclavicular joint in the absence of a good history may mimic sternoclavicular dislocation. The most commonly seen abnormality seen in the emergency department is osteomyelitis of the medial clavicular head. The physician must consider this etiology in any patient presenting with pain, swelling, and erythema of the sternoclavicular area.[145] This abnormality is particularly common in IV drug abusers.[146,147] Radiographic assessment of patients with osteomyelitis of the sternoclavicular area reveals either periosteal elevation, osteolytic lesions with markedly irregular borders and, occasionally, hypersclerotic lesions in cases of chronic osteomyelitis.[148] This distinction from sternoclavicular joint injury is important because the treatment of choice is surgical debridement and IV antibiotic therapy.

## SCAPULA
### Anatomy

The scapula is an integral part of the kinematic function of the shoulder. Situated on the superior lateral aspect of the posterior thorax, it is relatively protected from injury due to its relationships with the surrounding thick musculature (supraspinatus, infraspinatus, and subscapularis muscles). Anatomically, the scapula includes a body (the larger triangular component), a spine (the nearly horizontal linear posterior projection), the neck, the acromion, and the coracoid. The most common scapular injury is the scapular fracture although rarer injuries may occur.

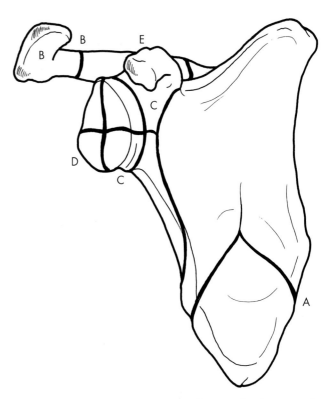

**Fig. 8-14.** The classification system for scapular fractures. **A,** Fracture extending through the scapular body. **B,** Fracture extending through the acromion. **C,** Fracture of the scapular neck. **D,** Fracture of the glenard fossa. **E,** Fracture of the coracoid. Please see the text for a complete description.

### Scapular fractures

Scapular fractures belong to one of five distinct classes (Fig. 8-14): scapular body fractures, acromion fractures, scapular neck fractures, glenoid fossa, and coracoid process fractures.

**Scapular body fractures.** Fractures of the scapular body are fortunately rare, accounting for only 1% of all fractures presenting to emergency departments.[149,150] These fractures are generally seen in patients between 40 and 60 years of age sustaining high-energy impact.

*Mechanism of injury.* Scapular body fractures occur most commonly from a direct blow. This usually results from motor vehicle accidents[151,152] and has also been seen in players of high-impact sports, such as professional football players.[153] Scapular body fractures also result from a variety of unusual mechanisms of injury. Scapular fractures have also occurred as a result of electrical shock;[154,155,156,157] some of these have been bilateral.[158,159,160] Patients suffering from generalized tonic-clonic seizures may suffer a relatively occult scapular body fracture.[161,162,163,164] Avulsion mechanisms may account for the remainder of scapular body fractures. These avulsion fractures are not commonly associated with other life-threatening injuries and appear to result from a variety of causes. Water-skiing,[165] jogging with weighted wristbands,[166] and wheelchair racing[167] all may cause avulsion

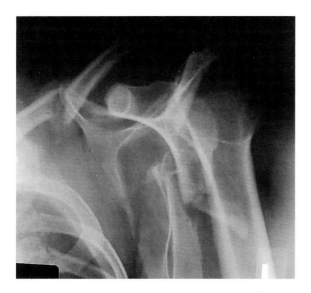

**Fig. 8-15.** A transscapular radiograph of a patient with a scapular body fracture (Type A).

fractures of the medial aspect of the scapular body. Rarely, avulsion mechanisms occur elsewhere on the scapular body,[168,169,170,171] including the superior margin.[172] These avulsion mechanisms are more common in patients suffering from osteoporosis or in those who have received radiation therapy.[173]

*Physical examination.* Examination of the scapular body is relatively straightforward. The scapula at rest extends from the spinous process, located approximately at T-2, to the apex, located at approximately T-7. The entire margin of the scapular body can be easily palpated. Fractures of the scapular body are difficult to palpate directly due to the thick overlying supraspinatus and infraspinatus musculature.

*Radiographic examination.* Proper diagnosis of scapular fracture requires adequate radiographic imaging. This imaging must be undertaken in at least two orthogenic planes. The traditional AP and transscapular views are the most commonly used views and are usually sufficient. Remember that standard AP chest x-rays reveal approximately half of all scapular body fractures.[174] The transscapular view is probably the most helpful single view[174,175] (Fig. 8-15). Additional views may be obtained if these standard two views are suggestive but not diagnostic. The most commonly used additional plane radiographic view is the apical oblique view.[70] A CT scan may be required when the suspicion for fracture is high, and standard radiographs are not diagnostic.[108]

*Treatment.* Most authors advocate closed, conservative treatment for fractures of the scapular body,[129,176,177]; however, recent work suggests that a more aggressive approach may result in better outcomes.[178] Simple shoulder immobilization with a sling and swath dressing is appropriate for a patient receiving closed, conservative therapy. Pay particular attention to adequate pain control which may

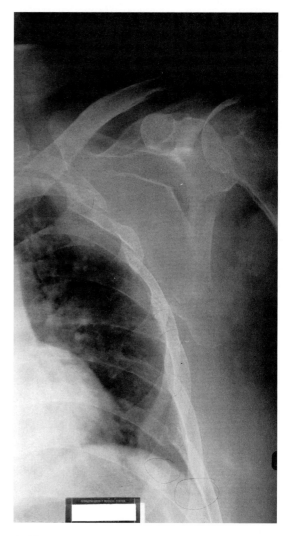

**Fig. 8-16.** Radiograph image demonstrates a displaced fracture of the scapular body (Type A) associated with ipsilateral rib fractures.

require suprascapular nerve block. Although conservative closed management is adequate for most patients, many authors advocate open reduction for a variety of presentations. However, open reduction yields a relatively high complication rate.[179] Fracture fragments that have undergone a large degree of displacement, simultaneous fracture of the clavicle, or neurovascular complications, require open reduction and fixation.[180] Some authors advocate open reduction for patients presenting with simultaneous AC separation.[45] Recently, authors advocating a more aggressive approach raised controversy regarding which type of scapular fractures are best treated in an open manner.[181,182,183] Consider open plating of scapular fractures presenting in young active patients with large degrees of displacement of the fracture fragments.[184]

*Associated injuries.* A number of injuries are associated with scapular fractures. Some of these injuries are life-threatening and result from the same high-energy mechanism that causes the scapular body fracture.[185] Pneumothorax is the most commonly associated injury,[176,186] and may be seen in as many as 45% of all patients undergoing serial chest x-ray.[187] The chest x-ray reveals hemopneumothorax in as many as 16% of patients with scapular body fractures.[152] Fig. 8-16 reveals multiple rib fractures in a patient with a type A scapular fracture. Almost 25% of patients presenting with scapular body fracture have a concomitant skull fracture,[152] with an associated cerebral contusion in approximately 20%. Injuries to the immediate surrounding structures may be multiple. Subclavian artery laceration,[188] lung contusion,[176] and rib fracture,[186] have all been described. Vertebral fracture with spinal cord injury is also associated with scapular fractures[189] and usually as thoracic spine fractures.[190] These varied, associated life-threatening injuries help explain the unusually high mortality rate of 10% in patients presenting with scapular body fractures.[191] Additionally, the physician must keep in mind that scapular body fractures presenting in children may be the only evidence of child abuse.[192]

There are also many orthopedic injuries that are associated with scapular body fractures. An ipsilateral fracture of the clavicle may be seen which constitutes a double instability of the shoulder[108] and requires open fixation.[109] Shoulder dislocations, in particular luxatio erecta, have been associated with this injury.[49] Other fractures around the shoulder joint itself associated with scapular body fractures include fracture of the coracoid[193] and ipsilateral proximal humeral fracture.[194] Rarely, a compartment syndrome develops about the infraspinatus muscle.[195] Fracture displacement may cause entrapment of the suprascapular nerve,[196,197] which results in deep, poorly localized pain and weakness of the supraspinatus and infraspinatus musculature.[198] Fragment displacement may also cause paralysis of the dorsal nerve of the scapula[199] resulting in paralysis of the rhomboids and levator scapulae muscles. Also, sternoclavicular dislocation has been reported with scapular body fracture.[137] The most common late complication of scapular fracture is nonunion, resulting in what is known as a "snapping scapula."[200]

**Acromion fractures.** Fracture of the acromion constitutes a Class B fracture of the scapula (Figure 8-14). The mechanism of injury in acromion fracture is usually due to a direct blow, although it rarely occurs as a result of a stress fracture,[201] or avulsion mechanism.[202] Acromion fractures, when isolated, are more common in children[203] and may occur as a result of superior dislocation of the shoulder.

*Physical examination.* The examination of the acromion is straightforward. Locate the acromion by palpating the clavicle and following it distally to the union at the AC joint. Alternatively, follow the spine of the scapula laterally to its end point at the AC joint. Patients with a fractured acromion complain of pain and tenderness over the acromial region. Active flexion of the ipsilateral elbow recruits the biceps and exacerbates the pain. Additionally, child abuse occasionally presents with fractures of the acromion as the only physical sign.[204]

*Radiographic examination.* Radiographic examination of the acromion requires the two orthogonal views and begins with the standard AP and lateral techniques described above. Acromial fractures should be distinguished from an os acromiale, which is a rare finding.[205]

*Treatment.* Treatment of acromial fractures usually includes conservative management with immobilization of the ipsilateral extremity in a sling and swath dressing.[43,206] Consider surgical fixation in patients who demonstrate large displacement of the fracture fragments. Complications of acromial fracture include restricted ROM due to loss of the acromial space with inferior displacement and pseudoarthrosis, which is rare and requires late surgical repair.[207]

*Associated injuries.* Injuries associated with acromial fracture are fortunately rare, and include AC dislocation,[43] luxatio erecta,[49] and axillary nerve deficit.[208]

**Scapular neck.** Fractures of the scapula neck constitute Class C scapular fractures (Fig. 8-14). These fractures are uncommon and usually result from an extreme lateral-to-medial force applied over the humeral head (Fig. 8-10).

*Physical examination.* Patients present with the ipsilateral arm adducted and supported by the contralateral arm. Medial pressure over the humeral head worsens the patient's symptoms.

*Treatment.* Treatment of scapular neck fractures is straightforward. Conservative treatment begins with immobilization of the ipsilateral extremity with ROM exercises beginning in 48 hours.[209] Consider open treatment for patients displaying marked displacement of the fracture fragments,[210] or when the fracture extends intra-articularly.[211,212,213] Complications of scapular neck fractures include restrictive range-of-motion and degenerative arthritis.

*Disposition.* Patients with closed injury requiring only immobilization may be discharged home with early follow-up care. Open injury or injury requiring open treatment require consultation.

*Associated injuries.* Injuries associated with glenoid neck fractures include proximal humeral fractures and shoulder dislocations, but axillary artery laceration has also been reported.[214]

**Glenoid fossa.** Fractures involving the glenoid fossa constitute Class D type scapular fractures (Fig. 8-14). These fractures can be of two types. Type I includes a fracture of the glenoid rim only, which can be extremely difficult to diagnose radiographically.[215] A type II fracture involves a single or comminuted fracture of the glenoid fossa itself.

*Mechanism of injury.* Class D fractures usually result from a direct blow exerted from a lateral-to-medial orientation on the humeral head. Occasionally, Class D fractures result from falls onto a flexed elbow or extreme triceps contraction resulting in inferior rim avulsion.

*Radiographic examination.* The radiographic examination for Class D fractures begins with the standard AP and transscapular views described above. Additionally, the posterior oblique view occasionally demonstrates fractures not apparent on either the AP or transscapular view.[71]

*Treatment.* Treatment of Class D fractures is straightforward. Patients with undisplaced fractures undergo a conservative immobilization of the ipsilateral extremity with early ROM exercises. Consider surgical treatment for open fractures, highly comminuted intra-articular fractures,[211,212,213] or fractures with marked displacement of the fragments.

**Coracoid process fractures.** Fractures of the coracoid process constitute Class E fractures of the scapula[206] (Fig. 8-14). Class E fractures occurring in isolation are relatively rare,[43,216,217] but these isolated injuries do appear more commonly in children.[203] The coracoid process supports muscular insertions for the coracobrachiales, the short head of the biceps, and the pectoralis minor, as well as the ligamentous origins for the coracoacromial, coracoclavicular, and coracohumeral ligaments.

*Physical examination.* Examination of the coracoid process is more difficult than examination of the acromion process. The coracoid may be palpated approximately 2.5 cm below the junction of the lateral one third and the medial two thirds of the clavicle. Patients with coracoid fractures will have pain and tenderness over this area and will demonstrate these symptoms with adduction, flexion of the ipsilateral elbow, and supination of the forearm. The mechanism of injury to the coracoid is usually by direct blow,[218] but also results from a fall to the ipsilateral elbow,[218] avulsion mechanism,[171,219] or by stress fracture.[220]

*Radiographic examination.* Radiographic examination of coracoid injury begins with the standard AP and transscapular views outlined above. Occasionally, additional views such as the posterior cephalad angulation view may be required to visualize otherwise occult fractures.[221]

*Treatment.* Treatment of coracoid fractures begins conservatively by immobilizing the ipsilateral extremity. This can be accomplished using the shoulder immobilizer or a sling and swath dressing. Consider open treatment if there is significant ipsilateral orthopedic injury, particularly clavicular fracture or shoulder dislocation,[222] open fractures, or fractures with marked displacement of fragments.

*Associated injuries.* Injuries associated with coracoid fractures are generally orthopedic in nature. Among these, ipsilateral AC separation is the most common.[44,46,223,224,225,226] Ipsilateral shoulder dislocation may also occur[222,227,228] and, specifically, luxatio erecta.[229] Occasionally, ipsilateral clavicular fracture can be seen[230,216] which may require open repair.

*Disposition.* Patients with uncomplicated closed injury may be discharged with early orthopedic follow-up. Patients with open fracture or fracture with associated injury require consultation.

**Miscellaneous scapular abnormalities.**

*Dislocation of the scapula.* Dislocation of the scapula is a rare injury[231] that results from a backwards fall onto an outstretched arm.[232] This mechanism may result in a *locked scapula*[233] where the scapular tip is locked into the intercostal space.[234]

*Physical examination.* The physical examination reveals marked resistance to active and passive motion of the ipsilateral arm. Tenderness is exacerbated by lateral-to-medial pressure on either the humeral head or scapular body.

*Radiographic examination.* Radiographic examination my reveal an intercostal location of the scapular tip.

*Treatment.* Treatment of this type of scapular dislocation requires unlocking the scapula by applying traction to the hyperabducted arm, followed by immobilization of the ipsilateral upper extremity. Specifically, seek evidence for significant associated injuries including rib fracture and pneumothorax.

*Scapular thoracic disassociation.* Scapular thoracic disassociation[235,236,237,238,239,240] is a rare orthopedic injury. It almost always results from an extremely high-energy motor vehicle accident and is the forerunner of traumatic four-quarter amputation.[241,242] Although this injury most frequently presents with simultaneous multiple trauma, it may present as an isolated injury.[243]

*Radiographic examination.* Radiographic examination begins with the standard AP and lateral x-rays described above. These reveal a lateral displacement of the entire scapula when visualized in the AP projection.[243]

*Treatment and disposition.* This injury is always associated with significant surrounding soft-tissue disruption and with significant neurovascular damage.[244,245] As a result, this injury mandates arteriography.[246] Do not treat this injury in the emergency department. Instead, resuscitate the patient and consult with a trauma surgeon.

*Scapular osteomyelitis.* Scapular osteomyelitis is extremely rare. It is very difficult to diagnose because of the significant soft-tissue encasement of the scapula with thick muscular bodies. These overlying structures obscure the physical findings of erythema and inflammation. Generalized immunosuppression or IV drug abuse may predispose to this illness, and scapular osteomyelitis, when missed, has resulted in fatal dissemination.[247]

*Scapular winging.* Patients occasionally present to the emergency department with complaints of scapular winging.[248,249,250,251]

*Physical examination.* The patient demonstrates winging of the scapula which is exacerbated when the patient leans forward against a wall with outstretched arms. This injury is usually nontender.

*Mechanism.* Scapular winging invariably results from injury to the long thoracic nerve. This injury may be minor and may go relatively unnoticed,[252] or may be the result of low-energy repetitive injury such as scapular winging that is seen in competitive archers.[253] This injury has also been associated with the posttraumatic phase of shoulder dislocation[254] or from the result of a direct blow to the top of the shoulder with downward traction of the arm.[255]

*Treatment.* Treatment of scapular winging involves surgical repair and requires referral to an appropriate surgeon.[256]

## DISCUSSION

The scapula, clavicle, and associated articulations comprise a complex structure required for the proper functioning of the upper extremity. Injuries and abnormalities about the scapula and clavicle can be particularly debilitating if not properly diagnosed and treated. Fortunately, the vast majority of these injuries can be adequately diagnosed and initially treated by the emergency physician.

## REFERENCES

1. Kent BE: Functional anatomy of the shoulder complex: a review. *Phys Ther* 1971; August 51(8): 947.
2. Teubner E, Gerstenberger F, Burgert R: Kinematic consideration of the shoulder girdle and its consequences on common surgical methods. *Unfallchirurg.* 1991; 94: 471-477.
3. Cadenat FM: The treatment of dislocations and fractures of the outer end of the clavicle. *Internat Clin* 1917; I:145-169.
4. Rosenorn M, Pedersen EB: The significance of the coracoclavicular ligament in experimental dislocation of the acromioclavicular joint. *Acta Orthop Scand* 1974; 45: 346-358.
5. Meixner J: Diagnosis and treatment of dislocations with para-articular fractures of the acromioclavicular joint in childhood. *Zentralbl Chir* 1983; 108: 793-797.
6. Eidman DK, Siff SJ, Tullos HS: Acromioclavicular lesions in children. *Am J Sports Med* 1981; 9: 150-154.
7. Nguyen V, Williams G, Rockwood C: Radiography of acromioclavicular dislocation and associated injuries. *Crit-Rev-Diagn-Imaging* 1991; 32: 191-228.
8. Flinn RM, MacMillan CL Jr, Campbell DR, Fraser DB: Optimal radiography of the acutely injured shoulder. *J Can Assoc Radiol* 1983; 34: 128-132.
9. Zanca P: Shoulder pain: Involvement of the acromioclavicular joint. Analysis of 1,000 cases. *Am J Roentgenol Radium Ther Nucl Med* 1971, 112:493-506.
10. DeSmet AA: Anterior oblique projection in radiography of the traumatized shoulder. *Am J Roentgenol* 1980; 134: P 515-8.
11. Bossart PJ, Joyce SM, Manaster BJ, Packer SM: Lack of efficacy of 'weighted' radiographs in diagnosing acute acromioclavicular separation. *Ann Emerg Med* 1988; 17: 20-24.
12. Falstie Jensen S, Mikkelsen P: Pseudodislocation of the acromioclavicular joint. *J Bone Joint Surg Br* 1982; 3: 368-369.
13. Black GB, McPherson JA, Reed MH: Traumatic pseudodislocation of the acromioclavicular joint in children: a fifteen-year review. *Am J Sports Med* 1991; 19: 644-646.
14. Fenkl R, Gotzen L: Sonographic diagnosis of the injured acromioclavicular joint: a standardized examination procedure. *Unfallchirurg* 1992; 95: 393-400.
15. Bearden JM, Hughston JC, Whatley GS: Acromioclavicular dislocation: method of treatment. *J Sports Med* 1973: 1(4). P 5-17.
16. Schwarz N, Kuderna H: Inferior acromioclavicular separation: report of an unusual case. *Clin Orthop* 1988; (234): 28-30.
17. Nixon JR, Corry IS: Inferomedial fracture dislocation of the acromioclavicular joint. *Injury* 1988; 19(3): 211-213.
18. McPhee IB: Inferior dislocation of the outer end of the clavicle. *J Trauma* 1980; 20: P 709-710.
19. Patterson WR: Inferior Dislocation of distal end of the Clavicle. *J Bone Joint Surg* 1967; 49a:1184-1186.
20. Nieminen S, Aho AJ: Anterior dislocation of the acromioclavicular joint. *Ann-Chir-Gynaecol* 1984; 73: 21-24.
21. Verhaven E, Casteleyn PP, DeBoeck H, Handelberg F, Haentjens P: Opdecam P: Surgical treatment of acute type-V acromioclavicular injuries: a prospective study. *Acta–Orthop–Belg.* 1992. 58(2) P176-87.
22. Verhaven E, DeBoeck H, Haentjens P, Handelberg-F, Casteleyn PP, Opdecam P: Surgical treatment of acute type-V acromioclavicular injuries in athletes. *Arch Orthop Trauma Surg* 1993; 112: 189-192.
23. Richards RR: Acromioclavicular joint injuries. *Instr-Course-Lect.* 1993; 42: 259-269.
24. Eskola A, Vainionpaa S, Korkala S, Santavirta S. Gronblad M, Rokkanen P: Four-year outcome of operative treatment of acute acromioclavicular dislocation. *J Orthop Trauma* 1991; 5: 9-13.
25. Walch G: Traumatic acromio-clavicular pathology. *Rev-Prat.* 1990 Apr 11. 40(11). P 999-1002.
26. Heitemeyer U, Hierholzer G, Schneppendahl G, Haines J: The operative treatment of fresh ruptures of the acromioclavicular joint (Tossy III). *Arch Orthop Trauma Surg* 1986; 104: 371-373.
27. Rahmanzadeh R, Voigt C, Fahimi S: Surgical treatment of acromioclavicular joint injury. *Helv Chir Acta* 1991; 57: 805-814.
28. Zaricznyj B: Reconstruction for chronic scapuloclavicular instability. *Am J Sports Med* 1983; 11. P 17-25.
29. Tsou-P-M. Percutaneous cannulated screw coracoclavicular fixation for acute acromioclavicular dislocations. *Clin Orthop* 1989; 243: 112-121.
30. Eberle C, Fodor P, Metzger U: Hook plate (so-called Balser plate) or tension banding with the Bosworth screw in complete acromioclavicular dislocation and clavicular fracture. *Z-Unfallchir-Versicherungsmed* 1992; 85: 134-139.
31. Golser K, Sperner G, Thoni H, Resch H: Early and intermediate results of conservatively and surgically treated lateral clavicular fractures. *Aktuel Traumatol* 1991; 21: 148-152.
32. Morimoto K, Mori E, Nakagawa Y: Calcification of the coracoacromial ligament: a case report of the shoulder impingement syndrome. *Am J Sports Med.* 1988; 16(1). 80-81.
33. Chen YM, Bohrer SP: Coracoclavicular and coracoacromial ligament calcification and ossification. *Skeletal Radiol* 1990; 19: 263-266.
34. Quinn SF, Glass TA: Posttraumatic osteolysis of the clavicle. *South Med J* 1983; 76: 307-308.
35. Scavenius M, Iversen BF: Nontraumatic clavicular osteolysis in weight lifters. *Am J Sports Med* 1992; 20: 463-467.
36. Seymour EQ: Osteolysis of the clavicular tip associated with repeated minor trauma to the shoulder. *Radiology* 1977; 123: 56.
37. Murphy OB, Bellamy R, Wheeler W, Brower TD: Post-traumatic osteolysis of the distal clavicle. *Clin Orthop* 1975; (109): 108-114.
38. Brunet ME, Reynolds MC, Cook SD, Brown TW: A traumatic osteolysis of the distal clavicle: histologic evidence of synovial pathogenesis: a case report. *Orthopedics* 1986; Apr. 9(4). P 557-9.
39. Cotta H, Correll J: The post-traumatic frozen shoulder. *Unfallchirurgie* 1982; 8: 294-306.
40. Wurtz LD, Lyons FA, Rockwood-C-A Jr: Fracture of the middle third of the clavicle and dislocation of the acromioclavicular joint: a report of four cases. *J Bone Joint Surg Am.* 1992; 74: 133-137.
41. Lancourt JE: Acromioclavicular dislocation with adjacent clavicular fracture in a horseback rider: a case report. *Am J Sports Med* 1990; 18: 321-322.
42. Balvanyossy P, Devay K: A case of acromioclavicular dislocation associated with clavicular fracture. *Magy Traumatol Orthop Helyreallito Sebesz* 1988; 31: 229-232.
43. Martin Herrero T, Rodriguez Merchan C, Munuera Martinez L: Fractures of the coracoid process: presentation of seven cases and review of the literature. *J Trauma* 1990 30: 1597-1599.
44. Lasda NA, Murray DG: Fracture separation of the coracoid process associated with acromioclavicular dislocation: conservative treatment: a case report and review of the literature. *Clin Orthop* 1978; (134): 222-224.
45. Barentz JH, Driessen AP: Fracture of the coracoid process of the

scapula with acromioclavicular separation: case report and review of the literature. *Acta-Orthop Belg* 1989; 55:499-503.

46. Wilson KM, Colwill JC: Combined acromioclavicular dislocation with coracoclavicular ligament disruption and coracoid process fracture. *Am J Sports Med* 1989; 17: 697-698.

47. Santa S: Acromioclavicular dislocation associated with fracture of the coracoid process. *Magy-Traumatol-Orthop-Helyreallito-Sebesz* 1992; 35: 162-167.

48. Montgomery SP, Loyd RD: Avulsion fracture of the coracoid epiphysis with acromioclavicular separation: report of two cases in adolescents and review of the literature. *J Bone Joint Surg Am.* 1977; 59: 963-965.

49. Davids Jr, Talbott RD: Luxatio erecta humeri: a case report. *Clin Orthop* 1990; (252): 144-149.

50. Sturm JT, Perry JF Jr: Brachial plexus injuries from blunt trauma, a harbinger of vascular and thoracic injury. *Ann Emerg Med* 1987; 16: 404-406.

51. Meislin RJ, Zuckerman JD, Nainzadeh N: Type III acromioclavicular joint separation association with late brachial-plexus neurapraxia. *J Orthop Trauma* 1992; 6: 370-372.

52. Harrington MA Jr, Keller TS; Seiler JG III, Weikert DR, Moeljanto E, Schwartz HS: Geometric properties and the predicted mechanical behavior of adult human clavicles. *J Biomech* 1993; 26: 417-426.

53. Loder RT, Mayhew HE: Common fractures from a fall on an outstretched hand. *Am Fam Physician* 1988; 37: 327-338.

54. Stanley D, Trowbridge EA, Norris SH: The mechanism of clavicular fracture: a clinical and biochemical analysis. *J Bone Joint Surg Br* 1988; 70:461-464.

55. Seeley DG, Browner WS, Nevitt MC, Genant HK, Scott JC, Cummings SR: Which fractures are associated with low appendicular bone mass in elderly women? The Study of Osteoporotic Fractures Research Group. *Ann Intern Med* 1991; 115: P 837-42.

56. Finelli PF, Cardi JK: Seizure as a cause of fracture CM. In: *Neurology* 1990; 40: 725-726.

57. Peen I: The vascular complications of fractures of the clavicle. *J Trauma* 1964; 4:819, 1964.

58. Post M: Current concepts in the treatment of fractures of the clavicle. *Clin Orthop* 1989; (245): 89-101.

59. Conwell HE: Fractures of the clavicle. *JAMA;* 90:838, 1928.

60. Brunner U, Habermeyer P, Schweiberer L: Special status of lateral clavicular fracture. *Orthopade.* 1992; 21: 163-171.

61. Edwards DJ, Kavanagh TG, Flannery MC: Fractures of the distal clavicle: a case for fixation. *Injury* 1992; 23: 44-46.

62. Riddervold HO: Easily missed fractures. *Radiol Clin North Am* 1992; 30: 475-494.

63. Pantano LC, Grenga E, Masala R, Morandini S: Congenital Pseudoarthrosis of the clavicle. *Pediatr-Med-Chir* 1988; 10. 445-447.

64. Russo MT, Maffuli N: Bilateral congenital pseudarthrosis of the clavicle. *Arch Orthop Trauma Surg* 1990; 109: 177-178.

65. Richter H: Congenital clavicular pseudarthrosis. *Zentralbl-Chir* 1991; 116. 151-154.

66. Morin LR, Fossey FP, Besselievre A, Loisel JC, Edwards JN: Congenital pseudarthrosis of the clavicle. *Acta Obstet Gynecol-Scand* 1993; 72: 120-121.

67. Ogden JA: Distal clavicular physeal injury. *Clin-Orthop* 1984; (188): 68-73.

68. Levin B: The unilateral wavy clavicle. *Skeletal Radiol* 1991; 20: 192. Comment. *Skeletal-Radiol.* 1990; 19: 519-520. Comment.

69. Riemer BL, Butterfield SL, Daffner RH, O'Keeffe RM Jr: The abduction lordotic view of the clavicle: a new technique for radiographic visualization. *J Orthop Trauma* 1991; 5: 392-394.

70. Sloth C, Just SL: The apical oblique radiograph in examination of acute shoulder trauma. *Eur-J-Radiol* 1989; 9: 147-151.

71. Kornguth PJ, Salazar AM: The apical oblique view of the shoulder: its usefulness in acute trauma. *Am-J-Roentgenol* 1987; 149: 113-116.

72. Weinberg B, Seife B, Alonso-P: The apical oblique view of the clavicle: its usefulness in neonatal and childhood trauma. *Skeletal Radiol* 1991; 20. 201-203.

73. Dugdale TW, Fulkerson JP: Pneumothorax complicating a closed fracture of the clavicle: a case report. *Clin Orthop* 1987; 221: 212-214.

74. Meeks RJ, Riebel GD: Isolated clavicle fracture with associated pneumothorax: a case report. *Am J Emerg-Med* 1991 9: 555-556.

75. Costa MC, Robbs JV: Nonpenetrating subclavian artery trauma. *J Vasc Surg* 1988; 8: 71-715.

76. Koss SD, Goitz HT, Redler MR, Whitehill R: Nonunion of a midshaft clavicle fracture associated with subclavian vein compression: a case report. *Orthop Rev* 1989; 18: 431-434.

77. Lim EV, Day LJ: Subclavian vein thrombosis following fracture of the clavicle: a case report. *Orthopedics* 1987; 10: 349-351.

78. Kanbar MS: Subclavian vein thrombosis following fracture of the clavicle: a case report. *Orthopedics* 1988; 11: 1372, 1374. Letter.

79. Williams J, Jehle D, Cottington E, Shufflebarger C: Head, facial, and clavicular trauma as a predictor of cervical-spine injury. *Ann Emerg Med* 1992; 21: 719-722.

80. Unger JM, Schuchmann GG, Grossman JE, Pellett-JR: Tears of the trachea and main bronchi caused by blunt trauma: radiologic findings. *Am J Roentgenol* 1990; 154: 1122-1123. Comment. *Am J Roentgenol* 1989; 153: 1175-1180. Comment.

81. Baumgartner F, Sheppard B, deVirgilio O, et al: Tracheal and main bronchial disruptions after blunt chest trauma: presentation and management. *Ann Thorac Surg* 1990; 50: 523, 569-574. Comment.

82. Suzuki Y, Fjuimori S, Sakai M, Ohkawa S, Ueda-K: A case of pacemaker lead fracture associated with thoracic outlet syndrome. *PACE-Pacing-Clin-Electrophysiol.* 1988; 11: 326-330.

83. Schuger CD, Mittleman R, Habbal B, Wagshal A, Huang SK: Ventricular lead transection and atrial lead damage in a young softball player shortly after the insertion of a permanent pacemaker. *PACE-Pacing-Clin-Electrophysiol.* 1992; 15: P1236-1239.

84. Magney JE, Flynn-D-M, Parsons-J-A, et al: Anatomical mechanisms explaining damage to pacemaker leads, defibrillator leads, and failure of central venous catheters adjacent to the sternoclavicular joint. *Pacing Clin Electrophysiol* 1993; 16(3 Pt 1):373-376, 445-457. Comment.

85. Inoue Y, Nezu R, Nakai S, Takagi Y, Okada A: Spontaneous partial fracture of the catheter of a totally implantable subcutaneous infusion port. *J Parenteral Nutr* 1992; 16: 75-77.

86. Hayes CW, Conway WF, Walsh JW, Coppage L, Gervin AS: Seat belt injuries: radiologic findings and clinical correlation. *Radiographics* 1991; 11: 23-36.

87. Eilenberger K, Janousek A, Poigenfurst J: Heart arrest as a sequela of clavicular fracture. *Unfallchirurgie* 1992; 18: 186-188.

88. Ablin DS, Greenspan A, Reinhart MA: Pelvic injuries in child abuse. *Pediatr Radiol* 1992; 22: 454-457.

89. Sperry K, Pfalzgraf R: Inadvertent clavicular fractures caused by "chiropractic" manipulations in an infant: an unusual form of pseudoabuse. *J Forensic Sci* 1990; 35: 1211-1216.

90. Rivara FP, Kamitsuka MD, Quan L: Injuries to children younger than 1 year of age. *Pediatrics.* 1988; 81: 93-97.

91. Dannohl C, Meeder PJ, Weller S: Costoclavicular syndrome: a rare complication of clavicular fracture. *Aktuel Traumatol* 1988; 18: 149-151.

92. Della-Santa DR, Narakas AO: Fractures of the clavicle and secondary lesions of the brachial plexus. *Z-Unfallchir-Versicherungsmed* 1992; 85: 58-65.

93. Connolly JF, Dehne R: Delayed thoracic outlet syndrome from clavicular non-union: management by morseling. *Nebr Med J,* 1986; 71: 303-306.

94. Jupiter JB, Leffert RD: Non-union of the clavicle: associated complications and surgical management. *J Bone Joint Surg Am.* 1987 69: 753-760.

95. Dellon AL: The results of supraclavicular brachial plexus neurolysis (without first rib resection) in management of post-traumatic "thoracic outlet syndrome." *J Reconstr Microsurg* 1993; 9: 11-17.

96. Karwasz RR, Kutzner M, Kramme WG: Late brachial plexus lesion following clavicular fracture. *Unfallchirurg* 1988; 91: 45-47.

97. Jahn R, Friedrich B: Damage to the arm plexus caused by atypical callus formation following clavicular fracture. *Unfallchirurg* 1989; 92: 227-228.

98. Della-Santa D, Narakas A, Bonnard C: Late lesions of the brachial plexus after fracture of the clavicle. *Ann Chir Main Memb Super* 1991; 10: P 531-540.

99. Andersen K, Jensen PO, Lauritzen J: Treatment of clavicular fractures: figure-of-eight bandage versus a simple sling. *Acta Orthop Scand* 1987; 58: 71-74.

100. Reichenbacher D, Siebler G: Early secondary lesions of the brachial plexus, a rare complication following clavicular fracture. *Unfallchirurgie* 1987; 13: 91-92.

101. Connolly JF, Dehne R: Nonunion of the clavicle and thoracic outlet syndrome. *J Trauma* 1989; 29: 1127-1132, 33.

102. Rumball KM, Da Silva VF, Preston DN, Carruthers CC: Brachial-plexus injury after clavicular fracture: case report and literature review. *Can J Surg* 1991; 34: 264-266.

103. Matz SO, Welliver PS, Welliver DI: Brachial plexus neuropraxia complicating a comminuted clavicle fracture in a college football player: Case report and review of the literature. *Am J Sports Med* 1989, 17: 581-583.

104. Gebuhr P: Brachial plexus involvement after fracture of the clavicle. *Ugeskr Laeger* 1988 150: 105-106.

105. Thomas CB Jr, Friedman RJ: Ipsilateral sternoclavicular dislocation and clavicle fracture. *J Orthop Trauma* 1989; 3: 355-357.

106. Elliott AC: Tripartite injury of the clavicle: a case report. *S Afr Med J* 1986; 70: 115.

107. Wang KC, Hsu-K-Y, Shih-C-H: Brachial plexus injury with erect dislocation of the shoulder. *Orthop-Rev.* 1992; 21: 1345-3467.

108. Kohler A, Kach K, Platz A, Friedl HP, Trentz O: Extended surgical indications in combined shoulder girdle fracture. *Z-Unfallchir-Versicherungsmed* 1992; 85: 140-144.

109. Herscovici D Jr, Fiennes AG, Allgower M, Ruedi TP: The floating shoulder: ipsilateral clavicle and scapular neck fractures. *J Bone Joint Surg Br* 1992; 74: 362-364.

110. Bartosh RA, Dugdale TW, Nielsen R: Isolated musculocutaneous nerve injury complicating closed fracture of the clavicle: a case report. *Am J-Sports-Med* 1992; 20: 356-359.

111. Karwasz R, Przuntek H: Late neurologic complications of clavicular fractures. *Med-Klin* 1988; 83: 406-407.

112. Stanley D, Norris SH: Recovery following fractures of the clavicle treated conservatively. *Injury* 1988 19 162-164.

113. Eskola A, Vainionpaa S, Myllynen P, Patiala H, Rokkanen P: Outcome of clavicular fracture in 89 patients. *Arch Orthop Trauma-Surg* 1986; 105: 337-338.

114. Nordqvist A, Petersson C, Redlund-Johnell I: The natural course of lateral clavicle fracture. Fifteen (11-21) year follow-up of 110 cases. *Acta Orthop Scand* 1993; 64: 87-91.

115. Palarcik J: Clavicular fractures (group of patients treated in the Traumatological Research Institute in 1986-1989). *Czech Med* 1991; 14: 184-90.

116. Ballmer FT, Gerber C: Coracoclavicular screw fixation for unstable fractures of the distal clavicle: a report of five cases. *J Bone Joint Surg Br* 1991; 73: 291-294.

117. Poigenfurst J, Baumgarten-Hofmann U, Hofmann J: Unstable fractures of the lateral end of the clavicle and principles of their treatment. *Unfallchirurgie.* 1991; 17: 131-139.

118. Zaslav KR, Ray S, Neer CS II: Conservative management of a displaced medial clavicular physeal injury in an adolescent athlete. A case report and literature review. *Am J Sports Med* 1989; 17: 833-836.

119. Schuind F, Pay Pay E, Andrianne Y, Donkerwolcke M, Rasquin C, Burny F. External fixation of the clavicle for fracture or non-union in adults. *J Bone Joint Surg Am.* 1988; 70: 692-695.

120. Schuind F, Pay Pay E, Andrianne Y, Donkerwolcke M, Rasquin C, Burny F: [Osteosynthesis of the clavicle using an external fixator]. *Acta-Orthop-Belg* 1989; 55: P 191-196.

121. Connolly JF: Non-union of fractures of the mid-shaft of the clavicle: treatment with a modified Hagie intramedullary pin and autogenous bone-grafting. *J Bone Joint Surg Am* 1992; 74: 1430-1431. Letter.

122. Schwarz N, Hocker K: Osteosynthesis of irreducible fractures of the clavicle with 2.7-MM ASIF plates. *J Trauma* 1992; 33: 179-83.

123. Curtis RJ Jr: Operative management of children's fractures of the shoulder region. *Orthop Clin North Am* 1990; 21: 315-324.

124. Freeland A: Unstable adult midclavicular fracture. *Orthopedics* 1990; 13: 1279-1281.

125. Gaudernak T, Poigenfurst J: Simultaneous dislocation-fracture of both ends of the clavicle. *Unfallchirurgie* 1991; 17: 362-364.

126. Parkes JC, Deland DP: A three-part distal clavicle fracture. *J Trauma* 1983; 23: 437-438.

127. Pizio Z, Czuduk T, Olejnik Z: Fixation of multi-fragment fracture of the clavicle using an external stabilizer "Zespol." *Chir-Narzadow-Ruchu-Ortop-Pol* 1989; 54: 341-343.

128. Leung KS, Lam TP: Open reduction and internal fixation of ipsilateral fractures of the scapular neck and clavicle. *J Bone Joint Surg Am.* 1993; 75(7). P 1015-1018.

129. Klein P, Sommerer G, Link W: Shoulder girdle injury in childhood. Operation or conservative procedure? *Unfallchirurgie* 1991; (1). 14-18.

130. Neviaser RJ: Injuries to the clavicle and acromioclavicular joint. *Orthop Clin North Am* 1987; 18: 443-438.

131. Eskola A, Vainionpaa S, Myllynen P, Patiala H. Rokkanen P: Surgery for ununited clavicular fracture. *Acta Orthop Scand* 1986, Aug. 57: 366-367.

132. Boehme D, Curtis RJ Jr, DeHaan JT, Kay SP, Young DC, Rockwood CA Jr: Non-union of fractures of the mid-shaft of the clavicle: treatment with a modified Hagie intramedullary pin and autogenous bone-grafting.

133. Poigenfurst J, Rappold-G, Fischer-W: Plating of fresh clavicular fractures: results of 122 operations. *Injury* 1992. 23: 237-241.

134. Schunk K, Strunk H, Lohr S, Schild H: Fractures of the clavicle: classification, diagnosis, therapy. *Rontgenblatter* 1988; 41: 392-396.

135. Ivey M, Britt M, Johnston RV Jr: Reflex sympathetic dystrophy after clavicle fracture case report. *J Trauma* 1991; 31: 276-279.

136. Habernek H, Hertz H: Origin, diagnosis and treatment of sternoclavicular joint dislocation. *Aktuel Traumatol* 1987; 17: 23-28.

137. Fery A, Sommelet J: Sternoclavicular dislocations: observations on the treatment and result of 49 cases. *Int Orthop* 1988; 12: 187-195.

138. Ogden JA, Conlogue GJ. Bronson ML: Radiology of postnatal skeletal development: the clavicle. *Skeletal Radiol* 1979; 4(III): 196-203.

139. Hobbs DW: Sternoclavicular joint: a new axial radiographic view. *Radiology* 1968; 90:801-802.

140. Leighton D, Oudjhane K, Ben-Mohammed-H: The sternoclavicular joint in trauma: retrosternal dislocation versus epiphyseal fracture. *Pediatr Radiol* 1989; 20: P 126-127.

141. Lewonowski K, Bassett GS: Complete posterior sternoclavicular epiphyseal separation: a case report and review of the literature. *Clin Orthop* 1992; (281): 84-88.

142. Prime HT, Doig SG, Hooper JC: Retrosternal dislocation of the clavicle: a case report. *Am J Sports Med* 1991; 19: 92-93.

143. Wasylenko MJ, Busse EF: Posterior dislocation of the clavicle causing fatal tracheoesophageal fistula. *Can J Surg* 1981; 24: 626-627.

144. McKenzie JM: Retrosternal dislocation of the Clavicle: a report of two cases. *J Bone Joint Surg* 1963; 456: 138-141.

145. Granick MS, Ramasastry SS, Goodman MA, Hardesty R: Chronic osteomyelitis of the clavicle. *Plast Reconstr Surg* 1989; 84: 80-804.

146. Goldin RH, Chow AW, Edwards JE, Louie JS, Guze LB: sternoclavicular septic arthritis in heroin users. *New Engl J Med* 1973; 289:616-618.

147. Friedman RS, Perez HD, Goldstein IM: Septic arthritis of the sternoclavicular joint due to gram-negative Microorganisms. *Am J Sci* 1981; 282:91-93.

148. Jurik AG, Moller BN: Chronic sclerosing osteomyelitis of the clavicle: a manifestation of chronic recurrent multifocal osteomyelitis. *Arch Orthop Trauma Surg* 1987; 106: 144-151.

149. Rao JP, Femino FP: Repair of a glenoid fracture using a powered stapler. *Orthop-Rev.* 1992 Dec 21(12). P 1449-52.

150. Deltoff MN, Bressler HB: Atypical scapular fracture: a case report. *Am J Sports Med* 1989; 17: P 292-295.

151. Imatani RJ: Fractures of the scapula: a review of 53 fractures. *J Trauma* 1975; 15: 473-478.

152. McGahan JP, Rab GT, Dublin A: Fractures of the scapula. *J Trauma* 1980; 20: 880-883.

153. Cain TE, Hamilton WP: Scapular fractures in professional football players. *Am J Sports Med* 1992; 20: 363-365.

154. Henneking K, Hofmann D, Kunze K: Scapula fractures following electrical accidents. *Unfallchirurgie* 1984; 10: 149-151.

155. Ai SH: Electric injury with a secondary fracture of the scapula. *Chung-Hua-Cheng-Hsing-Shao-Shang-Wai-Ko-Tsa-Chih* 1985; 1:252.

156. Simon JP, Van Delm I, Fabry G. Comminuted fracture of the scapula following electric shock: a case report. *Acta-Orthop-Belg 1991*; 57: 459-460.

157. Dumas JL, Walker N: Bilateral scapular fractures secondary to electrical shock. *Arch Orthop Trauma Surg.* 1992; 111 287-288.

158. Cser I, Vajda A, trans: Bilateral fracture of the scapulae caused by a convulsive seizure. *Arch Orthop Unfallchir* 1976; 86: 227-233.

159. Tarquinio T, Weinstein ME, Virgilio RW: Bilateral scapular fractures from accidental electric shock. *J Trauma* 1979; 19: 132-133.

160. Beswick DR, Morse SD, Barnes AU: Bilateral scapular fractures from low-voltage electrical injury. *Ann Emerg Med.* 1982 Dec. 11(12). P 676-7.

161. Peraino RA, Weinman EJ, Schloeder FX: Unusual fractures during convulsions in two patients with renal osteodystrophy. *South Med J* 1977; 70: 595-596.

162. Mathews RE, Cocke TB, DAmbrosia RD: Scapular fractures secondary to seizures in patients with osteodystrophy: Report of two cases and review of the literature. *J Bone Joint Surg Am* 1983; 65: 850-853.

163. Diraimondo CR, Powers TA, Diraimondo CV, Stone WJ: Scapular fractures resulting from grand mal seizures in chronic hemodialysis patients. *J Tenn Med Assoc* 1986; 79: 411-414.

164. Wertheimer C, Mogan J: Bilateral scapular fractures during a seizure in a patient following subtotal parathyroidectomy. *Orthopedics* 1990; 13: 656-659.

165. Banerjee AK, Field S: An unusual scapular fracture caused by a water skiing accident. *Br-J-Radiol* 1985; 58: 465-467.

166. Veluvolu P, Kohn HS, Guten GN, et al: Unusual stress fracture of the scapula in a jogger. *Clin-Nucl-Med.* 1988 13(7). P 531-2.

167. Fink-Bennett DM, Benson MT: Unusual exercise-related stress fractures: two case reports. *Clin Nucl Med* 1984; 9: 430-434.

168. Ishizuki M, Yamaura I, Isobe Y, Furuya K, Tanabe K, Nagatsuka Y: Avulsion fracture of the superior border of the scapula: report of five cases. *J Bone Joint Surg Am* 1981; 63: P 820-2.

169. Heyse-Moore GH, Stoker DJ: Avulsion fractures of the scapula. *Skeletal Radiol* 1982; 9: 27-32.

170. Williamson DM, Wilson-MacDonald J: Bilateral avulsion fractures of the cranial margin of the scapula. *J Trauma* 1988; May. 28(5). P 713-4.

171. Binazzi R, Assiso J, Vaccari V, Felli L: Avulsion fractures of the scapula: report of eight cases. *J Trauma* 1992; 33: 785-789.

172. Houghton GR: Avulsion of the cranial margin of the scapula: a report of two cases. *Injury* 1979; 11: 45-46.

173. Riggs JH III, Schultz GD, Hanes SA: Radiation induced fracture of the scapula. *J-Manipulative-Physiol-Ther* 1990; 13: 477-481.

174. Harris RD, Harris JH Jr: The prevalence and significance of missed scapular fractures in blunt chest trauma. *Am J Roentgenol* 1988; 151: 747-750.

175. Rubin SA, Gray RL, Green WR: The scapular "Y": a diagnostic aid in shoulder trauma. *Radiology* 1974; 110: 725-726.

176. Guttentag IJ, Rechtine GR: Fractures of the scapula: a review of the literature. *Orthop Rev* 1988; 17: P 147-58.

177. Santa S, Varga Z, Antal S, Szabo J: Experience with the management of scapula fractures. *Magy-Traumatol-Orthop-Helyreallito-Sebesz* 1992; 35: 269-278.

178. Nordqvist A, Petersson C: Fracture of the body, neck, or spine of the scapula: A long-term follow-up study. *Clin-Orthop* 1992; (283): P 139-144.

179. Schmidt M, Armbrecht A, Havemann D: Results of surgical management of scapula fractures. 78th Annual Meeting of the Swiss Society of Accident Surgery and Occupational Diseases. *Z-Unfallchir-Versicherungsmed* 1992; 85: 186-188.

180. Leutenegger A, Ruedi-T: Fractures of the scapula and injuries of the acromioclavicular joint. The traumatized shoulder and its sequelae. *Z-Unfallchir-Versicherungsmed* 1993; 86: 22-26.

181. Vecsei V, Dann K: Surgical management of shoulderblade fractures. *Aktuel Traumatol* 1990; 20: P 277-282.

182. Schuhr EU, Neumann S: Surgical treatment of scapula fracture. *Zentralbl-Chir* 1988; 113: 705-709.

183. Fleischmann W, Kinzl L: Philosophy of osteosynthesis in shoulder fractures. *Orthopedics* 1993; 16: 59-63.

184. Barany I, Kazacsay F: Possibilities of surgical management of fractures of the scapular corpus. *Magy-Traumatol-Orthop-Helyreallito-Sebesz* 1992; 35: 68-72.

185. McGinnis M, Denton JR: Fractures of the scapula: a retrospective study of 40 fractured scapulae. *J Trauma* 1989; 29: 1488-1493.

186. Thompson DA, Flynn TC, Miller PW, Fischer RP: The significance of scapular fractures. *J Trauma* 1985; 25: P 974-977.

187. McLennan JG, Ungersma J: Pneumothorax complicating fracture of the scapula. *J Bone Joint Surg Am.* 1982; 64. P 598-599.

188. Halpern AA, Joseph R, Page J, Nagel DA: Subclavian artery injury and fracture of the scapula. *JACEP* 1979; 8: 19-20.

189. Folman Y, el Masri W, Gepstein R, Messias R: Fractures of the scapula associated with traumatic paralysis: a pathomechanical indicator. *Injury* 1993; 24: 306-308.

190. Argenson C, Boileau P, dePeretti F, Lovet J, Dalzotto H: Fractures of the thoracic spine (T1-T10): apropos of 105 cases. *Rev Chir Orthop* 1989; 75: 370-386.

191. Armstrong CP, Van der Spuy J: The fractured scapula: importance and management based on a series of 62 patients. *Injury* 1984; 15: 324-329.

192. Kogutt MS, Swischuk LE, Fagan CJ: Patterns of injury and significance of uncommon fractures in the battered child syndrome. *Am J Roentgenol Radium Ther Nucl Med* 1974; 121: 143-149.

193. DeRosa GP, Kettelkamp DB: Fracture of the coracoid process of the scapula: case report. *J Bone Joint Surg Am* 1977; 59: 696-697.

194. Maggi G, Fusaro I, Prioli L: Detachment of the short head of the biceps brachii and paralysis of the musculo-cutaneous nerve in traumatic dislocation of the scapula and humerus (description of a case). *Chir Organi Mov* 1985; 70: 389-392.

195. Landi A: Schoenhuber R, Funicello R, Rasio G, Esposito M: Compartment syndrome of the scapula: definition on clinical, neurophysiological and magnetic resonance data. *Ann Chir Main Memb Super* 1992; 11: 383-388.

196. Edeland HG, Zachrisson BE: Fracture of the scapular notch associated with lesion of the suprascapular nerve. *Acta Orthop Scand* 1975; 46: 758-763.

197. Habermeyer P, Rapaport D, Wiedemann E, Wilhelm K: Incisura scapulae syndrome. *Handchir-Mikrochir-Plast-Chir* 1990; 22: 120-124.

198. Habermeyer P, Brunner U, Wiedemann E, Wilhelm K: Compression syndromes of the shoulder and their differential diagnosis. *Orthopade* 1987; 16: 448-457.

199. Malessy MJ, Thomeer RT, Marani E: The dorsoscapular nerve in traumatic brachial plexus lesions. *Clin Neurol Neurosurg* 1993; 94 Suppl. P. 517-23.

200. Percy EC, Birbrager D, Pitt MJ: Snapping scapula: a review of the literature and presentation of 14 patients. *Can J Surg* 1988; 31: 248-250.

201. Schils JP, Freed HA, Richmond BJ, Piraino DW. Bergfeld JA, Belhobek GH: Stress fracture of the acromion. *Am-J-Roentgenol* 1990; 155: 1140-1141. Letter.

202. Rask MR, Steinberg LH: Fracture of the acromion caused by muscle forces: a case report. *J Bone Joint Surg Am* 1978; 60: 1146-1147.

203. Starke W: Isolated fractures of the shoulder blade in childhood and adolescence. *Aktuel-Traumatol* 1988; 18: 73-75.

204. Kleinman PK, Spevak MR: Variations in acromial ossification simulating infant abuse in victims of sudden infant death syndrome. *Radiology* 1991; 180: 185-187.

205. Fery A, Sommelet J: Os acromiale: significance, diagnosis, pathology: apropos of 28 cases including 2 with fracture separation. *Rev Chir Orthop* 1988; 74: 160-672.

206. Ogawa K, Toyama Y, Ishige S, Matsui K: Fracture of the coracoid process: its classification and pathomechanism. *Nippon-Seikeigeka-Gakkai-Zasshi*. 1990; 64: 909-919.

207. Mick CA, Weiland AJ: Pseudoarthrosis of a fracture of the acromion. *J Trauma* 1983; 23: 248-249.

208. McGahan JP, Rab GT: Fracture of the acromion associated with an axillary nerve deficit: a case report and review of the literature *Clin-Orthop*. 1980 Mar-Apr. (147). P 216-8.

209. Oni OO, Hoskinson J: The 'stove-in shoulder': results of treatment by early mobilization. *Injury* 1992; 23: 444-446.

210. Ada JR, Miller ME: Scapular fractures: analysis of 113 cases. *Clin Orthop*. 1991; 269:174-180.

211. Hardegger FH, Simpson LA, Weber BG: The operative treatment of scapular fractures. *J Bone Joint Surg Br* 1984; 66:725-731.

212. Gagey O, Curey JP, Mazas F: Recent fractures of the scapula: apropos of 43 cases. *Rev Chir Orthop Reparatrice Appar Mot* 1984; 70: 443-447.

213. Leung KS, Lam TP, Poon KM: Operative treatment of displaced intra-articular glenoid fractures. *Injury* 1993; 24: 324-328.

214. Stein RE, Bono J, Korn J, Wolff WI: Axillary artery injury in closed fracture of the neck of the scapula: a case report. *J Trauma* 1971; 11: 528-531.

215. Varriale PL, Adler ML: Occult fracture of the glenoid without dislocation: a case report. *J Bone Joint Surg Am*. 1983; 65: 688-689.

216. Casteleiro-Gonzalez R, Vega-Talles R, Atienza-Lopez J. Assiso-Cassarrubios J: Isolated fractures of the coracoid process: presentation of 5 cases and review of the literature. *Chir Organi Mov* 1987; 72: 55-61.

217. Gil JF, Haydar A: Isolated injury of the coracoid process: case report. *J Trauma* 1991; 31: 1696-1697.

218. Zilberman Z, Rejovitzky R: Fracture of the coracoid process of the scapula. *Injury*. 1981 Nov. 13(3). P 203-6.

219. Benton J, Nelson C: Avulsion of the coracoid process in an athlete: report of a case. *J Bone Joint Surg Am* 1971; 53:356-358.

220. Sandrock AR: Another sports fatigue fracture: stress fracture of the coracoid process of the scapula. *Radiology* 1975; 117:274.

221. Goldberg RP, Vicks B: Oblique angled view for coracoid fractures. *Skeletal Radiol* 1983; 9: 195-197.

222. Wong Chung J, Quinlan W: Fractured coracoid process preventing closed reduction of anterior dislocation of the shoulder. *Injury* 1989; 20: 296-297.

223. Carr AJ, Broughton NS: Acromioclavicular dislocation associated with fracture of the coracoid process. *J Trauma* 1989; 29: 125-126.

224. Schaefer RK, Bassman D, Gilula LA: Roentgen rounds #93: Third degree acromioclavicular dislocation with a fracture of the left coracoid process base. *Orthop-Rev* 1987; 16: 945-947.

225. Smith DM: Coracoid fracture associated with acromioclavicular dislocation: a case report. *Clin Orthop* 1975; (108): 165-167.

226. Bernard TN Jr, Brunet ME, Haddad RJ Jr: Fractured coracoid process in acromioclavicular dislocations: report of four cases and review of the literature. *Clin Orthop* 1983; (175): 227-232.

227. Wong Pack WK, Bobechko PE, Becker EJ: Fractured coracoid with anterior shoulder dislocation. *J Can Assoc Radiol*. 1980; 31: 278-279.

228. Garcia-Elias M, Salo JM. Non-union of a fractured coracoid process after dislocation of the shoulder: a case report. *J Bone Joint Surg Br*. 1985; 67: 722-723.

229. Benchetrit E, Friedman B: Fracture of the coracoid process associated with subglenoid dislocation of the shoulder: a case report. *J Bone Joint Surg Am* 1979; 61: 295-296.

230. Baccarani G, Porcellini G, Brunetti E: Fracture of the coracoid process associated with fracture of the clavicle: description of a rare case. *Chir Organi Mov* 1993; 78: 49-51.

231. Ainscow DA: Dislocation of the scapula. *J R Coll Surg Edinb*. 1982; 27: 56-57.

232. Walker JS, Walker BB: Scapular dislocation (locked scapula). *Ann Emerg Med*; 1990; 19: 29-31.

233. Ward WG, Weaver JP, Garrett WE Jr: Locked scapula: a case report. *J Bone Joint Surg Am*. 1989; 71: P 1558-1559.

234. Nettrour LF, Krufky EL, Mueller RE, Raycroft JF: Locked scapula: intrathoracic dislocation of the inferior angle: a case report. *J Bone Joint Surg Am* 1972; 54: 413-416.

235. Rubenstein JD, Ebraheim NA, Kellam JF: Traumatic scapulothoracic dissociation. *Radiology* 1985; 157: 297-298.

236. Kelbel JM, Jardon O-M: Huurman WW: Scapulothoracic dissociation: a case report. *Clin Orthop* 1986; (209): 210-214.

237. Morris CS, Lloyd T: Case report 642: traumatic scapulothoracic dissociation in a child. *Skeletal-Radiol* 1990; 19: 607-608.

238. Oni OO, Hoskinson J, McPherson S: Closed traumatic scapulothoracic dissociation. *Injury* 1992; 23: 138-139.

239. Ebraheim NA, An HS: Jackson WT, et al: Scapulothoracic dissociation. *J Bone Joint Surg Am*. 1988; 70: 428-32.

240. An HS, Vonderbrink JP, Ebraheim NA, Shiple F, Jackson WT: Open scapulothoracic dissociation with intact neurovascular status in a child. *J Orthop Trauma* 1988; 2: 36-38.

241. Pollono F, Nava A, Carli M: Complete traumatic interscapulothoracic amputation. *Arch Sci Med (Torino)* 1971; 128: 205-209.

242. Layton TR, Villella ER, Marrangoni AG: Traumatic forequarter amputation. *J Trauma* 1981; 21: 411-2.

243. Ebraheim NA, Pearlstein SR, Savolaine ER, Gordon SL: Jackson-WT, Corray T: Scapulothoracic dissociation (closed avulsion of the scapula, subclavian artery, and brachial plexus): a newly recognized variant, a new classification, and a review of the literature and treatment options. *J Orthop Trauma* 1987; 1: 18-23.

244. Oreck SL, Burgess A, Levine AM: Traumatic lateral displacement of the scapula: a radiographic sign of neurovascular disruption. *J Bone Joint Surg Am*. 1984; 66: 758-763.

245. Sampson LN, Britton JC, Eldrup-Jorgensen J, Clark DE, Rosenberg JM, Bredenberg CE: The neurovascular outcome of scapulothoracic dissociation. *J Vasc Surg* 1993; 17: 1083-1089.

246. Nagi ON, Dhillon MS: Traumatic scapulothoracic dissociation: a case report. *Arch Orthop Trauma Surg*. 1992; 116: 348-349.

247. Handorf CR: Fatal subscapular staphylococcal abscess. *South Med J* 1983; 76: 271.

248. Foo CL, Swann M: Isolated paralysis of the cereus anterior. *J Bone Joint Surg* 1983; 65(5): 552-556.

249. Mah JY, Otsuka NY: Scapular winging in young athletes. *J Pediatr Orthop* 1992; 12: 245-247.

250. Schultz JS, Leonard JA Jr: Long thoracic neuropathy from athletic activity. *Arch Phys Med Rehabil* 1992; 73: 87-90.

251. Burdett-Smith P: Experience of scapula winging in an accident and emergency department. *Br J Clin Pract* 1990; 44: 643-644.

252. Packer GJ, McLatchie GR, Bowden W: Scapula winging in a sports injury clinic. *Br J Sports Med*. 1993; 27: 90-91.

253. Shimizu J, Nishiyama K, Takeda K, Ichiba T, Sakuta M: A case of long thoracic nerve palsy, with winged scapula, as a result of prolonged exertion on practicing archery. *Rinsho-Shinkeigaku*. 1990; 30: 873-876.

254. Jerosch J, Castro WH, Geske B: Damage of the long thoracic and dorsal scapular nerve after traumatic shoulder dislocation: case report and review of the literature. *Acta Orthop Belg 1990*; 56: 625-627.

255. Gozna ER, Harris WR: Traumatic winging of the scapula. *J Bone Joint Surg Am.* 1979; 61: 1230-1233.

256. Iceton J, Harris WR: Treatment of winged scapula by pectoralis major transfer. *J Bone Joint Surg Br* 1987; 69: 108-110.

257. Agre JC, Ash N, Cameron MC, House J: Suprascapular neuropathy after intensive progressive resistive exercise: case report. *Arch Phys Med Rehabil* 1987; 68:236-238.

258. Breen TW, Haigh JD: Continuous suprascapular nerve block for analgesia of scapular fracture. *Can J Anaesth* 1990; 37:786-788.

259. Brower AC, Neff JR, Tillema DA: An unusual scapular stress fracture. *Am-J-Roentgenol* 1977; 129: 519-520.

260. Euler E, Habermeyer P, Kohler W, Schweiberer L: Scapula fractures: classification and differential therapy. *Orthopade* 1992; 21: 158-162.

261. Holzgraefe M, Klingelhofer J, Eggert S, Benecke R: Chronic neuropathy of the suprascapular nerve in high performance athletes. *Nervenarzt* 1988; 59:545-548.

262. Kopecky KK, Bies JR, Ellis JH: CT diagnosis of fracture of the coracoid process of the scapula. *Comput-Radiol* 1984; (5): 325-327.

263. Larde D, Benazet JP, Benameur C, Ferrane J, trans: Value of the transscapular view in radiological of shoulder trauma. *J Radiol* 1981; 62: 277-282.

264. Moskowitz E, Rashkoff ES: Suprascapular nerve palsy. *Conn Med 1989*; 53: 639-640.

265. Post M, Mayer J: Suprascapular nerve entrapment: diagnosis and treatment. *Clin Orthop* 1987; (223): 126-136.

266. Post M: Current concepts in the diagnosis and management of acromioclavicular dislocations. *Clin-Orthop* 1985; 200: 234-247.

267. Ringel SP, Treihaft M, Carry M, Fisher R, Jacobs P: Suprascapular neuropathy in pitchers. *Am-J-Sports-Med* 1990; 18: 80-86.

268. Shabas D, Scheiber M: Suprascapular neuropathy related to the use of crutches. *Am J Phys Med* 1986; 65: 298-300.

269. Thielemann FW, Kley U, Holz U: Isolated injury of the subscapular muscle tendon. *Sportverletz Sportschaden.* 1992; 6: 26-28.

270. Wilkes RA, Halawa M: Scapular and clavicular osteotomy for malunion: case report: *J Trauma* 1993; 34. 309.

# The Shoulder

*Karen A. Quaday*

The shoulder is often called "a universal joint" because of its impressive degree of mobility. This permits an individual to lift heavy weights, throw a baseball at great speed, and scratch most of one's back. Unfortunately, this variety in function comes at a sacrifice in stability. The relatively large humeral head must be seated properly in the shallow glenoid fossa, and the surrounding soft tissues must operate smoothly to obtain optimal shoulder performance. So many factors may disturb the delicate equilibrium between mobility and stability that it is a wonder that more people do not have shoulder problems.

Acute shoulder complaints may be divided into three categories: acute (traumatic), chronic, and referred pain (Table 9-1). Trauma may cause fractures, dislocation, subluxation, bursitis, sprain, tendinitis, rotator cuff tears, and other problems such as arthritis. Chronic shoulder pain or dysfunction may be related to a rotator cuff tear, instability, impingement, adhesive capsulitis, avascular necrosis, arthritis, and musculoskeletal tumors. Pain referred to the shoulder occurs in a variety of diseases including cervical, pleural, cardiac, hepatic, and those with splenic pathology.

As is true in so many areas of medicine, understanding the anatomy, obtaining the history, and performing a thorough physical examination provide the diagnosis in most cases. Further testing, such as radiologic studies, should confirm the diagnosis and may give supplemental information. It is sad to think that in this day of advanced technology, radiographs and other tests are sometimes substituted for an appropriate history and physical. An example of "progress gone wrong" is the lost art of diagnosing posterior shoulder dislocations by physical examination. Recent literature has claimed that as many as 50% of posterior dislocations are missed initially, and yet the largest series of posterior dislocations was reported by Dr. Malgaigne almost a half century before the medical application of radiographs. Thus, a working knowledge of

**Table 9-1.** Most common causes of shoulder pain and/or dysfunction

| Acute | Chronic | Referred pain |
|---|---|---|
| Fracture | Impingement | Cervical spine disease (spondylosis) |
| Glenohumeral dislocation | Rotator cuff tear | Brachial plexus compression or injury |
| Glenohumeral subluxation | Adhesive cellulitis | Pleuritis |
| Acromioclavicular dislocation | Avascular necrosis | Pneumonia |
| Rotator cuff tear | Paget's disease | Lung tumor |
| Subacromial bursitis | Musculoskeletal tumor | PE/lung infarction |
| Tendinitis | Instability | Myocardial ischemia |
| Sprain/Strain | Arthritis | Pericarditis |
| Contusion | Osteomyelitis | Splenic injury |
| Arthritis | | Hepatic injury |
| | | Hepatitis |
| | | Cholecystitis |
| | | Diaphragmatic irritation |

Key: PE = Pulmonary embolism

anatomy and basic examination of the shoulder are essential to making the proper diagnosis.

## ANATOMY

The three joints of the shoulder are the sternoclavicular, acromioclavicular, and glenohumeral joints. Because the sternoclavicular and acromioclavicular joints are discussed elsewhere (see Chapter 8), this discussion will focus on the glenohumeral joint. The glenohumeral joint is considered a ball-and-socket joint but it has more mobility than is typical for this type of joint. It moves in virtually all planes. This mobility, although highly desirable, comes at the sacrifice of stability. Consequently, the shoulder is the most commonly dislocated major joint in the body.[1]

### Stability of glenohumeral joint

The key to stability of the glenohumeral joint is the soft tissues that maintain the intimate relationship of the humeral head and the glenoid fossa (Fig. 9-1). The articular surface of the humeral head is three to four times that of the glenoid fossa. Therefore, only a small area of the humeral head articulates with the fossa at any time. Also, the glenoid fossa is usually extremely shallow or may be nearly flat, resulting in its having less bony depth with which to "cup" the humeral head. These factors place great demands on the adjacent soft tissues to support this joint. The capsule, glenoid labrum, ligaments, and surrounding musculotendinous structures hold the humeral head in proper position. These stabilizing soft tissues are so vulnerable that a

sudden force to the shoulder can overwhelm them, causing dislocation or subluxation.

Another important factor for stabilization is the ability of the scapula to move along the chest wall. When an axial load is applied to the arm, the forces transmitted up to the scapula are dissipated as it recoils on the thorax (Fig. 9-2). In fact, the movement of the scapula on the thorax is essential for maintaining an optimal relationship between the humeral head and glenoid fossa.[2]

### Capsule and glenoid labrum

The capsule, glenoid labrum, and several ligaments are loosely defined as *static stabilizers*. The capsule is thin, inelastic, and is approximately twice the size of the humeral head. It originates on the rim of the glenoid fossa and inserts in the proximal humeral neck. There are two important extensions of the capsule. One covers the synovial sheath of the long head of the biceps tendon as it traverses the bicipital groove. The other extension is a bursa adjacent to the subscapularis below the coracoid process (Fig. 9-3).

The glenoid labrum is a fibrous rim that circumvents the articular rim of the glenoid fossa thus creating more depth and stabilizing the humeral head in proper position. This area is critical to checking the forward and backward movement of the humeral head that occurs during elevation and rotation. Injury to the anterior labrum is so predictive of recurrent shoulder dislocations that it is called the *Bankart essential lesion* (Fig. 9-4). The labrum is also an interconnection between the glenoid, capsule, articular cartilage, glenohumeral ligaments, and long head of the biceps tendon. The glenohumeral ligaments and the long head of the biceps tendon are contiguous with the glenoid labrum.[3]

### Ligaments and tendons

The glenohumeral ligaments, the transverse ligament, and the coracohumeral ligament all act as static stabilizers. The glenohumeral ligaments are actually one ligament divided into three parts. It is primarily located anteriorly and is contiguous with the capsule and glenoid labrum. These ligaments act as deterrents to dislocation of the humeral head. A series of tendons surrounds the joint blending with the capsule and maintaining the humeral head inside the fossa during movement (e.g., abduction). These dynamic stabilizers are referred to collectively as the *rotator cuff* (Fig. 9-5). These four tendons work as a single unit to seat the humeral head properly, thus permitting the deltoid muscle to move the arm efficiently. Their integrity is crucial to normal function. The four muscles involved are the subscapularis, infraspinatus, teres minor, and supraspinatus. The subscapularis is located anterior to the joint and prevents anterior dislocation. Inserting on the lesser tuberosity, it moves the humeral head inferiorly, anteriorly, medially and, in certain positions, rotates it internally. The remaining three muscles are all external rotators. They are located more posteriorly and insert on the greater tuberosity. The supraspinatus also moves the humerus superiorly

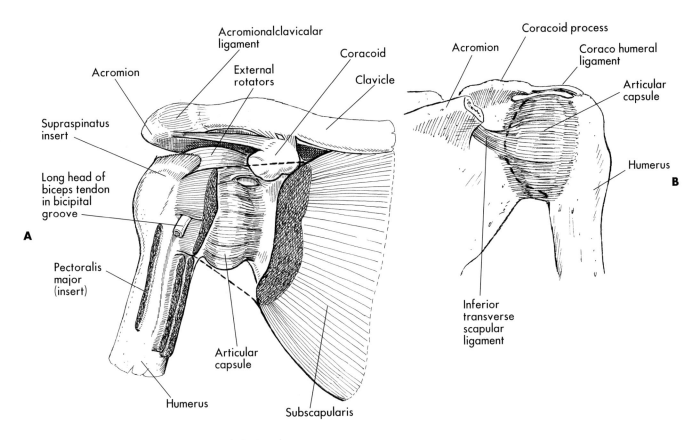

Anterior view

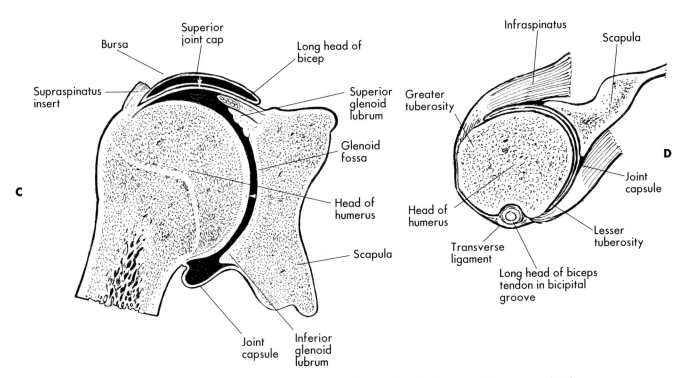

**Fig. 9-1.** Normal shoulder anatomy. **A,** anterior, **B,** posterior, **C,** deeper, and **D,** cross-sectional views.

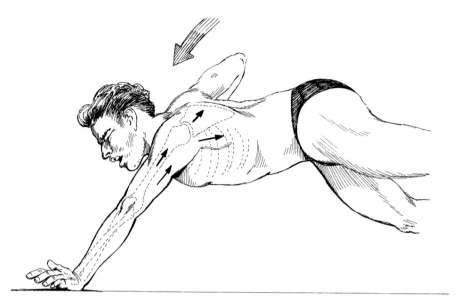

**Fig. 9-2.** Scapular mobility on the thorax is an important factor in shoulder stabilization.

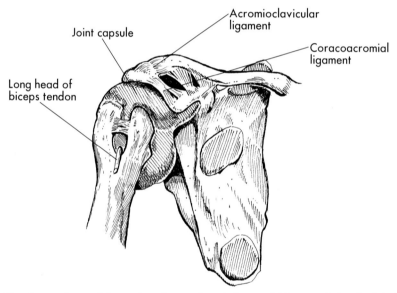

**Fig. 9-3.** Glenohumeral synovial capsule and extensions (subacromial bursa and sheath of the long head of the biceps tendon).

and posteriorly. It is the most commonly injured tendon of the rotator cuff.

The long head of the biceps tendon works with the subscapularis to depress the humeral head. It originates on the posterior glenoid labrum, crosses superiorly over the joint, and passes through the bicipital groove.[3] In an anterior dislocation, it may interpose, preventing relocation of the humeral head. It may also create shoulder pain when inflamed.

**Proximal humerus**

The proximal humerus should be mentioned briefly. As already stated, the humeral head is quite large. It may be damaged in trauma, especially during dislocation. The greater tuberosity is located superiorly and posteriorly on the shaft near but below the humeral head. It is often a mechanical deterrent to reduction of a dislocation. It is also the point of insertion of the supraspinatus, infraspinatus, and teres minor muscles. The greater tuberosity may be avulsed with trauma to the rotator cuff. The lesser tuberosity is the site of insertion of the subscapularis and is less frequently avulsed. Between the two tuberosities anteriorly is the bicipital groove, which contains the long head of the biceps tendon. It is covered by the transverse humeral ligament, an extension of the synovium of the glenohumeral joint, and is of variable depth. Shallower grooves

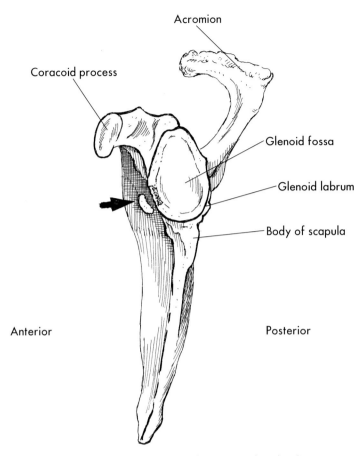

**Fig. 9-4.** Lateral view of a scapula with an arrow denoting the labral tear called the *Bankart essential lesion.*

may predispose to subluxation of the tendon. Tenderness in the groove may be due to biceps tendinitis.

### Deltoid

The major muscle that moves the shoulder joint is the deltoid. It is involved in abduction, flexion, and extension. It originates on the lateral third of the clavicle, scapular spine, and acromion and inserts on the lateral shaft of the humerus. It is innervated by the axillary nerve, which may be injured during anterior dislocations. The deltoid muscle relies heavily on the ability of the rotator cuff muscles to stabilize the humeral head in the glenoid fossa. Therefore, the inability of the joint to abduct well may be due to axillary nerve injury with subsequent deltoid weakness, dislocation, or rotator cuff tears. The pectoralis muscles move the arm medially and insert in the humerus.

### Coracoacromial arch

The coracoacromial arch is the focus of attention in the diagnosis of *impingement.* This area is below the coraco-acromial ligament and bordered by the coracoid and acromion (Fig. 9-3). The arch is a rigid space through which the subacromial bursa, rotator cuff, and proximal humerus must move. The subacromial bursa is a large synovial membrane—attached superiorly to the coracoacromial ligament and acromion, laterally to the deltoid, and inferiorly to the rotator cuff and greater tuberosity—that extends anteriorly and posteriorly around the proximal humerus. This bursa facilitates movement of the rotator cuff and proximal humerus under the coracoacromial arch. If the bursa is damaged, glenohumeral stability

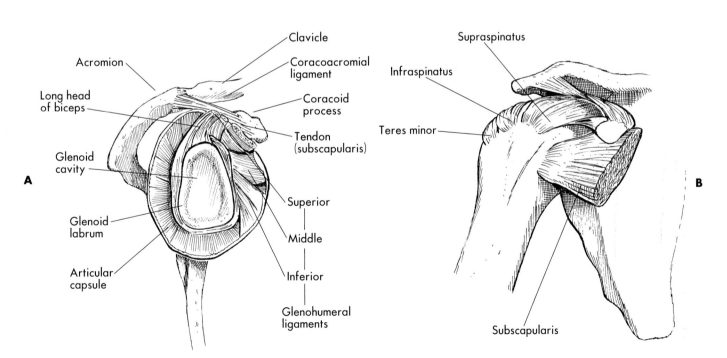

**Fig. 9-5. A** and **B,** The rotator cuff (subscapularis, supraspinatus, infraspinatus, and teres minor) nearly surrounds the glenohumeral joint and stabilizes it during movement.

will be compromised. Subacromial space pathology includes bursitis, rotator cuff tear, and impingement.

## HISTORY

No examination is complete without obtaining an adequate history. Important information includes age, handedness, and activity level as well as pain, location, onset, duration, and radiation. If traumatic in onset, the mechanism of injury offers a wealth of information. If previously dislocated, the duration of dislocation, radiographic findings, method of reduction, and length of immobilization may give clues to prognosis.

The age of the patient is helpful, because certain age groups have specific diagnoses and prognoses. Elderly patients are more likely to have degenerative changes of the rotator cuff, glenohumeral joint, and acromioclavicular joint. Furthermore, neoplastic processes are more likely to be involved in these patients. Impingement is also more often seen in the older population. However, younger patients have an increased chance of recurrent dislocations.

Quality of the pain may suggest a differential diagnosis. The dull ache that occurs at night or at rest is classic for rotator cuff tears. A burning pain is often described by patients with acute calcific bursitis. Deep burning pain posteriorly with radiation down the arm or paresthesias in the arm is indicative of cervical disc disease, as is pain in the shoulder with certain neck movements. Pain that a patient describes as "catching" or making a noise during passive range of motion (ROM) points to bursal irritation, intra-articular loose bodies, or labral lesions. The cause of the pain that occurs with increasing activity is usually the rotator cuff tendons. The overhand throwing motion is particularly painful. Pain that is relieved by salicylates may be from an osteoid osteoma. Chronic shoulder pain associated with decreased mobility may lead to adhesive capsulitis, thus confusing the situation with a second diagnosis.

The mechanism of any trauma is of significant interest because certain injury patterns exist. For example, the axial loading in adduction, internal rotation, and forward flexion that occurs when falling forward usually results in a posterior dislocation. Forces on the hand transmitted through an extended elbow onto a shoulder that is adducted, externally rotated, and posteriorly extended tend to cause an anterior shoulder dislocation. Unfortunately, many patients are not reliable historians regarding the mechanism of injury.

## EXAMINATION

No substitute exists for a systematic physical examination of the shoulder. Excessive dependence on radiographic evaluation, for example, often leads to a misdiagnosis of posterior dislocation. The physical examination should include comparison with the unaffected shoulder, if possible, and the patient must be undressed. Inspection, palpation, range of motion, strength, stability, and neurovascular status must be evaluated if the diagnosis is to be accurate.

If possible, watch the patient remove his or her shirt. Often valuable information can be obtained when the patient is least aware that he or she is being observed. Visualize the shoulders first by standing behind (and over) the patient when he or she is seated on a low stool. Look for asymmetry, atrophy, and deformity. Rotator cuff tears with atrophy of the supraspinatus may cause prominence of the scapular spine, as will lesions of the suprascapular nerve. Next, inspect the patient from the front at his or her level (seated). Again, note any asymmetry. In Sprengel's deformity from a third-degree acromioclavicular separation, for example, the lateral clavicle rides superiorly. Prominence of the acromion may be seen with an axillary nerve lesion, resulting in deltoid muscle atrophy. Asymmetry may be observed with acute fracture, dislocation, and chronic problems such as rotator cuff tears and nerve injuries.

### Palpation and tests

Palpation should include the sternoclavicular joint, the acromioclavicular (AC) joint, the glenohumeral joint, the scapulothoracic juncture (joint), humeral tuberosities, the intertubercular groove, and the space below the acromion. Check for tenderness, crepitation, deformity, and temperature abnormality. Tenderness may reflect fracture, dislocation, or sprain. Crepitation suggests bursitis, loose bodies, or labral tears. Skin coolness may be a subtle clue to thoracic outlet syndrome, whereas increased skin temperature suggests acute inflammation. The AC joint may be tender in injuries to the AC ligament, arthritis, or impingement. The subacromial space is involved in impingement; therefore, palpate inferior to the acromion for tenderness and crepitus.

With biceps tendinitis, the intertubercular groove is tender at rest or when performing Speed's test or Yergason's test. Speed's test produces pain in the groove when the

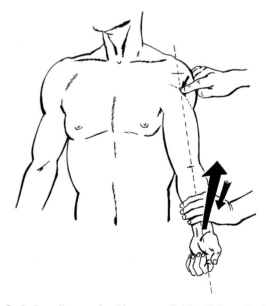

**Fig. 9-6.** Speed's test for biceps tendinitis elicits pain in the bicipital groove with forward flexion against resistance (arm adducted, elbow extended, and wrist supinated).

patient, with the elbow extended and wrist supinated, must forward flex the shoulder against resistance (Fig. 9-6).[4] Yergason's test is done with the elbow flexed at 90°, arm adducted; the wrist is then supinated against resistance (Fig. 9-7).[5] Also, the intertubercular groove should be palpated in

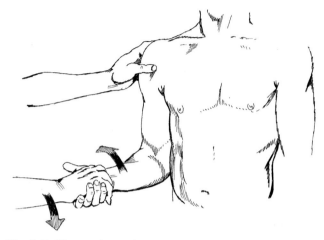

**Fig. 9-7.** Yergason's test for biceps tendinitis causes pain in the bicipital groove with supination against resistance (adducted arm and elbow flexed).

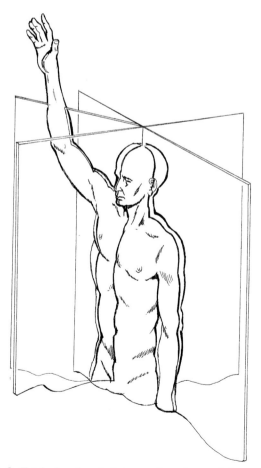

**Fig. 9-8.** Total elevation is between the planes of forward flexion and abduction.

90° abduction during internal and external rotation to assess any subluxation of the long head of the biceps tendon.

### Range of motion

Range of motion (ROM) should be compared with the unaffected shoulder, if possible. Active ROM should be done sitting and rhythm observed. If this is abnormal, the patient should be then reassessed passively and preferably supine. Both active ROM and passive ROM are decreased in fractures, dislocations, and adhesive capsulitis. Passive ROM may be nearly normal if the patient has musculotendinous disorders such as rotator cuff tears.

For diagnostic purposes, only three major motions need to be assessed: total elevation, total internal rotation, and total external rotation. Total elevation is a better assessment of true function than either abduction or forward flexion.[6] It is the angle of the arm to the thorax in a plane between the coronal and sagittal planes (Fig. 9-8). Total internal rotation is defined as the vertebral level that the thumb can reach (Fig. 9-9). Total external rotation is assessed with the elbow

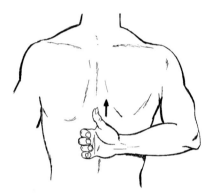

**Fig. 9-9.** Total internal rotation is defined by vertebral level that the thumb can reach.

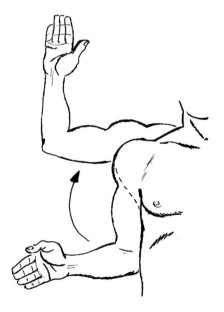

**Fig. 9-10.** Total external rotation is noted in two positions: adduction with elbow flexed and 90° abduction with elbow flexed.

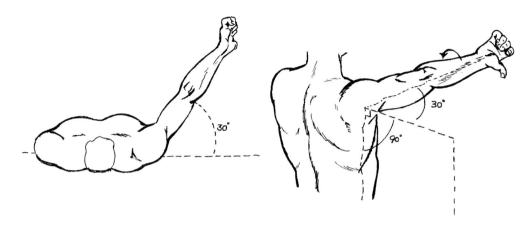

**Fig. 9-11.** Supraspinatus strength test is performed in 90° abduction and 30° forward flexion. The thumb is internally rotated so that it is pointing downward.

flexed and the shoulder in adduction and again with 90° abduction (Fig. 9-10).

The strength of abduction, forward flexion, and internal and external rotation should be assessed and compared with the unaffected shoulder. Weak or limited degrees of abduction and external rotation are seen with dislocations, rotator cuff disease, and neurologic deficits (axillary and supraspinatus nerves). A common test for rotator cuff integrity is the supraspinatus strength test that essentially isolates the supraspinatus muscle (with some assistance from the deltoid). The test is performed in 90° abduction with 30° forward flexion (i.e., near the plane of total elevation), and then the patient internally rotates so that the thumb is pointing down (Fig. 9-11). The observer applies downward force on the arm. Inability to resist this downward force is a positive test suggesting the most common tear of the rotator cuff—the supraspinatus. The "drop arm test" is another check for a rotator cuff tear. Passively abduct the shoulder to 90° and ask the patient to slowly lower the arm to the side in the same arch. (Do not permit the patient to slip into forward flexion.) The inability to lower the arm slowly or the development of pain suggests a rotator cuff tear.

### Impingement

Impingement is pressure on the rotator cuff as it passes under the coracoacromial arch and is associated with limitation and pain on abduction and external rotation. There may also be subacromial crepitus. The diagnosis is suggested by pain with abduction to 90° and proven with one of the following three tests. First, internal rotation and forced forward flexion cause pain when the greater tuberosity is pressed against the acromion.[7] The Hawkin's test is performed by passively placing the arm in 90° forward flexion and then forcing internal rotation, which compresses the supraspinatus tendon in the coracoacromial arch.[8] The final test is Neer's test. This test is positive when pain on abduction is relieved by the local infiltration of 10 ml of 1%

xylocaine beneath the anterior acromion.[9] These tests are helpful in making the diagnosis of impingement, which is usually a chronic problem (see the discussion of impingement under soft-tissue injuries below). Other causes of painful abduction and external rotation include dislocation, subluxation, labral lesion, and capsular pathology.

### Instability

Instability is usually not assessed as an acute condition, but a brief mention here is appropriate. This must be assessed with the patient comfortable and relaxed and using the unaffected shoulder for comparison. Anterior and posterior instability may be determined in two ways. The drawer test is done with the patient seated, hand in lap, and examiner behind the patient. The clavicle and scapula are stabilized with one of the examiner's hands and the other hand grasps the proximal humerus pushing medially to seat the humeral head in a neutral position. Then, without releasing either hand, the humeral head is directed forward to check for anterior instability and posteriorly to check for posterior instability, with a brief stop in a neutral position between the two movements. A normal shoulder has a firm end point and no pain, subluxation, apprehension, or noise. A snap or klunk may be elicited in patients with labral tears. The same findings may be demonstrated with the other test, which is performed with the patient supine and the shoulder abducted 90° and externally rotated. The shoulder should be off the edge of the table. The examiner grasps the proximal humerus and moves it anteriorly and posteriorly as in the drawer test. Again, instability of the shoulder is usually a chronic complaint.

### Neurovascular status

The neurovascular status of the upper extremity should be assessed. The brachial, radial, and ulnar pulses should be symmetrical. Major axillary vessel injury may be suggested by ecchymosis or expanding axillary hematoma as well as by distal pulse deficits. The brachial plexus may be injured

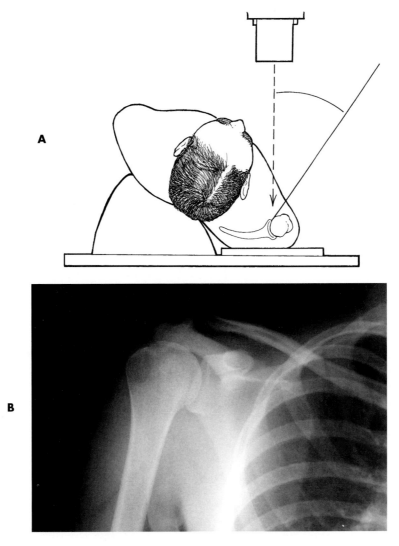

**Fig. 9-12.** **A** and **B,** Normal AP shoulder x-ray.

during shoulder trauma, resulting in a variety of nerve deficits. A routine neurologic examination should include the axillary, musculocutaneous, median, ulnar, and radial nerves. The axillary nerve innervates the deltoid muscle, allowing strong abduction and normal sensation over the lateral upper arm. The musculocutaneous nerve innervates the biceps, brachialis, and coracobrachialis muscles and provides cutaneous branches to the lateral aspect of the proximal forearm. The median, ulnar, and radial nerves can be assessed by testing sensation in the hand and the movement of the thumb (see Chapters 14 and 15).

If the examination is normal and the complaint is shoulder pain, a source of referred pain should be sought. The most common cause of referred pain to the shoulder is cervical spine pathology.[10] Spurling's test for cervical root irritation is positive when pain or radiculopathy is elicited by downward pressure on the head (axial loading) with the chin rotated toward the affected shoulder. Other causes of referred pain include pleural, pulmonary, cardiac, splenic, and hepatic diseases.

## RADIOLOGIC EVALUATION

After a thorough examination, radiographs of the shoulder may confirm the diagnosis or reveal additional unsuspected problems. A basic tenet of radiology is that a minimum of two views (at right angles to each other) is necessary to evaluate an area adequately. Many orthopedists routinely recommend three views of the shoulder. The anteroposterior (AP) and lateral views are a minimum, with the axillary view being the most common third view. There are also special views for specific situations. X-rays with weights are generally not necessary for the acute evaluation of the glenohumeral joint.

### AP view

The AP view is not a true AP view in the plane of the thorax as was done years ago. The glenohumeral joint is assessed best by a beam directed perpendicular to the plane of the scapula, which is 45° lateral. Thus, the AP view is an AP of the glenohumeral joint (Fig. 9-12). This view identifies the joint space easily in normal shoulders and can be done with the patient being supine, seated, or even while wearing a sling. The cassette is placed against the scapula and the beam is centered and directed at right angles to the coracoid process. This single view demonstrates most fractures and dislocations. Other diagnoses that may be evident include calcific tendonitis (calcium in the tendons), calcific bursitis (cloudiness inferior to the acromion), degenerative joint disease (narrow joint space and sclerotic articular surfaces), and rotator cuff tears (humeral-acromial interval less than or equal to 5 mm).[11,12]

### Lateral view

The best lateral view is also not a true lateral (i.e., transthoracic) but is really 60° anterior oblique. It is easy to do, easy to read, reproducible, and requires no additional positioning of a potentially painful shoulder. With the patient standing (preferably), the cassette is placed against the anterolateral deltoid and the beam is directed parallel to the spine and perpendicular to the cassette. The image has been described as the "Y" view[13] because the body of the scapula is vertical and the coracoid process forms an upper branch anteriorly, and the scapular spine and acromion form another branch posteriorly. The juncture is a circular density, which is the glenoid fossa with the humeral head overlapping it (Fig. 9-13). It is easy to see subcoracoid (anterior) dislocations and subacromial (posterior) dislocations based on the position of the humeral head.

### Axillary view

The axillary view is usually done with the patient lying supine, arm abducted, cassette superiorly, and the beam directed between the arm and chest, perpendicular to the cassette (Fig. 9-14). This may be difficult if the patient is unable or unwilling to abduct the arm. Therefore, a special cassette is available that can be placed in the axilla. The beam is then directed from above the shoulder. This view provides information on subtle fractures of the humeral head, coracoid process, glenoid fossa, and lesser tuberosity.[14,15]

### Other views and tools

There are numerous other views that may be obtained under special circumstances. The West Point axillary lateral view is a modification of the axillary view and demonstrates glenoid rim fractures.[11] The apical oblique view is used to check subtle posterolateral humeral fractures as well as glenoid rim fractures.[16,17] Acromion images may be indicated in the consideration of impingement syndrome.[11] Most of these less common views are unnecessary to diagnose most acute conditions.

Although magnetic resonance imaging (MRI) may make it obsolete, arthrography is still done in most institutions for the assessment of rotator cuff tears (Fig. 9-15). MRI may be less sensitive for detecting healed tears and partial tears with impingement. It is diagnostic for adhesive capsulitis if the volume of the joint space is markedly decreased. Recurrent dislocations with instability may be suggested by enlarged joint volumes. Arthrography is done preoperatively for an anterior dislocation to rule out an associated rotator cuff tear. Arthrography is also often combined with computed tomography.

Computed tomography (CT) scanning may be helpful

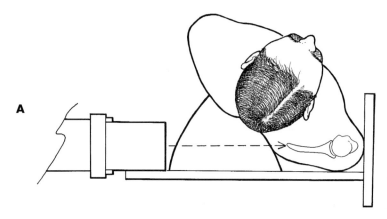

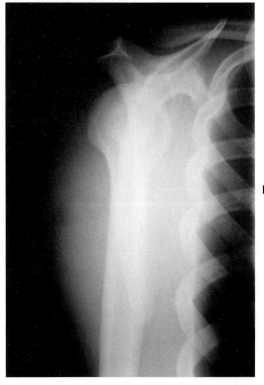

**Fig. 9-13. A** and **B,** Normal "Y" view of shoulder.

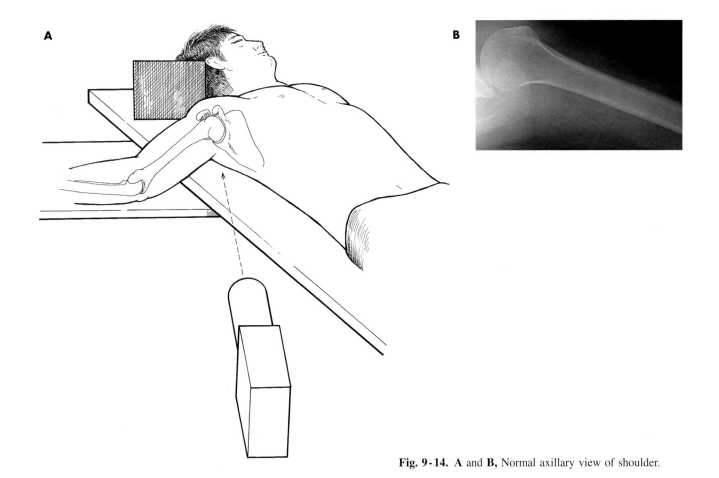

**Fig. 9-14. A** and **B,** Normal axillary view of shoulder.

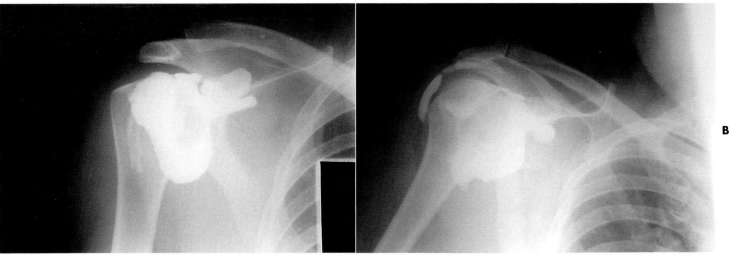

**Fig. 9-15.** Arthrography of shoulder: **A,** Normal and **B,** with classic subdeltoid and subacromial extravasation seen with complete rotator cuff tears. (Also noted are Hill-Sachs and Bankart lesions consistent with recurrent anterior dislocations.)

with or without arthrography in some situations. It is extremely accurate and sensitive for humeral head and scapular fractures.

Although it is still under investigation, MRI shows tremendous promise as a tool for shoulder evaluation. It is easy and reliable but, unfortunately, expensive. MRI is accurate at diagnosing most rotator cuff tears and tendinitis as well as providing helpful preoperative information.[18-20]

Ultrasound has been referred to as the "poor man's MRI." It is safe, fast, painless, and inexpensive, but is operator-dependent and difficult to perform. Most centers do not have the expertise to accurately and reliably use ultrasound for shoulder evaluation. However, in such centers, ultrasound studies have a 91% correlation with surgical findings, especially for rotator cuff tears.[21]

Arteriograms are indicated in patients with any evidence of vascular compromise or injury. The two most common reasons for arteriography in shoulder problems are the evaluation of thoracic outlet obstruction and quadrilateral space syndrome.

## DISLOCATIONS

The glenohumeral joint is the most commonly dislocated major joint in the body. By definition, dislocation is the complete separation of articular surfaces, as compared with subluxation, in which there is only a transient abnormal movement of the humeral head in the glenoid fossa. Shoulder dislocations and subluxations may be traumatic or atraumatic; voluntary or involuntary; and either acute, chronic, or recurrent.

There are four general classifications of shoulder dislocations, based on the final position of the humeral head in relation to the glenoid fossa. In order of decreasing frequency, these are anterior, posterior, inferior, and superior. All four are associated with specific fractures and soft-tissue injuries such as rotator cuff tears. Neurovascular compromise also may occur in all types but rarely in posterior dislocations. *Apprehension* is a condition in which

---

> **Indications for operative management of glenohumeral dislocations**
>
> Open dislocation
> Irreducible due to interposing structures (fracture fragment, tendon, joint capsule)
> Unstable relocation
> Displacement >5-10 mm of avulsed greater or lesser tuberosity
> Large glenoid rim fracture
> Intrathoracic dislocation
> Most posterior dislocations

a patient anticipates or dreads a subluxation or dislocation. This is usually noted with specific types of activities, movements, or positions and can be very disabling.

In general, the mechanism of injury and the examination will suggest the diagnosis and radiographs will confirm it. The Y view is especially important. Most dislocations can be managed by closed reduction but open dislocations, certain fracture patterns, irreducible (e.g., due to interposing structures) and unstable relocations will need to be taken to the operating room for reduction by an orthopedic surgeon (see box on this page).

### Anterior dislocations

By far, the largest proportion of shoulder dislocations are anterior, accounting for over 90% of all shoulder dislocations. The mechanism is usually a fall on an outstretched hand with an arm that is abducted, extended, and externally rotated (Fig. 9-16). Direct trauma to the posterolateral aspect of the shoulder may also cause an anterior dislocation. The differential includes fracture, contusion, and rotator cuff tear.

There are four types of anterior shoulder dislocations defined by the position of the humeral head. In all four types, the head of the humerus rests directly on the anterior

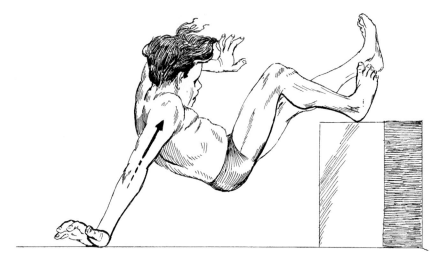

**Fig. 9-16.** Typical mechanism of anterior shoulder dislocation.

scapular neck. Subcoracoid dislocations are by far the most common (90%). The humeral head is anterior and inferior to the coracoid (Fig. 9-17). Approximately 7% of anterior shoulder dislocations are in the subglenoid position, which is more inferior and anterior to the fossa (Fig. 9-18). It is

distinctly different from an inferior dislocation, in which the humeral head has no contact with the scapula, and the subglenoid type of posterior dislocation, in which the humeral head is on the posterioinferior aspect of the glenoid rim. The last two types of anterior shoulder dislocations

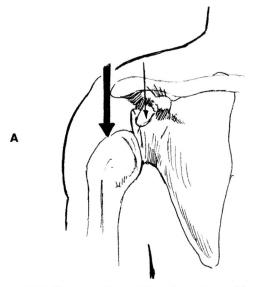

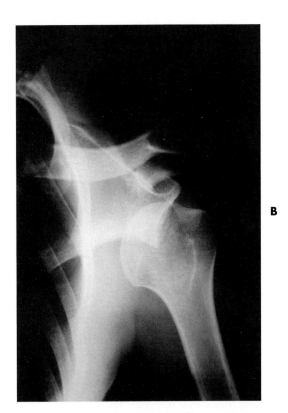

Fig. 9-17. A and B, Subcoracoid shoulder dislocation with fracture of the coracoid.

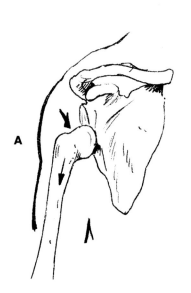

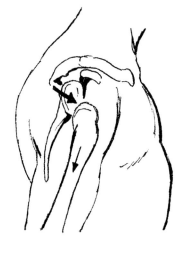

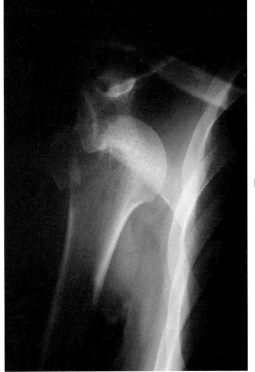

Fig. 9-18. A and B, Subglenoid anterior shoulder dislocation.

are extremely rare and usually seen in patients with severe multiple trauma. The subclavian variety is present when the humeral head is medial to the coracoid and inferior to the clavicle. In the appropriately named intrathoracic type, the humeral head extends through the ribs and into the thoracic cavity. Again, anterior dislocations are most likely subcoracoid or, less commonly, subglenoid.

Patients must be exposed because asymmetry is usually obvious. The arm is held slightly abducted and externally rotated with elbow flexed and forearm being supported in some manner (e.g., contralateral hand). The humeral head is palpable anteriorly. There is marked limitation of active external and internal rotation. A neurovascular examination may show evidence of nerve injury, but vascular trauma is unusual. In particular, the axillary nerve should be assessed by pinprick over the deltoid muscle, and the contractility of the deltoid muscle assessed as well. These findings however may be unreliable (Fig. 9-19).

**Radiography.** Radiography should be done before reduction, not only to confirm the diagnosis but also to identify any fractures. The AP, Y, and axillary views are sufficient. Exception to this may be taken for patients with recurrent dislocations and minimal or no trauma. However, if reduction is not easily done, then x-rays may demonstrate the reason (e.g., interposing fracture fragment). Radiographs done after reduction are usually recommended. Some authors have suggested that if the relocation is obviously successful and the initial views were adequate to detect subtle fractures, then taking films after reduction is not necessary.[22] This approach requires some caution because relocation may cause fractures, especially in elderly patients.

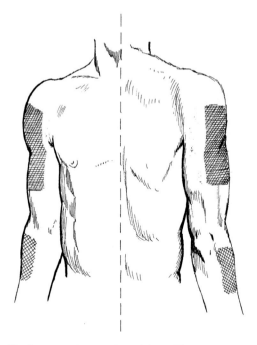

**Fig. 9-19.** Cutaneous innervation of the axillary and musculocutaneous nerves.

After assessing the patient's neurovascular status and reviewing the radiographs for obvious indications for open reduction (box on page 190), an attempt at closed reduction should be made. There are many different techniques available, each with its own advantages and disadvantages. The best technique would be one that is easy, quick, effective, without complications, and likely to require a minimum of drugs and assistance. Several techniques reportedly meet these criteria. Regardless of which technique is chosen, the most dislocations will be successfully reduced on the first attempt, even if associated with small fractures. Only 5% to 10% of closed reductions for anterior dislocations typically require general anesthesia.[23] These are usually open, chronic (more than a few days old), irreducible due to interposing structures, or associated with large anterior glenoid rim fractures or major displacement of a fractured greater tuberosity. Interposing structures are a definite block to successful closed reduction. Such structures include the joint capsule, greater tuberosity fractures, or long head of the biceps tendon. Major fractures of the anterior glenoid rim decrease stability and increase the risk of degenerative changes in the joint in the future. A greater tuberosity fracture that is displaced more than 1 cm should be reduced separately because it will shorten the rotator cuff muscles that attach there and lead to decreased overall strength.[23]

**Early shoulder reduction.** Early shoulder reduction is very important. As time passes, spasm increases, which makes reduction more difficult. Decompression of neurovascular structures is also an early goal. In addition, the longer the softer humeral head is pressed against the harder anterior scapular neck, the more likely there will be a large bony defect in the humeral head. This compression fracture (called *Hill-Sachs deformity*) may predispose to future dislocations. Therefore, after the appropriate radiographs are completed, closed reduction should be done as soon as possible.

The type of anterior shoulder dislocation has little significance in the method of reduction.[23] There are two general techniques for relocating the glenohumeral joint: traction and leverage (Table 9-2). Combinations of these exist as well. *Traction* reductions rely on traction to over-

**Table 9-2.** Techniques for reduction of anterior shoulder dislocation

| Traction | Leverage |
|---|---|
| Hippocratic | External rotation |
| Milch | Kocher |
| Eskimo | |
| Stimson | |
| Pick and Lippert | |
| (Scapular manipulation*) | |

*Scapular manipulation is a technique usually used in combination with one of the traction methods.

come muscle spasm that is locking the humeral head on the anterior scapular neck. By stretching these muscles enough to counter the spasm, the humeral head is lifted off the scapula and the rotator cuff muscles relocate it in the glenoid fossa. *Leverage* techniques also depend on some traction to lift the humeral head from its locked position on the anterior scapula but then to lever it into place. There are concerns that leverage methods cause unnecessary stress on periarticular structures and may be more likely to cause fractures of the glenoid rim and humeral shaft. *Scapular manipulation* is a technique described by Bosley and Miles in 1979[24] and further advanced by Anderson and colleagues in 1982.[25] It promises to reverse the mechanics of the original injury by focusing on repositioning the glenoid rather than the humeral head. Scapular manipulation is used in addition to a traction technique (i.e., Stimson).

Regardless of which method is used, most reductions are successful on the first attempt. Delays in presentation, fractures, interposing structures, and excessively muscular patients may have less success. Most authors believe that there is no relationship between reduction technique and future instability of the joint,[26] but some authors disagree. This latter group points to the increased incidence of recurrence with the Milch, Lacey, and Kocher methods.[27,28] Unfortunately, reported studies vary with the age of the patient, mechanism of injury, duration of dislocation, associated fractures, and soft-tissue injury as well as the use of medications before reduction. All these factors may play a role in predicting success and future instability. It is important to note that all techniques need to be performed slowly and gently but firmly to be successful and to minimize complications.

Premedication is somewhat controversial and depends on which technique will be attempted. Proponents of certain methods boast of painless reductions without medications. Other methods are quite painful and require analgesia with or without muscle relaxants. A less common and more technically difficult option is a suprascapular nerve block (described at the end of this chapter). If narcotics or other agents (e.g., muscle relaxants) are given, the patient must not be left unattended. As a general rule, these drugs are more appropriately given intravenously. In this way, the drugs have a shorter half-life, can be more easily titrated, and allow vascular access if complications occur (e.g., respiratory depression requiring naloxone administration). There should be pulse oximetry, oxygen, cardiac monitor, and suction and airway management equipment available if narcotics or benzodiazepines are given.

An alternative to this approach is to use nitrous oxide, which is an effective and safe analgesic as well as a mild sedative. Its effects in this application last less than 5 to 10 minutes. It is administered by the patient via a hand-held mask with a demand valve in a 50:50 mixture with oxygen. The risk of overmedicating the patient is decreased because a drowsy patient is unlikely to maintain the tight seal necessary to continue delivery. It is imperative that the mask not be affixed to the patient for this reason. Pulse oximetry should probably be monitored in these patients during and for 5 to 10 minutes after administration; however, hypoxia is extremely rare in this concentration.[29] Contraindications to the use of nitrous oxide include patients with significant chronic obstructive pulmonary disease, pneumothorax, bowel obstruction, alteration of mental status, shock, and pulmonary edema (see box on this page). These patients should not be left unattended while receiving nitrous oxide and should be monitored for a brief period after its administration.

The traction technique for shoulder reduction is used in a variety of methods. There are four subclasses, but all of these involve applying longitudinal traction on the abducted arm—with or without the elbow flexed—in order to relax the biceps muscle. Some techniques add external rotation to displace the greater tuberosity that may be blocking reduction. With the greater tuberosity located more posteriorly, the thinnest possible presentation of the humeral head is offered to the glenoid fossa.

The abduction method of shoulder dislocation described by Hippocrates is one of the oldest traction techniques known. It is associated with more neurovascular complications than are other methods and is less successful in the more common variety of anterior shoulder dislocations (subcoracoid) than other methods. The abduction method does work well for subglenoid type dislocations and, if done carefully, results in fewer neurovascular complications than once thought. The technique involves applying longitudinal traction on the abducted arm with additional external and internal rotation, if necessary, to disengage the impacted humeral head. To provide countertraction, the physician may place a stockinged foot in the axilla and then extend his knee and hip while pulling on the patient's arm, wrist, or hand. The foot may lift the humeral head off the scapula to facilitate reduction. It is absolutely crucial to place the foot over both the anterior and posterior axillary folds, thus maintaining the heel out of the axilla completely in order to prevent neurovascular injury. The alternative is to wrap a sheet around the patient's chest and under the axilla and have an assistant pull on the sheet toward the patient's contralateral ear (Fig. 9-20). Two other modifications include flexing the elbow to relax the biceps muscle and having an assistant lift the humeral head anteriorly off

---

**Contraindications to use of nitrous oxide**

Altered sensorium
Hypotension
Decompression sickness
Chronic obstructive pulmonary disease
Pneumothorax
Bowel obstruction
Severe maxillofacial injuries
Pulmonary edema or diminished cardiac reserve

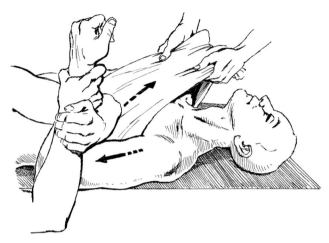

**Fig. 9-20.** A modification of the traction-countertraction technique for shoulder reduction initially described by Hippocrates.

the glenoid. Once reduced, the arm should be adducted and immobilized. Neurovascular assessment after reduction is mandatory and radiographs should be obtained to confirm reduction and reevaluate for fractures.

**Techniques.** Milch's technique was first described in 1938 as a modification of Cooper's technique.[30] Lacey modified it further. Milch's method is done with the patient supine, elbow flexed at 90°, and the physician standing at the affected side. It involves essentially three steps. First, the arm should be moved slowly into full abduction while an assistant presses on the medial and inferior aspect of the humeral head toward the fossa to prevent inferior displacement. If spasm occurs, movement should stop until the muscles relax. The second step involves extending the elbow and gradually applying in-line traction. If necessary, the arm may be externally rotated and more pressure applied on the humeral head. As the humeral head slips into

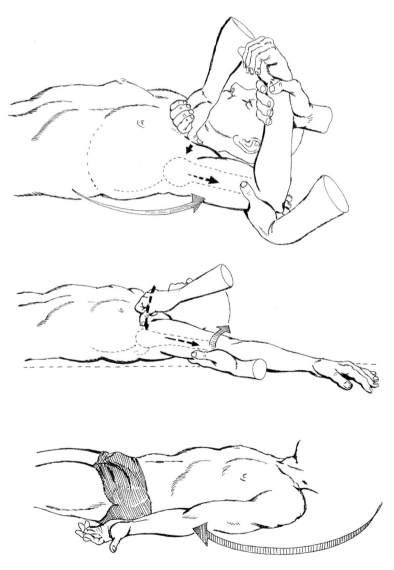

**Fig. 9-21.** The Milch technique is a three-step maneuver.

place, the arm should be adducted gradually (Fig. 9-21). These movements put most muscles around the shoulder into a plane parallel with the humeral axis. Proponents of this method argue that it is effective (over 90% fast), and usually accomplished without medications or complications.[31,32] It may also be a preferred method in patients with heavier builds. Lacey modified it to a prone position with the elbow flexed.[33] In either method, radiographs and neurovascular evaluation after reduction are recommended.

The Eskimo method (Greenland) is an extremely painful technique. The patient lies on the ground in a decubitus position with the unaffected shoulder down. The physician (usually with an assistant) stands over the patient and virtually lifts him off the ground by the affected arm (Fig. 9-22). It is reportedly successful 80% of the time, but may be associated with more damage to periarticular structures.[34] Premedication is obviously a necessity with this technique as are radiographs after reduction.

The gentler but slower methods of reduction are the forward-flexion techniques. These involve the slow stretching and relaxation of shoulder girdle musculature to permit spontaneous natural reduction. (Cole adapted Stimson's technique for reducing hip dislocations for the shoulder; for some reason, Cole's technique is credited to Stimson.) The patient is prone with the affected shoulder slightly off the cart and the arm hanging in forward flexion (Fig. 9-23). Originally, it was believed that the weight of the arm alone would be sufficient to reduce the shoulder, but most proponents now recommend that 5 to 10 lb of weight be hung from the arm in some manner. The smaller weights should be used for thin or elderly patients and heavier weights for more muscular patients or those with a delay in presentation. No pain medications are usually necessary, but the procedure can take up to 30 minutes to be successful. This technique is highly effective and relatively atraumatic. Several modifications have been proposed. Pick[35] and Lippert suggested placing the elbow in flexion to relax the biceps and decrease stretch on neurovascular structures. The weight is then hung from the elbow (Fig. 9-24). If these methods are unsuccessful, external rotation may help. Again, this movement displaces the greater tuberosity posteriorly, presenting a thinner profile to the glenoid. Radiographs after reduction are recommended to confirm successful reduction and assess for fractures.

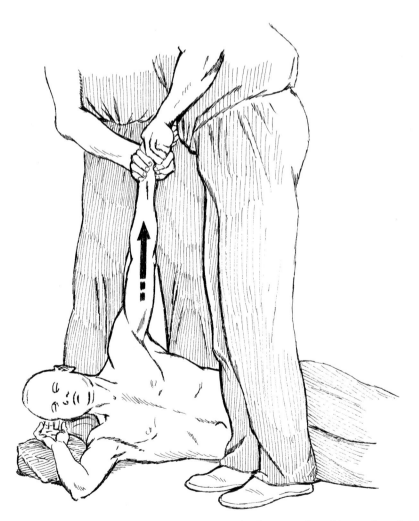

**Fig. 9-22.** The Eskimo method will require the strength of two people and is usually painful.

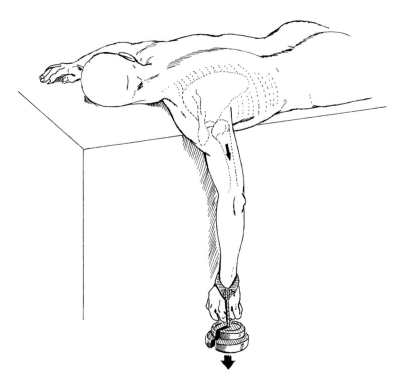

**Fig. 9-23.** Stimson's method affects reduction by the use of weights and gravity overcoming muscle spasm.

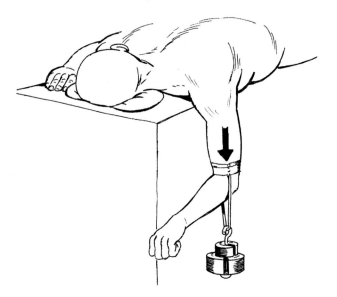

**Fig. 9-24.** A popular modification of Stimson's method is to hang the weights from the flexed elbow.

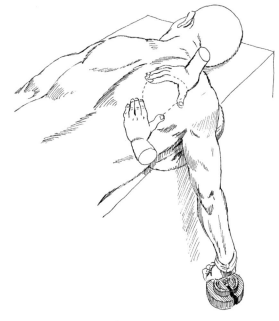

**Fig. 9-25.** Scapular manipulation is usually done in conjunction with a traction method such as Stimson's.

Scapular manipulation should be mentioned at this point. It is based on the idea of reversing the mechanics of the dislocation by returning the glenoid to its proper anatomic relationship with the humeral head.[24,25] It is quick, easy, and relatively atraumatic. It is very effective with success rates reported as high as 96%.[36]

Complications with this technique are rare. Positioning is identical to the above-mentioned Stimson technique. Patients may be premedicated and manipulation done im-

mediately after the weights are attached, or the physician may wait 5 to 10 minutes to allow the muscles to stretch and relax. Manipulation is done by stabilizing the superiomedial edge of the scapula with one hand while directing the tip of the scapula medially (Fig. 9-25). Radiographs after reduction are suggested, as is a repeat neurovascular examination, although complications are unusual.

Leverage techniques are centuries old and were diagrammed on an Egyptian tomb in 1200 BC. These techniques are typically successful and may be preferred for more muscular patients. There are two commonly used methods: the external rotation method and Kocher's technique. The former is gaining more popularity because it is fast and simple. Kocher's technique has been associated with increased complications compared with other methods and usually requires analgesics. This technique is losing favor with most clinicians.

The external rotation method (also called Hennepin's method) was described by Liedelmeyer in 1977.[37] It again relies on the fact that external rotation presents the smallest profile of the humeral head to the fossa, thus facilitating reduction. It is highly effective, fast, simple, and relatively painless. The patient lies supine with the arm adducted and elbow flexed. The physician holds the elbow in place and grasps the wrist while externally rotating the forearm slowly (Fig. 9-26). Gravity and the weight of the forearm should be the true determinants of how fast the forearm falls. The physician should not force the arm. There is usually no traction applied. Occasionally, patients cannot ascertain relocation, but active internal and external rotation is restored. Follow-up radiographs should be done, as well as a repeat neurovascular assessment. Complications are rare.[38]

Kocher's method has been nearly abandoned by emergency physicians because of its high incidence of complications. Other disadvantages include the need for significant strength or force and the amount of pain, which mandates premedication of these patients. The key to successful reduction with a minimum of complications is slow, gentle traction. The technique requires four steps. The patient lies supine with the elbow flexed and arm adducted. Gentle in-line traction is applied and the shoulder is externally rotated maximally. Then the arm is adducted across the chest until the elbow nears the midline. The final step is to internally rotate so that the hand touches the unaffected shoulder (Fig. 9-27). In this way, the humerus is levered against the thoracic wall. Cromwell added traction during adduction. Complications include vascular tears, spiral fracture of the humeral neck, and rotator cuff tears. This method may be preferred in patients with heavier builds and those with marked spasm or delay in presentation, but in elderly or thin patients it may cause significant damage to periarticular structure.[23] Some authors believe that Kocher's technique also is associated with an increased risk of recurrence.[27,28] Its overall success rate is comparable to other methods with lower complication rates.[39] Therefore, there are few advocates of this technique.

Again, all these techniques have had some success and require slow, gentle movements. Studies comparing the techniques are not well controlled for age, history of recurrence, degree of trauma (associated injuries), duration of dislocation, and drug usage. Thus, it is difficult to identify just one obviously better technique. Fig. 9-28 is a proposed approach if there is no obvious need for open reduction (e.g., interposing structure, large glenoid fracture, markedly displaced fracture of the greater tuberosity, or open fracture). Techniques such as the Kocher and Hippocratic methods have been virtually abandoned due to their higher rate of complications without offering any real advantage.[23]

Neurovascular evaluation and radiographs are recommended after reduction. A recent study suggested that routine radiographs after reduction may not be necessary in anterior shoulder dislocations.[22] It is true that successful reduction can usually be determined by the patient's resumption of active internal and external rotation. Acute, excessive external rotation should be avoided. However, fractures may be caused by reduction or simply better identified on films afterward. Therefore, further studies need to be done before this routine practice is discarded.

After reduction, the shoulder should be immobilized in a sling and swathe or shoulder immobilizer (Fig. 9-29). The goal is adduction and internal rotation. The patient should extend the elbow and externally rotate the arm to neutral (0° external rotation) several times a day to prevent stiffness. Isometric exercises are recommended, especially for the internal rotators. Duration of immobilization is controversial. Most orthopedists immobilize a patient less than 40 years of age for 3 to 6 weeks in an attempt to decrease the risk of recurrence. Older patients are less likely to dislocate again and more likely to develop complications associated with prolonged immobilization (e.g., adhesive capsulitis). Thus, patients over 40 years of age are usually immobilized for 1 to 3 weeks. Patients with previous dislocations are sometimes only immobilized for a week.

**Complications.** Complications associated with anterior dislocations include fractures, rotator cuff tears, and neurovascular injuries. Three fractures are more common: Hill-Sachs, glenoid rim, and greater tuberosity. The Hill-Sachs deformity (Fig. 9-30) is a posterolateral humeral head compression fracture best seen on an AP view with internal rotation. Its incidence is said to be as high as 40% in initial dislocations and 70% in recurrent ones. There is a relationship between larger defects of the humeral head and increased instability. As this defect rotates into glenoid fossa during normal abduction and external rotation, the joint becomes mechanically less stable. Less common is an anteroinferior glenoid rim fracture called an *osseous Bankart lesion* (Fig. 9-31). Bankart initially referred to the avulsion of the anterior glenoid labrum in recurrent anterior shoulder dislocations as the *essential lesion.* The bony rim involvement was subsequently named. Both entities may lead to increased anterior instability and subsequent recurrence if healing is incomplete.[40] Surgery is indicated if defects are large or prevent reduction. These lesions occur in approximately 5% to 10% of anterior dislocations. This is the same incidence reported for fractures of the greater tuberosity. As rotator cuff tendons are stressed, they may tear or avulse the tuberosity. Displacement of 5 to 10 mm of

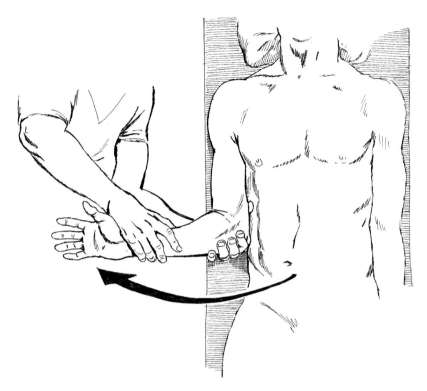

**Fig. 9-26.** The external rotation method is best performed with the patient supine, thus allowing gravity to lever the humeral head into anatomic position.

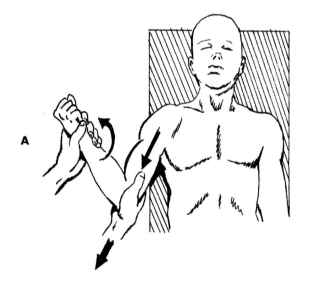

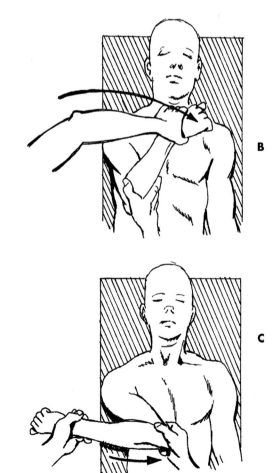

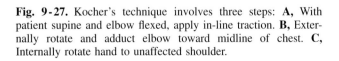

**Fig. 9-27.** Kocher's technique involves three steps: **A,** With patient supine and elbow flexed, apply in-line traction. **B,** Externally rotate and adduct elbow toward midline of chest. **C,** Internally rotate hand to unaffected shoulder.

Anterior Dislocation
(Without obvious reason for reduction under general anesthesia)

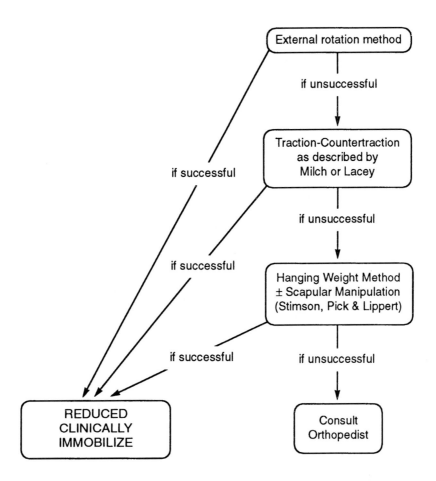

Kocher and Hippocratic methods are specifically excluded due to increased complications.

**Fig. 9-28.** Proposed algorithm for approaching anterior shoulder dislocations without an obvious indication for operative management.

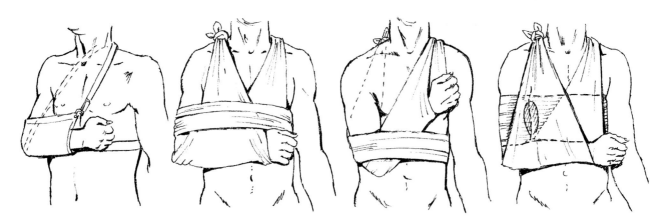

**Fig. 9-29.** Various types of shoulder immobilization.

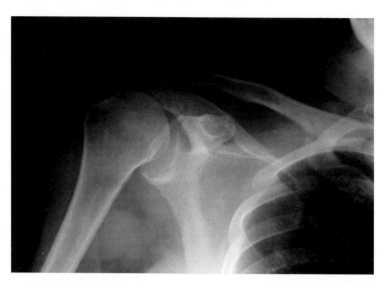

**Fig. 9-30.** X-ray with Hill-Sachs deformity associated with anterior shoulder dislocations.

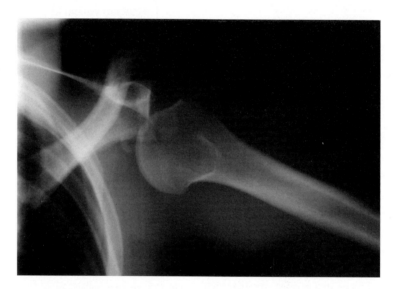

**Fig. 9-31.** Fracture of the anteroinferior glenoid rim is called an *osseous Bankart lesion.* This is seen in anterior shoulder dislocations and is associated with increased instability.

the greater tuberosity usually requires surgery to prevent weakness of the rotator cuff muscles.

Rotator cuff tears are often present, especially in older age groups. The overall incidence of rotator cuff injuries may be as high as 55% of all anterior dislocations. In fact, it has been reported to be as high as 80% in patients over 60 years of age. Patients have a slow recovery and continued pain and weakness of the external rotation and abduction (see the section below on Rotator Cuff Tears). Although a rotator cuff tear should be suspected initially, prolonged recovery is highly suggestive of a rotator cuff tear or axillary nerve injury.

Vascular injuries are more common in elderly patients, but are still quite rare. They can occur during dislocation or reduction, especially if excessive force is used. The mechanism is transsection, avulsion of a major branch, or intralu-

minal thrombus. Distal pulses should be checked before and after reduction. An arteriogram should be considered if there is a pulse deficit, pallor, pain, cyanosis, coolness, neurologic deficit, bruit, expanding axillary hematoma, or shock. Pressure may be applied near the first rib and clavicle to attempt temporary hemostasis if bleeding is suspected.

Neurologic deficits also occur during dislocation or reduction and therefore need to be evaluated afterward. Incidence increases with age, degree of trauma, and duration of dislocation. The reported incidence is as high as 30%, but 5% to 10% is more likely. Axillary nerve injuries are the most common.[2,41] Sensation over the deltoid muscle and the muscle's contractility are reasonable screens, albeit not sensitive ones. The brachial plexus is just inferior to the joint and therefore also vulnerable to injury. The most

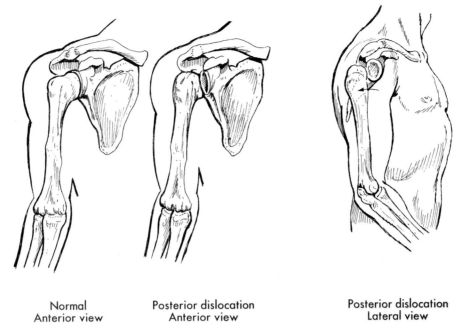

Normal
Anterior view

Posterior dislocation
Anterior view

Posterior dislocation
Lateral view

**Fig. 9-32.** Anatomically it is easy to see why posterior shoulder dislocations are often missed on initial AP shoulder x-rays.

common mechanism is traction or neuropraxia. Full recovery is expected in 1 to 2 months. Axonotmesis is less common but does occur. This is transsection of the axons, although the neural sheath is intact. Recovery is slower but usually complete. Full transsection, or neurotmesis, is rare in shoulder dislocations. Because the majority of nerve injuries are secondary to traction, early reduction decompresses the neural structures, thus decreasing injury and improving prognosis. Consideration should be given to axillary nerve injury if recovery is delayed.

Recurrence is usually more common in those patients with severe trauma, glenoid rim fractures, large defects in the humeral head, and younger age groups.[26] Longer duration of immobilization and early rehabilitation exercises may also be helpful in reducing future instability. Studies have shown that, in general, the method of reduction is probably less of a factor than previously believed (if it is any influence at all).[2,26] Also, the type of immobilization and dominant versus nondominant extremity do not predict future recurrence. Interestingly, there may be two distinct patterns of injury. In younger patients, the glenohumeral ligament and the glenoid labrum, with or without bony involvement, are commonly injured and heal poorly, leaving a vulnerable area anteriorly. This may account for the increased incidence of recurrence in younger patients. Older patients are more likely to stretch the ligament and capsule or tear the rotator cuff (or even avulse the greater tuberosity), but this injury will not affect future stability. In fact, a greater tuberosity fracture is one factor associated with less recurrences.[2] Recurrent dislocations are most likely to occur in the first 2 years following the initial dislocation. The incidence in patients under 20 years of age is 55% to 95% versus 5% to 15% in patients over 40 years of age.[2,26] Some studies have shown that instituting aggres-

sive rehabilitation exercises in younger patients has resulted in an incidence approaching that of the older age groups. *Occasional recurrers* are patients who have shoulder dislocations several years apart. These patients rarely need surgery. *Frequent recurrers* have several dislocations a year and may benefit from operative repair of any labral or capsular pathology.[2]

**Posterior dislocations**

Posterior dislocations account for less than 5% of all shoulder dislocations, which is fortunate, because the literature suggests that up to 50% of them are missed at initial evaluation. In fact, the diagnosis should be considered whenever external rotation is lost after a fall. The mechanism is an axial load on an adducted, internally rotated, and forward flexed arm (Fig. 9-2); a direct blow to the anterior shoulder; or causes severe muscular contractions (e.g., seizure or electrical injury). This last scenario causes posterior dislocation as the result of powerful internal rotators (latissimus dorsi, pectoralis major, and subscapularis) overpowering the weaker external rotators (teres minor and infraspinatus).

A patient with a posterior shoulder dislocation presents with the arm in a sling position and always internally rotated. There are subtle visual clues to the diagnosis. There is usually ecchymoses over the deltoid and suprascapular areas, prominence of the coracoid process and posterior shoulder (humeral head), and flattening of the anterior shoulder and deltoid curve. Patients are unable to externally rotate or elevate the arm above 90°.

There are three types of posterior dislocations: subacromial, subglenoid, and subspinous. The subacromial type is present in 98% of cases. The humeral head is posterior to the glenoid and inferior to the acromion (Fig. 9-32). The other two varieties are quite rare. Posterior to the glenoid fossa, the humeral head is inferior to the glenoid in the subglenoid type and medial to the acromion and inferior to the scapular spine in the subspinous type. Radiographs including AP, lateral (Y), and axillary views are necessary to confirm the dislocation and diagnose other associated injuries. The AP view may appear normal or there may be simply some overlap of the humeral head on the glenoid. The Y or axillary view gives the diagnosis and identifies any defect of the humeral head (Fig. 9-33). As the humeral head dislocates posteriorly, it stretches the strong anterior muscles, which then pull it back toward its normal position, abutting the softer humeral head against the hard posterior rim of the glenoid fossa. This causes a compression defect on the anteromedial articular surface of the humeral head and is called the *reverse Hill-Sachs lesion* or *trough sign* (Fig. 9-34).[42] Other associated injuries include fractures of the posterior rim of the glenoid fossa and the greater and lesser tuberosities as well as capsular and labral tears.

These injuries are often missed on initial radiographs but usually well visualized by CT scanning.[43] It is logical to see why neurovascular injuries are rare with posterior dislocations because all neurovascular structures are anterior and inferior to the glenohumeral joint.

**Treatment.**   Treatment usually requires general anesthesia. Spasm of the strong anterior muscles may impact the humeral head on the posterior scapular neck. If attempting closed reduction, strong sedation and muscle relaxation must be used. The patient should be supine. Humeral fractures can occur during relocation, especially if the process is not done gently and during internal rotation. Therefore, while maintaining internal rotation, slow in-line traction must be applied to the adducted arm. Usually, the humeral head needs to be lifted off the glenoid by an examiner's hand during traction. If reduced, a radiograph afterward is necessary. Some orthopedists will immobilize the shoulder in a sling and swathe for 3 to 4 weeks, but this places the shoulder in internal rotation, which is probably

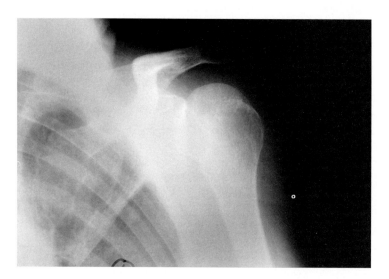

**Fig. 9-33.** X-ray of posterior shoulder dislocation.

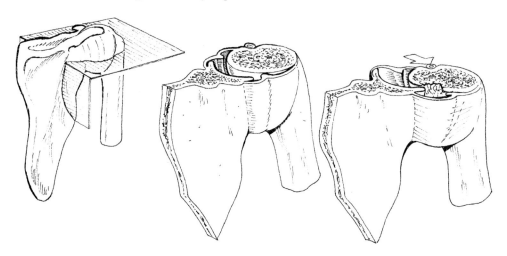

**Fig. 9-34.** Reverse Hill-Sachs lesion is a compression defect on the anteromedial aspect of the humeral head seen with some posterior shoulder dislocations.

not appropriate.[44] Some orthopedists place the shoulder in abduction, extension, and slight external rotation or a shoulder spica.[45] Surgery is indicated for open dislocations, instability, inability to reduce the shoulder (failed closed dislocations), large fractures of the posterior glenoid, or significant displacement of an avulsed lesser tuberosity. Eventual rehabilitation of external rotator muscles is necessary.

### Inferior dislocations

*Luxatio erecta* is another term for inferior dislocation of the shoulder. It was first described in 1859, but is accounts for less than 1% of all shoulder dislocations. It occurs more often in the elderly patient who has forced hyperabduction. The humerus is forced against the acromion, which acts as a fulcrum, to lever the humeral head out of the fossa, thereby tearing the capsule and rotator cuff. This is different than the anterior subglenoid and posterior subglenoid dislocations mentioned earlier because there is no contact between the humeral head and glenoid rim in inferior dislocations.

The patient with luxatio erecta is not difficult to diagnose. In severe pain, this patient classically is fully abducted, has his or her elbow flexed, and has the forearm on or behind his or her head. The humeral head is easily palpated on the lateral thorax. Neurovascular compromise is very common because these structures are inferior to the joint.

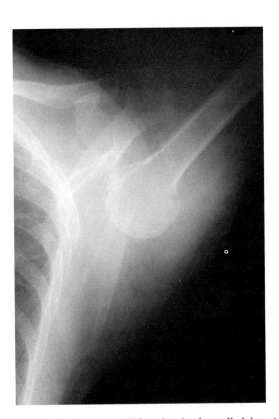

**Fig. 9-35.** Inferior shoulder dislocation is also called *luxatio erecta.*

AP and lateral (Y) radiographs easily demonstrate the dislocation (Fig. 9-35). Fractures of the inferior glenoid, greater tuberosity and acromion, as well as severe soft-tissue injury and rotator cuff tears, can occur.[46]

With analgesia, closed reduction can be done using in-line traction. An assistant is necessary to apply countertraction with a sheet over the injured shoulder and across the thorax while the physician applies in-line traction during slow adduction (Fig. 9-36). A radiograph after reduction is indicated as well as a repeat neurovascular assessment. Fortunately, most deficits are relieved by reduction. (Arteriography is indicated if any evidence exists of continued vascular insufficiency.) A shoulder immobilizer or sling and swathe should be applied. The patient should follow-up with an orthopedic surgeon in 1 week. Occasionally, severe capsular damage and interposing structures prevent closed reduction. These patients need operative repair as do those with open inferior dislocations.

### Superior dislocations

Superior dislocations are extremely rare but do occur. The mechanism is a severe force directed upward and forward on an adducted arm. Typically, the humeral head is superior to the fossa with the arm adducted and shortened (Fig. 9-37). The patient has significant pain and restricted movement, and neurovascular injuries are usually present. X-rays usually demonstrate other associated pathology such as fractures of the acromion, clavicle, coracoid process, and humeral tuberosities; rotator cuff tears; and other soft-tissue injuries. Fortunately, closed reduction is usually easily accomplished with analgesia. Radiographs and neurovascular assessment afterward are necessary.

## SOFT-TISSUE INJURIES
### Contusions and sprains

Shoulder sprains and contusions occur by the same mechanism as dislocations and are self-limited. The patient has pain and occasionally swelling but less disability (i.e., near normal ROM) and a normal radiograph. Treatment involves analgesics, cold compresses, and immobilization for 1 week. At that time, a reassessment should be made and gradual active ROM exercises should be initiated.

### Acute traumatic subacromial bursitis

Subacromial bursitis is associated with forces pressing the humeral head against the acromion. This places pressure on the subacromial bursa, which becomes inflamed. If aspirated, the bursa may yield a bloody fluid. Patients have pain that is often described as burning and can be temporarily relieved with the infiltration of 10 ml of 1% xylocaine (positive Neer's and Hawkin's tests; see the sections Examination and Impingement). The differential for subacromial bursitis includes subluxation and dislocation as well as a rotator cuff tear. The treatment for bursitis is rest for 3 to 6 weeks, heat and stretching, and strengthening exercises. In an acute episode, steroid injection should be avoided.

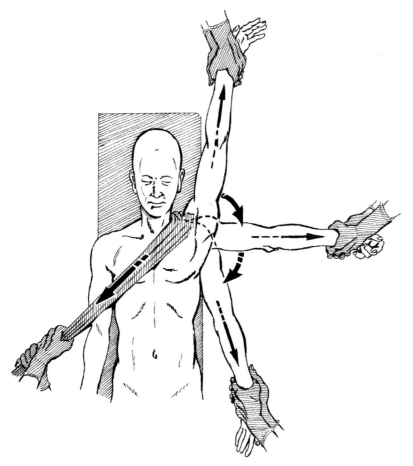

**Fig. 9-36.** Reduction of inferior dislocation of the shoulder. While an assistant provides counter-traction, the physician applies in-line traction as he slowly adducts the arm.

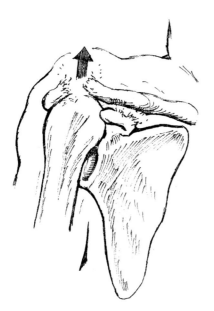

**Fig. 9-37.** Superior dislocation is usually associated with fractures and severe soft-tissue injuries.

Without proper rehabilitation, the patient may develop impingement in the future.

### Tendinitis

*Biceps tendinitis* is defined as anterior shoulder pain with a positive Speed's or Yergason's sign (see Examination). Tendinitis is usually the result of trauma and is often a part of impingement. Glenohumeral instability may be obscured by the presence of tendinitis. Therefore, tests for instability should be done in all patients with the diagnosis of biceps tendinitis. There are essentially two forms of biceps tendinitis: calcific and noncalcific. Radiographs distinguish these diagnoses. If the radiograph shows an amorphous cloudiness in the area of the subacromial bursa or supraspinatus tendon, the diagnosis, of course, is bursitis or calcific tendinitis. This cloudiness reflects crystals of basic calcium phosphate (e.g., calcium hydroxyapatite) that are deposited within the rotator cuff and biceps tendon (Fig. 9-38). This creates inflammation and pain. These crystals can then gain access into the bursa, causing more pain and inflammation. Over a period of weeks, the calcium is reabsorbed and the symptoms resolve even if untreated.

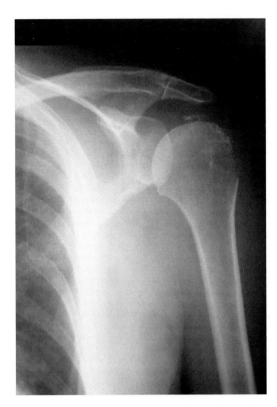

**Fig. 9-38.** Calcium deposits in the rotator cuff and biceps tendon make the diagnosis of calcific tendinitis easier.

Initially, there is pain during active ROM as well as a deep ache in the shoulder. There is tenderness over the tendon. Occasionally, calcifications are seen in an asymptomatic individual. Calcific tendinitis tends not to be related to acute trauma and is more suggestive of impingement. Noncalcific tendinitis may have a normal radiographic appearance and is difficult to differentiate from a rotator cuff tear.

Treatment for both forms of biceps tendinitis includes rest from painful activity (restricted abduction), nonsteroidal anti-inflammatory agents (NSAIDs), and, eventually, exercises to increase strength of the internal and external rotators. In true impingement, the occasional use of steroids in the subacromial space or in the intertubercular groove may be helpful but should only be done by an experienced clinician committed to long-term follow-up.[6,7] Unfortunately, this may weaken the tendon enough to cause spontaneous rupture. It is extremely important that patients limit activity for 2 to 3 weeks after a steroid injection. If, after 6 months, conservative therapy fails, surgery may be indicated.

### Rotator cuff tears

Although rotator cuff tears are usually chronic, they are associated with acute trauma. Delays in their treatment are associated with decreased functional recovery. The rotator cuff is essentially four muscles whose tendons surround the glenohumeral joint, thus controlling internal and external

rotation as well as assisting the deltoid muscle in abduction. The supraspinatus, infraspinatus, teres minor, and subscapularis work as a single unit to stabilize the humeral head in the glenoid fossa during most movements. The supraspinatus is the most frequently diagnosed rotator cuff tear. Tears tend to occur near its insertion (perhaps because of a relatively avascular zone described there).[47] Occasionally, teres minor and infraspinatus tendons are involved, but rarely is the subscapularis tendon torn (except when unnecessary forces are used in closed reduction of anterior dislocations). Be aware that the long head of the biceps tendon may rupture and present in a similar way to a rotator cuff tear.

Rotator cuff tears occur by direct blows or indirect forces such as a fall on an outstretched hand. Five injury patterns of rotator cuff tears have been described[48]:

1. Chronic with or without history of trauma
2. Anterior dislocation
3. Avulsion fracture of the greater tuberosity
4. Any dislocation with an avulsion fracture of the greater tuberosity
5. Severe injury without fracture or dislocation.

By far, the most common of these is the chronic variety (95%) that is associated with impingement (see Impingement). That is not surprising because the diagnosis is often missed acutely in the presence of a dislocation.

Physical examination offers clues to a rotator cuff tear by weakness of abduction. The differential diagnosis is subacromial bursitis, tendinitis of the long head of the biceps tendon or rotator cuff muscles, subluxation, dislocation, and fractures. There are several tests to assess the integrity of the rotator cuff. The supraspinatus strength test, as described earlier, essentially isolates this tendon. It involves maintaining 90° abduction, 30° forward flexion, and maximal internal rotation against resistance (Fig. 9-11). The "drop arm test" is performed by passively abducting the arm to 90° and asking the patient to lower it slowly in the same plane (i.e., without forward flexing). If pain develops or the patient is unable to lower the arm slowly, a rotator cuff tear is indicated. If either test is positive, 10 ml of 1% xylocaine should be infiltrated anteriorly and inferior to the acromion. If the pain is relieved, but the patient still cannot actively abduct, the diagnosis of rotator cuff tear is made (Neer's test).[9]

Radiographs show no calcification but may reveal a narrowed acromiohumeral distance (less than 5 to 6 mm).[11,12] The lack of interposing tendon between the acromion and humeral head, in addition to the unopposed action of the deltoid muscle, causes slight subluxation superiorly of the humerus. This is often apparent on radiographs done after reducing an anterior dislocation. To confirm a rotator cuff tear in a patient who is not improving with conservative management or one in whom a large tear is suspected, MRI or arthrography should be done to demonstrate extravasation of dye from the glenohumeral

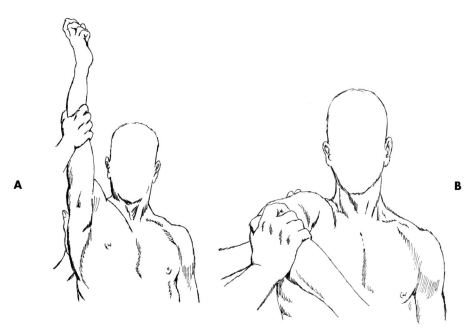

**Fig. 9-39.** Tests for impingement are **A,** passively forward flexing the arm while it is internally rotated and **B,** passively internally rotating the arm while it is forward flexed to 90°. If either maneuver creates pain, impingement is the leading diagnosis and Neer's test should be done.

joint. The latter is invasive and the former, although expensive, offers more accuracy and information on other structures. Many orthopedists who do not suspect large tears may try 10 to 14 days of immobilization and reevaluation before ordering these tests.

Treatment of a small tear is usually immobilization in a sling for a few weeks. The patient should be rechecked before beginning muscle strengthening and ROM exercises. Large tears usually require surgery and delays may result in poor functional recovery.[48,49]

### Impingement

Subacromial space pathology was called impingement by Neer in 1972.[50] He described it as a mechanical conflict under and against the rigid coracoacromial arch. This is defined by the coracoid process, anterior edge of the acromion, and the coracoacromial ligament. The supraspinatus, long head of the biceps tendon, and the subacromial bursa as well as the proximal humerus must pass through this area. Impingement is increased pressure on these structures that causes pain and inflammation. Long-term impingement results in fibrosis of the bursa and eventually tendon destruction and rupture (i.e., rotator cuff tear). Impingement occurs more in overhead movements with various degrees of internal rotation (e.g., pitching, tennis). This forces the long head of the biceps tendon and supraspinatus tendon against the anterior edge of the acromion. Impingement also results from congenital hooking of the anterior acromion, bony spurs of the anterioinferior acromion, and fibrotic thickening of the coracoacromial ligament.

The diagnosis is suggested by limited abduction due to pain and a positive impingement test. One test is to forcibly forward flex and internally rotate the arm, pressing the greater tuberosity against the acromion to elicit pain.[50] Hawkin's test is performed by passively forward flexing to 90° and then internally rotating, thus pressing the supraspinatus tendon against the rigid coracoacromial arch (Fig. 9-39).[8] When one or both of these tests result in pain, Neer's test is indicated. Inject 10 ml of 1% xylocaine

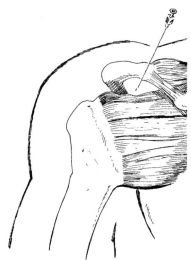

**Fig. 9-40.** Neer's test involves the injection of 10 ml of 1% xylocaine inferior to the anterior edge of the acromion. Then, the tests for impingement are repeated. If pain and mobility are improved, the diagnosis is impingement.

inferior to the anterior edge of the acromion and then recheck these two maneuvers. If pain and mobility are improved, impingement is diagnosed (i.e., a positive Neer's test)[30] (Fig. 9-40). MRI may give more specific anatomic information.[51]

There are three stages of impingement as delineated by Neer.[9] Stage I is seen in young athletes with positive Neer's and Hawkin's tests. The signs are edema and hemorrhage, usually as a result of overly aggressive training. There is inflammation of the subacromial bursa or tendinitis of the supraspinatus. This is a reversible phase when treated with cold compresses, rest, NSAIDs, and physiotherapy. After a few weeks, rehabilitation exercises to strengthen shoulder internal rotators and external rotators should be started to prevent future problems. Stage II is the result of chronic overuse and the normal degenerative changes of aging. The patients are usually between 25 to 40 years of age. Joint mobility is maintained, but patients complain of pain with normal activities and at night. Neer's and Hawkin's tests are again positive. During this phase, fibrosis and tendinitis are present. Treatment is the same as for Stage I but longer. If conservative treatment fails after 12 to 18 months, surgery should be considered. Stage III is seen in the middle-aged sportsman with a long history of tendinitis. The patient has nocturnal pain and limited ROM. Impingement tests for these patients will be positive. The anterior acromion may have bony spurs or erosion on the radiograph. Both findings suggest wear on the underlying supraspinatus tendon, which eventually ruptures. The only options are surgery or (if there is no rotator cuff tear) a brief trial of steroids.[7]

**Labral tears**

The biceps tendon may originate from the glenoid labrum and be contiguous with the superior portion of the structure. When stimulated, the biceps tendon may tear the labrum off the glenoid rim. Labral tears are also associated with dislocations and subluxations. Of tears of the glenoid labrum, 80% occur in the anterosuperior portion near the origin of the long head of the biceps tendon.[3] Tears usually represent a degenerative process seen in elderly patients. Symptoms include pain, tenderness over the glenohumeral joint, and a "popping" or "catching" of the glenohumeral joint, especially in full abduction. Physical examination is usually not diagnostic; arthroscopy can be used to diagnose the condition.[44] Labral tears require the assistance of an orthopedic specialist because conservative therapy may not be successful.

**INVASIVE TECHNIQUES**

Invasive shoulder procedures include arthrocentesis, subacromial bursa injection, and supraspinatus nerve block. Emergency arthrocentesis of the shoulder joint is relatively uncommon; joint infection would be one indication. There are two approaches: anterior and posterior. Most physicians have more success with the posterior approach. The patient

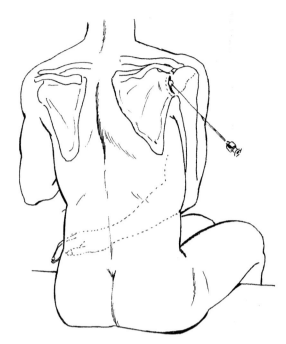

**Fig. 9-41.** Posterior approach to shoulder arthrocentesis is done with the patient seated and arm adducted and internally rotated as much as possible.

is seated with the arm adducted and internally rotated. After skin preparation, a two-inch 20-gauge needle is introduced inferior to the posterolateral aspect of the acromion and directed anteromedially. The joint is usually aspirated within one inch of the skin (Fig. 9-41). The anterior approach is done with the arm slightly abducted and slightly externally rotated. A two-inch, 20-gauge needle is used after appropriate skin preparation. It is placed just inferolateral to the coracoid process and directed posteromedially. The joint should be located at a depth of less than one inch (Fig. 9-42).

The subacromial space is located immediately inferior to the acromion. Blood or inflammatory effusion may be aspirated in trauma or calcific bursitis, respectively. Neer's test involves injecting 10 ml of 1% xylocaine in this area to diagnose impingement (Fig. 9-40). In an acute exacerbation, there is no reason to inject steroids into the bursa. This should probably be limited to chronic, recurrent impingement and done by experienced clinicians who will provide long-term follow-up.

Suprascapular nerve block may be used to relieve acute shoulder pain and has been advocated as an adjunct in shoulder reductions. It is extremely safe but does require skill. The goal is to anesthetize the suprascapular nerve as it passes through the suprascapular notch. A 1½-inch needle with 5 to 10 ml of xylocaine should be used, and the patient should be in a sitting position. Lines should be drawn along the spine of the scapula and the lower border of the scapula. A line from the scapular tip should be drawn cephalad bisecting the line drawn over the scapular spine. At approximately 1.5 cm superiorly and medially from where these two lines meet, the needle should be inserted. It is crucial that aspiration before injection is done. If the scapula is encountered, the needle should be partly withdrawn and reintroduced medially and somewhat more caudally until the suprascapular notch is entered (Fig. 9-43). If the needle is not inserted more than 1.5 cm, the thoracic cavity should not be violated, thus avoiding the

development of pneumothorax. Again, this technique has become a lost art, but offers safe analgesia for the glenohumeral joint and surrounding shoulder structures.

## MISCELLANEOUS

Acromioclavicular (AC) separation is in the differential of any patient with a direct blow to the shoulder. Palpation of the AC area reveals tenderness. Deformity of the AC joint suggests more significant ligamentous injury (Grade II or III) (see Chapter 8 for more details).

Adhesive capsulitis is seen primarily in patients immobilized for a period of time. The mechanism is unclear. Patients complain of pain and restricted motion in all planes. Routine radiographs are normal. Arthrography is diagnostic, revealing a very small joint space. Early mobilization of the shoulder, such as pendulum or pocketbook swing, should prevent this (Fig. 9-44).

Arthritis also occurs in the shoulder causing pain and general restriction of motion. Arthritis rarely is isolated to the shoulder, making the diagnosis more obvious. All forms of arthritis have been reported to involve the shoulder (see box on page 209). Arthritis is associated with rotator cuff tears and may be a direct cause of tendon rupture. Treatment depends on the type of arthritis.

Primary osseous tumors of the shoulder are extremely rare, as are soft-tissue tumors. The diagnosis of osteoid osteoma should be considered when shoulder pain is relieved by salicylates. Metastases and Paget's disease are more common but are usually apparent on plain radiographs. Further testing with CT, MRI, or a radionuclide

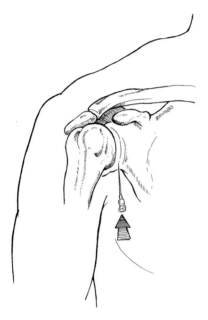

**Fig. 9-42.** Anterior approach to arthrocentesis is done with the arm abducted slightly and externally rotated.

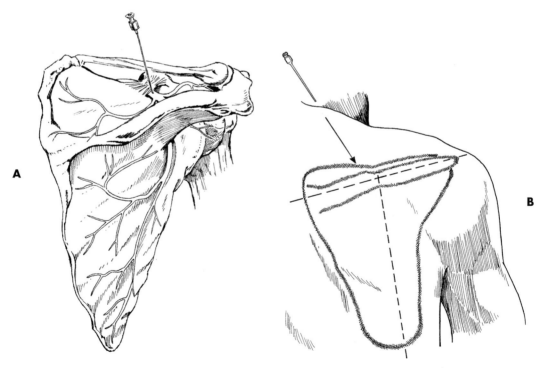

**Fig. 9-43.** The suprascapular nerve (**A**) may be anesthetized at the point where it passes through the suprascapular notch (**B**).

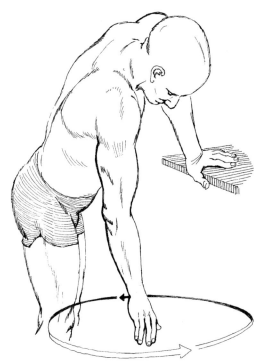

**Fig. 9-44.** Early range-of-motion exercises may prevent adhesive capsulitis.

---

**Arthritic causes of shoulder pain**

Infective arthritis
Crystalline arthropathy (gout or pyrophosphate)
Osteoarthritis
Rheumatoid arthritis
Idiopathic destructive arthritis
Neuropathic arthritis

---

bone scan may be necessary. Any tumor that presses on or erodes into the brachial plexus can cause shoulder pain (e.g., Pancoast's tumor).

Neurovascular compression around the shoulder unrelated to trauma is unusual but does cause shoulder pain. The subclavian vessels and brachial plexus may be compressed near the first rib and clavicle. This is often called *thoracic outlet syndrome.* Various physical abnormalities may cause this problem; treatment depends on the specific etiology. The diagnosis is suggested by a pulse change or pain or paresthesia of the upper extremity with certain movements. For example, Adson's test is done with the patient seated and head extended and rotated toward the affected side. The radial pulse is palpated as the patient takes a deep breath. If the pulse diminishes, the test is positive. The hyperabduction test is positive if there is a decrease in pulse or if the patient's symptoms are reproduced when the patient takes a deep breath while standing, with head extended and shoulder passively abducted. The quadrangular space syndrome involves compression of the posterior circumflex humeral artery or the axillary nerve. This is an extremely rare cause of shoulder pain. Both diagnoses (thoracic outlet syndrome and quadrangular space syndrome) are made by arteriography.

Pain referred to the shoulder is not uncommon. The cervical spine is the major source, specifically due to C4, C5, or C6 nerve-root compression. Pleurisy, cardiac ischemia, and diaphragmatic irritation are just a few of the many causes of referred pain. Whenever the examination and radiographs are normal and the patient is complaining of shoulder pain, a thorough search should be done for a nonorthopedic cause (Table 9-1).

Rehabilitation exercises should be started early for most traumatic shoulder problems. Limited motion exercises include pendulum or pocketbook swings (Fig. 9-44). The patient leans forward, supporting his or her weight with the normal hand on a piece of furniture waist high. Then, with a lightweight object in the affected hand, the arm is gently swung forward and back for 1 to 2 minutes, then side to side for 1 to 2 minutes, then clockwise and counterclockwise for 1 to 2 minutes. If done early and regularly, this reduces the risk of a "frozen shoulder" (i.e., adhesive capsulitis). Isometric exercises should be done early as well in shoulder injuries. Other exercises to develop full ROM and muscle strengthening should be done in consultation with an orthopedist. For example, strengthening the subscapularis muscle may deter recurrent anterior shoulder dislocations. Exercising internal and external rotators may prevent rotator cuff tears. These are not indicated for acute episodes. Significant healing must have occurred before these exercises may be done safely.

## DISCUSSION

The glenohumeral joint has an impressive degree of mobility, but this comes at a cost in stability. So many structures are intimately related and vital to its performance that it is surprising that more individuals do not have shoulder problems. Acute trauma may cause contusions, sprains, fractures, dislocations, subluxations, and rotator cuff tears. Applying one's knowledge of shoulder anatomy as well as performing a complete examination are crucial to making the diagnosis in most shoulder injuries. Conservative management with early limited-motion exercises will usually produce excellent results.

**REFERENCES**

1. Rowe CR: Anterior dislocation of the shoulder, *Surg Clin North Am* 43:1609, 1963.
2. Rowe CR, Sakellarides HT: Factors related to recurrences of anterior dislocations of the shoulder, *Clin Orthop* 20:40-48, 1961.
3. Andrews JR, Carson WG Jr, and McLeod WD: Glenoid labrum tears related to the long head of the biceps, *Am J Sports Med* 13:337-341, 1985.
4. Crenshaw AH, Kilgore WE: Surgical treatment of bicipital tenosynovitis, *J Bone Joint Surg* 48A:1496-1502, 1966.
5. Yerganson RM: Supraspinatus sign, *J Bone Joint Surg* 13:60, 1931.

6. Jobe FW, Bradley JP: The diagnosis and nonoperative treatment of shoulder injuries in athletes, *Clin Sports Med* 8:419-438, 1989.

7. Neer CS, Welsh RP: The shoulder in sports, *Orthop Clin North Am* 8:583-591, July 1977.

8. Hawkins RJ, Kennedy JC: Impingement syndrome in athletes, *Am J Sports Med* 8:151-158, 1980.

9. Neer CS: Impingement lesions, *Clin Orthop* 173:70-77, March 1983.

10. Neviaser RJ: Anatomic considerations and examination of the shoulder, *Orthop Clin North Am* 11:187-195, 1980.

11. Pope TL Jr, Chen MYM: Imaging the acutely painful shoulder, *Emerg Med* 122-139, September 15, 1992.

12. Weiner DS, Macnab I: Superior migration of the humeral head, *J Bone Joint Surg* 52B:524-527, 1970.

13. Rubin SA, Gray RL, and Green WR: The scapular "Y": a diagnostic aid in shoulder trauma, *Technical Notes* 110:725-726, 1974.

14. DeSmet AA: Axillary projection in radiography of the nontraumatized shoulder, *Am J Radiol* 134:511-514, 1980.

15. Flinn RM, MacMillan CL Jr, Campbell DR, et al: Optimal radiography of the acutely injured shoulder, *J Can Assoc Radiol* 34:128-32, 1983.

16. Garth WP Jr, Slappey CE, and Ochs CW: Roentgenographic demonstration of instability of the shoulder: the apical oblique projection, *J Bone Joint Surg* 66A:1450-1453, 1984.

17. Kornguth PJ, Salazar AM: The apical oblique view of the shoulder: its usefulness in acute trauma, *Am J Radiol* 149:113-116, 1987.

18. Boorstein JM, Dalinka MK, Kneeland JB, et al: Magnetic resonance imaging of the shoulder, *Curr Probl Diag Radiol* 7–27, January/February, 1992.

19. Heron CW: Imaging the painful shoulder, *Clin Radiol* 41:376-379, 1990.

20. Tsai JC, Zlatkin MB: Magnetic resonance imaging of the shoulder, *Radiol Clin North Am* 28:279-291, 1990.

21. Mack LA, Gannon MK, Kilcoyne RF, et al: Sonographic evaluation of the rotator cuff, *Clin Orthop* 234:21-27, 1988.

22. Harvey RA, Trabulsy ME, and Roe L: Are postreduction anteroposterior and scapular Y Views Useful in anterior shoulder dislocations? *Am J Emerg Med* 10: March 1992.

23. Riebel GD, McCabe JB: Anterior shoulder dislocation: a review of reduction techniques, *Am J Emerg Med* 9:180-188, March 1991.

24. Bosley R, Miles J: Scapular manipulation for reduction of anterior inferior dislocations, Presented at the American Association of Orthopedic Surgeons: June, 1979.

25. Anderson D, Zvirbulis R, and Ciullo J: Scapular manipulation for reduction of anterior shoulder dislocations, *Clin Orthop* 164:181-183, 1982.

26. Simonet WT, Cofield RH: Prognosis in anterior shoulder dislocation, *Am J Sports Med* 12:19-24, 1984.

27. McMurray TB: Recurrent dislocation of shoulder, *J Bone Joint Surg* 43B:402, 1961.

28. Rowe CR: Prognosis in dislocation of the shoulder, *J Bone Joint Surg* 38A:947-977, 1965.

29. Stewart R: Nitrous oxide sedation/analgesia in emergency medicine, *Ann Emerg Med* 14:139-148, 1985.

30. Milch H: Dislocation of the shoulder, *Surgery* 3:732-738, 1938.

31. Garnavos C: Technical note: Modifications and improvements of the Milch technique for the reduction of anterior dislocation of the shoulder without premedication, *J Trauma* 32:801-803, 1992.

32. Johnson G, Hulse W, and McGowan A: The Milch technique for reduction of anterior shoulder dislocations in an accident and emergency department, *Arch Emerg Med* 9:40-43, 1992.

33. Lacey T, Crawford HB: Reduction of anterior dislocations of the shoulder by means of the milch abduction technique, *J Bone Joint Surg* 34A:108-109.

34. Poulsen SR: Reduction of acute shoulder dislocation using the eskimo technique, *J Trauma* 29:1392-1383, 1988.

35. Pick RY: Treatment of the dislocated shoulder, *Clin Orthop* 123:76-77, 1988.

36. Kothari RU, Dronen SC: Prospective evaluation of the scapular manipulation techniques in reducing anterior shoulder dislocations, *Ann Emerg Med* 21:1349-1352, 1992.

37. Leidelmeyer R: Reduced! A shoulder subtly and painlessly, *J Emerg Med* 9:233-234, 1977.

38. Plummer D, Clinton J: The External rotation method for reduction of acute anterior shoulder dislocation, *Emerg Med Clin North Am* 7:165-175, 1989.

39. Jeyarajan R, Cope AR: Anaesthesia for reduction of anterior dislocations of the shoulder, *Arch Emerg Med* 9:71, 1992.

40. Bankart ASB: The pathology and treatment of recurrent dislocation of the shoulder, *J Bone Joint Surg* 26:23-29, 1939.

41. Neviaser RJ, Neviaser TJ, and Neviaser JS: Concurrent rupture of the rotator cuff and anterior dislocation of the shoulder in the older patient, *J Bone Joint Surg* 70A:1308-1311, 1988.

42. Neustadter LM, Weiss MJ: Trauma to the shoulder girdle, *Seminar in Roentgenology* 26:331-343, 1991.

43. Wadlington VR, Hendrix RW, and Rogers LF: Computed tomography of posterior fracture-dislocations of the shoulder: Case reports, *J Trauma* 32:113-115, 1992.

44. Brown DE: Shoulder injuries, *Primary Care* 19:265-281, 1992.

45. Samilson RL, Miller E: Posterior dislocations of the shoulder, *Clin Orthop* 32:69-86, 1964.

46. Kothari K et al: Luxatio erecta, *Skeletal Radiol* 11:47-49, 1984.

47. Rathbun JB, Macnab I: The microvascular pattern of the rotator cuff, *J Bone Joint Surg* 52B:540-553, 1970.

48. Neviaser RJ: Tears of the rotator cuff, *Orthop Clin North Am* 11:295-306, 1980.

49. Bassett RW, Cofield RH: Acute tears of the rotator cuff, *Clin Orthop* 175:18-24, 1983.

50. Neer CS: Anterior acromioplasty for the chronic impingement syndrome in the shoulder, *J Bone Joint Surg* 54A:41, 1972.

51. Seeger LL, Gold RH, Bassett LW, et al: Shoulder impingement syndrome: mr Findings in 53 shoulders, *Am J Radiol* 150:343-347, February 1988.

52. DiChristina DG: Imaging rounds, *Orthop Rev* 21:507-512, 1992.

53. Fields KB, Rasco T, Kramer JS, et al: Rehabilitation exercises for common sports injuries, *Am Fam Physician* 45:1233-1243, March 1992.

54. Pirrallo RG, Bridges TP: Luxatio erecta: a missed diagnosis, *Am J Emerg Med* 8:315-317, 1990.

# Fractures of the Humeral Shaft

*Steven Sterner*

Fractures of the shaft of the humerus are relatively uncommon, accounting for approximately 1% of all fractures.[1] These fractures are both interesting and gratifying to care for because treatment modalities are numerous and highly effective when used in the appropriate circumstance. Most fractures can be treated effectively with closed techniques, but in some cases open reduction with internal fixation is preferred. Significant shortening and angulation are well tolerated in the humerus because of the great mobility of the shoulder joint. Complications are uncommon and are readily treated.

## ANATOMY

The humerus bone connects the trunk with the articulating forearm and hand. It is designed more for pulling and hanging than for load bearing. The humeral shaft extends from the insertion of the pectoralis major muscle to the supracondylar ridges above the elbow joint.[1]

The humerus is surrounded by muscle contained in two compartments. The anterior compartment holds the biceps brachii, coracobrachialis, and brachialis anticus muscles. The posterior compartment holds the triceps brachii.[2] These compartments are relatively roomy; compartment syndromes here are rare.[3] A neurovascular bundle containing the brachial artery, brachial vein, median nerve, and ulnar nerve travels along the median border of the biceps muscles. The radial nerve travels in the posterior compartment proximally, before coursing tightly around the lateral distal humerus to finish anteriorly. In this area (Fig. 10-1), the radial nerve is especially vulnerable to injury.[4,5]

A supracondylar process is variably present on the anteromedial aspect of the distal humerus. This is the origin of the ligament of Struthers that inserts on the medial epicondyle of the elbow. The brachial artery and median nerve traverse the space between this ligament and the humerus. This process can be rarely fractured.

The location of a fracture in relation to muscular attachments determines the degree and direction of distraction of bony fragments. If the fracture occurs above the attachment of the pectoralis major muscle, the proximal humerus is pulled laterally and superiorly by the supraspinatus muscle. If the fracture occurs below the attachment of the pectoralis major muscle but above the attachment of the deltoid muscle, the proximal humerus is pulled medially by the pectoralis muscle. In any fracture occurring distal to the attachment of the deltoid muscle, the proximal humerus is pulled laterally by the deltoid. The biceps and triceps muscles pull the distal humerus in a proximal direction, causing shortening in virtually all complete fractures of the humeral shaft (Fig. 10-2). Although rotation may occur to some degree, it is usually not marked and is difficult even to appreciate.

## MECHANISM OF INJURY

Humeral fractures tend toward a bimodal age distribution. In the younger group, men 16 to 24 years of age predomi-

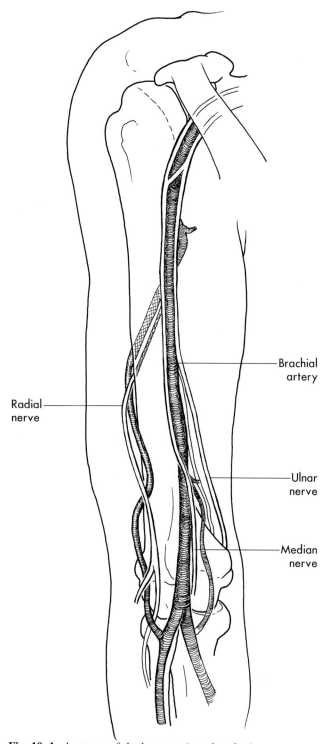

Radial
nerve

Brachial
artery

Ulnar
nerve

Median
nerve

**Fig. 10-1.** Anatomy of the humerus (anterior view).

nate. Most fractures are caused by either motor vehicle accidents or missile injuries (i.e., gunshot wounds).[4,6] Humeral fractures have also been associated with the throwing action, particularly in baseball pitchers. It is felt that stress fractures occur accompanied by pain, then suddenly progress to a complete shaft fracture during a throw.[7] These fractures tend to occur between the middle and distal thirds of the humerus. In the older group, women 56 to 65 years

of age predominate, with fractures typically caused by falls.[4,6] Pathologic fractures become more common with increasing age as well.

In older children, pathologic fractures through unicameral bone cysts are not rare. These cysts usually develop close to the proximal humeral metaphysis.[7a] Figure 10-3 shows an unfractured unicameral cyst in the humerus of a 12-year-old. When these cysts fracture, a fracture fragment often falls into the cyst as if a "fallen leaf."

Direct trauma, such as that experienced in a motor vehicle accident, tends to cause a bending action that results in a transverse or minimally oblique fracture. Falls tend to cause axial loading and torsion, resulting in oblique or spiral fractures.[6] Most humeral fractures are closed, but the rate of open fracture may be as high as 28% in some patient populations.[4] Most open fractures are caused by gunshot wounds (Fig. 10-4), but many are due to high-speed trauma.[4]

## ASSOCIATED INJURIES

The most common injury associated with humeral fracture is radial nerve palsy, which is reported to occur in 5% to 20% of fractures.[4,5,6,8] Radial nerve injury is associated with fractures of the middle third (72%) or distal third (28%) of the humerus.[17] Most are primary nerve injuries occurring at the time of fracture; however, secondary radial nerve palsy occurring after manipulation and reduction has been reported.[4,5,6,9,10] The radial nerve may suffer contusion, laceration, or traction injury. Spontaneous recovery of function occurs in most patients but may take up to 6 months.[4,5,20,10,12]

Median nerve and ulnar nerve injuries are rarely seen; usually these are associated with penetrating injuries.[14] Brachial artery laceration or contusion with thrombosis is seen in about 3% of patients.[4]

## DIAGNOSIS
### History

The history in the patient with a fracture of the humerus is not crucial to diagnosis and treatment of that fracture. Typically, the patient complains of pain in the arm or shoulder. The mechanism may lead the physician to suspect a certain type of fracture, but more importantly, it must lead the physician to suspect and search for other injuries. In addition to pain, other important symptoms should be elicited, such as neurologic deficit or difficulty breathing.

### Physical examination

The upper arm in the patient with a fracture of the humeral shaft is typically tender and swollen, and possibly shortened. If it is a complete fracture, abnormal mobility is demonstrated. The physician must palpate the anterior and posterior compartments, searching for tenseness or other sign of compartment syndrome. Circulation is assessed by evaluating capillary refill in the hand and by palpating pulses in the brachial, radial, and ulnar arteries. Neurologic examination includes a test of motor and sensory function

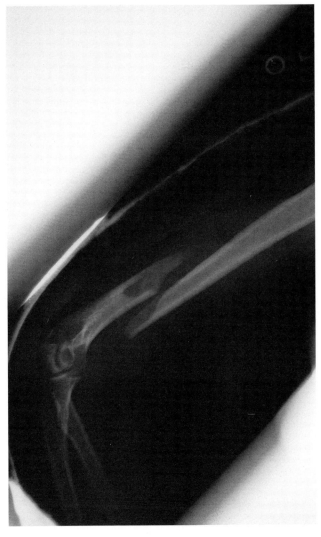

**Fig. 10-2.** Distal humeral shaft fracture.

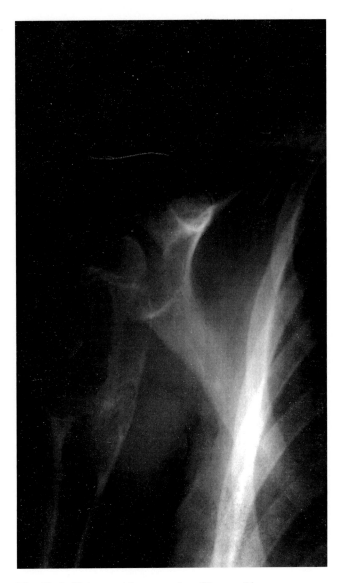

**Fig. 10-3.** Unicameral bone cyst in a 12-year-old.

in the areas served by the radial, median, and ulnar nerves. It is most important to carefully evaluate and document these functions before any manipulation. In particular, management of radial nerve palsy is conservative if the deficit was caused by the original injury but is likely to be surgical if the deficit occurred later as a result of treatment.[4,5,6]

### Radiography

Radiographic studies should include at least two views of the entire shaft of the humerus, including the shoulder and elbow joints. The radiographs should confirm the diagnosis and lend additional information as to type, location, angulation, and displacement of the fracture. In addition, unsuspected fractures of the shoulder or elbow may be identified.

### TREATMENT

As with many fractures, a multitude of treatment options for humeral fractures exists. General principles to follow include: 1) traction to bring the bone and fragments back to length and to align fracture surfaces; 2) reduction of angulation; 3) immobilization to allow healing; and 4) early mobilization of the shoulder and elbow joints to prevent loss of range of motion. Weight bearing is not a consideration with the humerus. Alignment need not be perfect because of the extreme mobility of the shoulder joint; however, one cannot help but believe that good alignment, if it is readily attainable, is preferable to poor alignment (Fig. 10-5). It is helpful that gravity assists in attaining alignment and length in the hanging arm. Muscles surround the humerus, supporting it and aiding in alignment. If nothing is done to immobilize the fractured humerus, the incidence of nonunion is high.[4,13] However, if any of the following treatment modalities is used, incidence of nonunion is low.

### First consideration: extent of injury

In the emergent treatment of a humeral fracture, the first consideration is if the patient has isolated or multiple

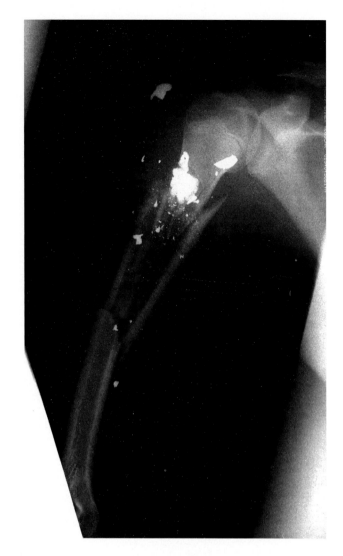

**Fig. 10-4.** Typical open humeral fracture from gunshot penetrating injury.

injuries. More serous injuries take precedence over the care of simple fractures. In the multiply injured patient, it is appropriate to quickly splint the humerus fracture, planning more definitive treatment for a later time. One indication for open reduction with internal fixation (ORIF) is a multiply injured patient with multiple impediments to mobilization.[4,9,11,14,15,16,17,18] If fixed surgically and early, the humeral fracture is less of an impediment to mobilization of the patient, and the sooner the patient can be mobilized, the fewer problems the patient will experience.

### Next consideration: open or closed fracture

The next consideration in the emergent situation is to determine if the humeral fracture is open or closed. Open fractures are nearly always treated with ORIF.[4,9,11,14,15,16,17] If the fracture is closed, other indications for ORIF may be present. If the fracture is pathologic, ORIF may be indicated for diagnosis or to improve the likelihood of union. Vascular disruption is an indication for surgery. If an intra-articular fracture requiring ORIF is present on the same arm, ORIF of the humerus may be necessary as well.

If a radial nerve that was intact prior to closed reduction becomes injured during reduction, radial nerve exploration is indicated for possible repair and ORIF of the fracture.[4,5,6]

Radial nerve palsy alone is not an indication for primary nerve exploration. Most radial nerve palsies resolve spontaneously within weeks to months. It is recommended that nerve exploration be reserved for those few cases that do not recover in 3 to 4 months. Late nerve reconstruction has been shown to restore useful function in 92% of radial nerve palsies.[5]

Severely comminuted fractures and those in which closed reduction simply does not result in adequate alignment are also candidates for ORIF.[1,4,6,9,10,11,15,16,17]

### For most patients: closed treatment

In most patients, the above factors are not present and closed treatment is the modality of choice. A number of closed modalities are available. In the emergent treatment of a humeral fracture, swelling is either a real or potential problem. For this reason, circumferential splints or casts should be avoided.

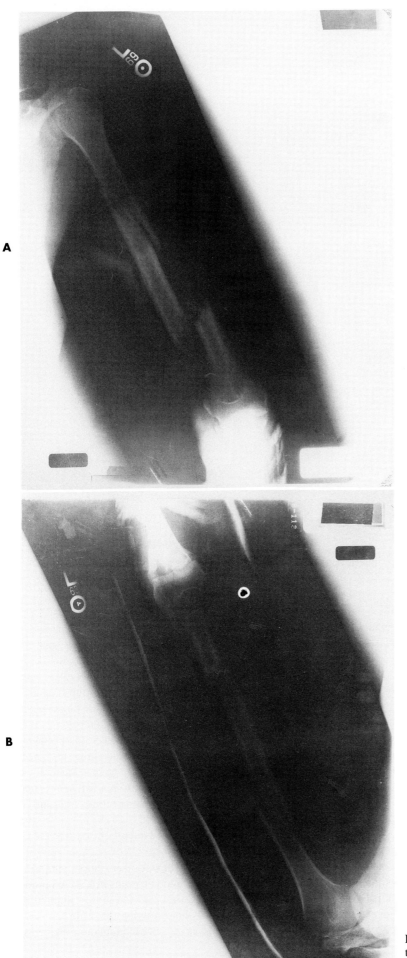

**Fig. 10-5. A**, Comminuted midshaft humerus fracture. **B**, Comminuted midshaft humerus fracture immobilized with sugar-tong splint.

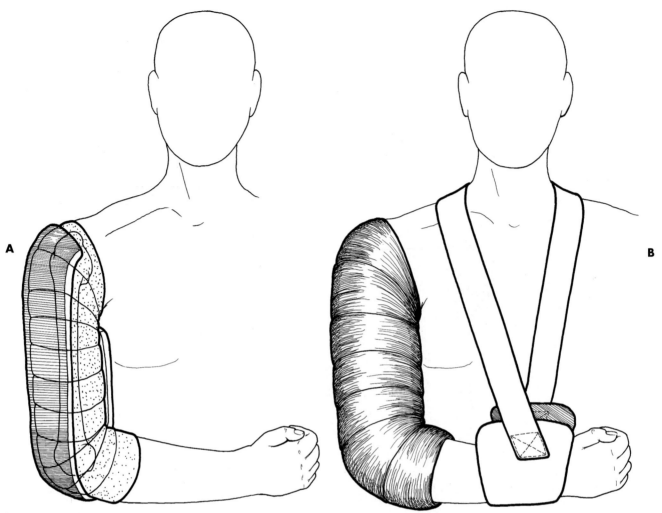

**Fig. 10-6.** **A,** Sugar-tong splint applied over a layer of padding. **B,** Splint secured with elastic wrap and arm supported in 90° of flexion with collar and cuff.

**Sugar-tong splint.** Most likely the best initial modality is the sugar-tong splint (Fig. 10-6).[4,10,11,12,20] A plaster or fiberglass splint is placed in a U shape as high as possible in the axilla, down around and beneath the elbow and up the upper arm, ending over the top of the shoulder. The arm is supported in 90° or less of flexion, by means of a sling or a collar and cuff. This splint provides adequate immobilization of the fracture site as well as some traction by gravity through the weight of the splint. It is not circumferential; therefore, swelling can increase or decrease without effect. The elbow joint is allowed some movement so it is not completely immobilized.

After 7 to 14 days, when swelling is no longer a problem, another type of splint or cast may be applied, or the sugar-tong splint may be used until the fracture is healed.[4,10,11] An advantage of the sugar-tong splint is that it is individually made of plaster or fiberglass, which is readily available anywhere and can be made to fit a patient of any size or shape. Because it is not circumferential and is custom-fit, there is little risk of pressure-induced ischemia or skin breakdown.

**Hanging cast.** Another highly reported treatment modality for humeral fractures is the hanging cast (Fig. 10-7).[1,4,6,11,13,19] The hanging cast was popularized by Caldwell in 1933. A circular plaster or fiberglass cast is applied from at least one inch proximal to the fracture site extending to the wrist, with the elbow at 90° flexion and the forearm in neutral position. A sling is fixed to the cast by a loop at the wrist.[13] The arm must always be dependent to apply traction, so the patient must sleep sitting up. The cast should be heavy enough to apply gentle traction, thus pulling the fracture to length, but not so heavy that it distracts the bony fragments, which could interfere with healing.

The hanging cast was the standard closed treatment for humeral fractures for many years. However, recently it has received criticism. It is believed inconvenient and uncomfortable for the patient to spend months in a seated position. The cast has also been criticized for rigidly immobilizing the elbow and for causing a hinging effect on the fracture site. This leads to more posterior angulation and delayed union.[11]

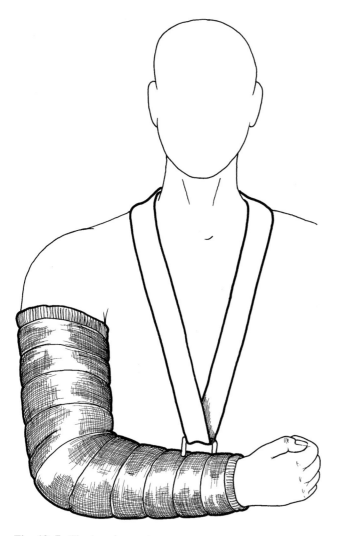

**Fig. 10-7.** The hanging cast.

**Other splints and modalities.** Other more convenient splints have been described. A molded, two-piece, anterior-posterior functional brace first described in 1977 was said to be more comfortable and effective than the hanging cast (Fig. 10-8).[18] Initially, the patient is treated with a sugar-tong splint for an average of 11 days. Then the brace is applied until the fracture is healed. The splint consists of two pieces. One is applied anteriorly and the other posteriorly, so that when strapped together they form a circular brace from 1.3 cm above the medial epicondyle to 2.5 cm below the axilla. The brace is lightweight, allows the patient to lie flat, and allows full range of motion at the elbow and shoulder. Initially, the arm is supported by a sling but range-of-motion exercises can be initiated almost immediately. Within a few weeks, the patient can touch his or her face. The brace can be discontinued at a median 8.5 weeks. Only one nonunion was reported out of 51 total fractures[18]; this occurred in a patient with a pathologic fracture from metastatic cancer.

Use of a prefabricated interlocking brace was reported in 1988 by Zagorski.[12] In a series of 233 patients, 85% had

angulation of less than 8°. Shortening was minimal (mean shortening, 4 mm). Only three nonunions occurred, and 95% were judged to have an excellent functional result.

Other treatment modalities include sling and swath, shoulder spica casting, and thoracobrachial casting.[4,6,8] Although these may be appropriate for the occasional unusual case, their use seems unwarranted for most fractures. Skeletal traction by way of an olecranon pin has been used for some fractures, mostly in nonambulatory patients, but has been associated with delayed union.[6]

**Open reduction for nonresponsive fractures**

For fractures not responding to closed modalities and for fractures with other indications discussed previously, ORIF is the main treatment. ORIF options include primarily plate fixation or intramedullary fixation.

Several methods of fixing humeral fractures with various plates have been described.[9,14,17,20] An advantage of plate fixation is early rigid immobilization, allowing early patient mobilization (Fig. 10-9). This is especially important in patients with multiple injuries. An increased incidence of radial nerve injury has been reported.[4,9] Leaving a plate permanently in place has been recommended because of concern for nerve injury at the time of plate removal.[9] However, other reports note very low incidences of nerve injury.[14,17,20] A disadvantage here is an increased risk of nonunion. However, this risk is difficult to assess, because ORIF is often reserved for more difficult fractures, where closed treatment is expected to fail. ORIF also poses an increased yet low risk of infection.[14,16,17,20]

A technique of closed intramedullary rod fixation has been described by Brumback[9] with low risk of infection or nerve injury and 94% union rate in 10.5 weeks. Kristiansen[16] has reported a technique for transcutaneous reduction using Steinman pins and external fixation with a Hoffman-type neutralizing bar.

**DISCUSSION**

When faced with a fracture of the humerus, the emergency physician must first assess the patient for other injuries and prioritize care of all injuries. Next, the physician must determine if the fracture requires ORIF or can be managed closed. The most common indications for ORIF are open fracture and multiple injuries. If closed management seems likely, a sugar-tong splint should be applied. This is an excellent option because it can be used as long as required with good results, and it preserves the option of any other modality once acute swelling has subsided. After 7 to 14 days, a two-piece functional brace can be used, allowing the patient greater comfort and mobility. A hanging cast is another viable alternative, but may not be as convenient for the patient. Union in uncomplicated fractures usually occurs within 10 weeks. The most common complication, radial nerve palsy, almost always resolves spontaneously and should be followed for at least 3 to 4 months before nerve exploration is considered. Late nerve reconstruction is associated with excellent recovery.

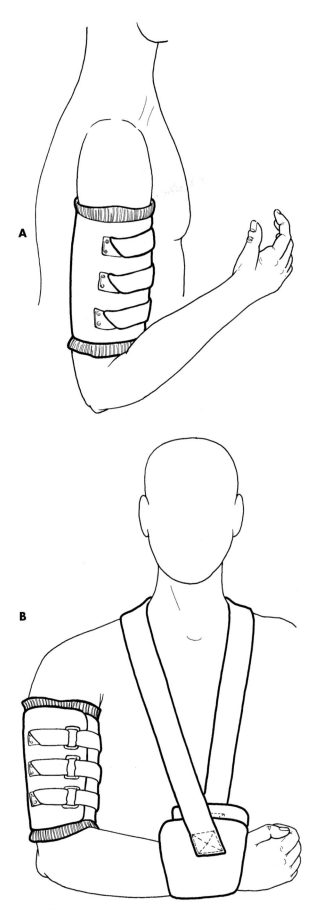

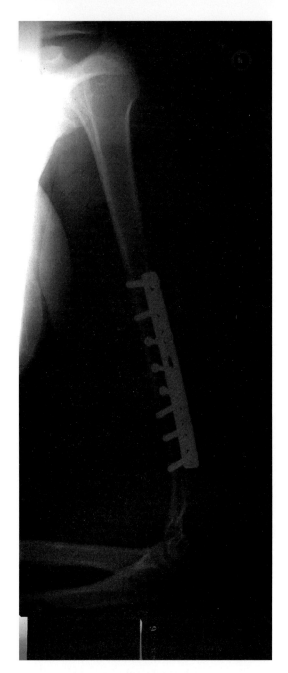

**Fig. 10-9.** Distal humeral shaft fracture with internal plate fixation.

**Fig. 10-8. A,** Prefabricated anterior-posterior functional brace (*lateral view*). **B,** Prefabricated anterior-posterior functional brace with arm supported (*anterior view*).

### REFERENCES

1. Epps CH, Grant RE: Fractures of the shaft of the humerus. In Rockwood CA and Green DP, eds: *Fractures in adults.* Philadelphia, JB Lippincott, 1991, pp. 843-868.

2. Agur AM, Lee MG: *Grant's atlas of anatomy,* edn 9, Baltimore, Williams and Wilkins, 1991, p. 389.

3. Mubarak SJ: Etiologies of compartment syndromes. In Mubarak SJ and Hargans AR, eds: *Compartment syndromes and Volkmann's contracture.* Philadelphia, WB Saunders, 1981, pp. 71-97.

4. Mast JW, Spiegel PG, Harvey JP et al: Fractures of the humeral shaft: A retrospective study of 240 adult fractures, *Clin Orthop* 112: pp. 254-262, 1975.

5. Samardzic M, Grujicic D, and Milinkovic ZB: Radial nerve lesions associated with fractures of the humeral shaft, *Injury* 21: pp. 220-222, 1990.

6. Bleeker WA, Nijsten MW, and ten Duis HJ: Treatment of humeral shaft fractures related to associated injuries, *Acta Orthop Scand* 62: pp. 148-153, 1991.

7. Branch T, Partin C, Chamberland P et al: Spontaneous fractures of the humerus during pitching, *Am J Sports Med* 20: pp. 468-470, 1992.

7a. Salter RB: *Textbook of disorders and injuries of the musculoskeletal system*, edn. 2, Baltimore, Williams and Wilkins, 1983, pp. 332-333.

8. Holm CL: Management of humeral shaft fractures: Fundamental nonoperative techniques, *Clin Orthop* 71: pp. 132-139, 1970.

9. Brumback RJ, Bosse MJ, Poka A et al: Intramedullary stabilization of humeral shaft fractures in patients with multiple trauma, *J Bone Joint Surg* 68A: pp. 960-969, 1986.

10. Dameron TB, Grubb SA: Humeral shaft fractures in adults, *South Med J* 74: pp. 1461-1467, 1981.

11. Klenerman L: Fractures of the shaft of the humerus, *J Bone Joint Surg* 48B: pp. 105-111, 1966.

12. Zagorski JB, Latta LL, Zych GA et al: Diaphyseal fractures of the humerus: Treatment with prefabricated braces, *J Bone Joint Surg* 70A: pp. 607-610, 1988.

13. Caldwell JA: Treatment of fractures in the Cincinnati General Hospital, *Ann Surg* 97: pp. 161-176, 1933.

14. Bell MJ, Beauchamp CG, Kellam JK et al: The results of plating humeral shaft fractures in patients with multiple injuries, *J Bone Joint Surg* 67B: pp. 293-296, 1985.

15. Healy WL, White GM, Mick CA et al: Nonunion of the humeral shaft, *Clin Orthop* 219: pp. 206-213, 1987.

16. Kristiansen B, Kofoed H: External fixation of displaced fractures of the proximal humerus, *J Bone Joint Surg* 69B: pp. 643-646, 1987.

17. Moda SK, Chadha NS, Sangwan SS et al: Open reduction and fixation of proximal humerus fractures and fracture-dislocations, *J Bone Joint Surg* 72B: pp. 1050-1052, 1990.

18. Sarmiento A, Kinman P, Galvin EG et al: Functional bracing of fractures of the shaft of the humerus, *J Bone Joint Surg* 59A: pp. 596-601, 1977.

19. Ciernik IF, Meier L, and Hollinger A: Humeral mobility after treatment with hanging cast, *J Trauma* 31: pp. 230-233, 1991.

20. Vander Griend R, Tomasin J, and Ward EF: Open reduction and internal fixation of humeral shaft fractures, *J Bone Joint Surg* 68A: pp. 430-433, 1986.

# The Elbow Joint

*Albert K. Tsai*
*Ernest Ruiz*

The elbow is a remarkable joint because of its flexibility, durability, and strength. It is frequently in a position to be injured during falls and other traumatic events. It is also subject to overuse because of its important role in so many occupational, recreational, and daily living activities. Elbow injuries frequently are seen first in the emergency department. Consequently, it behooves the emergency physician to be prepared for such injuries in order to preserve the integrity of this joint.

## INCIDENCE

Elbow fractures are common injuries in adults and children. Of all fractures in children, 65% to 75%[1-3] involve the upper extremities and about 7% to 9% of these are fractures about the elbow. Eighty-six percent of elbow fractures in children involve the distal humerus. Supracondylar humeral fractures are the most common, followed by lateral condylar fractures and medial epicondylar fractures. T-condylar and medial condylar fractures are rare. Elbow fractures are more common in boys than in girls and usually occur during the summer months.

## OBJECTIVE

The objective of this chapter is to provide the emergency physician with the knowledge necessary to manage elbow injuries safely and effectively. This entails:

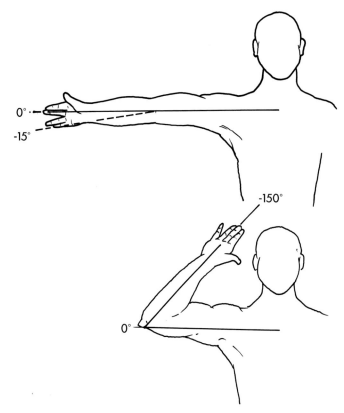

**Fig. 11-1.** Normal range of motion of the elbow. The activities of daily living require at least 130° of flexion and extension to 30°.

1) the ability to differentiate injuries that require immediate orthopedic consultation from injuries that can be managed nonoperatively in the emergency department with orthopedic or other appropriate follow-up; and

2) the ability to perform certain emergency maneuvers in order to reduce the elbow or return it to a configuration preserving vascular integrity and neurologic function in the upper extremity.

## ANATOMY
### Range of motion

The elbow contains three articulations: the humeroradial, the humeroulnar, and the radioulnar. The humeroradial and radioulnar articulations provide the rotatory motion necessary for hand dexterity. The humeroulnar articulation provides stability while also facilitating flexion and extension of the forearm. At least 130° of flexion along with extension to at least 30° are needed for activities of daily living. Fifty degrees of supination and pronation are also necessary. When these functions are limited, some compensation is provided by neck, shoulder, and truncal positioning. There is also a normal degree of outward angulation of the extended forearm at the elbow called the *carrying angle*. This angle ranges from 5° to 20° in adults, with women having more angulation than men. In childhood, boys have a carrying angle of about 5.5° and girls about 6° with wide variation. Normally,

the range of flexion-extension is 0° to 150° with the forearm supinated. Up to 15° of hyperextension may be normal for some individuals (Figs. 11-1 and 11-2). When the elbow is flexed to 90° with the hands in neutral position (thumbs up), the normal range of supination and pronation of the wrist is 90° in both directions. When the patient has preexisting limitations of movement of the shoulder or neck, the disability caused by any loss of motion at the elbow is magnified.

### Bony landmarks

In full elbow extension the epicondyles of the humerus and the tip of the olecranon of the ulna lie in the same horizontal plane. When the elbow is placed in full flexion the outer border of the capitellum becomes prominent laterally just distal and anterior to the lateral epicondyle.

The landmarks that locate the area of the joint capsule most accessible for aspiration are the radial head, the tip of the olecranon, and the lateral epicondyle. These form a triangle through which the slightly ballottable anconeus muscle can be palpated under the tricipital aponeurosis (Fig. 11-3). The anconeus muscle arises from the lateral epicondyle and inserts on the lateral border of the ulnar shaft.

### The bones of the elbow

The distal end of the humerus is triangular with medial and lateral columns forming the sides of the triangle. These columns terminate in supracondylar ridges called epi-

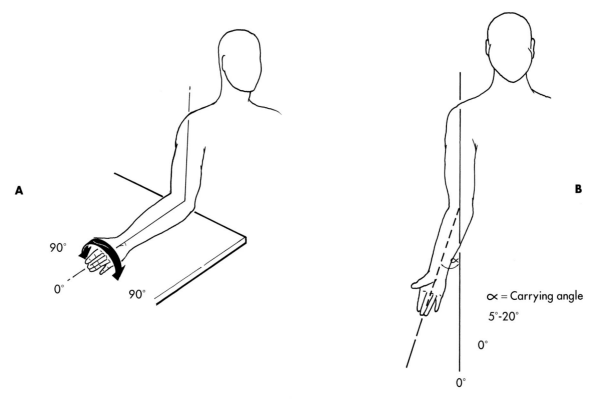

**Fig. 11-2.** **A,** Normal range of motion of the elbow. The activities of daily living require 50° of supination and pronation. **B,** The normal carrying angle. On average, women have a larger carrying angle than men. There is much less difference in carrying angle between sexes in children.

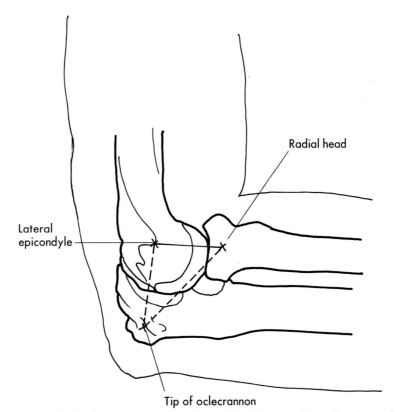

**Fig. 11-3.** Bony landmarks for aspiration of the elbow joint. This triangle overlies the portion of the joint capsule that is least overlaid with muscles, tendons, nerves, and blood vessels. Only the tricipital aponeurosis and the anconeus muscle cover the capsule in this triangle.

condyles. A prominence of variable size is located supra-condylarly on the anteromedial aspect of the humerus, giving rise to a fibrous band that attaches to the medial epicondyle. This band forms a tunnel through which the median nerve and brachial artery pass to cross the elbow joint anteriorly (Fig. 11-4). The medial epicondyle is larger than the lateral epicondyle. The lateral epicondyle has a roughened surface from which the superficial extensor muscles of the forearm arise (Fig. 11-5A). The medial epicondyle is the origin of the flexor muscles of the forearm; it also has a smooth posterior surface where it comes in contact with the ulnar nerve (Fig. 11-5B). The articular surface of the medial condyle is the trochlea, which is spool-like with prominent medial and lateral ridges that provide stability to its ulnar articulation. Posteriorly, the groove angles laterally, producing the carrying angle when the elbow is extended. The articular surface of the lateral condyle is the capitellum, which is hemispherical and projects anteriorly to articulate with the concave surface of the radial head. The capitellum is in contact with the radial head to only a minor degree with full range of motion of the elbow. The articular surfaces of the trochlea and the capitellum are directed downward and forward at an angle of about 30° (Fig. 11-6).

The proximal end of the radius forms the radial head and neck proximal to the radial tuberosity where the biceps muscle inserts. The head of the radius articulates with the lateral side of the coronoid process of the ulna as well as with the capitellum. The proximal end of the ulna consists of the olecranon and coronoid processes, which form the trochlear notch that articulates with the trochlea of the humerus.

### Ligaments

The medial (or ulnar) collateral ligament of the elbow is shown in Fig. 11-7. The anterior portion of this ligament is attached to the medial epicondyle and the coronoid process; it is taut in extension. The posterior portion fans out from the inferior surface of the medial epicondyle and is attached to the border of the trochlear notch of the ulna. This portion is relatively weak and is taut in flexion of the elbow.

The lateral (or radial) collateral ligament of the elbow is shown in Fig. 11-8. It arises from the lateral epicondyle and inserts into the annular ligament of the radius. The annular ligament (Fig. 11-9) provides a cup-shaped socket for the neck and head of the radius that prevents dislocation of the radial head distally.

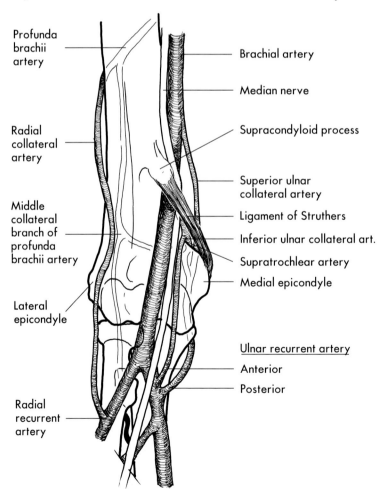

**Fig. 11-4.** The brachial artery and the median nerve approach the elbow through a tunnel formed by the ligament of Struthers. The elbow is generally well vascularized by collateral vessels.

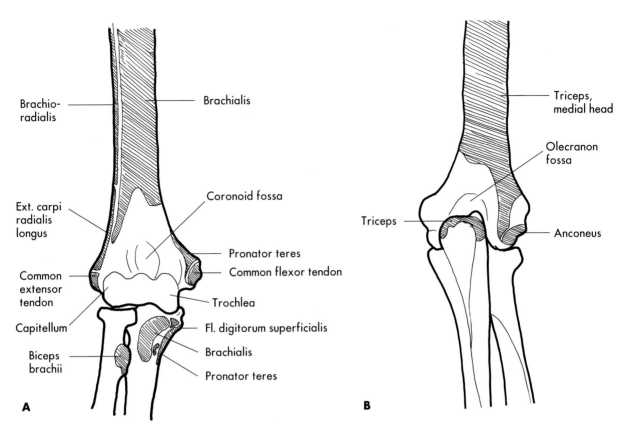

Brachio-radialis

Brachialis

Ext. carpi radialis longus

Coronoid fossa

Common extensor tendon

Pronator teres

Common flexor tendon

Capitellum

Trochlea

Biceps brachii

Fl. digitorum superficialis

Brachialis

Pronator teres

Triceps, medial head

Olecranon fossa

Triceps

Anconeus

**A**          **B**

**Fig. 11-5. A,** Anterior view of the right elbow joint showing muscle origins and insertions. **B,** Posterior view of the right elbow.

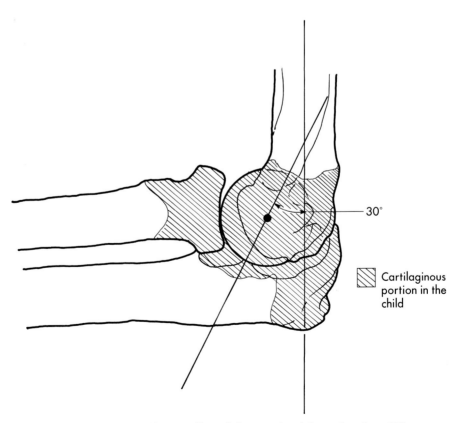

30°

Cartilaginous portion in the child

**Fig. 11-6.** The trochlea and the capitellum are directed downward and forward at about 30°.

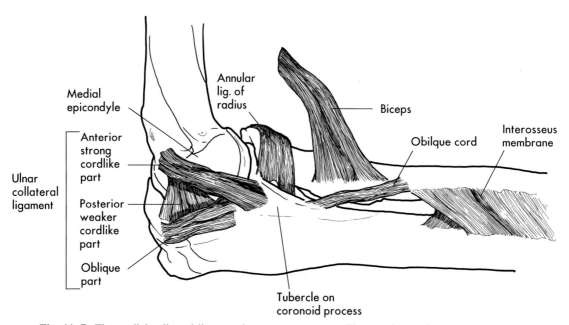

**Fig. 11-7.** The medial collateral ligament has two components. The anterior portion is subject to valgus stress the most during activities such as throwing a baseball. The posterior portion of the ligament is relatively weaker.

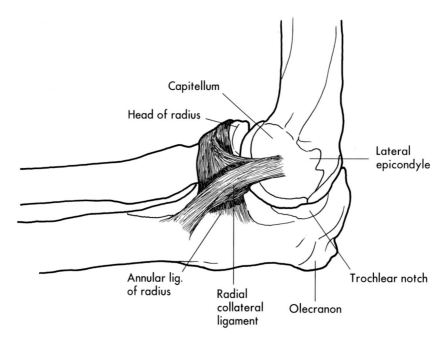

**Fig. 11-8.** The lateral collateral ligament reinforces and retains the annular ligament of the radius.

### The joint capsule

The joint capsule of the elbow consists of a fibrous and a synovial layer. Its dimensions are shown diagrammatically in Fig. 11-10 from an anterior perspective. Fat pads occupy the radial, coronoid, and olecranon fossae between the fibrous and synovial layers of the capsule.

### Stability

The wide range of motion required of the elbow limits the stabilizing architecture of its bones and ligaments. How-

ever, the muscles and fibrous attachments of the upper arm and forearm provide dynamic tension that holds the joint together, resisting forces that would otherwise dislocate or sublux the joint. Anteriorly, the biceps and brachialis muscles insert on the radial tuberosity and proximal ulna, respectively (Figs. 11-7 and 11-5A). The triceps aponeurosis inserts posteriorly on the olecranon and fans out over the joint (Fig. 11-11). Varus and valgus stresses to the elbow are counteracted by the muscles of the forearm originating in tendinous attachments to the epicondyles of the humerus as well as the collateral ligaments.

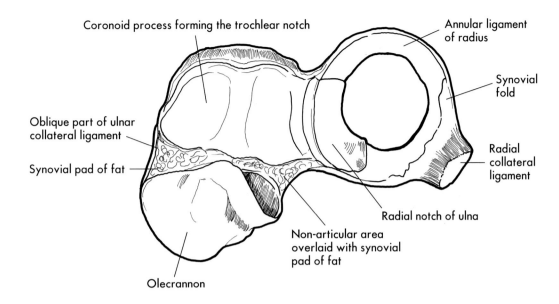

Coronoid process forming the trochlear notch

Annular ligament of radius

Synovial fold

Oblique part of ulnar collateral ligament

Synovial pad of fat

Radial collateral ligament

Radial notch of ulna

Non-articular area overlaid with synovial pad of fat

Olecrannon

**Fig. 11-9.** End-on view of the annular ligament of the radius. This ligament is cup-shaped and retains the head of the radius in its normal proximal position.

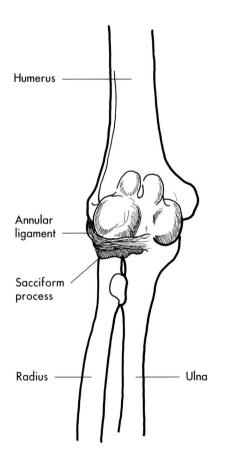

Humerus

Annular ligament

Sacciform process

Radius

Ulna

**Fig. 11-10.** Anterior view of the elbow joint showing the synovial joint capsule. The fat pads of the elbow joint lie between the synovial and outer fibrous capsules.

### Nerves

The radial nerve arises from behind the humerus at midshaft level and crosses the elbow joint laterally and anteriorly over the capitellum deep to the brachioradialis muscle where it divides into a deep interosseous branch and a superficial branch (Fig. 11-12). If the radial nerve is damaged at the elbow the brachioradialis is usually spared, but sensation is affected over the snuff box area of the hand and the dorsum of the thumb. Because the radial nerve innervates the extensor muscles of the forearm, wrist drop with ulnar deviation is seen when the elbow is flexed and the forearm pronated.

The median nerve crosses the elbow anteriorly medial to the biceps muscle behind the brachial artery. It dives under the pronator teres muscle with the ulnar artery branch of the brachial artery (Fig. 11-12). This nerve provides sensation to the tips of the thumb and index finger. Its muscular branches provide coarse hand movements including grasp. When the median nerve is damaged above the elbow crease, the index finger cannot be flexed because innervation of the flexor digitorum profundus is interrupted. This is called Ochsner's clasping test. When the anterior interosseus branch of the median nerve is damaged in the forearm, the interphalangeal joint of the thumb cannot be flexed when the metacarpophalangeal joint is splinted because innervation of the flexor pollicis longus is interrupted.

The ulnar nerve crosses the elbow posteriorly behind the medial epicondyle (Fig. 11-11). The medial epicondyle has a smooth groove in which the ulnar nerve lies. The ulnar nerve provides sensation to the palmar and dorsal aspects of the ulnar side of the hand. Damage to the ulnar nerve at the elbow results in a clawlike hand secondary to loss of

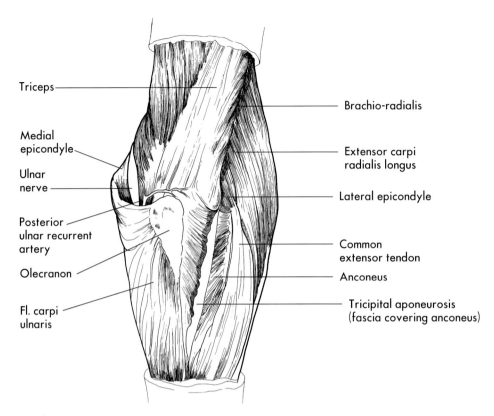

Triceps

Medial epicondyle

Ulnar nerve

Posterior ulnar recurrent artery

Olecranon

Fl. carpi ulnaris

Brachio-radialis

Extensor carpi radialis longus

Lateral epicondyle

Common extensor tendon

Anconeus

Tricipital aponeurosis (fascia covering anconeus)

**Fig. 11-11.** Posterior view of the elbow showing how the tricipital aponeurosis and tendinous origins of forearm muscles firmly wrap the joint, providing tension bracing.

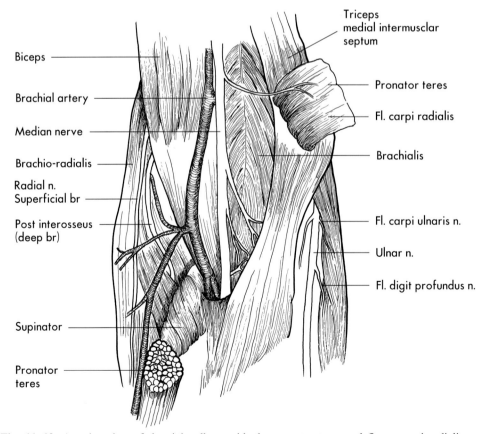

Biceps

Brachial artery

Median nerve

Brachio-radialis

Radial n. Superficial br

Post interosseus (deep br)

Supinator

Pronator teres

Triceps medial intermusclar septum

Pronator teres

Fl. carpi radialis

Brachialis

Fl. carpi ulnaris n.

Ulnar n.

Fl. digit profundus n.

**Fig. 11-12.** Anterior view of the right elbow with the pronator teres and flexor carpi radialis muscles retracted to reveal the nerves and arteries that cross the joint anteriorly.

function of the intrinsic muscles of the hand as well as of the flexors of the fingers and wrist.

### Blood vessels

The brachial artery crosses the elbow with the median nerve medial to the biceps muscle and tendon (Figs. 11-4 and 11-12). At the level of the insertion of the biceps tendon it divides into the radial and ulnar arteries. Interruption of the brachial artery at the elbow results in almost complete devascularization of the forearm and hand. When blood flow through the brachial artery is compromised, the forearm and hand undergo ischemic muscle wasting, which results in a condition known as Volkmann's ischemic contracture. The elbow is a well-vascularized joint because of extensive collateralization of the branches of the brachial artery (Fig. 11-4). However, in children the secondary ossification centers of the trochlea and epicondyles are served by small terminal arteries that put these centers at risk of avascular necrosis when injured. This occurs because blood vessels do not traverse the metaphyseal junction and articular surfaces, and they do not penetrate the elbow joint capsule. The centers at risk have only small surface areas that can accept blood vessels given these restrictions.

### Development

The humerus is ossified at birth to the level of the condyles. Ossification of the bones of the elbow generally proceeds more rapidly in girls, with ossification of the olecranon and lateral epicondyle occurring about a year earlier in girls than in boys. Figure 11-13A shows the approximate ages of the radiographic appearances of the secondary ossification centers of the elbow as described by Ogden.[4] Figure 11-13B shows the approximate ages of radiographic phy-

seal closure of these ossification centers, also described by Ogden.[4] The ossification centers can be multiple and can appear as psuedofracture fragments on elbow radiographs in children.

Physeal injury to the distal humerus occurs relatively early with respect to physeal injuries of other bones. These injuries occur most commonly in girls between the ages of 4 and 5 years, and between 5 and 8 years in boys. Conversely, physeal injuries to other bones occur between the ages of 10 and 13 years.

### RADIOLOGY

It is relatively difficult to picture the elbow radiographically, so several views are required to display all of its parts adequately. A routine series should include at least

1) an anteroposterior (AP) view with the elbow in extension and the forearm supinated;
2) a lateral view with the elbow in 90° of flexion and the forearm in supination; and
3) a capitellum view with the elbow flexed at 90°, the forearm in supination, and the x-ray beam angled at 45° off of true lateral.

Normal examples of these views are shown in Fig. 11-14. Several other views can be obtained to observe specific areas. A medial oblique view shows the coronoid process without superimposition. A lateral oblique view shows the radial head without superimposition. An axial projection with acute elbow flexion shows the olecranon process. When the patient cannot fully extend the elbow, separate AP views of the distal humerus and proximal ulna and radius will usually suffice.

The fat pad occupying the coronoid fossa of the humerus can be seen on the lateral view of the elbow. The fat pad has a concave configuration projecting out of the fossa (Fig. 11-14).

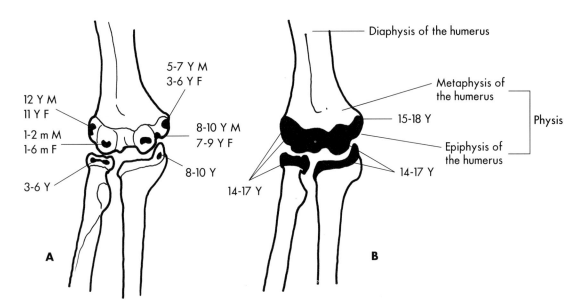

**Fig. 11-13. A,** The secondary ossification centers of the elbow with the approximate ages of radiographic appearance. Girls develop ossification of the distal humeral epiphyses earlier than boys. **B,** The age of physeal closure for the epiphyses of the elbow.

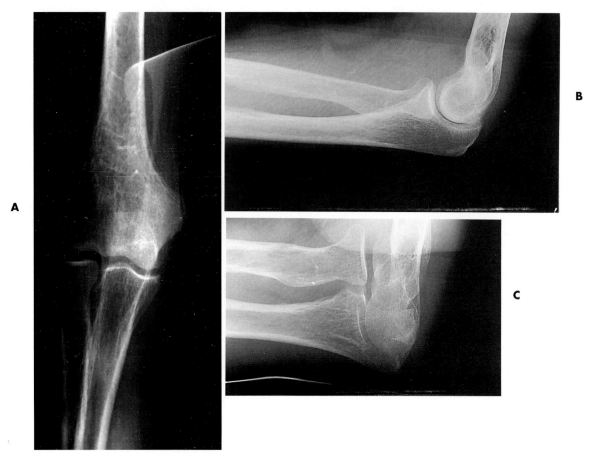

**Fig. 11-14. A**, Normal anterposterior view. **B**, Normal lateral view. Note that the anterior fat pad occupying the coronoid fossa can be seen with its normal concave appearance. The posterior fat pad occupying the olecranon fossa is normally not seen. The supinator line formed by the fascial investment of the supinator muscle is marked with an arrow. **C**, The capitellum view displays the capitellum without superimposition of the trochlea.

When the content of the elbow joint is increased, as in a fracture communicating with the joint, the anterior fat pad is displaced superiorly and anteriorly so that it becomes convex in appearance. This appearance is sometimes called the "sail sign" and is a sensitive indicator for fracture. The fat pad occupying the olecranon fossa of the humerus normally cannot be seen on a lateral view. When it projects outward and becomes visible, there is a high incidence of fracture. It can be seen in 74% of children with elbow fractures. When it is seen, 76% to 82% of adults will have a fracture and 42% of children will have a fracture.[5-11] Abnormal anterior and posterior fat pad findings can be seen in Fig. 11-15.

On the lateral view, a fascial plane can be seen overlying the supinator muscle ventrally. This is called the *supinator line*. When this line is elevated, blurred, or thickened there is a high incidence of radial head fracture. When this sign is present (Figs. 11-14 and 11-15), only 10% of cases will not have a fracture.[12]

A radiocapitellar line drawn through the central long axis of the proximal radial shaft normally extends through the central portion of the capitellar ossification center (Fig. 11-16). This line is especially important in children in whom the lack of calcified bone makes radiographic interpretation difficult.

Another very useful line for evaluating the elbow in children is the anterior humeral line. This line, which can be seen on lateral view, is drawn along the anterior surface of the shaft of the humerus and should pass through the middle third of the ossification center of the capitellum (Fig. 11-17).

If a line is drawn along the top of the coronoid process of the ulna, it should just barely cross through the superior margins of the capitellum and the trochlea (Fig. 11-17). This is called the coronoid line.

## SOFT TISSUE CONDITIONS AROUND THE ELBOW

Although a discussion of arthritic and rheumatoid conditions is not within the scope of this text, there are several painful overuse syndromes involving the elbow that are presented frequently to the emergency physician. Brief descriptions of some of these syndromes follow.

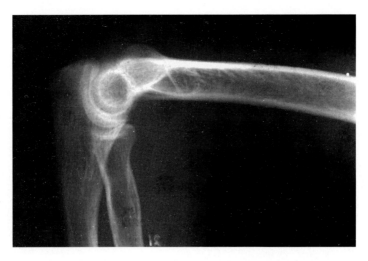

**Fig. 11-15.** Lateral view of the elbow with a radial head fracture. The anterior fat pad displays the sail sign. The posterior fat pad has become discernable. The supinator line is obscured.

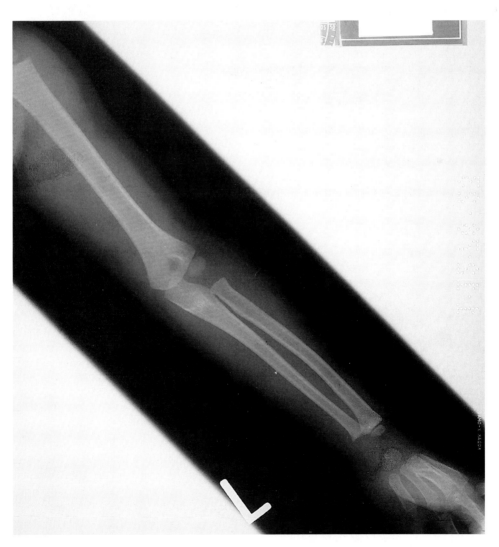

**Fig. 11-16.** Anteroposterior view of a normal elbow in a child. The radiocapitellar line extends through the central portion of the ossification center of the capitellum.

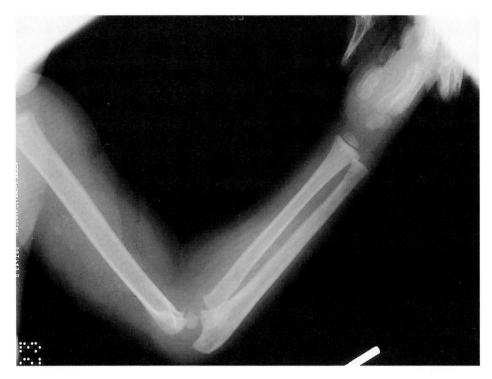

**Fig. 11-17.** Lateral view of a normal elbow in a child. The anterior humeral line (*closed arrow*) passes through the middle third of the ossification center of the capitellum. The coronoid line (*open arrow*) passes through the periphery of the capitellum and trochlea.

## Lateral epicondylitis (tennis elbow)

This condition is characterized by point tenderness either over or just distal to the lateral epicondyle. There is no limitation of movement of the elbow joint. Pain is elicited by forced flexion of the extended wrist (Cozen's test) or pronation of the forearm with the elbow in extension and the wrist flexed (Mill's maneuver).

## Baseball elbow

Acute fracture and dislocation of the elbow can occur in baseball but chronic musculoskeletal problems associated with throwing are more prevalent. A throwing injury has three components: medial tension overload (in the young), lateral compression (in the old), and extension overload.

Injury secondary to medial tension overload can involve the muscles. Such injuries are caused by strain of the common flexor-pronator muscle group, and can range anatomically from microtears to severe ruptures. Patients with these injuries should be immobilized, treated symptomatically along with ice locally, and referred for orthopedic follow-up or physical therapy for graded exercise (since myostatic contracture is a known complication). A more severe injury results in avulsion fracture of the medial epicondyle. This condition is diagnosed by the gravity stress test, which is performed with the patient in the supine position and the shoulder rotated externally. The elbow is flexed to 15° to 20° to free the olecranon from the fossa. With the weight of the forearm providing the valgus force,

a radiograph showing the medial epicondyle is obtained, and the ulnar nerve is assessed. Patients with a separation of more than 0.5 to 1 cm are referred to the orthopedist for possible open reduction and internal fixation (ORIF). Lastly, the medial collateral ligament can be ruptured, requiring surgical repair.

With extreme lateral compression, fracture of capitellum can result. These fractures affect those over 10 years of age and are caused by a repeated valgus stress compressing the capitellum and resulting in osteochondral fractures. The loose bodies may require excision because they are known to cause permanent functional loss in the elbow. Referral to the orthopedist is indicated.

Olecranon hypertrophy results from extension overload. This is created by stress fractures of the olecranon secondary to overuse of the triceps. It can result in reactive hyperosteoses, fixed flexion contracture, and loose bodies in the olecranon fossa, which might benefit from surgical removal.

## Olecranon bursitis

The olecranon bursa, like the prepatellar bursae, are particularly prone to inflammation. The olecranon bursa lies on the extensor aspect of the elbow over the olecranon and does not communicate with the joint space. This superficial location allows the bursa to be exposed to recognized and unrecognized local trauma, which precipitates inflammation. Bursitis can also occur from irritation caused by an underlying olecranon bone spur or the extension of regional infections. These injuries present with a swollen bursa and peribursal cellulitis. Range of motion of the elbow is painless except at the extreme of flexion. Bursal tenderness, extensive cellulitis, obvious overlying wounds, fever, and an impaired host defense would suggest septic bursitis; while a patient with concurrent gouty arthritis, a history of rheumatoid arthritis, or recent intrabursal injection have a higher likelihood of nonseptic bursitis.[13] Using septic precautions, an 18- or 20-gauge needle is introduced into the bursal cavity from a lateral distal approach. The fluid is sent for crystals and joint fluid analysis including culture.

Classification into septic versus nonseptic bursitis is difficult, even with findings on joint fluid analysis. Glucose concentration, gram stain, cell count, and differential cannot distinguish conclusively between the two entities. Nontoxic patients who can be treated as outpatients should be placed in a well-padded posterior splint with the elbow flexed, started on anti-staphylococcal anti-infectives and nonsteroidal anti-inflammatories, and arrangements should be made for orthopedic or rheumatologic follow-up within 2 days. All others will require admission for intensive therapy, which may include intravenous and intrabursal medication, serial bursal aspiration, percutaneous suction and continuous irrigation, and surgical incision and drainage. Known complications include bacteremia, extension of the infection into the elbow joint, and development of a chronic draining sinus.

## FRACTURES OF THE DISTAL HUMERUS
### Supracondylar fractures

Supracondylar fractures are classified into two types: a) extension, in which the distal fragment is displaced posterior to the shaft of the humerus; and b) flexion, in which the fragment is displaced anteriorly (Fig. 11-18A). The extension-type injury is more common. These fractures do not involve the joint and generally occur in the extremes of age. Sixty percent of these fractures are found in patients under 15 years of age.

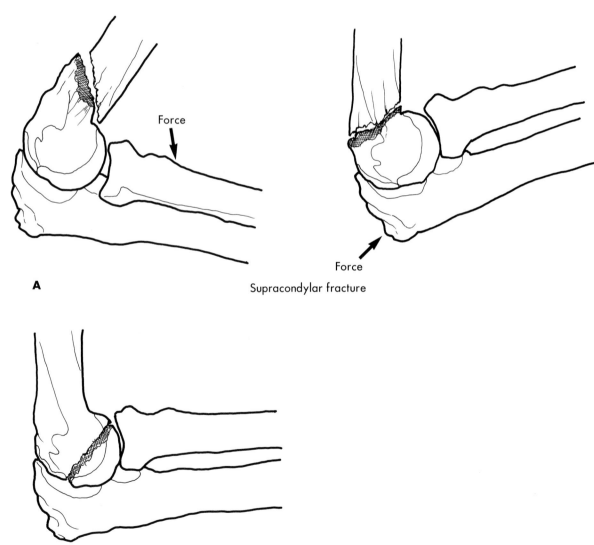

**A**

Supracondylar fracture

**B**  Transcondylar

**Fig. 11-18. A,** Extension- and flexion-type supracondylar fractures. **B,** Transcondylar fractures.

Supracondylar fractures are the tenth most commonly found fracture type in children.[3] There is a higher incidence of complications with these fractures, including a greater rate of loss of reduction, nerve injury, surgical intervention, and poor results than in any other extremity fracture. The peak age of occurrence is 5 to 8 years. They are open in 1% of the cases. Nerve injury occurs in 7.7%, with the most common being radial nerve injury in extension-type fractures and ulnar nerve injury in flexion-type fractures. In both adults and children, the incidence of flexion-type supracondylar fractures is rare (2%). Vascular injury requiring surgical intervention occurs in 0.5% of the cases. Associated ipsilateral injuries occur at a rate of 1% to 13%, and consist of fractures of the radial shaft, humeral diaphysis, olecranon, and elbow dislocation.[14]

**Extension-type fractures.** Extension-type fractures are the result of hyperextension injury to the elbow secondary to a fall on the outstretched hand or a direct blow to the elbow. The fracture extends obliquely from the posterior humerus proximally to the anterior humerus distally. The distal fragment is displaced posteriorly and proximally with the elbow flexed.

The predisposition to extension-type supracondylar fractures in children is due to the developmental ligamentous laxity in children, which allows hyperextensibility. With hyperextensibility, the linear force along the elbow is converted to a bending force, with the fulcrum at the olecranon forcing the distal humerus to fail anteriorly in the supracondylar region. The fracture is described classically as starting proximal-posterior and extending obliquely to anterior-distal as in adults. The edges of the torn anterior periosteum of the humerus may be caught in the fracture line, preventing full reduction. Posteromedial displacement and internal rotation of the distal fragment with resultant displacement of the medial spike of the proximal fragment anteriorly is noted in 75% of cases.[15–17] Conversely, posterolateral displacement with external rotation of the distal fragment results in anterior displacement of the lateral spike of the proximal fragment. The differential diagnosis of this type of fracture in children is between supracondylar or distal humeral physis fracture.

The fracture is unstable and gives rise to intense pain and swelling. On examination, these fractures can be confused with posterior elbow dislocation, but the spatial relationship of the three bony landmarks of the elbow is maintained. Neurovascular evaluation is essential because the radial nerve is often involved.[18]

The pediatric patient can present with an S-shaped extremity when the fracture is complete. But, more commonly they present with signs of hemorrhage anteriorly as the distal end of the proximal fragment has penetrated into the brachialis muscle. Dimpling of the skin (as the spike of the proximal fragment lodges in the dermal layer) is a sign that the fracture will be difficult to reduce. Conversely, there may be a palpable elbow joint effusion and this, along with localized tenderness over the supracondylar region,

may be the only finding in fractures with minimal displacement. The neurovascular examination is important. The neurologic examination should assess both motor and sensory nerves. Vascular integrity should be judged by signs of ischemia to the forearm, eg, pain with passive extension of fingers. Associated fractures from the sternoclavicular joint to the wrist should be sought. Dislocation of the elbow should be distinguished by noting the preservation of the relationship between epicondyle and olecranon. Further differentiation should be sought (by the location of maximum tenderness) from lateral condylar physis fracture, avulsion of the medial epicondyle, and radial neck fracture.

**Radiographic findings.** Radiographic findings are classified as follows:

1) nondisplaced: positive fat pad with a transverse fracture line seen on the AP view;
2) minimally displaced: decrease in the angulation of the articular surface with the long axis of the humerus seen on the lateral view with a transverse fracture line seen on the AP view;
3) moderately displaced: fracture in which a distal fragment can lie medially or laterally in relationship to the humeral shaft; and
4) markedly displaced: fracture in which a distal fragment is displaced posterior and proximal with possible axial rotation or angulation.

Classification in the pediatric population is different. They are classified into three types: type I includes nondisplaced fractures; type II includes displaced fractures (with an intact posterior cortex); and type III includes fractures that are displaced posteromedially or posterolaterally (with no cortical contact).

The anterior humeral line is useful in identifying minimal hyperextension of the distal fragment. In children this line is abnormal in 95% of minimally displaced supracondylar fractures.[19-21]

With the exception of nondisplaced or minimally displaced fractures in adults and type I fractures in children, prompt reduction is desirable. Soft tissue swelling often occurs after reduction of displaced fractures. This swelling can result in vascular compromise, so admission for close observation is necessary. Orthopedic consultation is advisable.

**Management.** Management of supracondylar fractures by emergency physicians should occur in two instances. First, when impairment of circulation is identified, temporary reduction is undertaken immediately to restore the pulse. Under these conditions, adequate anesthesia is obtained by regional block of the involved limb and longitudinal traction is applied with the elbow extended to unlock fragments with careful hyperextension. Reduction is achieved by forward pressure on the distal fragment and backward pressure on the proximal end. The fragments are then locked in place with elbow flexed at a point 5° to 10° before the radial pulse disappears. The forearm is pronated to correct for medial displacement and supinated in instances of lateral displacement.

The second instance in which the emergency physician should undertake fracture management is at the other extreme. These are cases of closed fractures without neurovascular compromise that are nondisplaced or minimally displaced (condyle shaft angulation no greater than 20°) and associated with minimal soft tissue swelling. Such fractures do not require reduction. Immobilization in a long-arm splint with follow-up arranged in 1 to 2 days is needed. Complications of these fractures are Volkmann's ischemia and varus or valgus angulation. Similarly, no reduction is needed in type I fractures in the pediatric population. In these fractures with minimal soft tissue swelling, the arm is placed in a posterior splint for 3 weeks and the patient seen in follow-up within 1 to 2 days. Type II and type III fractures in children and fractures in adults that are moderately or markedly displaced will require closed or open reduction and cast immobilization. Percutaneous pin fixation may be needed. Open reduction is also indicated in open fracture cases and when closed reduction is unsuccessful (ie, the distal portion of the proximal fragment is "button-holed" through the brachialis muscle), and in cases of severe vascular compromise (especially as a result of multiple reduction attempts).

Results are poor in 4% to 6% of pediatric cases. Such poor results are most likely in cases of severe displacement, incomplete reduction, major soft tissue damage, or a history of previous elbow injury. Around 5° of loss in range of motion is to be expected. With posteromedial and posterolateral displacement of the distal fragment, injuries to the radial and median nerves, respectively, are seen. Median nerve injury is associated with vascular injury. Injury to the isolated anterior interosseous branch of the median nerve can occur; this is manifested by motor deficits of the flexor pollicis longus and flexor digitorum longus tendons of the thumb and index finger, respectively. Surgical exploration is indicated when there is arterial compromise with manipulation because the median nerve and artery may be trapped in the fracture fragments. Vascular injury occurs in less than 0.5% of the cases, mostly when there is posterolateral displacement of the distal fragment.[22-24] Vascular injury is also more common when the fragment is rotated externally. Myositis ossificans is rare, and is associated with open reduction, multiple attempts at manipulative closed reduction, and vigorous manipulation in the rehabilitative phase. Cubitus varus (loss of the carrying angle) occurs as a complication in 9% to 58% of cases.[25-26] Predisposing factors include rotation of the distal fragment leading to subsequent coronal tilt or angulation, impaction of the medial supracondylar column, and lateral opening of the fracture site. Varus deformity gives rise to decreased external rotation, which is well compensated for at the shoulder. There is an anterior prominence laterally caused by the lateral spike of the proximal fragment. This prominence is accentuated by hyperextension, which can be important cosmetically. Decubitus valgus, conversely, has an incidence of 2%. This complication is associated with postero-lateral displacement in extension-type supracondylar fractures. It can cause significant elbow extension loss as well as tardy ulnar nerve paralysis. Osteoarthritis occurs in less than 2% of the cases. In addition, infection can occur in patients undergoing pinning and open reduction.

**Flexion-type fractures.** Flexion-type fractures are quite rare, comprising only 2% to 4% of supracondylar fractures. They are a result of direct trauma to the posterior aspect of the flexed elbow, which results in anterolateral displacement of the distal fragment. The fracture extends obliquely on the lateral view, from the anterior proximal aspect to the posterior distal aspect. The distal fragment is displaced anteriorly and flexed at the elbow. The posterior periosteum is torn but the anterior periosteum may remain attached, having separated only from the anterior surface of the proximal fragment. The posteromedial spike of the proximal fragment gives rise to ulnar nerve damage and is sometimes impaled into the triceps. Vascular injury is rare. On presentation the elbow is flexed with a decrease in olecranon prominence posteriorly. A sharp proximal fragment may be seen piercing the triceps tendon and skin. The plane of the triangle formed by the bony landmarks is shifted anterior to the humerus. Radiographic findings on the AP view may be misleading because only a transverse fracture line can be seen. On the lateral view, however, the findings range from anterior angulation of the distal fragment with or without cortical defect posteriorly to distal fragment displacement anteriorly and proximally.

These fractures are classified into three types. Type I fractures are either nondisplaced or minimally displaced. The condylar shaft angle is not increased by more than 10° to 15°. In type II fractures some integrity of the anterior cortex exists. In type III, the fragments are completely displaced.

Management of type I fractures consists of placing the involved arm in a posterior splint without reduction by the emergency physician. Follow-up with an orthopedist should take place within a week. Management of types II and III fractures should involve an orthopedist because reduction with traction, closed manipulation or open reduction and immobilization by percutaneous pinning, open pinning, and extension casting or casting with the elbow in flexion are options to be considered. Of the three major nerves around the elbow, the ulnar nerve is most likely to be injured.[27-29] Loss in range of motion, stiffness, and cubitus valgus are also complications of this injury.

### Distal humeral metaphyseal-diaphyseal fractures

It is fortunate that these fractures are rare because they are difficult to manage due to the fact that it is hard to secure the metaphyseal segments with percutaneous pins. Pronation produces a valgus angulation and supination a varus angulation of the distal fragment. Management should involve an orthopedist for possible skeletal traction. Coaptation humeral and forearm splints are also possibilities.

### Transcondylar (dicondylar) fractures

These fractures pass through both condyles and are located within the joint capsule (Fig. 11-18B). They are very similar to supracondylar fractures in that there are extension and flexion variations. As with supracondylar fractures, the flexion type with anterior displacement is again the most unusual.[29] They occur more commonly in the elderly. The fracture line is crescent-shaped or transverse, passing just proximal to the articular surface or the old epiphyseal line and entering the coronoid and olecranon fossae.

Orthopedic consultation is prudent because these fractures are difficult to manage due to the small distal fragment, which causes problems with reduction and union. Furthermore, due to their intracapsular location, reduction may be complicated by radiohumeral and ulnohumeral dislocation.

### Fractures involving the entire distal humeral physis

The peak age of occurrence for fractures involving the entire metaphyseal-epiphyseal junction is 6 or 7 years. Little is known about the mechanism of this injury. Rotary shear force is said to account for cases associated with birth injury, and in the very young as a result of a hyperextension injury or child abuse.[30-34] Because the fracture has a broad surface and does not involve the articular surface, tilting of the distal fragment and loss of motion are not seen. Avascular changes may be a consequence of fracture in this region because the blood supply of the medial ridge of the trochlea courses through the physis. These patients present with a swollen elbow and a history of trauma. On palpation the relationship of the epicondyles and the olecranon is maintained. Crepitus, which is muffled, is believed to be caused by the cartilaginous ends rubbing together. On imaging the displacement is consistently posteromedial with respect to the distal humerus, with a normal relationship between the radius and ulna.

Physeal fractures are classified according to DeLee et al.[31] into three types. Type A fractures occur before the secondary ossification center of the lateral condylar epiphysis appears. In type B there is definite ossification of the lateral condylar epiphysis. A small flake of metaphyseal bone may be attached to the fragment. In type C fractures, a large metaphyseal fragment, most commonly lateral, is present. DeLee's type C fractures can be differentiated from a supracondylar fracture by not having a smooth contour of the distal metaphysis; a fracture of the lateral condylar physis by misalignment of the lateral condylar epiphysis and proximal radius; and an elbow dislocation by posterolateral displacement of the forearm and misalignment of the lateral condylar physis and proximal radius. Further studies may be required for delineation, including comparison films, arthrography, magnetic resonance imaging, and ultrasonography. Management is best left to the orthopedist who may try skin traction, closed reduction in extension, or open reduction and immobilization with a splint or cast, either with or without pins. The emergency physician should be

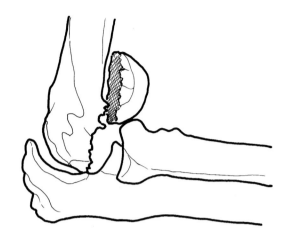

**Fig. 11-19.** Posadas fracture.

aware of the association of child abuse with Delee's type A fracture in patients younger than 3 years of age. Neurovascular injury and nonunion are rare, and if they do occur, secondary cubitus varus is seen.

### Posadas fracture

The mechanism of injury in Posadas fracture is trauma to the flexed elbow. Anatomically, there is dislocation of the radius and ulna from the anteriorly displaced dicondylar fragment. The coronoid process becomes wedged between the anteriorly displaced dicondylar fragment and the proximal fragment. They present similar to a simple dislocation with the elbow in extension and supination, lying along the longitudinal axis of the humerus.[35] On lateral radiographic view, this fracture may be mistaken for a transcondylar fracture with anterior displacement (Fig. 11-19). Because management is controversial, with complication of pseudarthrosis of the ulna with the distal portion of the humerus a possibility, orthopedic consultation is advised.

### Intercondylar T- or Y-fractures

These fractures are rare and usually occur in adults. The hallmark is a vertical component through the articular surface, most commonly through the trochlear sulcus into the humeral fossae. Prognosis is determined largely by condylar separation.

The splitting of the condyles is thought to be due to a wedgelike action of the proximal ulnar articular surface against the trochlea of the humerus when the patient attempts to break a fall with an outstretched hand. In children, a direct blow to the posterior portion of the elbow can cause this injury. When this occurs with the elbow in flexion the condyles are usually displaced anterior to the humeral shaft. Conversely, when the elbow is in extension, which is more commonly the case, the condyles are usually posterior to the humeral shaft. In either case, both condyles are separated distally and the articular surfaces rotated outward. The patient presents with the forearm held in pronation with apparent shortening. There is soft tissue swelling and widening in the condylar region. The condyles move independently of each other and the humeral shaft and, when approximated, will spring apart when the pressure is released. The massive swelling and extensive displacement mimics the supracondylar fracture.

With radiologic studies, which may include computed tomography or arthrography, classification of these fractures is possible using the Riseborough and Radin[36] criteria. Type I is an undisplaced fracture between the capitellum and trochlea; type II involves separation of the capitellum and trochlea without appreciable rotation of the fragments in the frontal plane; type III involves separation of the fragments with rotary deformity; and type IV involves severe comminution of the articular surface with wide separation of the humeral condyles. Misclassification of these fracture as supracondylar fractures occurs if the physician does not search for the vertical fracture component.

In adults, management of fracture types I and II by the emergency physician is possible while type III and IV fractures necessitate orthopedic consultation. Reduction with condylar control and immobilization using a posterior splint, supplemented by medial and lateral reinforcements with the elbow at 90°, and follow-up within 1 week is appropriate for fracture types I and II.

Known complications from this type of fracture include loss of elbow function due to excessive anterior tilting of the condyles, nonunion of the fragments, fibrosis and ankylosis of the joint from prolonged immobilization, and neurovascular injury.

Although the articular cartilage is usually intact in the pediatric patient presenting with this injury, orthopedic consultation is advised. Management is influenced by condylar separation and stability of the supracondylar columns. Methods of reduction include traction, closed or open reduction, and immobilization by pinning or casting.

## FRACTURES OF THE HUMERAL CONDYLES

Fractures in this region can be classified into three categories. Type A fractures involve the condyles and are accompanied by gross swelling, joint instability, and limitation of motion. Type B fractures involve the articular portion only. They are characterized by minimal swelling, a stable joint, loss of motion, and fracture fragments not influenced by muscle forces. Type C fractures involve the epicondyle or supracondylar process only, and are characterized by local tenderness with some swelling, some joint instability if the epicondyles are involved, and fragments displaced by muscle forces.

During the growth period, the distal humerus is the second most common site for physeal injury, the first being distal radius. The fracture pattern is dependent on both age and mechanism. The most vulnerable period for this fracture is just before puberty when the epiphysis is weakest.[37] Physeal injuries seen within the first year of life commonly

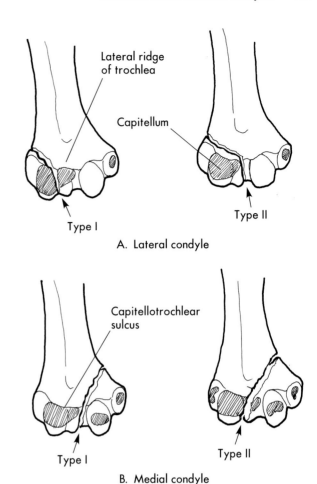

**Fig. 11-20.** Milch's classification of condylar fractures.

involve the entire distal humerus. At approximately 6 years of age, the lateral condyle is usually involved in these fractures. The medial condyle is usually involved at around 8 to 12 years of age, and the medial epicondyle at around 11 to 16 years of age. These fractures are associated with posterolateral elbow dislocation.

Condylar fractures are uncommon in adults and when present are frequently associated with fractures of both bones of the forearm. These fractures must be classified into Milch type I or II[38] (Fig. 11-20). The distinction is that in type I fractures, the lateral trochlear ridge remains with the intact condyle, thereby maintaining mediolateral stability. The converse is true for type II fractures, in which the lateral trochlear ridge does not remain with the intact condyle, thereby losing the mediolateral stability. It is important to realize that all type II fractures require open reduction and internal fixation.

### Lateral condylar fractures

Fractures of the condyles more commonly involve the lateral condyle (Fig. 11-21). These fracture patients present with a history of either falling on an outstretched arm, allowing compressive forces to be transmitted axially via the bones of the forearm to the lateral condyle or of a direct

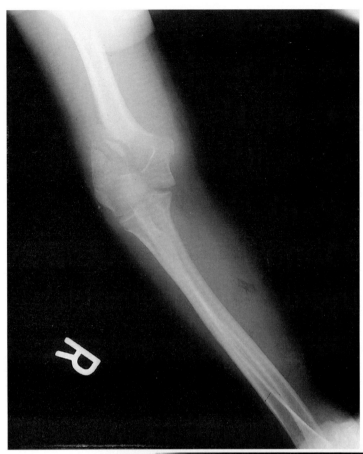

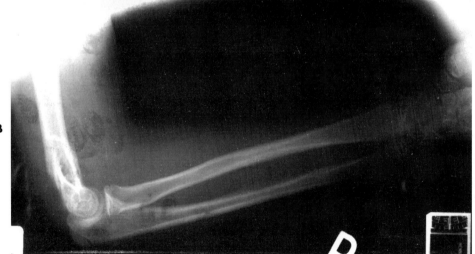

**Fig. 11-21.** Lateral condylar fracture. **A,** Anteroposterior view. **B,** Lateral view.

force over the posterior aspect of the flexed elbow, exposing the condyle laterally. On examination the patient has loss of carrying angle, swelling over the lateral condyle, and widening of the intercondylar distance without shortening. On palpation of the lateral condyle, tenderness, crepitation, and motion are noted. This can be accentuated with rotation of the radius. Loss of range of motion is noted. There may be swelling with accompanying tenderness over the medial collateral ligament. Ulnar nerve deficit should be sought. Radiographic findings consist of a fracture line extending obliquely lateral (type I) or medial (type

II) to the capitellotrochlear sulcus to the supracondylar ridge. The fragment is displaced by the extensor muscles of the forearm. Lateral translocation of the ulna associated with type II fractures and concomitant fracture of the capitellum should be noted.

Reduction for type I fractures is accomplished by direct realignment of the fragment with the forearm supinated, and the elbow in extension and adduction. A long-arm splint with supinated forearm, flexed elbow, and dorsiflexed wrist completes the immobilization process. Follow-up should be arranged within 2 to 3 days. Failed closed reduction of type I and type II fractures necessitates open reduction and internal fixation by an orthopedist as soon after the injury as possible. Complications associated with this fracture are joint instability, traumatic arthritis, limitation of joint motion, cubitus valgus, and ulnar neuropathy.

## Medial condylar fractures

Fractures of the medial condyle can also result from a fall either on the outstretched arm with the elbow forced into varus or on the apex of the flexed elbow. The most common is a type I fracture originating at the depth of the trochlear groove that ascends obliquely toward the supracondylar ridge. A type II fracture originating in the capitellotrochlear sulcus will result if the main force is applied by the rim of the radial head.

When the medial epicondyle is manipulated, movement of the condyle is noted. This movement is accentuated when the elbow is extended because this stretches the forearm flexor muscle, further displacing the fragment distally. With medial displacement of the radial head in a type II injury, the lateral condyle and capitellum gain relative prominence. There may be signs of ulnar nerve injury and lateral collateral ligament involvement.

Because closed reduction is difficult to achieve and maintain, orthopedic involvement is warranted in most cases. The exception is a closed nondisplaced type I fracture without neurovascular involvement. These fractures can be immobilized in a posterior splint with elbow flexed, forearm pronated, and wrist flexed. Referral for follow-up should be made within 2 to 3 days because known complications include restricted joint motion, traumatic arthritis, cubitus varus from nonunion with the fragment displaced proximally, and ulnar nerve symptoms.

## Fractures involving the lateral condylar physis

The peak age of occurrence for fractures involving the lateral condylar physis is around 6 years. The incidence is 16.9% of all distal humeral fractures and 54.2% of all distal humeral physeal injuries. Associated ipsilateral injuries include resultant translocation of the elbow, olecranon greenstick fracture, ulnar shaft fracture, medial epicondyle fracture, and elbow dislocation.

The mechanism of injury in the pediatric patient is an axially transmitted force resulting from a fall on an outstretched arm. This force results in either a Salter-Harris type II fracture without involvement of the lateral condylar epiphysis, or a Salter-Harris type IV fracture through the capitulotrochlear groove, which is the less common of the two. Pull on the origins of the extensor carpi radialis longus and brachioradialis muscles as well as the lateral collateral ligament tears the elbow capsule when the fragment is displaced. Only valgus angulation (Salter-Harris IV) is seen in fractures that traverse the lateral condylar epiphysis but do not include the lateral ridge of the trochlea in the distal fragment. In cases in which the fragment involves the lateral ridge, translocation and dislocation in addition to valgus angulation (Salter-Harris II) can be seen.

Radiographically, the initial classification of lateral condylar fractures is Milch's type I (Salter-Harris type IV) and Milch's type II (Salter-Harris type II). Displacement of the fragment is further classified into four types.[39] Type 1 fractures are relatively undisplaced with an intact articular surface and no lateral translocation of the ulna. The fracture can be seen in one radiographic view only. The intactness of the articular surface is evaluated by the lateral view when looking for nondisplacement of the ulna. In type 2, the fracture extends through the articular surface and allows for lateral translocation of the ulna. Although it can be seen in two radiographic views, the fracture displacement is less than 2 mm. Type 3 fractures are similar to type 2 fractures, but displacement is greater than 2 mm. In type 4, the fragment is rotated and displaced both laterally and proximally. Translocation of both the radius and ulna can be seen.

Soft tissue swelling around the injury site can be used as a guide to the likelihood of late displacement. The major pitfall is to mistake these fractures for fractures of the entire distal humeral physis. With fractures of the entire distal humeral physis the relationship of the lateral condylar ossification center and radius remains intact and displacement is posteromedial. Arthrography may be helpful.

These fracture patients present with soft tissue swelling over the lateral aspect of the distal humerus. In type 1 displacement, local tenderness and pain are increased by forced flexion of the wrist. In type 2 and type 3 displacement, local crepitation on pronation and supination is also seen. Tests for radial nerve involvement should be performed.

In cases in which the fracture line is barely perceptible on radiography, ie, type 1 displacement with minimal local soft tissue swelling and absence of crepitation on elbow or forearm motion, no reduction is necessary. Immobilization is provided by a posterior splint with the elbow flexed at least 90° and the forearm in some pronation. Orthopedic follow-up should occur within 3 to 5 days. Closed fracture reduction in patients with Milch's type I with displacement that is less than 24 to 48 hours old can be accomplished with the elbow extended and the forearm in supination. Unlike adults, children should be immobilized in a long-arm splint with the elbow in hyperflexion with pronation of the forearm.[40] All patients should have orthopedic consultation immediately. The orthopedist may elect to perform closed or open reduction (about 60% of the cases), and may use various immobilizing techniques such as figure-of-eight casting, long-arm casting, percutaneous pinning, sutures, pins, nails, or screws.

Orthopedic consultation should be obtained liberally because complications can result in nonunion with resultant weakness or pain in the elbow, loss in range of motion, cubitus valgus, and tardy ulnar nerve palsy. Physeal arrest, which usually does not give rise to significant angular or length deformities, malunion, avascular necrosis, or myositis ossificans, can occur. Even with acceptable reduction, complications do occur. For example, lateral spur formation due to the periosteal flap associated with the distal fragment can give rise to a pseudovarus deformity, even though there is no functional disability. The rate of cubitus varus deformity can be as high as 40% and is thought to be a combination of inadequate reduction and stimulation of lateral physis growth caused by the fracture. Cubitus valgus, less common than cubitus varus, is caused by epiphysiodesis of the lateral physis, which does not result in clinical or functional disability. Finally, delayed union occurs even with satisfactory alignment of the fracture fragments. This can be a result of poor vascular supply to the fragment, inhibition of the repair process by synovial fluid, or constant tension forces generated by the muscles attached to the fragment.

### Fractures involving the medial condylar physis

Fractures in this region can be divided into two types. Intra-articular fractures involve the trochlear articular surface in some manner, while extra-articular fractures include the medial metaphysis and medial epicondyle.

These fractures comprise less than 1% of all distal humeral fractures in children,[41] with peak occurrence between 8 and 14 years of age. They are associated with olecranon greenstick fractures and posterolateral elbow dislocation. Child abuse should be included in the differential diagnosis.

There are two possible histories for patients presenting with these fractures:

1) falling directly on the point of the flexed elbow (with the speculation that the sharp edge of the semilunar notch of the olecranon splits the trochlea, directly resulting in the more common Salter-Harris II fracture); or

2) falling on an outstretched arm with the elbow extended and the wrist dosiflexed, producing an avulsion fracture with a valgus stress (Salter-Harris IV). The fragment rotates anteriorly in the sagittal plane due to the pull of the forearm flexor muscles.

In general, the distal metaphyseal fragment includes the medial epicondyle and the common flexor origin of the muscles of the forearm. The flexor muscles rotate the fragment so the fracture surface is facing anteriorly and medially. The capsule is disrupted anteriorly lateral to the common flexor origin. If the blood supply to the medial ridge of the trochlea, which traverses the surface of the medial condylar physis, is disrupted by the fracture line in this region, a "fishtail" deformity may develop. This in turn gives rise to joint instability and varus deformity.

The patient presents with medial swelling and ulnar nerve paresthesia. It is important to differentiate between fracture of the medial condylar physis, which is intra-articular, from fracture of the medial epicondylar physis, which is extra-articular, because both have similar presentations. The distinguishing feature is that intra-articular lesions have both valgus and varus instability while extra-articular injuries have valgus instability only.

Classification of medial condylar physis fractures is made by examining the fracture line radiologically. Milch's type I fracture is a Salter-Harris type II with the fracture line running between the common physeal line, separating medial and lateral condylar ossification centers, and traversing the apex of the trochlea. Milch's type II is a Salter-Harris type IV fracture with the fracture line traversing the medial aspect of the lateral condylar ossification center, ending in the capitulotrochlear groove. The fracture fragments can include varying amounts of the metaphysis, including the ossification center of the medial epicondyle.

Displacement of the fracture is next assessed, and is classified as follows.[42] In Kilfoyle type I, the fracture line extends down to the physis. This is not a serious injury unless there is greenstick crushing of the medial supracondylar column. This is seen in younger patients. In Kilfoyle type II, the fracture line extends into the physis and the fragment remains undisplaced. In Kilfoyle type III, the condylar fragment is displaced and rotated.

In cases in which ossification of the medial condyle is not apparent an arthrogram may be needed to make the diagnosis. A case of fracture of the medial epiphysis with the presence of metaphyseal ossification, especially in association with posteromedial elbow dislocation is one situation in which arthrography should be considered.

Kilfoyle's type I fracture without involvement of the medial supracondylar column and Kilfoyle's type II fracture do not need reduction. In these fractures, a posterior splint is applied with the elbow in flexion. Follow-up is arranged with an orthopedist within 1 week. Other fractures of the medial physis should result in orthopedic consultation. Open reduction and pin immobilization may be needed. Complications include misdiagnosis of the fracture as a medial epicondylar fracture, decubitus varus due to a disturbance of the vascular supply affecting the medial ridge of the trochlea, nonunion or delayed union, decubitus valgus, and ulnar neuropathy.

### Articular surface fractures

**Fractures of the capitellum.** Fractures of the capitellum (Fig. 11-22) are rare and occur mostly in women. In children, the incidence is 1 in 2,000 elbow fractures.

The fracture lines are seen in the coronal plane with fragments consisting primarily of articular cartilage with varying amounts of subchondral bone. They are without soft tissue attachment and lie free in the joint; they are produced by shearing forces or compressive wedging involving the capitellum and trochlea. In 31% of children with these injuries a proximal radial injury is present.[43] These fractures are classified into two types. Type I (Hahn-Steinthal) involves a large part of the osseous portion and may contain part of the adjacent ridge of the trochlea. Type II (Kocher-Lorenz) involves the articular cartilage with minimal osseous involvement. The involved cartilage is often a piece of articular cartilage from an underlying osteochondritis dissecans injury.

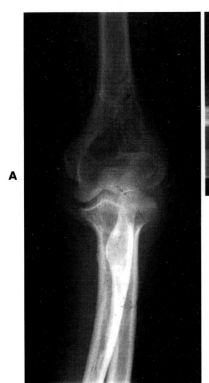
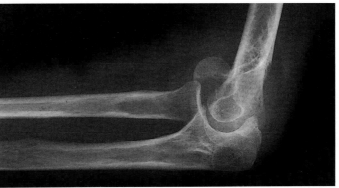

**Fig. 11-22.** Capitellum fracture. **A,** Anteroposterior view. **B,** Lateral view.

These fractures can be associated with ulnar collateral ligament rupture and radial head fracture. The presenting history is of a fall broken with the wrist and elbow in slight flexion or of direct trauma to a flexed and pronated elbow. Because the acute symptoms are caused by distension of the joint capsule, there may be a delay in presentation with respect to time of injury. On examination, there is limitation of flexion and extension due to fragments in the various fossae and minimal swelling. With the elbow in extension, a fragment may be palpable along with crepitation anterior to the radial head. Findings of radial head and medial collateral ligament tenderness may be present when these associated injuries are present. The AP view is useful in demonstrating the degree of associated trochlear involvement. The lateral view may show the fragment anterior to the main fragment of capitellum and proximal to the radial head.

Small fragments may require an oblique or capitellar view for visualization. If the fragment is nondisplaced, the elbow is immobilized in a posterior splint with the elbow flexed and the forearm pronated. Closed reduction can be attempted for displaced fractures in children and young adults, especially in type I fractures. Reduction is achieved by traction of the forearm with the elbow extended and varus stress to open the elbow laterally in order to allow direct manipulation of the fragment. The fragment is held in position by the radius with the elbow flexed and the forearm pronated. Follow-up is arranged within 1 week. All others need emergency orthopedic involvement. Reduction and immobilization may include closed reduction with pin immobilization or open reduction with wire or screw

reattachment and even excision. Known complications are ulnar neuropathy, joint instability, avascular necrosis, degenerative arthritis, loss in range of motion, and delayed distal radioulnar joint symptoms.

**Fractures of the trochlea.** Fractures of the trochlea are usually associated with elbow dislocation. Isolated fractures involving only the articular surface are extremely rare. They present with pain, elbow effusion associated with restriction of motion, and crepitus. These fractures should be suspected in the older child with a dislocated elbow in whom there is some widening of the joint following reduction. The fragment is found radiologically lying on the medial side of the joint just distal to the medial epicondyle.

Orthopedic involvement is necessary because management is by open reduction and fixation for all cases except those that are nondisplaced. Nondisplaced fractures require posterior splinting and follow-up within 1 week.

### Epicondylar fractures

Primary isolated epicondylar fractures are uncommon in adults. In children, epiphyseal separation via avulsion is the norm. In this section, fractures of the two epicondyles as well as those of the supracondylar process will be addressed.

Fractures of the lateral epicondyle are extremely rare (Fig. 11-23) because most fractures in this area involve the lateral condyle, with which it is almost level. Symptomatic cases are immobilized.

Fractures of the medial epicondyle are more common compared with fractures of its lateral counterpart. In some adults, fusion has never occurred, predisposing them to

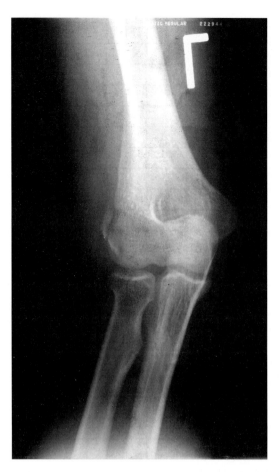

**Fig. 11-23.** Lateral epicondylar fracture seen in the anteroposterior view.

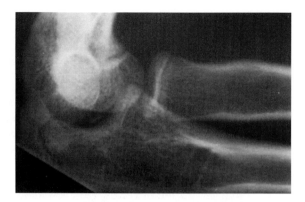

**Fig. 11-24.** Entrapped medial epicondylar fragment in an elbow joint.

avulsion fractures. Most commonly, these fractures are associated with posterolateral elbow dislocation, which is rare after 20 years of age. A direct blow to the medial aspect of the elbow, often with the elbow flexed, as well as avulsion, are common causes. The fragment is displaced anteriorly and distally by the flexor muscles of the forearm. Either pain over the medial epicondyle, which is accentuated by active elbow flexion and wrist pronation, or flexion accompanied by tenderness and crepitation locally, is usually present. Radiographic findings of fragments lying at the level of the joint should prompt a diagnosis of joint incarceration.[44] Minimally displaced fractures should be immobilized with the elbow and wrist flexed and the forearm pronated. Follow-up should be arranged within 1 week. In other cases (eg, fragments lying within the joint) (Fig. 11-24) and in moderately to severely displaced fragments open reduction by an orthopedist is indicated. Complications include elbow instability with valgus stress, wrist flexor weakness, nonunion, delayed motion predisposed to joint stiffness, and ulnar and median nerve symptoms.

### Medial epicondylar apophysis fractures

In the pediatric population, medial epicondylar fractures are the second most common fractures of the elbow, following

those involving the lateral condylar physis. The incidence is 14.1% of all distal humerus fractures and 11.5% of all fractures occurring in the elbow region, peaking at 11 and 12 years of age. These fractures are associated with elbow dislocation in 30% to 55% of cases and are incarcerated in the joint in the spontaneously relocated elbow in 14% of cases. They are also seen with radial neck fractures from valgus angulation, greenstick fractures of the olecranon, and coronoid process fractures.

The major cause is posterolateral dislocation of the elbow where the ulnar collateral ligament provides the avulsion force. They can also be caused by a direct blow to the posteromedial aspect of the elbow or through avulsive forces due to falling on outstretched arm or throwing a baseball (via the flexor muscles). The patient presents with a myriad of symptoms and signs depending on the degree of displacement of the medial epicondyle. These range from some swelling, localized tenderness, and palpable crepitus over the medial epicondyle to a palpable and freely mobile fragment suggestive of a displaced fragment. Some can even present with a block to motion, especially in extension, which is a sign of entrapment of fragment in the joint.

On radiographic examination, the undisplaced fracture has some loss of soft tissue planes medially. Minimally displaced fractures have loss of smooth sclerotic margins and increased apophyseal width. Those classified as significantly displaced have greater than 5 mm of separation, yet are proximal to the true joint surface.

Entrapment should be considered if the fragment is at the joint level in the absence of an apophyseal center in children older than 4 to 6 years of age. In these cases the fragment may be hidden by the distal humerus or proximal ulna. This is more apt to occur in younger children because the joint capsule extends up to the apophyseal line of the medial epicondyle in that age group. The presence of a fat pad finding is not consistent, because some fractures are wholly extra-articular and some elbow dislocations can result in capsule rupture, thus not allowing accumulation of hemarthrosis. Significant hemarthrosis in a minimally displaced fracture or a significant piece of metaphyseal bone accompanying the medial epicondylar fragment can be a sign of physeal fracture of the medial condyle, which may require arthrography for clarification.

Classification of acute medial epicondylar apophysis injuries is as follows. Type 1 injuries are undisplaced. Type 2 are minimally displaced. Type 3 are significantly displaced and can occur with or without elbow dislocation. Type 4 injuries involve entrapment of a fragment in the joint with elbow either relocated or dislocated. Type 5 injuries occur through the epicondylar apophysis either with or without displacement.

No reduction is needed for nondisplaced, minimally displaced, or moderately displaced fractures. The involved extremity is placed in a posterior splint with follow-up with an orthopedist within 1 week to ensure early motion. When the fragment has been incarcerated in the dislocated elbow joint within the last 24 hours, the emergency physician needs to actively intervene. Valgus stress on the elbow is applied with the forearm supinated and wrist and fingers dorsiflexed.[45] The incarcerated fragment is manipulated out of the joint initially before elbow relocation is attempted. The arm is placed in a posterior splint. Further management of these cases and acute management of all other cases in which there is significant displacement is left to the consulting orthopedist. Reduction by either closed (especially in injuries associated with elbow dislocation) or open (in cases of valgus instability or ulnar nerve dysfunction, unextractable incarceration in the joint, and fracture through the epicondylar apophysis) methods is possible.

Immobilization for these fractures may employ percutaneous pins in cases of closed reduction or pins, screws, and sutures in cases of open reduction. In cases of comminuted fractures, excision is sometimes used. Complications of these injuries include the failure to recognize incarceration of a fragment within the joint cavity; ulnar neuropathy, which is attributed to direct injury with an incidence of 10% to 16% (and rising to 50% in cases in which a fragment is entrapped in the joint);[46] delayed ulnar neuropathy associated with elbow dislocation; median nerve injury; nonunion, which occurs in 50% of cases with significant displacement; loss of terminal 5° to 10° of extension in 20% of the cases; myositis ossificans with vigorous manipulation; medial prominence creating a false impression of an increased carrying angle; and a low incidence of decreased carrying angle.

### Supracondylar process fractures

The supracondylar process is located on the anteromedial surface of humerus, 5 cm proximal to the elbow. Fractures of this process are rare, and usually are caused by direct trauma. The ligament of Struthers joins the process to the medial epicondyle, forming a fibro-osseous arch through which the median nerve and sometimes brachial artery pass. Attached to this arch are the lower fibers of coracobrachialis and the upper fibers of pronator teres. Patients present with pain that worsens with active extension of the elbow with the forearm in pronation or supination and localized tenderness on palpation. An oblique view of humerus may be required for visualization.

Management involves simple immobilization until the patient is pain-free, followed by early motion. Excision is reserved for median nerve compression. Complications that should be expected are symptoms and signs of median nerve and brachial artery compression.

## DISLOCATIONS OF THE ELBOW

The elbow is the third most commonly dislocated joint following the shoulders and fingers. The dislocation must be relocated as quickly as possible because of pain, swelling, progressive articular cartilage damage, and vascular injuries. Dislocations are described according to how the radius and ulna are displaced with respect to the distal humerus and each other. Posterior or posterolateral dislocations are the most common, comprising of 80% to 90% of all dislocations. Divergent and isolated radial and ulnar dislocations are rare.

The general classification of dislocations are:
1) primary elbow dislocation, including posterior, medial/lateral, anterior, and divergent;
2) dislocation of radial head;
3) dislocation of ulna; and
4) subluxation of the head of the radius.

In children, the incidence of elbow dislocation is 3% to 6% of elbow injuries, with the peak age of incidence being 13 to 14 years when the physes are closing. Eighteen percent of all elbow dislocations occur in the first decade of life while 29% happen in the second decade. This is in sharp contrast to supracondylar fractures, which peak at the age of 5 to 7 years. In 60% of the cases,[47] there are associated fractures. Medial epicondyle involvement is most common, but the proximal radius, coronoid process, and, rarely, olecranon, trochlea, lateral condyle, and lateral epicondyle can also be involved. Most pediatric dislocations are posterior types and involve disruption of the radioulnar joint or isolated dislocation of the radius. Fractures involving the proximal ulna are very rare.

### Primary elbow dislocation

**Posterior dislocation.** Posterior dislocation, the most common type, results from a fall onto an outstretched hand with the arm extended and abducted. The coronoid process either slips posteriorly to lie in the olecranon fossa or is jammed into the distal end of humerus, which drives through the anterior joint capsule and tears the brachialis muscle anteriorly. Both collateral ligaments are torn. The final position is dependent on relative forces, of which posterolateral is the most common (Fig. 11-25). The patient presents with the forearm in mid-flexion with a full antecubital fossa and a shortened appearance. Posteriorly, the olecranon tents the skin with a "sucked in" appearance between the edges of the triceps. The triangular relationship

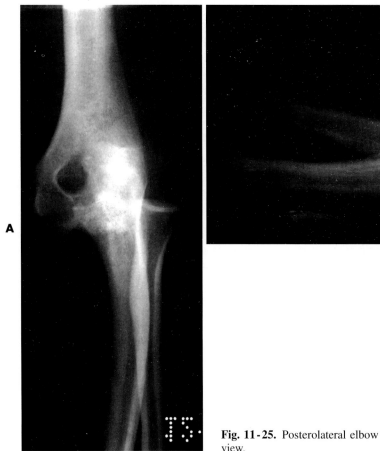

**Fig. 11-25.** Posterolateral elbow dislocation. **A,** Anteroposterior view. **B,** Lateral view.

of the bony landmarks is lost. In posterolateral dislocation the radial head is prominent posteriorly on palpation. Initial neurovascular examination is essential. When evaluating films of dislocation, special attention should be given to the presence of possible associated fractures.

Fractures of the coronoid process can occur as isolated injuries but are most often associated with posterior dislocation of elbow due to avulsion via the attachment of the brachialis muscle when the elbow is hyperextended. This results in an oblique fracture line with the distal end of fragment pointing anteriorly. When associated with posterior dislocation the fragment is more comminuted and, as with all coronoid fractures, the intra-articular tip may be free. Early open reduction and internal fixation is indicated in cases in which fragments interfere with joint motion. In the remaining cases, especially with large fragments, immobilization in the flexed position is suggested. Consultation with the orthopedist is advisable prior to discharge in cases of posterior dislocation with associated fractures.

Reduction is initiated by providing complete muscle relaxation. With countertraction on the humerus and traction applied distally at the wrist and proximal forearm, medial or lateral displacement is corrected first. With continued traction and flexion of the elbow, the coronoid process is disengaged and lifted over the humerus. Flexion and extension through the full range of motion ensure joint stability and rule out mechanical blockage. A postreduction

neurovascular examination is important. The elbow is immobilized in a long-arm splint flexed to at least 90° unless limited by circulatory status. Discharge instruction includes elevation, ice, and circulation, movement, and sensory checks with follow-up with an orthopedist in 3 to 4 days. Immediate orthopedic consultation is advised in cases in which closed gentle reduction under adequate anesthesia fails or if the patient has associated injuries requiring operative repair. Patients should be advised of the known complications of limitation of full elbow extension and joint instability.

The majority of closed elbow dislocations in children, barring entrapment of the medial epicondylar apophysis, do not require surgery for adequate reduction. Management by the emergency physician starts with documentation of a complete neurovascular examination, especially of median nerve function. Dislodgement of the medial epicondylar apophysis is attempted if present (see section on medial epicondylar apophysis). This is followed by hypersupination to dislodge the radial head from the posterolateral aspect of the lateral distal humerus with the elbow flexed to 70° to 80°. Force is then transmitted along the long axis of the humerus to overcome muscular contraction, followed by a force along the long axis of the forearm, which allows the radial head and coronoid process to pass from posterior to anterior of the distal humerus. After reduction, a post-neurovascular examination is repeated and full range of motion ensured. The elbow is immobilized in a posterior splint with elbow at 90° in mid-pronation with referral to an orthopedist in 1 to 4 days. Immediate consultation with the orthopedist for possible open reduction is mandatory in cases of an inability to obtain closed reduction, open dislocation, associated neurovascular injury, or associated fractures.

**Medial and lateral dislocations.** Medial and lateral dislocations are commonly caused by a fall on an out-stretched arm. It is a very rare injury in children. In some cases of lateral dislocation, the greater sigmoid notch is found articulating with the capitulotrochlear sulcus, giving rise to some preservation of flexion and extension. Compared with lateral dislocation, medial dislocation is usually a subluxation with lesser accompanying soft tissue damage. The elbow is widened with preservation of the relative lengths of the upper arm and forearm. The AP view of the elbow reveals the medial or lateral displacement of the ulna. Reduction is carried out with the forearm in mild extension with stabilization of the upper arm. Straight medial or lateral pressure is exerted with care not to produce a posterior dislocation. Immobilization and follow-up instruction is identical to that for posterior dislocations. Indications for orthopedic consultation from the emergency department are also similar. The inability to reduce a lateral dislocation can be caused by the anconeus muscle interposing in the joint space.

**Anterior dislocation.** Anterior dislocation is caused by a blow to the flexed elbow that drives the olecranon forward. The dislocation is most likely to be open and cause vascular injury. This injury is also associated with stripping of soft tissue with complete avulsion of the triceps mechanism. The arm is shortened while the forearm is lengthened and supinated with the elbow in full extension. Anteriorly, there is tenting of the biceps tendon and brachialis muscle. Posteriorly, the olecranon fossa and trochlea are palpable. This injury is rare in children. Radiographically, the olecranon can be seen impinging on the anterior aspect of the humerus.

Reduction is accomplished by partial extension and distal traction, along with backward pressure on the forearm. Orthopedic consult is advised.

**Divergent dislocation.** Divergent dislocation is rare. It is divided into two types: anteroposterior and mediolateral, the latter of which is very rare. Because both types involve radial head reduction that is hard to maintain, orthopedic consultation should be used liberally after emergent reduction by the emergency physician.

In anteroposterior dislocations, the humerus is forced distally onto the forearm, which is pronated with the elbow extended. The coronoid process is thus lodged in the olecranon fossa (posterior dislocation) and the radial head in the coronoid fossa (anterior dislocation); this is associated with tearing of the interosseous membrane and disruption of the orbicular and collateral ligaments. Presentation is similar to that of posterior dislocation except that the radial head is palpable in the antecubital fossa. Reduction is obtained by a simultaneous posterior reduction maneuver with direct pressure applied to reduce the radial head. The elbow is immobilized in a flexed position with the forearm supinated.

In mediolateral dislocations, the humerus is wedged between radius and ulna, creating a divergence. The elbow appears widened and the articular surface of the trochlea is palpable posteriorly. Reduction is carried out by traction with the elbow in extension while the proximal portions of radius and ulna are pressed together.

## Radial head dislocation

Dislocation of the radial head by itself is exceedingly rare. It is usually associated with fracture of the ulna (Monteggia's). This type of dislocation results from a fall on the pronated forearm with the elbow flexed by muscular contraction. Hyperextension of radial head is created through lever action, resulting in anterior displacement. It is recognized radiographically when the axis of the radial head does not pass through the capitellum. Reduction is obtained by gentle supination while the elbow is extended. Because it is usually unstable and may require open repair of the annular ligament, orthopedic involvement is recommended.

In children with radial head dislocation, the average age of presentation is 7 years. Many of these dislocations are associated with an occult fracture of the ulna or olecranon.[48] The dislocation is most commonly anterior, followed in incidence by lateral dislocation. The mechanism of injury is a fall on the outstretched arm.

Radiographically, the line through the long axis of the radius does not pass through the center of capitellum. In the majority of the acute cases, closed reduction is usually successful with the patient under anesthesia. Open reduction and repair of the annular ligament along with fixation using wires or pins for immobilization may also be used.

## Dislocation of the ulna

Isolated dislocation of the ulna is divided into two types: posterior and the rare anterior. Immediate orthopedic referral after relocation by the emergency physician is prudent. In posterior ulnar dislocation, angular force on the forearm, with the radial head acting as pivot, disrupts the medial collateral and orbicular ligaments. This results in the coronoid process becoming displaced posterior to the trochlea. The patient presents with the elbow in extension and varus. Reduction is by traction and valgus force to the elbow and supination of the forearm.

In anterior dislocation, again with the radial head acting as pivot, the ulna rotates forward with forearm abducted, resulting in the olecranon lying in the coronoid fossa. On presentation, the elbow is in flexion and valgus. The ulna is reduced with posterior pressure over the ulna with forearm pronated and varus force applied.

## Subluxation of the radial head

Subluxation of the radial head, or "nurse maid's elbow," is common, estimated to constitute 27.5% of all elbow injuries. The peak age of incidence is 2 to 3 years (range, 2 months to 7 years) with a recurrence rate reported to vary between 5% and 39%. The usual mechanism of injury is a longitudinal pull of an extended elbow with a pronated forearm. Anatomically it occurs when the orbicular ligament slips proximally but still covers the radial head partially. These patients present with a history of sustaining a longitudinal pull on the elbow. Initial pain, which resolves, can be referred to the wrist. This is followed by a period of disuse with the arm held at the side and the forearm pronated, which can lead to dependent edema. There is localized tenderness without evidence of joint effusion over the radial head and orbicular ligament. There is resistance with supination or flexion of the elbow. This classical history is present in two thirds of cases. The differential diagnosis is that of a supracondylar fracture, septic joint, or subluxated radial head. The radiographic findings are usually normal although an increase in the radiolucent interval between the radius and capitellum and more than 3 mm of lateral displacement of the radiocapitullar line have been associated with subluxation.[49] Films are indicated prior to reduction in cases in which the history and examination are not classical or when reduction is unsuccessful. Fractures distant from the elbow, eg, undisplaced fractures of the clavicle and torus fractures of the distal radius, can be confused with this condition. Reduction is accomplished by supination followed by flexion. Full supination and pronation should be attained after a successful reduction.

Immobilization in a sling is indicated if full use of the extremity is not observed in 5 to 10 minutes. Otherwise, follow-up is necessary with an orthopedist for possible immobilization in a long-arm cast only if the child is still symptomatic after 24 hours or has a history of subluxation (more than two or three times). Irreducible subluxation, which may require open reduction, is the only other indication for orthopedic involvement. There generally are no long-term complications caused by unreduced subluxation because they all seem to reduce spontaneously.

## OLECRANON FRACTURES

The large curved eminence of the olecranon lies in a subcutaneous location, susceptible to direct trauma. In conjunction with the proximal part of the coronoid process it forms the greater sigmoid notch, which provides stability in the AP plane to the elbow joint. The articular surface is interrupted by a "bare area" midway between the tip of the olecranon and the coronoid process. All fractures of the olecranon that are intra-articular disrupt the stability of the elbow. Nonfusion of the ossification centers and patella cubiti, which is a true accessory ossicle located in the triceps tendon at its insertion into the olecranon, may be mistaken for a fracture.

There are three main mechanisms of injury: direct force, indirect force, and combinations of the two. Direct force largely results in a comminuted fracture. The indirect force resulting from a fall on an outstretched hand with the elbow

flexed accompanied by strong contraction of the triceps may result in transverse or oblique fractures. With extreme force, a fracture-dislocation can result with the proximal fragment of the ulna displaced posteriorly and the radial head and distal ulnar fragment displaced anteriorly, accompanied by severe anterior soft tissue injury. With less force a transverse or oblique fracture entering the semilunar notch results. The amount of separation is influenced by the pull of triceps balanced by the soft tissue of the elbow joint and the periosteum of the olecranon.

These patients present with pain over the olecranon and a painful, limited range of motion of the elbow. If the fracture is intra-articular, there is swelling over the olecranon and signs of joint effusion on inspection. On palpation, a sulcus over the fracture site may be felt. These patients may have signs and symptoms of ulnar nerve injury (ie, inability to extend the elbow against gravity), especially in cases of comminuted fracture resulting from direct trauma or triceps mechanism disruption.

### Displaced and undisplaced fractures

Most of the radiographic findings are found on the lateral view with special attention paid to the degree of comminution, the extent of articular surface disruption in the semilunar notch, and the displacement of the radial head. The AP view is used to delineate the extent of the fracture in the sagittal plane. This view is most useful in cases in which an oblique fracture line is seen running dorsally and distally (Fig. 11-26), because these fractures may be accompanied by comminution in the sagittal plane or central depression on the articular surface. The fractures are divided into two general types:[50] undisplaced and displaced. Undisplaced fractures are defined as less than 2 mm of displacement with no or minimal increase in displacement on elbow

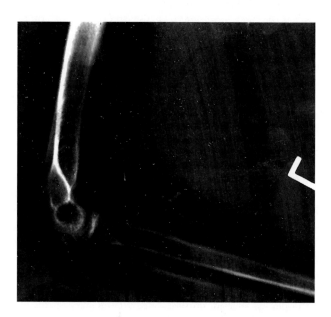

**Fig. 11-26.** Olecranon fracture seen in the lateral view.

flexion to 90° and an ability to extend against gravity. All other fractures are considered to be displaced.

Undisplaced fractures, as well as displaced fractures in the elderly (usually an avulsion fracture resulting in a transverse fracture that separates a small proximal fragment from the ulna), can generally be managed nonoperatively with closed reduction. In cases of undisplaced fractures, the arm is immobilized in a long-arm splint with the elbow in 45° to 90° of flexion. For displaced fractures in the elderly, immobilization is accomplished with a simple sling, avoiding flexion past 90°. Follow-up with an orthopedist within 3 to 5 days is warranted. All other displaced fractures usually require open reduction and internal fixation, which may include excision of the olecranon fragment, tension-band wiring, intramedullary devices, screws, and plates.

Known complications consist of decreased range of motion (usually extension) in up to 50%; posttraumatic arthritis associated with separations greater than 2 mm; nonunion occurring in 5%; and ulnar nerve symptoms in the form of numbness or paresthesias in 10%.

## Metaphyseal fractures

These fractures are rare, accounting for 4% to 6% of all elbow fractures. The peak age of incidence is 5 to 6 years. The incidence of associated injuries is high (48% to 77%); these include fracture or dislocation of the proximal radius, lateral condyle, and ulna shaft.

Two common mechanisms of injury are seen. First is a fall onto a semi-flexed elbow giving rise to flexion injuries. Tension provided by the muscles acting over the posterior cortex results in a transverse intra-articular fracture perpendicular to the long axis of the ulna. Second, extension injuries giving rise to a greenstick fracture can result from a fall on a hyperextended elbow with abduction or adduction of the forearm. The immature olecranon has a thin cortex and a thick periosteum predisposing it to greenstick fracture.

The patient presents with swelling, contusion, or abrasion over the olecranon. A separation may be palpable between fragments in flexion injury. Weakness or the inability to extend the arm is also seen.

In flexion injuries, the fracture line is perpendicular to the long axis of ulna. Conversely, the fracture is oriented longitudinally in extension injury. With the extension injury pattern, associated fractures of the radius and distal humerus need to be ruled out.

In injuries with insignificant displacement, with a non-palpable defect associated with flexion injury, or an intact posterior periosteum, no reduction is needed and the elbow is immobilized in a posterior splint at less than 75° to 80° of flexion. Follow-up with an orthopedist in 3 to 5 days should be arranged. All other cases should receive orthopedic consultation because 10% to 17% will have significant displacement requiring open reduction and internal fixation with sutures, screws, tension band wiring, and axial pins; all others will require complicated closed reduction. Known

complications of this fracture include an inability to reduce the fracture secondary to a proximal fragment trapped in the joint, delayed loss of reduction in cases treated closed, nerve injury of the ulna and posterior interosseous nerve in Monteggia III-type injury, Volkmann's ischemic contractures, nonunion, and reduced range of motion secondary to elongation of the tip of olecranon.

## Fractures involving the proximal apophysis of the olecranon

This is the rarest form of epiphyseal detachment because much of the triceps expansion attaches to the metaphysis distally. These fractures occur with hyperextension, by a direct blow or avulsion with the elbow flexed, or by recurrent tension forces across the apophysis in athletes. Acute injuries present with localized swelling and pain. Tenderness is localized over the defect between the apophysis and metaphysis. Muffled crepitation can be felt. The patient is unable to extend actively if the fragment is completely displaced. With radiologic findings these fractures fall into two classifications:

1) those through the apophyseal plate that may need arthrography for diagnosis if a secondary center has not developed and
2) Salter II, with a metaphyseal fragment included with proximal displacement.

Stress fractures are characteristic in that there are irregular apophysis and cystic changes. In cases of stress injuries, the emergency physician should advise rest in a posterior splint and referral for possible operative immobilization using a compressive device and bone graft. Other fractures are best managed by the orthopedist. Closed reduction is necessary in cases presenting before the development of a secondary ossification center and open reduction and immobilization with pins and compression wires are necessary for those with a developed secondary ossification center. Complications are ulnar shortening without functional problems and symptomatic proximal spurring from epiphyseal overgrowth.

## FRACTURES OF THE CORONOID PROCESS

This fracture is quite rare, being involved in only 1% to 2% of elbow fractures. It peaks in two age groups; 8- to 9-year-olds and 12- to 14-year-olds. Most fractures are associated with elbow dislocation but can also occur with fractures of the olecranon, medial epicondyle, lateral condyle, and radial neck. Isolated fractures are of the avulsion type by the brachialis. Anatomically, they do not develop a secondary center of ossification but ossify by the advancing edge of the metaphysis at the age of 6 years. A small avulsion tip fracture of the coronoid or a flap of articular cartilage with minimal osseous elements in the anterior joint cavity is seen. Oblique or radiocapitellar views may be necessary for better visualization. With the presence of an anterior and posterior fat pad, suspicion is high for a spontaneously relocated elbow dislocation. These are classified as follows:[51]

type I, which involve only the tip of the process;

type II, which involve more than the tip but less than 50% of the process; and

type III, which involve more than 50% of the process.

With type I and II injuries (usually an isolated avulsion), closed reduction is obtained with the elbow in extension. Immobilization is maintained by 100° of elbow flexion and full supination with follow-up with the orthopedist in 3 to 5 days. Type III injuries will require orthopedic involvement as open reduction and internal fixation is optimal because the elbow is unstable.

Complications with these injuries usually involve missed associated fractures, rarely of a free fragment in the joint. In the type III injury, instability of the joint may lead to recurrent dislocation.

## FRACTURES OF THE NECK AND HEAD OF THE RADIUS

The radial head takes part not only in elbow flexion and extension but also plays a part in forearm rotation. The decision for surgery following fractures to this area is complex because it is complicated by the preclusion of internal fixation due to anatomic limitations and postoperative complications with radial head excision. The decision to operate is influenced by the presence of concomitant injury (and its severity). Associated injuries are more common in high-energy trauma but also can occur after a simple fall. They are comprised of ligamentous injury of elbow, forearm, and wrist; posterior elbow dislocation, fracture of capitellum including the osteochondral variety, and distal radioulnar dissociation.

These injuries are caused sometimes by direct trauma but more often are the indirect result of a fall on an outstretched hand with a longitudinal thrust of the radius against the capitellum. The resultant fractures seen vary and include damage to the articular surface, depression of part of the head (chisel fracture), and angulated fracture of the head or neck. When these fractures are associated with elbow dislocation, significant soft tissue injury (tearing of the anterior capsule and brachialis muscle) occurs because the capitellum is displaced posteriorly.

Fractures of the radial head are classified into four types.[52] Type I includes fissure or marginal sector fractures without displacement. Type II includes marginal fractures with displacement including impaction, depression, and angulation. (The amount of tilt and percentage of head involvement is important.) Type III fractures are comminuted fractures involving the entire radial head. Type IV are fractures of the radial head in association with dislocation of the elbow.

In addition, two other variables are important in arriving at a management plan: mechanical block and other associated injuries. Mechanical block is assessed with the elbow in various degrees of flexion, noting severe crepitation with passive rotation. This can be performed after anesthesia. Half-percent marcaine intra-articularly, is administered following joint aspiration. Other associated injuries, eg, injury to the interosseus membrane, distal radioulnar joint injury, acute longitudinal radioulnar dissociation (Essex-Lopresti), and anteromedial elbow ligament disruption with or without fracture of the coronoid process associated with elbow dislocation, can also affect treatment plans.

Patients with isolated fracture of the radial head present with pain over the lateral side of the elbow, which limits active range of motion and is aggravated by forearm rotation. There is minimal swelling, well-localized tenderness over the radial head, and pain or crepitation with motion. If the radial head fracture is associated with elbow dislocation, there is substantial pain and swelling, which preclude palpation and range of motion. In all cases the forearm and wrist should be examined for acute radioulnar dissociation and the medial ligament of elbow palpated for signs of possible disruption.

Radiographic findings of undisplaced fractures may include only a positive fat pad sign. In these cases a radial head–capitellum view may be needed to visualize the fracture. This is an oblique view with the forearm in neutral rotation and the x-ray tube angled at 45° cephalad. Specifically, fractures of the capitellum and posterior elbow dislocation associated with or without coronoid process fractures should be sought. Fragments lying free within the joint space are suggestive of capitellum fracture because fragments from a comminuted radial head are rarely displaced proximally. Advanced imaging studies such as computed tomography may be used to delineate and quantify the extent of the fracture.

Management of type I (isolated and associated with posterior elbow dislocation) and type II (isolated, with fracture involving less than one quarter to one third of the radial head, with angulation less than 30° and depression less than 3 mm) fractures is straightforward. No reduction is needed. The elbow is placed in a sling with instructions for active motion as early as possible. There is some debate as to whether immediate joint aspiration is necessary to facilitate early active range of motion. Orthopedic follow-up should be arranged within 2 days. In all other types of radial head fractures, early orthopedic input is essential because treatment is controversial. Management of radial head fractures depends on the severity of the fracture and any associated injuries, and ranges from early motion, open reduction and internal fixation with screws and wires of the radial head, partial excision, and immediate and delayed excision to the use of a prosthesis. In cases of acute longitudinal radioulnar dislocation in which the ulna is most commonly being subluxated dorsally, reduction of the longitudinal translation is followed by splinting or pinning of the distal radioulnar joint with the forearm in supination. Use of a hinged orthosis with extension stops, repair of the lateral capsule, anteromedial ligament and brachialis insertion, and reduction and immobilization of the coronoid process may be undertaken in the management of type IV fractures.

Known complications of these fractures include minimal loss of extension and displacement leading to pain, contractures, and radiocapitellar arthrosis. In addition, with acute longitudinal radioulnar dissociation, there is radioulnar synostosis and loss of forearm motion; with elbow dislocation, joint stiffness, ankylosis, and instability may be present; with radial head excision, there may be damage to the posterior interosseous nerve, proximal translation of the radius with associated wrist problems, and joint instability; and with prosthestic replacement, material failure can result.

In children, fractures of the radial neck and head account for 5% to 8.5% of all elbow fractures and 14% to 20% of all proximal radius fractures. The average age of occurrence is 9 to 10 years with this type of injury; it is rare in the younger, skeletally immature child. Prognosis depends on the magnitude of the injuring force. Severe force is associated with elbow dislocation; other fractures, eg, olecranon fractures and avulsion fracture of the medial epicondylar apophysis; pronounced soft tissue injury; and significant displacement of the radial head. The objective is to attain a high-quality reduction of angulation of less than 15° to 45° and translocation of less than 3 to 4 mm. Because poor results can occur in 15% to 33% of cases, early orthopedic involvement is encouraged.

Because most of the radial neck is extra-articular, fractures to this area do not necessarily give rise to a fad pad sign. Patients with these injuries have minimal initial symptoms, followed by swelling and pain over hours. Pain is localized over the radial head or neck, or over the wrist; and is accentuated by passive pronation and supination or pressure over the proximal radius. In addition to regular views of the elbow, additional views in supination and pronation and a radiocapitellar view may be needed. When there is loss in smoothness of the metaphyseal margin, displacement of an unossified radial head, which can be confirmed by arthrography, can be suspected. Supinator fat pad and distal humeral fat pad displacement may be present. The fractures can then be classified using both the radiologic findings and mechanism of injury into the following:

*Primary displacement of the radial head.* This is the most common type, and includes valgus fractures and fractures associated with elbow dislocation. These are further classified into type A—Salter-Harris type I and II injuries of the proximal radial physis; type B—Salter-Harris type IV injuries of the proximal radial physis; type C—fractures involving only the proximal radial metaphysis; type D—reduction injuries with the radial head in the posterior aspect of the joint; and type E—relocation injuries with the radial head lying anteriorly in joint.

*Primary displacement of the radial neck.* These are divided into angular and torsional injuries.

*Stress injuries.* These fractures include osteochondritis dissecans of the radial head, and physeal injuries with neck angulation.

Management by the emergency physician is limited to isolated injuries resulting in less than 20° to 30° of angulation of the head. In these cases no reduction is required,[53–56] and the arm is immobilized using a collar and cuff or posterior splint with referral to an orthopedist within 3 to 5 days. All other fractures are managed by the orthopedist with closed or open reduction. The reductions are held with or without percutaneous pinning and long-arm casting with the elbow flexed and forearm pronated. Complications are numerous. Loss in range of motion is common, usually of either supination-pronation but affecting pronation comparatively more. Myositis ossificans is seen with synostosis of the proximal radioulnar joint. Nerve injuries in the form of partial ulnar nerve and posterior interosseus nerve injury have been documented, the latter being mainly associated with surgical exploration.

## REFERENCES

1. Beekman F, Sullivan JE: Some observations on fractures of long bones in children, *Am J Surg,* 51:722-738, 1941.
2. Hanlon CR, Estes WL: Fractures in childhood: a statistical analysis, *Am J Surg,* 87:312-323, 1954.
3. Landin LA: Fracture patterns in children. Analysis of 8682 fractures with special reference to incidence, etiology and secular changes in a Swedish urban population, 1950-1979, *Acta Orthop Scand* [suppl], 54, 1983.
4. Ogden JA: *Skeletal injury in the child.* Philadelphia, Lea & Febiger, 1982.
5. Bledsoe RC, Izenstark JL: Displacement of the fat pads in disease and injury of the elbow: a new radiographic sign, *Radiology,* 73:717-724, 1959.
6. Bohrer SP: The fat pad sign following elbow trauma: its usefulness and reliability in suspecting "invisible" fractures, *Clin Radiol.,* 21:90-94, 1970.
7. Jackman RJ, Rugh DG: The positive elbow fat pad sign in rheumatoid arthritis, *AJR,* 108:812-818, 1970.
8. Kohn AM: Soft tissue alterations in elbow trauma, *AJR,* 82:867-874, 1959.
9. Murphy WA, Siegel MJ: Elbow fat pads with new signs and extended differential diagnosis, *Radiology,* 124:659-665, 1977.
10. Norell HG: Roentgenologic visualization of the extracapsular fat: its importance in the diagnosis of traumatic injuries to the elbow, *Acta Radiol,* 42:205-210, 1954.
11. Smith DN, Lee JR: The radiological diagnosis of posttraumatic effusion of the elbow joint and its clinical significance: the "displaced fat pad" sign, *Injury,* 10:115-119, 1978.
12. Rogers SL, MacEwan DW: Changes due to trauma in the fat plane overlying the supinator muscle: a radiological sign, *Radiology,* 92:954-958, 1969.
13. McAfee JH, Smith DL: Olecranon and prepatellar bursitis: diagnosis and treatment. *West J Med,* 149:607-610, 1988.
14. Rockwood CA, Wilkins KE, and King RE: Fractures in children, ed 3, Philadelphia 1991, JB Lippincott Co.
15. Arnold JA, Nasca RJ, and Nelson CL: Supracondylar fractures of the humerus, *J Bone Joint Surg,* 59-A:589-595, 1977.
16. Aronson DD, Prager PI: Supracondylar fractures of the humerus in children: a modified technique for closed pinning, *Clin Orthop,* 219:174-184, 1987.
17. Pirone AM, Graham HK, and Krajbich JI: Management of displaced extension-type supracondylar fractures of the humerus in children, *J Bone Joint Surg,* 70-A:641-650, 1988.

18. Bertola L: On supracondylar fractures of the humerus in childhood, *Minerva Orthop,* 10:543, 1959.

19. Rogers LF: Fractures and dislocations of the elbow, *Semin Roentgenol,* 13:97-107, 1978.

20. Rogers LF, Malave S Jr, and White H: Plastic bowing, torus, and greenstick supracondylar fractures of the humerus: radiographic clues to obscure fractures of the elbow in children, *Radiology,* 128:145-150, 1978.

21. Silberstein MJ, Brodeur AE, and GraViss ER: Some vagaries of the capitellum, *J Bone Joint Surg,* 61A:244-247, 1979.

22. Fowles Jr, Kassab MT: Displaced supracondylar fractures of the elbow in children, *J Bone Joint Surg,* 56B:490-500, 1974.

23. Karlsson J, Thorsteinsson T, and Thorleifsson R: Entrapment of the median nerve and brachial artery after supracondylar fractures of the humerus in children, *Arch Orthop Trauma Surg,* 104:389-391, 1986.

24. Ottolenghi CE: Acute ischemic syndrome: its treatment; prophylaxis of Volkmann's syndrome, *Am J Orthop,* 2:312-316, 1960.

25. Edman P, Lohr G: Supracondylar fractures of the humerus treated with olecranon traction, *Acta Chir Scand,* 126:505-516, 1963.

26. Hoyer A: Treatment of supracondylar fracture of the humerus by skeletal traction in an abduction splint, *J Bone Joint Surg,* 34-A:623-637, 1952.

27. Aitken AP, Smtih L, and Blackette CW: Supracondylar fractures in children, *Am J Surg,* 59:161-171, 1943.

28. Hagen R: Skin-traction-treatment of supracondylar fractures of the humerus in children, *Acta Orthop Scand,* 35:138-148, 1964.

29. Ashurst APC: *An anatomical and surgical study of fractures of the lower end of the humerus,* (The Samuel D. Gross prize essay of the Philadelphia Academy.) Philadelphia, 1910, Lea & Febiger.

30. Akbarnia BA, Silberstein MJ, and Rende J: Arthrography in the diagnosis of fractures of the distal end of the humerus in infants, *J Bone Joint Surg,* 68-A:599-602, 1986.

31. DeLee JC, Wilkins KE, and Rogers LF: Fracture-separation of the distal humerus epiphysis, *J Bone Joint Surg,* 62:46-51, 1980.

32. Odgen JA: *Skeletal injury in the child,* Philadelphia, 1990, WB Saunders, pp. 386-391.

33. Paige ML, Port RB: Separation of the distal humeral epiphysis in the neonate: a combined clinical and roentgenographic diagnosis, *Am J Dis Child,* 139:1203-1205, 1985.

34. Willems B, Stuyck J, and Hoogmartens M: Fracture-separation of the distal humeral epiphysis, *Acta Orthop Belg,* 53:109-111, 1987.

35. Chutro P: Fracturas de la extremidad inferior del humero en los ninos. Buenos Aires, Theses J Peuser, 1904.

36. Riseborough EJ, Radin EL: Intercondylar T fractures of the humerus in the adult: a comparison of operative and nonoperative treatment in twenty-nine cases, *J Bone Joint Surg,* 51-A:130-141, 1969.

37. Peterson CA, Peterson HA: Analysis of the incidence of injuries to the epiphyseal growth plate, *J Trauma,* 12:275-281, 1972.

38. Milch H: Fractures and dislocations of the humeral condyles, *J Trauma,* 4:592-607, 1964.

39. Badelon O, Bensahel H, and Mazda K: Lateral humeral condylar fractures in children: a report of 47 cases, *J Pediatr Orthop,* 8:31-34, 1988.

40. Kini M: Fractures of the lateral condyle of the lower end of the humerus with complication, *J Bone Joint Surg,* 24:270-280, 1942.

41. Faysse R, Marion J: Fractures du condyle interne, *Rev Chir Orthop,* 48:473-477, 1962.

42. Kilfoyle RM: Fractures of the medial condyle and epicondyle of the elbow in children, *Clin Orthop,* 41:43-50, 1965.

43. Palmer I: Open treatment of transcondylar T-fracture of the humerus, *Acta Chir Scand,* 121:486-490, 1961.

44. Patrick J: Fracture of the medial epicondyle with displacement into the elbow joint, *J Bone Joint Surg,* 28:143-147, 1946.

45. Roberts NW: Displacement of the internal epicondyle into the joint, *Lancet,* 2:78-79, 1934.

46. Aitken AP, Childress HM: Intra-articular displacement of the internal epicondyle following dislocation, *J Bone Joint Surg,* 20:161-166, 1938.

47. Carlioz H, Abols Y: Posterior dislocation of the elbow in children, *J Pediatr Orthop,* 4:8-12, 1984.

48. Hume AC: Anterior dislocation of the head of the radius associated with undisplaced fracture of the olecranon in children. *J Bone Joint Surg,* 39-B:508-512, 1957.

49. Snyder HS: Radiographic changes with radial head subluxation in children, *J Emerg Med,* 8:265-269, 1990.

50. Colton CL: Fractures of the olecranon in adults: classification and management, *Injury,* 5:121-129, 1973.

51. Regan W, Morre B: Fractures of the coronoid process of the ulna, *J Bone Joint Surg,* 71-A:1348-1354, 1989.

52. Johnston GW: A follow-up of one hundred cases of fracture of the head of the radius with a review of the literature, *Ulster Med J,* 31:51-56, 1962.

53. Lindham S, Hugasson C: Significance of associated lesions including dislocation of fracture of the radius in children, *Acta Orthop Scand,* 50:79-83, 1979.

54. McBride ED, Monnet JC: Epiphyseal fracture of the head of the radius in children, *Clin Orthop,* 16:264-271, 1960.

55. Newman JH: Displaced radial neck fractures in children, *Injury* 9:114-121, 1977.

56. Vahvanen V: Fracture of the radial neck in children, *Acta Orthop Scand,* 49:32-38, 1978.

# Forearm Injuries

*Mary Carr*

Fractures of the forearm occur relatively frequently. When they occur, the affected individual must learn to cope with limited use of his or her arm during the healing phase. If the fracture heals poorly, the individual will face a lifetime of limited arm use. Unfortunately, a suboptimal result is a real possibility in most forearm fractures because a precise relationship between the radius and ulna is necessary to maintain function.

## ANATOMY

It is important to understand the anatomy of the forearm before discussing injuries sustained by it. Much of the following material has been gathered from the textbook *Essentials of Human Anatomy* by Woodburne.[1]

The radius and ulna compose the bony structure of the forearm (Fig. 12-1). Viewing the forearm anatomically, the ulna is relatively straight. Proximally, it has two large projections: the olecranon and coronoid processes. Between these two processes is the trochanteric notch. Into this notch fits the trochanteric process of the humerus. Distally, the head of the ulna is a rounded articular surface with a dorsal styloid process.

The ulna is the primary forearm bone involved in flexion and extension at the elbow. It also participates to a very small degree in abduction and adduction during supination and pronation.

The radius, by contrast, has a very important lateral bow that must be maintained if full supination and pronation are to be achieved. The proximal end of the radius has a disklike head, a narrower neck, and the radial tuberosity. Distally, the radius is expanded to a carpal articular surface anteriorly. Medially, there is a radial notch where the radius articulates with the ulna; and laterally, there is a radial styloid process, which is a projection of the radius downward beyond the radiocarpal articular surface.

The head of the radius moves on the capitellum (Fig. 12-2) of the humerus during flexion and extension. The radius rotates on the humerus and over the ulna during supination and pronation. Because the radius moves along with the ulna, supination and pronation are possible at all degrees of elbow flexion.

The radius and ulna are relatively parallel but articulate with each other proximally and distally. They are bound together proximally by the capsule of the elbow joint and the annular ligament (Fig. 12-3A), and distally by the capsule of the wrist joint, the anterior and posterior radioulnar ligaments, and the fibrocartilagenous articular disk. The proximal radioulnar articulation functions as a trochoid joint, which means its chief movement is rotation. In a trochoid joint one bone serves as a stable force (in this case the ulna) and the other bone (the radius) and its ligaments form a circle enclosing the stable bone. The annular ligament holds the radius against the ulna. Proximally, there is also an ulnohumeral and a radiohumeral joint, both of which are hinge joints. Distally, there is a stable radioulnar articulation and a radiocarpal joint (Fig. 12-3B). The radiocarpal joint lies between the radius and articular disk of the ulna proximally and the scaphoid, lunate, and triquetral carpal bones distally. This allows palmar flexion and dorsiflexion at the wrist and ulnar abduction. Malunion of either the radius or ulna can seriously compromise the function of any of these joints. The fibers of the interosseous membrane run obliquely in the space between the shafts of the radius and ulna (Fig. 12-4). These fibers originate proximally on the radius and insert distally on the ulna. This space is called the *interosseous space*.

**Ossification centers**

Diaphyseal centers for the radius and ulna are formed at about the eighth week of embryonic life (Fig. 12-5). Other

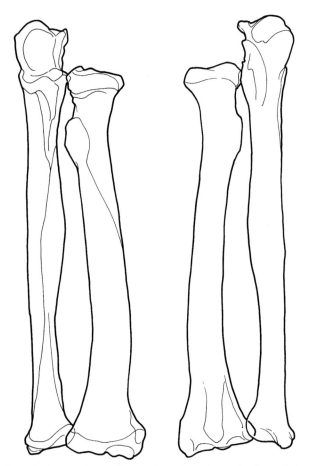

**Fig. 12-1.** Anterior and posterior views in supination of the bones of the forearm—the radius and ulna.

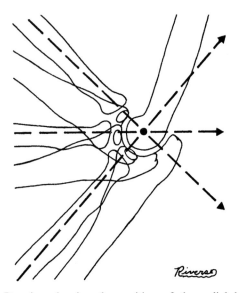

**Fig. 12-2.** Drawing showing the position of the radial head relative to the capitellum of the humerus in flexion and extension of the forearm. (Redrawn from Smith FM: *Clin Orthop* 50:7, 1967.)

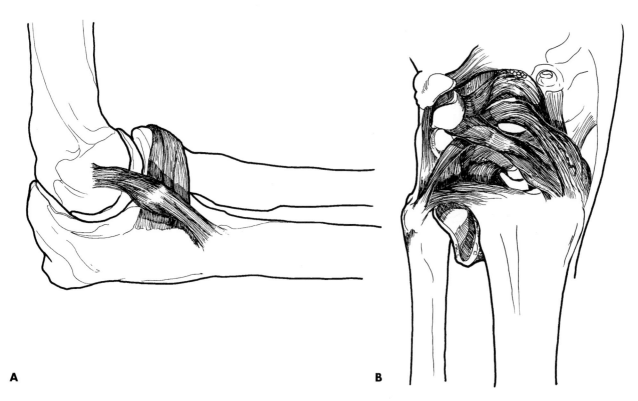

**A**

**B**

**Fig. 12-3. A,** Lateral view of the proximal articulation between the radial head and the capitellum. The annular ligament forms a cuplike aperature that retains the head of the radius during supination and pronation. This ligament is reinforced by the radial collateral ligament. **B,** The radiocarpal joint is held together by ligaments between the carpal bones and the radius and ulna. The ulna and radius articulation allows rotation of the radius around the ulna with a stabilizing ligamentous attachment of the radius to the ulnar styloid.

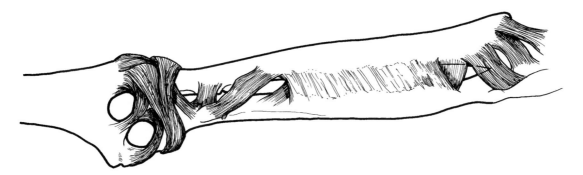

**Fig. 12-4.** An interosseous membrane spans the interosseous space. The fibers of this membrane cross diagonally from the radius proximally to the ulna distally.

ossification centers occur at several sites. The head of the radius appears at about 5 years of age and fuses with the diaphysis at age 15 years. The olecranon appears at age 9 years and fuses at 15 years. Distally, the radial epiphysis appears at age 6 months and fuses at 20 years. The ulnar epiphysis appears at age 7 years and fuses at age 21.

### Muscles

The muscles of the forearm are divided into an anterior compartment and a posterior compartment, which are separated by an antebrachial fascia. This antebrachial fascia is the origin for some of the muscles in the proximal two thirds of the forearm. At the wrist the antebrachial fascia is strengthened dorsally by the extensor retinaculum and anteriorly by the palmar carpal ligament.

Nineteen muscles are located in the forearm, most of which affect wrist and hand motion. These muscles can be divided into functional groups (see box on page 255). Any muscle group in the forearm can act as a strong deforming force once a fracture has occurred. The supinator, pronator teres, and pronator quadratus, however, are the muscles most likely to contribute to deforming forces on the fracture fragments.

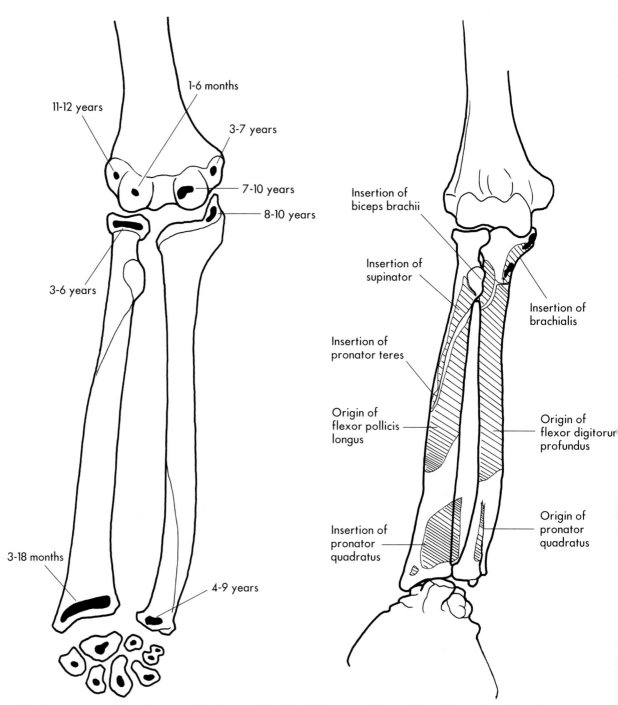

**Fig. 12-5.** The ossification centers of the forearm with the approximate age of appearance.

**Fig. 12-6.** Diagram of the origin and insertion of the forearm muscles on the radius and ulna.

The supinator muscle (Fig. 12-6) is a flat sheet of muscle that takes its origin on the lateral epicondyle of the humerus, the radial collateral ligament of the elbow, the annular ligament of the radius, and the supinator crest and fossa of the ulna. This muscle travels downward and laterally and wraps around and inserts on the radius. There is a superficial and a deep layer to this muscle. The deep radial nerve travels between these two layers, innervating the muscle.

The pronator teres (Fig. 12-6) originates on the medial epicondyle of the humerus and the medial side of the coronoid process of the ulna. The median nerve passes between these two origins. Muscle fibers travel obliquely across the forearm and insert on the lateral aspect of the radius at the middle portion.

The pronator quadratus (Fig. 12-6) is so named because of its quadrilateral shape. It arises on the anteromedial surface of the distal one fourth of the ulna. Its fibers travel

### Functional muscle groups of the forearm

**Anterior compartment**

Rotation of the radius on the ulna
    Pronator teres
    Pronator quadratus
    Supinator (located in the posterior compartment)
Flexion of the hand at the wrist
    Flexor carpi radialis
    Flexor carpi ulnaris
    Palmaris longus
Flexion of the digits
    Flexor digitorum superficialis
    Flexor digitorum profundus
    Flexor pollicis longus

**Posterior compartment**

Extension of the hand at the wrist
    Extensor carpi radialis longus
    Extensor carpi radialis brevis
    Extensor carpi ulnaris
Extension of the digits (excluding thumb)
    Extensor digitorum
    Extensor indicis
    Extensor digiti minimi
Thumb extensors
    Abductor pollicis longus
    Extensor pollicis brevis
    Extensor pollicis longus
Elbow flexor
    Brachioradialis

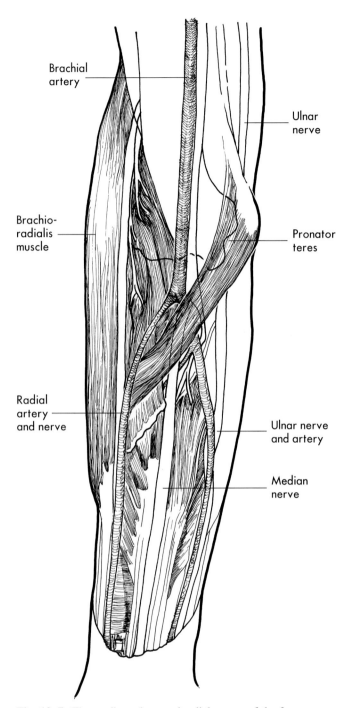

**Fig. 12-7.** The median, ulnar, and radial nerves of the forearm.

across and insert on the anterior surface of the distal one fourth of the radius.

The supinator, pronator teres, and pronator quadratus muscles exert their influence on the motion of the radius and ulna about each other. In general, only a few of the forearm muscles insert on the radius or ulna; most take their origin from the radius, ulna, or interosseous membrane and insert in the wrist or hand.

### Nerves

The nerves of the forearm are the median, ulnar, and superficial and deep branches of the radial nerve (Fig. 12-7). The median nerve supplies most of the motor function to the muscles in the anterior compartment. The ulnar nerve supplies function to the flexor carpi ulnaris muscle and the ulnar portion of the flexor digitorum profundus in the anterior compartment. The deep radial nerve supplies innervation to all the muscles of the posterior compartment.

### Vasculature

Blood supply (Fig. 12-8) in the forearm comes from branches off the radial and ulnar arteries, which are a division of the brachial artery at the level of the radial neck.

### GENERAL MANAGEMENT

Probably the most important point to remember when diagnosing a forearm fracture is that solitary fractures are rare. Fractures occur either at two or more sites or involve a fracture of one bone and accompanying ligamentous injury with or without dislocation. Careful scrutiny of the wrist and elbow is imperative because these are common sites of associated injury.[2]

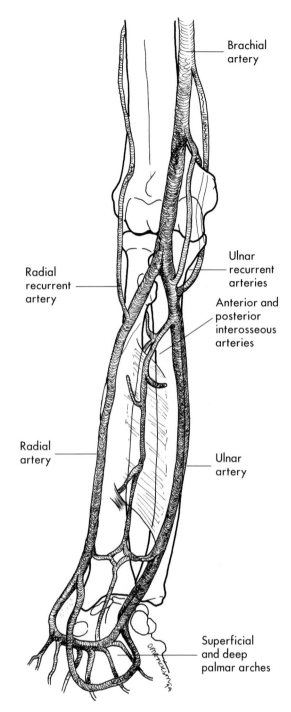

Radial recurrent artery

Radial artery

Brachial artery

Ulnar recurrent arteries

Anterior and posterior interosseous arteries

Ulnar artery

Superficial and deep palmar arches

**Fig. 12-8.** The arteries of the forearm.

When a fracture is noted in one or both of the forearm bones, the bones must be checked for loss of length, which can occur if the fracture fragments override each other or if the muscles cause deforming forces. When foreshortening is noted there is a high probability of associated injuries either proximally or distally. For example, in a radial fracture, some of the force may be transmitted through the interosseous membrane and may fracture the ulna at a similar site or more proximally or distally. The force may also be transmitted up or down the shaft of the bone to

cause ligamentous injury at the elbow or wrist. Proximally the ulna and humerus are strongly connected but the radial head is not. It may dislocate relative to the humerus or ulna. At the wrist the opposite is true: the radius has a much firmer attachment to the carpal bones while the ulna, with its smaller articular surface, may dislocate relative to the radius or the carpal bones.

For treatment of forearm fractures to be considered successful, function and length must be restored, union of the fracture must occur, and the integrity of the proximal and distal joints must be maintained. Because of the multiple articulations at the elbow and wrist, inadequate treatment or poor healing will result in limited function. This, combined with deforming forces exerted by forearm muscles, has caused many clinicians to prefer open reduction and internal fixation (ORIF) as the treatment of choice for forearm fractures.

Problems associated with ORIF for forearm fractures include infection, fibrosis, and scarring of the damaged tissues. Scarring is especially likely to occur in the interosseous membrane and annular ligaments of the elbow and wrist. Closed reduction, however, may result in malunion and ultimately some loss of function.[3] Because the radius has a lateral bow to it, and because hardware such as plates, screws, and nails tends to be straight, it is difficult to get a proper fit. Nonetheless, despite its drawbacks, ORIF is often the method of choice for treating forearm fractures in adults. Although the physiologic reason is not known, ORIF is best performed 24 hours after injury occurs. Hardware should be removed 12 to 18 months after fixation, with postremoval protection for an additional 4 to 6 weeks.[4] During this time, the patient is prohibited from engaging in contact sports or other potentially violent activities.

### Children

Children have a larger zone of plastic deformation than adults because children's bones are more porous and flexible as a result of larger haversian canals. Due to this inherent difference, children may present not only with fractures but also with bowing injuries. A cortex fractured on only one side is sometimes termed a *greenstick fracture*. If the cortex is wrinkled, it is referred to as a torus fracture (Fig. 12-17). Children presenting with these types of bowing injuries often require comparison views with the non-affected forearm to determine the degree of deformation that has occurred.

Many clinicians feel that in children younger than 5 years of age, bowing injuries with less than 20° of angulation will remodel with immobilization alone.[5] When there is no cortical disruption, no callus formation will be seen on follow-up radiographs and immobilization is usually needed only for a short time (up to 4 weeks). If callus formation occurs, indicating fracture through the cortex, immobilization for 4 to 6 weeks is generally optimal. In children older than 10 years of age,

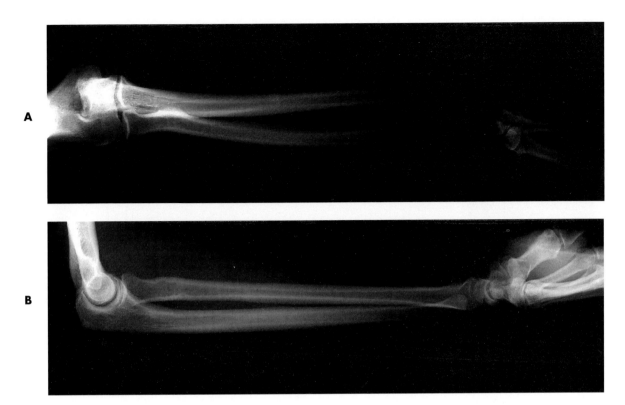

**Fig. 12-9. A** and **B**, Normal anteroposterior and lateral radiographic views of the forearm.

bowing injuries less than 10° can remodel without reduction. In children between 5 and 10 years of age, the body's ability to remodel bowing-type injuries probably ranges in between that of other age groups.

If a bowing defect falls outside the maximum degree that can remodel without reduction, the injury must be reduced. Closed reduction may be tried intraoperatively. The apex of the bow is placed on a fulcrum and 100% to 150% of the patient's body weight is applied for 2 to 3 minutes to slowly straighten the bow.[5] Care must be taken not to place this force on the growth plates.

### Radiographs

Radiography of an injured forearm must include both anteroposterior and lateral views (Fig. 12-9). Because of the possibility of occult fractures either proximally or distally, the wrist and elbow must be visualized. If the forearm films include these joints, additional elbow and wrist views may be unnecessary. If these joints are not well seen on the forearm views, however, or if an abnormality is suspected clinically or radiologically, these views may be necessary.

### RADIAL INJURY
### Proximal-third and middle-third radial fractures

Because fractures rarely occur in the proximal two thirds of the radius, the proximal one third and middle one third will be discussed as a single entity. When dealing with a proximal one-third radial fracture, it is important to remem-ber that supinating forces are exerted on the proximal fragment by the supinator and biceps brachii muscles. Middle-third radial fractures have pronating forces exerted on their fragments by the pronator teres muscle. These muscles tend to approximate the radius and ulna and decrease the interosseous space when a fracture has occurred (Fig. 12-10).

The supinator, biceps brachii, and pronator teres muscles may also act as deforming forces on the fracture fragments. Acutely this may cause shortening of the radius and a concomitant elbow or wrist injury. On a longer-term basis, these muscles may exert deforming forces on the fracture fragments even while the arm is immobilized in a cast. This will be discussed in more detail in the section on treatment.

**Mechanism.** Most commonly, proximal- and middle-third radial fractures occur as result of a direct blow to the radius. Because of the protection afforded by the surrounding muscle and its anatomic position, this area of the radius is the least prone to injury of any area in the forearm.

**Symptoms and physical findings.** At the fracture site, there is pain and tenderness to palpation, which may also be elicited by longitudinal compression of the radius. Deformity may not be as obvious as in other forearm fractures because of the significant amount of soft tissue surrounding this part of the bone. The elbow and wrist must be examined for tenderness on palpation because occult fractures are possible. The ulna should also be examined for tenderness because most injuries severe enough to fracture the radius at this level will also fracture the ulna.

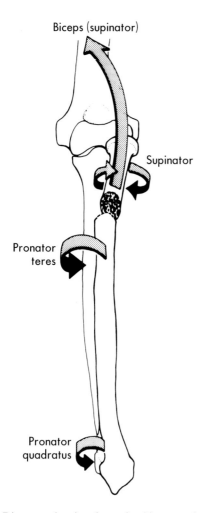

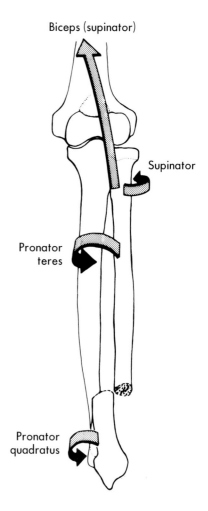

**Fig. 12-10.** Diagram showing how the biceps and supinator muscles pull the proximal fragment of a proximal radial fracture up and in supination while the distal fragment is pulled in pronation toward the ulna by the pronator teres muscle. (From Cruess RL: *Orthop Clin North Am* 4:969, 1973.)

**Fig. 12-11.** Diagram showing how the pronator teres muscle pulls the distal fragment toward the ulna in a distal shaft fracture of the radius. (From Cruess RL: *Orthop Clin North Am* 4:969, 1973.)

**Radiographs.** Routine anteroposterior and lateral views of the forearm are adequate to diagnose radial fractures. The high probability that there is associated elbow or wrist pathology may necessitate radiographs of these areas as well.

**Treatment.** The radius is a complex bone. Its angles and curves, especially the lateral bow, must be maintained for full supination and pronation to exist.

If a fracture occurs in the upper one third of the radius but below the insertion of the supinator muscle, a strong supinating force will exist on the proximal fragment and the distal fragment will have a pronating force exerted by the pronator teres. This will act to displace the fracture fragment (Fig. 12-11).

If the fracture occurs distal to the insertion of the pronator teres in the middle one third of the radius, the supinating and pronating forces are somewhat neutralized. In these fractures the proximal fragment of the radius is in a slightly supinated or neutral position. When closed treat-

ment is used the location of the radial fracture determines the degree of supination of the distal fragment needed to provide correct rotational alignment.

Undisplaced fractures, which are rare, should be placed in a long-arm cast or anterior/posterior splint with 90° of flexion at the elbow. The arm should be placed in mild supination if the fracture is below the insertion of the pronator teres muscle. Full supination is needed if the fracture occurs above this insertion.

Deforming forces by supinating or pronating muscles may require ORIF as definitive treatment. This is especially true of midshaft radial fractures and proximal-third radial fractures. If the proximal fracture fragment is small, ie, the proximal one fifth of the radius, internal fixation becomes difficult because the piece of bone cannot accommodate hardware. Closed reduction with full forearm supination is then performed with postreduction films. This form of reduction must be followed closely because of the tendency of muscles to cause loss of reduction. When the fragment cannot be reduced or the reduction cannot be maintained a medullary nail will be needed. ORIF for the other fractures consists of a plate and screws or a medullary nail.

**Complications.** Neurovascular injuries are very rare in fractures of the proximal two thirds of the radius. The primary complications are malunion or nonunion because of inadequate reduction or a loss of reduction while immobilized. Fractures that are initially nondisplaced may become displaced even while immobilized because of muscular forces exerted on the fragments. Failure to diagnose a concomitant injury at the elbow or wrist will result in loss of motion at that joint.

**Follow-up.** Careful regular and frequent follow-up is necessary with these fractures. Fractures treated by closed reduction require follow up radiographs on a weekly basis for the first few weeks to ensure that proper alignment is maintained. If a loss of reduction occurs, ORIF may be necessary.

**Children.** Children with proximal two-thirds radial fractures will need treatment similar to that of an adult. However, children tend to achieve more satisfactory results with closed reduction and immobilization than adults.

### Distal-third radial fractures

The distal one third of the radius is the area most prone to fracture because of its relative lack of soft tissue protection by overlying musculature.

**Mechanism.** A direct blow is the most common mechanism of injury in this type of radial fracture. A fall on an outstretched hand may also cause a fracture in this region. Although solitary fractures of the distal one third of the radius do occur, Goldberg et al.[2] reported that they are probably much rarer than previously thought. They noted a single distal radial fracture as the only injury in only 4% of their patients with forearm injuries. Solitary distal one-third radial fractures are most commonly the result of a direct blow to that portion of the forearm.

Radial fractures at the junction of the middle and distal thirds that also have a dislocation or subluxation of the distal radioulnar joint are sometimes known as Galeazzi fractures (Fig. 12-12). The Galleazzi fracture has other less common eponyms: the Piedmont fracture, fracture of necessity, and reverse Monteggia fracture. The injury to the radioulnar joint may be purely ligamentous, disrupting the triangular fibrocartilage complex, or the ligament may remain intact and the ulnar styloid may be avulsed. Rupture of the articular disk may also occur. These fractures are inherently unstable because of the distal radioulnar joint injury.

The triangular fibrocartilage complex is the main stabilizer of the distal radioulnar joint. For this joint to be dislocated or subluxed the triangular fibrocartilage complex must be ruptured. The components are not discretely identified as separate structures but are actually anatomic areas of the homogeneous triangular fibrocartilage complex.[6] Its components are the articular disk, the ulnar collateral ligament, the dorsal and volar radioulnar ligaments, the sheath of the extensor carpi ulnaris tendon, and the ulnocarpal meniscus (Fig. 12-3).

**Signs and symptoms.** Swelling and tenderness at the fracture site are the chief characteristics of this injury. A prominence of the head of the ulna may be noted especially in cases of ligamentous injury of the distal radioulnar joint or fracture of the ulnar styloid. If there is marked soft tissue swelling, however, a deformity may be obscured. Rarely does neurovascular damage occur.

**Radiographs.** The radial shaft fracture may be transverse or oblique, and often occurs between the insertions of the pronator teres and pronator quadratus muscles. Four reliable radiographic signs of injury to the distal radioulnar joint and the triangular fibrocartilaginous complex are 1) fracture of the ulnar styloid at its base, 2) widening of the joint space of the distal radioulnar joint articulation on anteroposterior view, 3) dislocation of the radius relative to

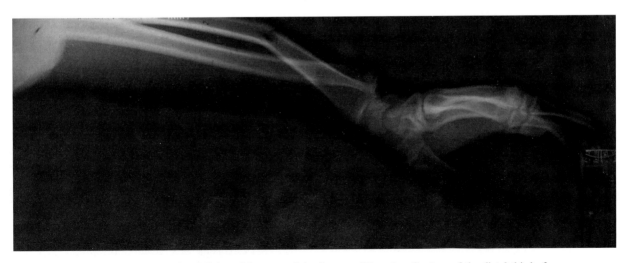

**Fig. 12-12.** Example of Galeazzi fracture of the forearm. There is a fracture of the distal third of the radius that is associated with a radioulnar dislocation at the wrist.

the ulna on lateral view, and 4) shortening of the radius greater than 5 mm on the anteroposterior view.[7]

**Treatment.** Results of closed reduction are poor because of displacement while in the cast. As Hughston[8] has pointed out, there are four major deforming forces that cause unsatisfactory results with closed methods:

1) gravity, which will cause subluxation or dislocation of the distal radioulnar joint (even through a cast) and angulation of the fractured radius;
2) rotation of the distal radial fragment by the pronator quadratus in a proximal and volar direction;
3) the brachioradialis, which rotates the distal fragment on the distal radioulnar joint causing shortening; and
4) rotation of the fracture by the thumb abductors and extensors, which also causes shortening.

Because of these considerations, ORIF is the preferred method of treatment. Until the definitive procedure is performed, the patient should be placed in a long-arm cast or anterior/posterior splint. The elbow should be flexed to 90°, and the forearm should be in pronation.

**Complications.** The complications for this type of fracture are the same as for those of any fracture being treated by open reduction, ie, infection, nonunion, and malunion. The most common complication is failure to diagnose the subluxation or dislocation of the distal radioulnar joint. This problem can be overlooked for years because patients may compensate for their inability to pronate and supinate by abduction and adduction at the shoulder.

**Follow-up.** Patients with distal-third radial fractures should be followed closely by the orthopedist who performs their surgery. If a solitary distal radial fracture is the diagnosis and the patient is treated conservatively in a cast, he or she should initially be followed closely for evidence of injury of the distal radioulnar joint.

**Children.** Galeazzi fracture dislocation is much less common in children than in adults. When they occur these fractures follow the same pattern as adult Galeazzi fractures.

There is a variant of Galeazzi fracture that occurs rarely in children. This is a fracture of the radius with a distal physeal separation of the ulna instead of dislocation of the radioulnar joint.[9] The mechanism appears to be the same as in adults. The ulnar physis avulses due to failure of the cartilaginous growth plate before failure of the triangular fibrocartilage complex. In children with open physes, the distal ulnar epiphysis can avulse before rupture of the triangular fibrocartilage complex, thus presenting as an epiphyseal fracture rather than a radioulnar dislocation. This occurs because the cartilaginous growth plate has less resistance to failure than the triangular fibrocartilage complex.

Schranz[10] found that distal radial fractures in children most apt to displace after immobilization in plaster were those fractures with dorsal angulation, bicortical breach, or dorsal fracture with volar cortical breach.

Radiographs should be taken within 1 week of the initial presentation and treatment in order to allow manipulation if the fracture angulation is unacceptable. This would be necessary if the angulation is greater than 10° for children over 10 years of age or greater than 20° for children under 5 years of age. Angulation between 10° and 20° needs reduction if the child is between the ages of 5 and 10 years.

## ULNAR INJURIES
### Proximal-third ulnar fractures

Fractures of the proximal third of the ulna may either exist as a single entity or can occur in association with a radial head dislocation. Ulnar fractures with a radial head dislocation are called Monteggia fractures, named after the Italian physician who initially missed the diagnosis in one of his patients. He went on to write about the entity in 1814. Today the diagnosis is still missed relatively frequently.

**Mechanism.** The ulna may be fractured by a direct blow. Solitary ulnar fractures are sometimes called *nightstick fractures,* because at the moment of impact, the arm is being held in a defensive posture to protect the head and face and an object is brought down hard directly against the ulna.

The mechanism of injury resulting in a Monteggia fracture has been much debated and disagreement persists. Furthermore, Bado[11] has since classified Monteggia fractures into four categories, each with different mechanisms of injury and each with the radial head dislocated in a different position (see section on diagnosis). Some authors have even added a fifth category for Monteggia fractures.[12]

**Signs and symptoms.** Pain and tenderness exist at the fracture site. If it is dislocated, the radial head may be palpated in the region of the elbow.

**Radiographs.** The ulnar fracture will probably not be missed on primary forearm views (Fig. 12-13). However, a concomitant dislocated radial head is often overlooked. If there is more than a few millimeters of displacement of the ulnar fracture, elbow and wrist films should be obtained.

If the radial head is in its normal position, a line drawn through the radial shaft and radial head should align with the capitellum of the humerus (see Fig. 12-2) in any projection. This sign was described by McLaughlin.[13]

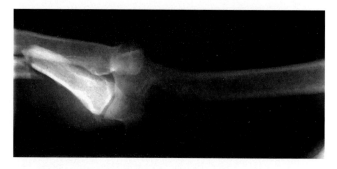

**Fig. 12-13.** Example of a Monteggia fracture with a proximal-third ulnar fracture in association with a radial head dislocation.

**Diagnosis.** The Bado classification of Monteggia fractures defines four groups of proximal ulnar fractures with radial head dislocation. Each group is defined by mechanism of injury and location of the radial head (Fig. 12-14).

Type 1 is the most common type of Monteggia fracture, occurring in 65% to 70% of such cases. It is an ulnar diaphyseal fracture with anterior dislocation of the fracture fragment, including dislocation of the radial head. The mechanism is a hyperpronation and extension injury. Type 2 fracture occurs in approximately 10% of cases. It is an ulnar fracture with posterior angulation and a posterior or posterolateral radial head dislocation. The mechanism is believed to be a hyperflexion injury. Type 3, which accounts for about 20% of Monteggia fractures, is an ulnar metaphyseal frac-

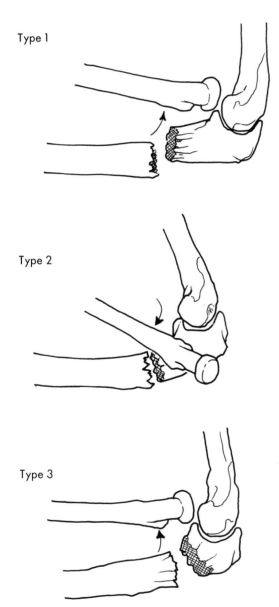

Type 1

Type 2

Type 3

**Fig. 12-14.** The Bado classification of Monteggia fractures. See text for description and incidence of these fractures. The rare type 4 fracture resulting from extreme pronation is not depicted.

ture with a lateral or anterolateral dislocation of the radial head. Lateral varus stress is the mechanism. Type 4, the rarest, is a fracture of the proximal third of the radius and ulna at the same level and an anterior dislocation of the radial head. Hyperpronation injury is the mechanism.

Solitary proximal ulnar fractures are diagnosed by a forearm radiograph. If there is less than 10° of displacement or less than 10° of angulation, the ulnar fracture may be the only injury. If the angulation or displacement exceeds 10° an accompanying injury is likely. A dislocated radial head must be considered.

**Treatment.** If the proximal ulnar fracture has less than 10° of angulation or displacement and there are no other accompanying forearm injuries the fracture can be treated by a long-arm cast with the elbow flexed to 90° and the forearm slightly supinated. The intact radius and interosseous membrane provide additional support in these cases. However, the proximal portion of the forearm is fleshier and follow-up radiography is needed to ensure that proper alignment is maintained in these fractures.

ORIF will be needed if the only injury is a proximal ulnar fracture but the displacement is greater than 10% of the ulnar shaft width or if the bone ends are separated by more than 5 mm.

The treatment of Monteggia fractures is somewhat controversial. Most authors feel that any of the four types of Monteggia fractures necessitate open reduction in adults.[14]

It may be possible to reduce the radial head without opening the joint. When the radial head cannot be reduced or the reduction cannot be maintained it is likely that the annular ligament is injured and is obstructing the repositioning of the radial head. Another possibility is that the joint capsule is blocking the reduction. If an open reduction is done, the annular ligament will probably need repair. It is essential to completely reduce the radial head. If the radial head is to stay relocated it is also essential to approximate the ulnar fragments.

Because of the high likelihood that orthopedic surgical intervention will be necessary in cases of Monteggia fractures, these patients will need a referral to an orthopedist within 48 hours for closed fractures. Until then the patient should be immobilized in a long-arm posterior splint with 90° of flexion at the elbow and the wrist in a neutral position.

**Prognosis.** The vast majority (approximately 95%) of adults have sequelae following a Monteggia fracture.[15] This may be due to the fact that adult Monteggia lesions are often the result of high-energy trauma, resulting in high numbers of open and comminuted fractures. A proportion of adults have other severe injuries; it may be that the associated injuries are actually causing the poor outcomes.

**Complications.** Complications include nonunion, infection, and loss of reduction of the fracture or the radial head. The deep branch of the radial nerve may be impinged by the radial head, causing paralysis of this nerve. This paralysis is manifested by weak hand and wrist extensors, and nearly always resolves without treatment. Exploration is not indicated unless motor function has not returned after 6 to 8 weeks. A persistent dislocation of the radial head is the usual feature of a missed dislocation, and may result in ankylosis and myositis ossificans.

**Follow-up.** At follow-up it is essential that adequate reduction still exists and that immobilization is adequate.

**Monteggia-equivalent lesions.** Some authors include many other lesions when categorizing Monteggia fractures. Those lesions do not fit into Bado's classification,[11] however, and are more accurately put in a separate category that may be called Monteggia-equivalent lesions. In an article by Karasick and Burk,[16] these injuries include entities such as radial head dislocation with olecranon fracture, radial neck fracture with proximal ulnar fracture, proximal radial fracture with ulnar diaphyseal fracture, and fracture of the radial neck with ulnar diaphyseal fracture.

In general, these lesions require ORIF for definitive treatment. Because both bones are involved it is likely that there is accompanying ligamentous injury or injury to the interosseous membrane. This, as well as the proximity of the injury to the fleshy portion of the forearm, causes loss of reduction easily. Individuals with these injuries should initially be placed in a long-arm cast with 90° of elbow flexion.

**Children.** Monteggia fractures occur in children much less often than in adults. The prognosis is good, provided the combined lesion is recognized. The usual reasons for missing such fractures are failure to consider them, or poor radiographs, especially of the elbow. In children this lesion is usually the result of low-energy trauma. Comminuted and open fractures are rarely encountered. Closed reduction should be attempted as the first line of treatment and usually gives excellent results.

Dislocation of the radial head with plastic deformation of the ulna occurs in children and is especially easy to miss. If elbow pain exists and radiographs fail to show a fracture, the radiocapitellar line must be assessed to rule out a radiocapitellar dislocation.

Children will likely require closed reduction performed with the patient under general anesthesia. A posterior long-arm splint followed by a long-arm cast should be used. There are reports of these fractures being missed for as long as 2 years. Delayed repairs have had variable results.

### Middle-third and distal-third ulnar fractures

Because the fractures that occur in the distal two thirds of the ulna are similar, they are discussed together.

**Mechanism.** A common mechanism causing fracture in the distal two thirds of the ulna is a direct blow to the ulna from a blunt object. This type is often called a *nightstick fracture* because the forearm is raised in a protective manner near the face and the arm is struck. Motor vehicle accidents can also cause nightstick fractures, as can excessive forced pronation or supination that occurs in a fall (Fig. 12-15).

**Signs and symptoms.** Pain and swelling occur at the fracture site. If the fracture is displaced, deformity will be noted.

**Radiographs.** Anteroposterior and lateral views of the

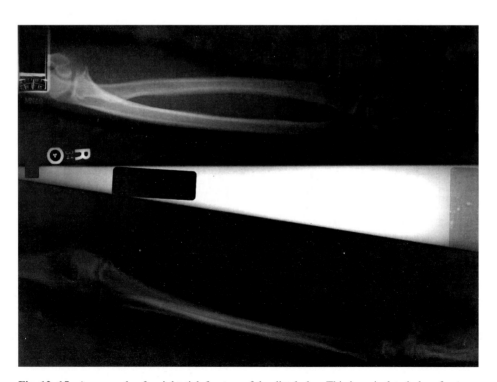

**Fig. 12-15.** An example of a nightstick fracture of the distal ulna. This is an isolated ulnar fracture.

forearm are adequate to visualize these fractures. If the fracture is displaced more than a few millimeters, wrist and elbow views should be included to rule out an associated subluxation, dislocation, or fracture in these areas.

**Diagnosis.** It is important to evaluate the displacement and angulation in these fractures because they affect treatment. In general, the greater the displacement or angulation the greater the force causing the injury.

In a cadaver study, Dymond[17] showed that if the fracture displacement is greater than one half the width of the shaft there is significant injury to the periosteum and the interosseous membrane. These fractures are apt to be unstable if treated closed. Hence, most of these fractures will need ORIF for definitive care. If the fracture is minimally displaced, ie, displacement is less than one half the width of the shaft, the periosteum, interosseous membrane, and intact radius can all act as stabilizing factors and additional immobilization in a cast or splint is all that is needed.

**Treatment.** Conservative treatment in a long-arm cast is usually sufficient for fractures with less than 50% or 5 mm of displacement and less than 10° of angulation. The elbow should be flexed at 90°, with the forearm in a neutral position. An anterior/posterior long-arm splint may also be used.

Some physicians have achieved good results in simple isolated ulnar fractures by providing minimal support for 7 to 10 days and then beginning early mobilization.[18] In high-energy fractures resulting in angulation greater than 10°, more than 50% displacement, or comminution, an orthopedic referral is necessary. These fractures heal best with ORIF.

**Prognosis.** Ulnar shaft fractures have had a reputation for nonunion, probably due to the fact that fractures that were displaced by more than 50% or angulated by more than 10° were treated in a cast alone and did not heal well. Only single, nondisplaced, and nonangulated ulnar fractures should be treated by cast or splint alone. These fractures may be amenable to early mobilization after 7 to 10 days. With comminuted, displaced, or angulated fractures ORIF is the preferred method of treatment. The hardware needs to be left on for 12 to 18 months, and vigorous activity should be curtailed for an additional 4 to 6 weeks after its removal.

**Complications.** Accompanying injuries are rare in fractures of the distal two thirds of the ulna. Occasionally, the deep branch of the radial nerve is injured, causing weakness of wrist and hand extensors. Nerve function usually returns without intervention.

**Follow-up.** As with all forearm fractures, it is essential that associated elbow or wrist injuries not be missed. These associated injuries are most likely to occur in fractures that are angulated more than 10° or displaced by more than 50% of the shaft width. Early follow-up with repeat radiographs is necessary to ensure proper reduction.

**Children.** The treatment of children with distal two-thirds ulnar fractures is similar to the treatment in adults.

Because children usually have low-energy injuries, the fractures are less likely to be angulated or displaced. Closed treatment is usually sufficient. ORIF will be necessary occasionally.

## RADIUS AND ULNA FRACTURES ("BOTH BONES")
### Mechanism

Concomitant fractures of the radius and ulna result from significant force. A motor vehicle accident or aggressive assault with a direct blow to the forearm may fracture the shafts of both the radius and ulna. Other causes include injury during sports activities or falls from a great height exerting longitudinal compressive forces (Fig. 12-16).

**Signs and symptoms.** Pain, deformity, and swelling are present in "both bones" fractures. Loss of sensory and motor function of the median, ulnar, or radial nerves is extremely rare but does occur, making a careful neurologic examination necessary. Patients with radial nerve injuries may have numbness on the dorsoradial aspect of the hand and weakness of the wrist and hand dorsiflexors. If the ulnar nerve is affected numbness will occur in the ulnar half of the ring finger and the little finger. Median nerve involvement is indicated by numbness on the index and long fingers and the volar aspect of the thumb. Both median and ulnar nerve palsy result in weakness of the wrist and hand flexors.

**Radiographs.** Because of the degree of force required to fracture both the radius and ulna it is common for one or both of the fractures to be displaced by more than 50% of the shaft width or angulated more than 10°. Comminuted fractures also occur regularly. When the bone fragments are angulated or displaced, injury also occurs to the interosseous membrane. The force may be transmitted along the membrane and may cause a proximal or distal injury such as elbow or wrist subluxation or dislocation.

**Treatment.** If the fracture is not angulated or displaced, it may be treated in a long-arm cast with the elbow at 90° flexion and the forearm in a neutral position. This is

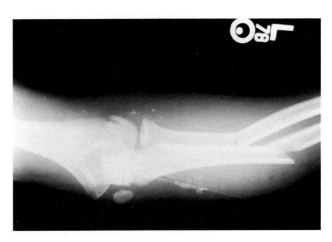

**Fig. 12-16.** Both bones of the forearm fracture in a child.

extremely rare, however. Most commonly, these fractures require ORIF to maintain the reduction.[19] Pending orthopedic consultation, the arm should be immobilized in a long-arm anterior/posterior or sugar tongs splint.

**Prognosis.** The greater the degree of displacement, angulation, or comminution the greater the likelihood of persisting functional deficits after the fracture has healed. The rare both bones fractures with neurovascular injuries are also prone to less than optimal functional and neurologic outcomes.

**Complications.** Lack of adequate reduction and nonunion are the most likely complications occurring with this type of fracture. Nonunion is most often the result of inadequate reduction or immobilization. Compartment syndrome can also occur.

**Follow-up.** It is very important to follow all patients with both bone fractures closely, especially those treated with immobilization alone. Eventual displacement of these fractures occurs when swelling subsides or muscles atrophy and the cast no longer fits properly. Fractures that initially appear reduced may lose their reduction because there is no internal stabilizing force since the radius, ulna, and interosseous membrane are all injured.

**Children.** Because of the special properties of children's bones relative to adults', they may suffer torus or greenstick fractures. Greenstick fractures are incomplete cortical fractures. Torus deformities (Fig. 12-17) are also known as bowing or plastic deformities. One or both bones may suffer plastic deformation, one bone may bow and the other break, or both may fracture. In a study by Carey et al.,[20] children under the age of 10 years fared extremely well when treated by closed reduction and a long-arm cast with the arm held in a neutral position. Children between the ages of 11 and 15 years had some residual angulation of their fractures with an average of 30° loss of supination and pronation but were pain-free at the fracture site. Carey et al. feel that the risk of infection from ORIF is not worth the

gain in rotational motion since the children seemed to be functionally intact despite the loss of motion. Theirs is not a universally held viewpoint; others believe ORIF is needed when there is angulation of 15° or more.

## OPEN FOREARM FRACTURES

Open fractures of the forearm are serious or potentially serious injuries that require immediate orthopedic consultation for irrigation, débridement, and repair. These fractures are caused by high-energy traumatic events such as motor vehicle accidents, gunshot injuries, or other violent events. There is extensive soft tissue injury that may also include neurovascular deficits. Fractures may be single or multiple but have a very high probability of being comminuted.

## COMPARTMENT SYNDROME

Closed fractures of the forearm, especially shaft fractures of both bones, may be accompanied by bleeding and bruising of the soft tissues. The fascial sheaths that contain the muscles have little room for additional fluid or swelling. If swelling occurs in the dorsal or volar compartments of the forearm the pressure in that compartment is increased and can lead to neurovascular damage or muscle necrosis.

### Signs and symptoms

Clinical signs and symptoms remain the basis for diagnosing compartment syndrome. Patients complain of excessive pain, characterized as deep and boring, that is out of proportion to their injury. It is important to remember that pulses are not necessarily lost. The pressure can be great enough to cut off capillary blood flow to muscles and nerves but a palpable radial or ulnar pulse persists. There is pain on passive extension or flexion of the fingers.[19] Sensation in the fingers is decreased and little or no function of the forearm exists. There may be a palpable induration of the compartment, and the skin may be warm and erythematous.

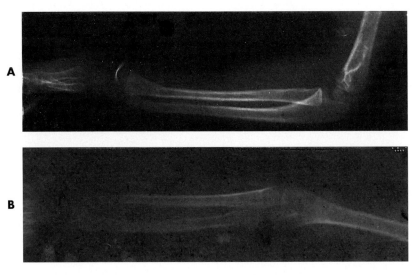

**Fig. 12-17.** **A** and **B**, Torus fracture of the distal radius in a child.

## Diagnosis

Tissue pressure more than 25 mm Hg is abnormal. These pressures can be measured with any of several tissue pressure-monitoring devices available. If these are not available an electronic pressure transducer used for arterial pressure monitoring can be connected to a 23G hypodermic needle. Pressures are obtained by introducing the needle into the deep fascia of the forearm.

McDougall and Johnston have described a method of measuring both the volar compartment and the dorsal compartment pressures using a single needle stick. With the arm in supination, the pressure is measured at the junction of the proximal and middle third of the forearm. The needle is introduced dorsally on the radial aspect of the ulna and directed towards the center of the forearm at that level. By keeping the needle near or against the ulna, nerves and arteries are avoided. Dorsal compartment pressure in the extensor carpi ulnaris or extensor pollicis longus muscle is measured before the needle enters the interosseous membrane. The needle is then advanced through the interosseous membrane where it will enter the flexor digitorum profundus muscle in the volar compartment. Volar compartment pressure is measured in the flexor digitorum muscle belly.[21]

## Treatment

The tissue pressure at which decompression should be performed has not been clearly established. Mubanak and Hargens[22] have suggested that a tissue pressure between 30 and 40 mm Hg indicates a need for decompression. Others feel that the clinical exam and the patient's symptoms are more important than tissue pressures. Decompression should be a full fasciotomy, which gives better and more consistent results than a limited or partial fasciotomy. Fasciotomy should extend from the elbow to the wrist.

Pressures between 20 and 40 mm Hg may be treated by elevation and immobilization of the forearm. These pressures need to be watched closely, however, for any further rise.

## Prognosis

Tissue pressures greater than 55 mm Hg are associated with permanent loss of function. The duration of the increased pressure is as important as the magnitude, and a delay in fasciotomy of over 12 hours has a high incidence of residual sequelae. These sequelae include weakness, loss of sensation, and diminished function of the forearm.

## Complications

Contractive deformities result from muscle necrosis. Failure to diagnose or treat such deformities in a timely manner will result in a permanent deficit.

## Follow-up

Patients who have compartment pressures that are high but not high enough to warrant fasciotomy need very close supervision. All constrictive dressings should be removed. If pressure increases or symptoms of pain, sensory deficit, or inability to passively extend the fingers occurs, fasciotomy needs to be performed.

## DISCUSSION

Fractures of the forearm are common injuries in all age groups. Other than open fractures, very few of these injuries involve neurovascular deficits. There is a low but real possibility of the occurrence of compartment syndrome, and care must be taken to avoid this complication. Many of these fractures will need ORIF for definitive care. Most importantly, a single fracture in the forearm may occur but both the radius and ulna and the elbow and wrist need to be scrutinized for additional injuries.

## REFERENCES

1. Woodburne RT: *Essentials of Human Anatomy,* ed 5, New York, 1973, Oxford University Press, pp. 93-109.
2. Goldberg HD, Young JWR, Reiner BI, et al: Double injuries of the forearm: a common occurrence, *Radiology* 185:223-227, 1992.
3. Sarmiento A, Ebramzadeh E, Brys D, et al: Angular deformities and forearm function, *J Orthop Res* 10:121-133, 1992.
4. Rumball K, Finnegan M: Refractures after forearm plate removal, *J Orthop Trauma* 4:124-129, 1990.
5. Nimityongskul P, Anderson LD, Sri P: Plastic deformation of the forearm: a review and case reports, *J Trauma* 31:1678-1685, 1991.
6. Palmer AK, Werner FW: The triangular fibrocartilage complex of the wrist: anatomy and function, *J Hand Surg* 6:153-162, 1981.
7. Aulicino PL, Siegel JL: Acute injuries of the distal radioulnar joint, *Hand Clin* 7:283-293, 1991.
8. Hughston JC: Fracture of the distal radial shaft: mistakes in management. *J Bone Joint Surg* 39:249-264, 1957.
9. Landfried MJ, Stenclik M, Susi JG: Variant of Galeazzi fracture-dislocation in children, *J Pediatr Orthop* 11:332-335, 1991.
10. Schranz PJ, Fagg PS: Undisplaced fractures of the distal third of the radius in children: an innocent fracture? *Injury* 23:165-167, 1992.
11. Bado JL: The Monteggia lesion: a review of 159 cases, *Clin Orthop* 50:71-86, 1967.
12. Dormans JP, Rang M: The problems of Monteggia fracture-dislocations in children, *Orthop Clin North Am* 21:251-256, 1990.
13. McLaughlin HL: *Trauma.* Philadelphia, 1959, WB Saunders, p 194.
14. Szabo RM, Skinner M: Isolated ulnar shaft fractures, *Acta Orthop Scand* 61:350-352, 1990.
15. Oveson O, Brok KE, Arreskov J, et al: Monteggia lesions in children and adults: an analysis of etiology and long-term results of treatment, *Orthopedics* 13:529-534, 1990.
16. Karasick D, Burk Jr D, Gross GW: Trauma to the elbow and forearm, *Semin Roentgenol* 4:318-330, 1990.
17. Dymond IW: The treatment of isolated fractures of the distal ulna, *J Bone Joint Surg* 66:408-410, 1984.
18. Goel SC, Raj KB, Srivastara TP: Isolated fractures of the ulnar shaft, *Injury* 22:212-214, 1991.
19. Rockwood, Green. *Fractures of the shafts of the radius and ulna,* Lewis D Anderson.
20. Carey PJ, Alburger PD, Betz RR, et al: Both-bone forearm fractures in children, *Orthopedics* 15:1015-1019, 1992.
21. McDougall CG, Johnston GHF: A new technique of catheter placement for measurement of forearm compartment pressures, *J Trauma* 31(10):1404-1407, 1991.
22. Mubanak SJ, Hargens AR: Acute compartment syndromes, *Surg Clin North Am* 63:539, 1983.

# CHAPTER 13

# The Wrist

*Robert Collier*

The wrist is one of the most complex joints in the human body. Anatomically, the wrist is not one joint, but a region that contains multiple joints interconnected by a network of ligaments working dynamically to allow many degrees of range of motion. Not surprisingly, the word *wrist* is etymologically derived from the Old English word *rist* which means to writhe or twist. Joints included in the wrist region that extend from the carpometacarpal joints to the proximal border of the pronator quadratus are termed radiocarpal, intercarpal, meniscocarpal, and radioulnar.[1] Commonly, the wrist is defined as the area from the distal radius and ulna to the distal row of carpal bones.

## FUNCTIONAL ANATOMY

The anatomy of the wrist (Fig. 13-1) is most easily understood by dividing the region into three areas: the distal radioulnar joint (DRUJ) and the proximal and distal carpal rows. The radial component of the DRUJ normally has a distal biconcave surface that is covered with articular cartilage and is divided by an anteroposterior crest creating

a scaphoid and a lunate sulcus.[1] The radial articular surface is angulated in two planes: anteroposteriorly with approximately 0° to 18° of volar tilt and transversely from lateral to medial with an inclination of 14° to 28°. This oblique, transverse angulation creates the radial styloid. The ulna articulates with the sigmoid notch, a depression on the medial aspect of the distal radius which forms the DRUJ. From a lateral plateau area at the head, it rises to form the ulnar styloid on the anatomic medial aspect of the bone.[2] From the medial radius, ulnar head, and styloid arises the triangular fibrocartilage complex (TFCC) which stabilizes the ulnar aspect of the carpal bones (Fig. 13-2). This fibrous ligament complex is a thick confluence of structures that is comprised of an articular disk (or the TFCC proper), a structure distal and ulnar to this called the *meniscus homolog,* and the radioulnar and ulnocarpal ligaments.[3] The TFCC connects to the pisiform and triquetrum.

The proximal carpal row from a radial to ulnar direction traditionally includes the scaphoid, lunate, triquetrum, and pisiform. The distal carpal row from a radial to ulnar direction consists of the trapezium, trapezoid, capitate, and the hamate. The articulation between the rows forms the midcarpal joint and the proximal row is thus interposed between the radiocarpal joint and the midcarpal joint. The distal carpal row articulates with the first through fifth metacarpal bases. Functionally, the proximal and distal carpal rows can be conceptualized topologically as a ring structure with the distal and proximal components closed on each end by the scaphoid radially and the triquetrum-pisiform complex on the ulnar aspect. Motions of either row or the connecting end links affect all other components of the ring and this interdependence helps to explain the dynamics of many wrist injuries.

The ligaments of the wrist are divided into two broad classifications: extrinsic and intrinsic. These dorsal and volar extrinsic ligaments attach and stabilize the radius and ulna to the carpus. The radial volar ligaments arise from the distal radial styloid in a V shape and connect as they sweep in an ulnar direction to the proximal and distal carpal rows. Similar ligaments arise from the TFCC complex and volar ulna and sweep in a radial direction stabilizing the ulnar aspect of the joint. These distal ligament complexes are also known as the arcuate ligaments. This complex includes the radioscaphocapitate ligament from the radial aspect and the ulnocarpal ligament from the ulnar aspect (Fig. 13-3). A similar but more proximal set of ligaments arises from the medial radius and radial aspect of the ulna to form an arc of ligaments only extending to the proximal carpal row. The lateral ligaments include the radiolunotriquetrial and radioscaphoid and the medial ulnolunate and ulnotriquetral ligaments. The anatomically significant Space of Poirer is created between the distal and proximal arcing ligament groups. This thinned area expands when the wrist is dorsiflexed and is the potential space of volar lunate dislocations. The thinner dorsal extrinsic ligaments extend primarily from the radius to the distal and proximal carpal

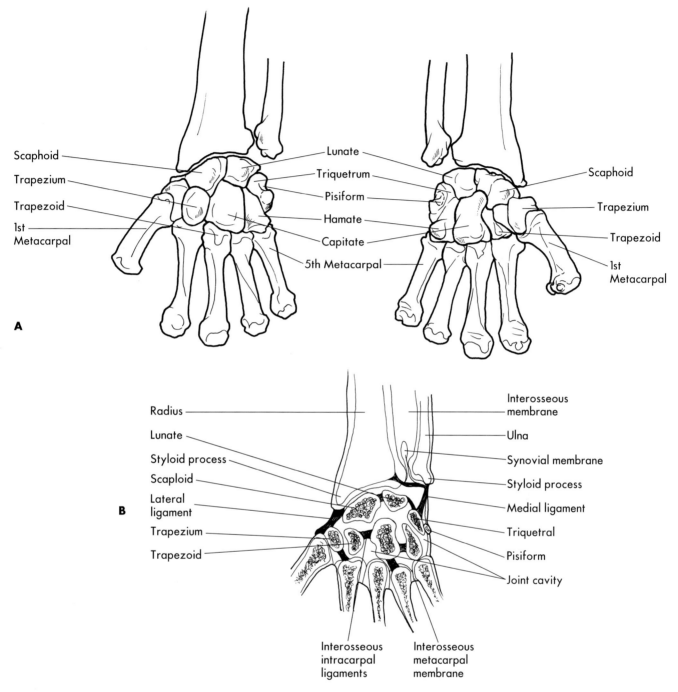

**Fig. 13-1. A,** A figure showing the normal anatomic relationship of the carpus to each other and to the radius, ulna, and metacarpus. The bones of distal carpal row from lateral to medial include the trapezium, trapezoid, capitate, and hamate. The proximal carpal row includes the scaphoid, lunate, triquetrum, and pisiform. **B,** A cross-section of the wrist showing the connecting ligaments.

rows. They stabilize the carpus dorsally and prevent ulnar and volar dislocation of the carpus on the volar sloping radiocarpal joint. The intrinsic ligaments are intra-articular, short ligaments that bind the distal and proximal carpal rows into functional units. Intrinsic ligaments between the rows are relatively longer and allow up to 30° of motion between the rows. Combined action of the intrinsic ligaments and volar extrinsic ligament attachments through the scaphoid on the radial side of the joint and the triquetrum on the ulnar side stabilize the midcarpal joint. The intrinsic scapholunate and the extrinsic radioscapholunate ligaments are the most important ligaments in assuring of carpal stability on the radial side of the wrist. The extrinsic ulnotriquetrial and ulnolunate ligaments combined with the intrinsic lunotriquetral ligament stabilize the ulnar aspect of the wrist.

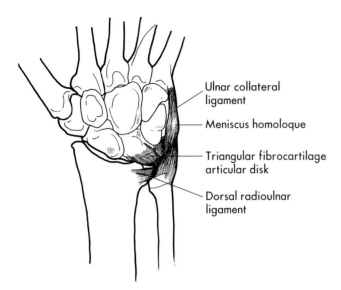

**Fig. 13-2.** The triangular fibrocartilage complex components which include the meniscus homolog, articular disc, ulnar collateral ligament, and radioulnar ligament.

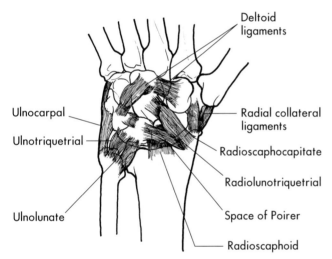

**Fig. 13-3.** The extrinsic volar ligaments of the wrist.

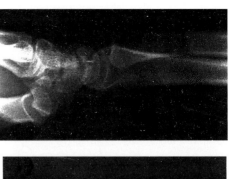

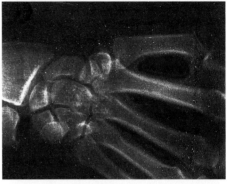

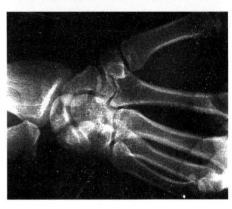

**Fig. 13-4.** Normal radiograph of the wrist with three views.

Other stabilizers include the flexor and extensor tendons as they enter the wrist under the flexor and extensor retinacula. Only one tendon actually inserts on the carpus and that is the flexor carpi ulnaris which attaches to the pisiform. Any motion of the radiocarpal joint or midcarpal joint is passive, mediated by the action of these tendons on the metacarpals and phalanges. Without the intrinsic and extrinsic carpal ligaments, the carpal joints would collapse with the forces generated by these tendons.

## RADIOGRAPHIC ANATOMY
### Adults

Figure 13-4 shows the normal radiographic anatomy of the wrist in the normal anteroposterior (AP) and lateral views. The AP view shows the scaphoid fitting smoothly in the scaphoid fossa of the radius and the lunate articulating with the medial radius in the lunate fossa. Ulnar to the scaphoid and lunate is the triquetrum superimposed over the pisiform. The distal pole of the scaphoid should be in close alignment with the trapezium, which is attached to the first metacarpal base, and the trapezoid, found at the base of the second metacarpal. The trapezoid and the concave ulnar surface of the scaphoid articulate with the capitate, the largest and most centrally located of the carpus. Medial (toward the ulna) to the capitate is the hamate, which is in association with the bases of the fourth and fifth metacarpal. The relationship between the radius, lunate, and capitate in the lateral view is an important anatomic feature. The central axis of each bone should be aligned along the longitudinal axis of the wrist. In the AP view, the scaphoid and lunate should not be more than 3 mm apart. Three arcs are described by the articulations of the proximal carpal row and the radioulnar surface, the proximal carpal row and its distal articulation, and the proximal articular surface of the capitate and hamate. Any loss of the contour of these arcs should make a physician suspicious of a fracture or dislocation.[4]

**Table 13-1.** Mean age and standard deviation at which ossification of each carpal bone occurs in boys and girls

|  | Boys mean, *months* | Standard deviation | Girls mean, *months* | Standard deviation |
|---|---|---|---|---|
| Capitate | 2.9 | 1.7 | 2.5 | 1.8 |
| Hamate | 4.2 | 2.7 | 3.1 | 2.2 |
| Triquetrium | 29.5 | 16.2 | 26.6 | 14.0 |
| Lunate | 43.5 | 14.7 | 36.1 | 17.3 |
| Scaphoid | 69.6 | 15.4 | 53.7 | 13.8 |
| Trapezoid | 72.0 | 16.1 | 51.8 | 12.3 |
| Trapezium | 72.7 | 13.1 | 51.6 | 16.4 |
| Pisiform | 94.5 | 13.1 | 120.0 | 12.1 |

## Children

The radiographic appearance of the wrist in children varies markedly with age. All of the carpus are radiolucent, cartilaginous structures at birth. Progressive ossification occurs with age as shown in Table 13-1.[5]

## EXAMINATION OF THE WRIST

The physical examination of the wrist follows traditional methods of inspection and palpation. Comparison with the opposite wrist is paramount when locating swelling and deformity. If the patient is not totally inhibited by pain, the physician should test the range of motion of the wrist and also compare this to the unaffected extremity. From a neutral forearm position, supination and pronation should be 80° in either direction. Dorsiflexion should reach approximately 60° to 80°, and palmar flexion should approach 90°. Radial deviation can range up to 25°; ulnar deviation is greater—up to 45°.

Palpation of the wrist should be done in an orderly fashion beginning on the dorsal surface and ending volarly. Figure 13-5 shows the important anatomic landmarks for the exam. The exam should progress radially and proximally and move ulnarly and distally. Areas of tenderness should be noted that may indicate underlying fractures, ligament injuries, arthritides, or tendinitis. Masses palpated may be due to ganglia, osteophytic protrusions, and tumors. With the wrist in ulnar deviation, the radial styloid can be palpated over the radial aspect. A prominence over the dorsum of the radius is called Lister's tubercle. Ulnar to this tubercle is the dorsal aspect of the DRUJ; moving still in an ulnar direction, the prominence of the ulnar head is appreciated. Palpation of the radially located anatomic snuffbox, a concavity created by the abductor pollicis longus and extensor pollicis longus reveals the scaphoid body. With the wrist held in flexion, palpation distal to Lister's tubercle on the radius reveals the proximal pole of the scaphoid. The lunate is difficult to palpate because it is surrounded both volarly and dorsally by tendons. Palpation dorsoulnarly and distal to the ulnar head reveals the triquetrum. Moving to the distal carpal row, the trapezium can be palpated just proximal to the first metacarpal base articulation. Ulnar from this is the trapezoid. Following the third metacarpal down to its base, one feels a depression in which the capitate can be palpated.

Palpation of the area just distal to the triquetrum can be used to assess hamate pathology. Fewer bone structures are palpable on the volar surface of the wrist. The pisiform is palpable in the most proximal part of the ulnar wrist, just as the hypothenar eminence becomes prominent. Distal and slightly radial to this is the nodular feeling called hook of the hamate, which is a process projecting from the distal volar surface of the bone. Surrounding all these landmarks are the various tendons that traverse the wrist as they slip under the dorsal and volar retinacula. Dorsally, extensor tendons and volar flexor tendons and on the radial aspect, the various thumb flexors, extensors, abductors, and adductors surround the carpus, stabilize, and provide motion through the wrist joint.

## MECHANISMS OF INJURY

The types of acute traumatic injuries to the wrist are a function of age, position of the wrist at the moment of impact, and magnitude and direction of the force vector transmitted through the carpometacarpal, midcarpal, and DRUJ. With the same amount of force and similar mechanism, an older adult may sustain a distal radius fracture, whereas the younger adult will have either a sprain or no injury. Similarly, a child might sustain an epiphyseal fracture. Lower energy forces usually result in distal radius fractures that are extrarticular. High energy forces result in intra-articular distal radius fractures with displacement and carpal ligament and bone injuries, including dislocations.

The most common mechanism is a fall on the outstretched forearm and hand that hyperextends, ulnarly deviates, and dorsiflexes the midcarpal joint. Shear forces on the volar aspect of the radius cause cortical disruption and result in fracture of metaphysis proximal to the joint. With increasing force, four patterns of injury occur through anatomic arcs found in the carpus and DRUJ. Figure 13-6 shows the four commonly described anatomic arcs. A greater arc injury is described that predictably results in scaphoid and capitate fractures, and associated perilunate dislocation. A lesser arc injury involves the scapholunate interval, the lunocapitate or midcarpal joint, and the lunotriquetrial articulation. Enough energy transmitted through these joints can ultimately cause a lunate dislocation. In a

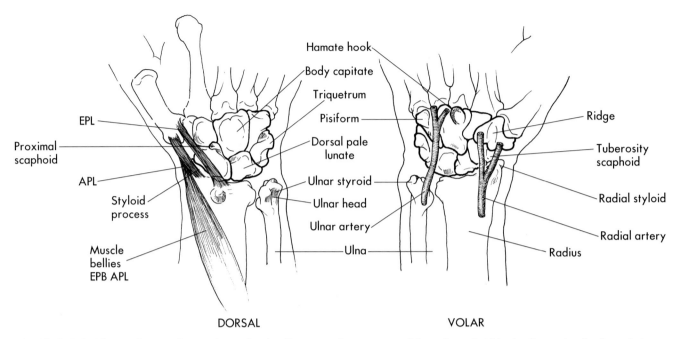

Fig. 13-5. Palpable prominences that can be used to localize anatomic structures of the wrist and aid in the diagnosis of wrist pathology.

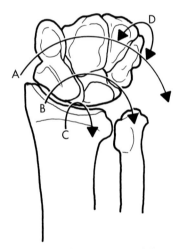

Fig. 13-6. Schematic showing common injury mechanisms through four different anatomic arcs. The text describes each injury pattern.

third arc of injury, the lunate can transmit a compression force on the distal radius that can, through what has been described as a die-punch mechanism,[6] cause a comminuted, intra-articular fracture of the distal radius. The fourth arc of injury is caused by extreme radial deviation and torsion on the carpal ring, and causes ligament injuries and associated fractures of the articulations of the triquetrum. Even without fracture of the carpus and radius or ulna, these arcs of injury can cause serious ligament injuries and can result in carpal instabilities, with associated chronic wrist pain and disability.[7]

Other less common mechanisms of injury include acute volar flexion, which results in volar displacement of distal radius fragments and direct compression over the dorsum or volar aspect of the joint. Severe trauma with open fractures and severe joint disruption occurs in situations such as industrial and farm accidents where heavy machinery is in use.

## DISTAL RADIUS FRACTURES

Much more is known about the mechanisms of injury to the wrist. Therefore, optimal treatment should be based on the particular pathology found, rather than that used only a few years ago when treatment was based on the rather arbitrary eponym-based historic classifications. These classifications are so established in orthopedic literature that they still must be used in any discussion of wrist fractures, but they must be used only as a broad way to classify these injuries; the specifics of the particular injury must be addressed. Optimal treatment in the management of distal radial fractures includes recognition of complicated injuries, accurate, stable anatomic reduction, and optimal immobilization, and open reduction if indicated.

### Colles' fractures

The most common type of wrist fracture in adults, the Colles' fracture, first described by and named after Scotch physician Abraham Colles, is classically defined as a fracture of the distal radius with dorsal displacement and associated ulnar styloid fracture, though this may be variable.[8]

**Anatomy and mechanism of injury.** The most important anatomic relationships in the wrist in regard to distal radius fractures are the previously mentioned ulnar inclination of the distal radius, its volar tilt and the precise neutral approximation of the DRUJ. Successful therapy of these fractures requires that these relationships are restored as accurately as possible. The distal radius has a lateral distal

**Table 13-2.** Frykman classification of distal radius fractures: Colles' fractures

| Type of fracture | Associated distal ulna fracture | |
|---|---|---|
| | Absent | Present |
| Extra-articular | Type I | Type II |
| Intra-articular/radiocarpal joint | Type III | Type IV |
| Intra-articular/radioulnar joint | Type V | Type VI |
| Intra-articular/both joints | Type VII | Type VIII |

**Table 13-3.** Melone classification of distal radius fractures (only intra-articular, four-part fractures)

| Fracture type | Description |
|---|---|
| Type I | Nondisplaced |
| Type II | Posterior or anterior displacement |
| Type III | Volar fragment with nerve impingement |
| Type IV | Rotation of fragments |

flair known as the *radial styloid*. This is the lateral border of the scaphoid fossa on the distal end of the radius that gives the radius its length in the longitudinal axis. The inclination in the coronal plane, radially to ulnarly directed, of the articular surface to the longitudinal axis of the radius is approximately 22° from a line drawn perpendicular to this axis. The volar tilt in the longitudinal axis is approximately 14°. Medial or ulnar to the scaphoid fossa is the lunate articulation with the distal radius in the concavity known as the lunate fossa. The ulna articulates with the radius at the sigmoid notch, a concavity on its ulnar metaphyseal surface. There should be no positive or negative variance of this relationship which implies that the length of the radius and ulnar are essentially equal at their medial articulation. The triangular fibrocartilage complex arises from the articular surface of this joint and attaches to the ulnar head and styloid. It stabilizes the ulnar aspect of the joint through articulations with the lunate and triquetrum. The most distal fibers of the TFCC attach to the base of the fifth metacarpal. The integrity of the TFCC is always at risk with distal radius fractures.

Colles' fractures usually result from a fall on the outstretched hand, which at impact, imparts a longitudinal compressive force that shears the radius volarly and propagates to the dorsum. Lower force injuries in older adults, especially in the relatively osteoporotic, result in extra-articular fractures with or without ulnar styloid involvement. In children, distal radial epiphysis fractures occur with or without metaphyseal injury. Higher-force injuries usually seen in young adults are believed to be caused by a die-punch mechanism that drives the proximal carpal row, especially the lunate, into the distal radius articular surface and invariably results in a comminuted, intra-articular fracture that may be unstable.[8]

**Classification systems.** Multiple classification systems of these fractures have been proposed to assess degree of injury, make therapeutic decisions, and predict complications. A feature common to all these systems is that the more displacement, comminution, and articular involvement present, the worse the prognosis and the higher the probability of instability and failure of closed reduction. Tables 13-2 and 13-3 list two commonly accepted classification methods, those of Frykmann and Melone[6,9] which are used to address therapeutic decisions and prognosis for healing and complications. Frykmann has eight different classifications, with each successive number implying a more extensive injury. Even numbers imply associated ulnar styloid fractures. Types I and II are extra-articular, and types III through VIII are articular. Types III and IV involve only the radiocarpal joint; Types V and VI the DRUJ; and VII and VIII involve both joints.[9] Melone classified strictly articular fractures and did not address the issue of the associated ulnar styloid fracture. He found that these types of fractures predictably fragment into four basic components: the radial shaft, the radial styloid, a dorsal medial fragment, and a volar medial fragment. Type I fractures were undisplaced and were stable when reduced. Type II fractures had displacement of the medial fragments and were usually unstable. Type III fractures had displacement of the medial complex and a fragment from the volar radial shaft which is displaced into the flexor and neurovascular compartments causing damage therein. Type IV fractures have marked displacement of the medial fragments with rotation and also always have associated soft-tissue injury.[6] Frykmann types III through VIII and Melone types II through IV almost always require more aggressive therapy to avoid complications and poor outcomes.

**Clinical presentation.** The patient invariably presents with a history of a fall or mechanism that acutely dorsiflexes the wrist. The hand is dorsally displaced in relation to the forearm and there is marked swelling with variable degrees of pain. The hand and wrist assume the classic configuration of a silverfork. Paresthesia may be present in the distribution of the median or ulnar nerve, and flexor tendon function may be compromised by entrapment. Marked swelling and increased tissue pressures can lead to a compartment syndrome and accelerate nerve involvement and create vascular compromise. Function of individual tendons, nerves, and capillary fill should be assessed recording the distribution of any paresthesia, and noting cyanosis or blanching.

**Radiographic findings.** Figure 13-7 shows an uncomplicated Frykman type I fracture with an extra-articular fracture of the distal radius and an associated ulnar styloid fracture. Note the dorsal angulation of the distal radial fragment. In general, AP radiographs will differ markedly from one type of Colles' fracture to another. Ulnar styloid fracture is variable. The distal radius will most commonly show a transverse fracture line proximal to the joint. The distal fragment may be either nondisplaced or dorsal to the

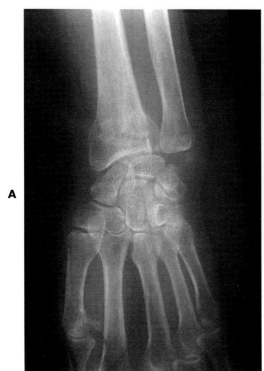

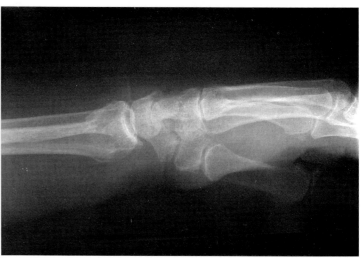

**Fig. 13-7. A,** Anteroposterior and **B,** lateral views of an uncomplicated Frykman type I distal radius fracture (Colles' fracture).

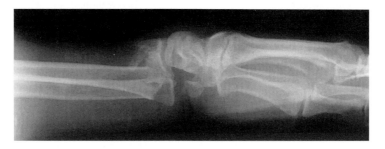

**Fig. 13-8.** Radiograph of a complicated, intra-articular fracture of the radius and ulna. Note the disruption of the distal radioulnar joint (DRUJ).

radius shaft. Complicated unstable fractures (Fig. 13-8) will be comminuted and displaced with loss of volar tilt and radius length. The ulnar head and the medial aspect of the articular surface of the radius should be well approximated at the sigmoid notch and should have equal length at that point. With associated disruption of the DRUJ, the ulna may appear to be longer or shorter than this corner of the radius. If it is longer, it is called positive ulnar variance; if shorter, it is called negative ulnar variance. Close scrutiny of this view should be executed to diagnose associated carpal fractures, dislocations, and instability syndromes. The lateral view shows the distal radius component dorsal to the longitudinal axis of the radius in displaced fractures. The lunate should still be in the lunate fossa and should be collinear with the capitate. Comminuted fractures may have displaced volar and dorsal medial fragments.

**Treatment.** Nondisplaced fractures or ones with minimal displacement, adequate length, and maintenance of volar tilt can be managed with initial splinting in a sugar-tong–type splint and then casted after maximal swelling occurs. Extra-articular displaced fractures (type I and II) can be treated with closed reduction with good results, whereas intra-articular fractures, though reducible by closed methods, have a high probability of instability and long-term complications if anatomically accurate reduction is not accomplished. These fractures are usually treated with open reduction and fixation either externally or internally. The best method of reduction for an uncomplicated displaced Colles fracture involves adequate anesthesia and attempts to reduce the fracture acutely in the emergency department. Anesthesia methods include a Bier block, axillary block, or conscious sedation. Hematoma block is

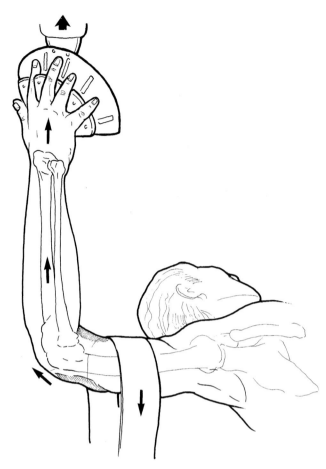

**Fig. 13-9.** Representation of use of finger-traps to assist in reduction and casting of a Colles fracture.

commonly used, but is not without controversy. Complications include a greater chance of post-reduction neuropathy, lidocaine toxicity, and inadequate anesthesia to accomplish the reduction.[8,10,11,12] After adequate anesthesia, the reduction is attempted with longitudinal traction applied through the hand and countertraction through the forearm. The fingers are placed in a trap and countertraction is applied with weight of approximately 2.5 to 5 kg in a traction sling (Fig. 13-9). The fracture is then manipulated by holding the distal forearm with the hands and using the thumbs on the distal fragment to reduce it in the opposite manner as it was displaced. The physician should feel the fracture fragment move volarly and the patient's wrist should appear more normal in contour. The goal is to reduce the fracture to a neutral or slightly volar tilt. A short-arm–sandwich or sugar-tong–type splint is applied in slight volar and ulnar deviation and the patient is sent for post-reduction films. Post-reduction films should be reviewed. Volar tilt angle, ulnar inclination that reflects length, and neutral ulnar variance at the DRUJ should be assessed. Unacceptable values for these parameters are clues pointing to unstable and potentially complicated fractures. Additionally, extreme dorsal angulation, displacement back to the original prereduction position,

marked comminution, intra-articular involvement, and shortening of 5 to 10 mm are all signs of more complicated and unstable fractures that will require more intervention and orthopedic consultation.[13] Melone type II and higher, or Frykman type III and higher are usually of this type and should be handled by orthopedics. Management usually consists of the use of pins and plaster, open reduction and internal fixation, or use of external fixation devices. Obviously, any fracture that is complicated by nerve or tendon entrapment also falls in this category.

### Smith's fractures

These fractures are essentially the opposite of the Colles fracture in mechanism and morphology. The distal radius fragment is volar to the radial shaft and it resembles what some have described as a garden spade.[14] The fracture was first distinguished from the Colles fracture by Robert William Smith, an Irish physician, around 1847.[14] Smith fractures are much more uncommon than Colles and represent only a small percentage of distal radius fractures.

**Anatomy and mechanism of injury.** The anatomical considerations are similar to those described previously for the Colles fracture. Extension into the radiocarpal and DRUJ portend complications and these relationships must be restored. The mechanism of injury is usually a fall that applies a force to the back of the hand. Motor vehicle accidents or cycling falls where the rider is thrown over the handle bars are the common scenarios for this type of injury. The shearing force is applied to the dorsum of the distal radius and it displaces volarly as the bone gives way.

**Classification.** Thomas[15] attempted to classify Smith fractures, though some authors feel that only an extra-articular fracture of this type should be called by this eponym.[14] Figure 13-10 shows Thomas classification. Thomas type I is a transverse extra-articular fracture that fits the original description of Smith. Type II fractures are oblique and extend from the proximal volar surface distally through the dorsal articular surface. Type III fractures are similar to Type II but run more directly into the joint space and are essentially the same as a Barton fracture-dislocation.

**Clinical presentation.** Patients with Smith fractures present with a history of high-energy trauma to the dorsum of the distal forearm and wrist. Marked swelling is present dorsally over the wrist, and the hand is displaced volarly from its usual neutral position. With extreme angulation, vascular compromise may be present, as well as median or ulnar neuropathy. Tendon involvement is possible, but not reported.

**Radiographic findings.** In the AP radiograph, type I Smith fractures will appear as a transverse fracture line, whereas types II and III may show only a double density of the volar fragment displaced below the distal radius. An associated ulnar styloid fracture may be present. Figure 13-11 is a lateral radiograph of a Smith type I fracture.

**Treatment.** A Smith-Thomas type I fracture can be treated with closed reduction just as a Colles fracture would

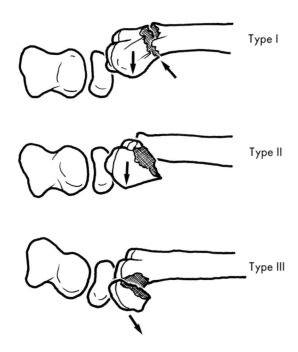

Type I

Type II

Type III

**Fig. 13-10.** Smith fractures classified as three types. A dorsal Barton fracture is equivalent to a type III Smith fracture.

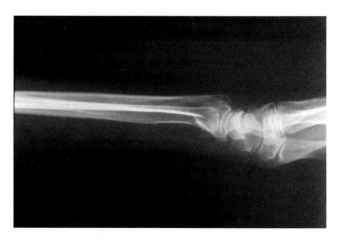

**Fig. 13-11.** Lateral radiograph of a Smith fracture with volar displacement of the distal radial fragment.

be. Longitudinal traction with the use of fingertraps and counterweights applied along the forearm and use of the thumbs to move the distal fragment dorsally into alignment is usually successful and can be accomplished in the emergency department setting. The reduced wrist is then immobilized in a long-arm splint with the forearm in supination. A cast should be applied in several days and the reduction maintained for 4 to 8 weeks.[14] Type II and type III (volar Barton fracture) fractures should be considered unstable and complicated and should be referred to orthopedic surgery for open reduction and internal fixation, usually with a volar buttress plate.

### Barton's fractures

Described in 1838 by John Rhea Barton, the fracture that bears his name is an intra-articular fracture-dislocation of the wrist of which there are of two types, dorsal and volar. The dorsal form is least common and involves a fragment of distal radius that is dorsally displaced, along with the carpus. The volar type is the opposite; it is essentially a Smith type III fracture, according to the classification system used by Thomas.

**Anatomy and mechanism of injury.** The anatomic considerations are essentially similar to those of the Colles' fracture, with concern of maintenance of all normal anatomic relationships. Because of the intra-articular aspect of these fractures, alignment of the distal radius articulations with the carpus in the scaphoid and lunate fossae, is important for restoration of normal wrist function. Disruption of the radioulnar joint is also possible in medial injuries and associated avulsion or instability of the ulnar side of the wrist through disruption of the TFCC is possible

as well. Associated carpal ligament injuries, fractures, and instability syndromes must be suspected due to the usually high-impact nature of these types of fractures. Mechanism of injury is usually a force applied to the dorsum of the wrist to create a volar Barton fracture and volar force in extension similar to the Colles' fracture mechanism in a dorsal Barton fracture. These fractures occur usually as a result of motor vehicle, motorcycle, and falling accidents.[14]

**Clinical presentation.** Clinical presentation is that of a very swollen, painful wrist after high-energy trauma. The hand appears dislocated from its radial and ulnar attachments in either a dorsal or volar direction. With extreme displacement, vascular compromise manifested by weak radial and ulnar pulses and poor capillary fill may be present. Paresthesia in the median and ulnar nerve distribution may also be present.

**Radiographic findings.** Figure 13-12 shows the type of displacement seen on the AP and lateral wrist views. Note the intra-articular extension. Radiographs must be examined carefully for any associated carpal fractures and dislocations. The relationships of the carpus to the distal fragment should appear to be a normal wrist from the point of the fracture.

**Treatment.** All Barton fractures are considered complicated and unstable. Closed reduction and casting will neither create a stable situation for healing nor will it allow proper alignment of the articular surface. Fragments of bone are usually in the fracture line and must be removed before using a volar buttress plate to maintain the reduction. Immediate consultation with an orthopedic surgeon is indicated when the diagnosis is made.

### Radial styloid fracture (Chauffeur fracture)

A Chauffeur fracture or radial styloid fracture is so named because it apparently occurred in the chauffeurs who, when attempting to turn the crank on older cars without starters, received a sudden torsing force, resulting in acute ulnar deviation to their wrists as the car engine backfired. The

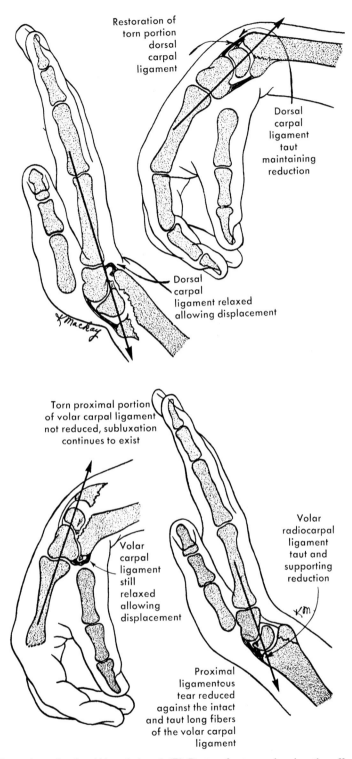

**Fig. 13-12.** Illustration of volar (**A**) and dorsal (**B**) Barton fractures showing the effects of the volar and dorsal radiocarpal ligaments. (From King RE: Barton's fracture-dislocation of the wrist. In Ahstrom JP Jr, ed: *Current practice in orthopaedic surgery,* vol 6. St. Louis, Mosby-Year Book, 1975.)

fracture is a triangular piece off the distal radius at its lateral flair known as the radial styloid.[16]

**Anatomy and mechanism of injury.** The radial styloid is a process of the distal, lateral radius and creates the lateral margin of the scaphoid fossa of the radial articular surface.

The radiocarpal ligaments are attached to its dorsal and volar surface. Acute ulnar deviation and possibly hyperextension stress these ligaments to the point of avulsing the styloid fragment. Because of these carpal attachments, there is a high incidence of associated scaphoid fracture and carpal instability syndromes. Most reported cases in modern times are secondary to motorcycle accidents and falls.[16]

**Clinical presentation.** These patients complain of pain and swelling of the wrist and are exquisitely tender over the radial styloid. No visible displacement is noted on clinical exam. Extensive swelling and diffuse wrist tenderness may be a clue to more extensive associated carpal injury.

**Radiographic findings.** The radial styloid will be separated from the radius by an oblique fracture from the mid-articular surface to the lateral metaphysis of the distal radius (Fig. 13-13).

**Treatment.** Because these fractures are intra-articular and complicated, orthopedic consultation for open reduction and screw fixation is the treatment of choice. During operative repair, injuries to the contiguous carpus can be evaluated and treated.[17]

### Fractures of the distal radial and ulnar epiphysis in children

Wrist fractures in children are usually through the distal radial epiphysis, the most common of epiphyseal injuries (25%). The childhood equivalent of the Colles fracture, distal radial epiphysis fractures are rarely comminuted, intra-articular, or associated with carpal injuries. Rarely, they will be very distal greenstick or torus fracture. These fractures are most common in patients between 6 and 12 years of age.

**Anatomy and mechanism of injury.** The distal radial epiphysis is visible on radiograph at approximately 1 year and the distal ulnar epiphysis at 6 to 7 years. The distal radial growth plate contributes 75% of the growth, especially in length, and the distal ulnar contributes 40% of the ulnar growth potential.[18]

The epiphysis, though stabilized by a strong periosteal connection, is very weak at the point of active growth which is a zone of cellular proliferation and provisional calcification. When fractured, the epiphyseal growth potential is usually not damaged because germinal layers stay attached and blood supply remains intact. Germinal layers can be interrupted if the mechanism of injury involves more of a crushing, compressive-type force than the more common shearing force that displaces the physis.[19]

Torus fractures, which are compression-induced buckle fractures, can occur just proximal to the epiphysis, as well as greenstick fractures, which are the result of lateral tension forces. The most common injury is a fracture through the radial epiphysis with a greenstick fracture of the distal ulna. The usual mechanism is that of a fall on the outstretched forearm with the wrist in hyperextension, though rarely the opposite occurs, creating a fracture similar in mechanism and deformity to a Smith fracture. Distal epiphyseal fractures are produced by compressive and shear-type forces. More compression longitudinally increases the probability of epiphyseal damage, as opposed to more laterally directed shearing forces, which displace the epiphysis from the metaphysis.

**Classification.** The general types of wrist fractures in children are torus, greenstick, and epiphyseal. A torus fracture represents a buckling fracture without angulation. A greenstick fracture describes a cortical break on the compression side and a bending without visible cortical break on the opposite; these are usually angulated. Epiphyseal fractures involve the distal growth plate. The Salter and Harris[20] classification of epiphyseal plate fractures is useful not only as a classification system but also as a prognostic tool. Type I fractures extend through the epiphyseal plate and usually leave a periosteal attachment. Type II involves the epiphyseal plate and a small fracture of the metaphysis. Type III is similar to type II, but the avulsion fracture is of the epiphysis. Salter type IV is an oblique fracture extending from the metaphysis, across and through the epiphysis. Finally, type V results from a compressing, longitudinal force that crushes the epiphyseal growth plate. Prognosis for complicated healing and bone growth arrest is poorer as the number of the fracture type increases. Figure 13-14 shows a Salter-Harris II fracture.

**Clinical presentation.** Undisplaced fractures may show no external signs of swelling especially early after presentation. Only exquisite point tenderness over the wrist may be present. Small children who cannot describe the location of their pain may only manifest their injury by lack of use. Displaced fractures of the distal radius will have the same silverfork deformity or garden spade appearance similar to the adult analogues of the Colles and Smith fractures, respectively. Neuropathies of the median and ulnar nerves are possible and sensory and motor function must be tested.

**Treatment.** Treatment of undisplaced fractures of the distal radius and ulna in children involves splinting the extremity in a lacer splint or volar forearm splint with close follow-up. Displaced physeal fractures must be reduced under hematoma block, Bier, or axillary block in older children and under conscious sedation or general anesthesia in small children. The reduction of a dorsally displaced fracture is accomplished by using the thumbs dorsally on the displaced physis and applying longitudinal and volar pressure to reverse the deformity and move it into alignment with the radial metaphysis. The dorsal periosteum is usually intact and opposes over-reduction. A long-arm splint or cast is applied with slight volar angulation and slight ulnar deviation. The forearm should be put in supination and post-reduction films taken. Inability to reduce the fracture may be secondary to a periosteal flap in the fracture line.[19] Salter III fractures and Salter IV fractures are intra-articular and require orthopedic consultation to evaluate the need for reduction and pinning.[21,22] Epiphyseal fractures that are unreduced after 10 days should not be manipulated, and attempts at reduction could injure the epiphyseal plate. Despite the best efforts to reduce these fractures, they can be complicated by growth problems. Parents of the young patient should be informed of this potential problem at the time of the visit.

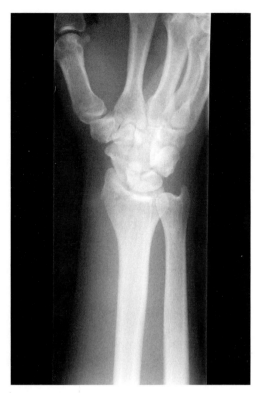

**Fig. 13-13.** A radial styloid fracture, also known as a Chauffeur fracture. Note the fracture line from the lateral aspect of the distal radius and its extension into the joint space. This fracture is mildly displaced.

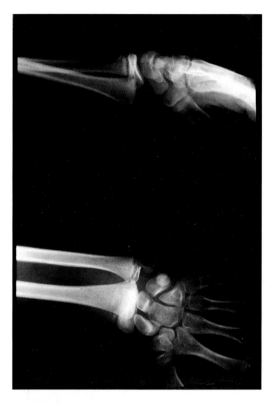

**Fig. 13-14.** Salter-Harris II fracture of the radius with a possible associated small greenstick fracture of the ulna. This would be a Salter-Harris I fracture but for a small bone fragment off the metaphysis seen in the anteroposterior (AP) view.

## MORE COMMON CARPAL FRACTURES

Fractures of the carpus are less common than those of the distal radius, but are very important types of wrist injuries, which if missed, can cause severe disability. These fractures are frequently not simple in that there may be associated dislocation and ligament injury that makes the wrist joint unstable.

### Scaphoid fractures

In both adults and children, the scaphoid is the most commonly fractured carpal bone. Scaphoid fracture is the second most common wrist injury, after fracture of the radius. The spectrum of injury ranges from a very classical clinical presentation to subtle presentations with minimal findings; the diagnosis being made by only clinical suspicion and mechanism of injury.

**Anatomy and clinical presentation.** The scaphoid is an integral part of the wrist anatomy and is the main stabilizer of the radial side of the carpal rows. It sits prominently in a line between the trapezoid and trapezium and the distal radius's scaphoid fossa. This makes the scaphoid highly susceptible to injury, especially with extreme dorsiflexion and ulnar deviation stresses. Because of ligament attachments to the lunate of the proximal carpal row and to the trapezoid, triquetrum, and capitate of the distal row, the scaphoid flexes in wrist flexion and radial deviation and extends in wrist extension and ulnar devia-

tion. These complex motions make the immobilization of a fractured scaphoid very difficult and also create an environment for associated carpal instabilities and other carpal fractures. Unstable or displaced fracture of the scaphoid breaks the link in the carpal ring and the midcarpal joint will collapse with the lunate becoming dorsiflexed in relation to the radius. In the parlance of carpal instabilities, this is known as a dorsal intercalated segment instability (DISI). Injuries to the scaphoid usually occur in the previously described greater arc.

The scaphoid is an oblong, almost peanut-shaped bone that obliquely attaches from volar to dorsal and from the distal carpal row to the proximal carpal row, as viewed from the radiolateral aspect of the wrist. The bone is anatomically divided into four regions: the distal tuberosity, the distal third, middle third, and proximal pole. Three groups of vessels that mostly perfuse the distal pole, tuberosity, and midscaphoid constitute the vascular supply. The proximal pole is devoid of its own blood supply, which accounts for a high incidence of avascular necrosis with improper or delayed treatment.[23] Figure 13-15 shows the anatomy of the scaphoid.

**Classification.** Usually, scaphoid fractures are classified according to the method of Russe into three groups: proximal third, middle third, and distal third, with tuberosity fractures placed in the distal third grouping. The distal and proximal thirds are called the poles, and the middle

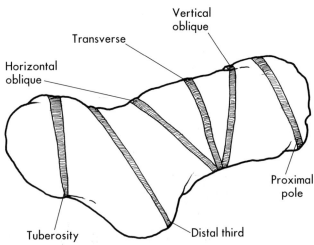

**Fig. 13-15.** The anatomic regions of the scaphoid. The scaphoid's blood supply is more abundant in the tuberosity, distal, and middle thirds that account for the higher incidence of avascular necrosis in the proximal pole of the bone.

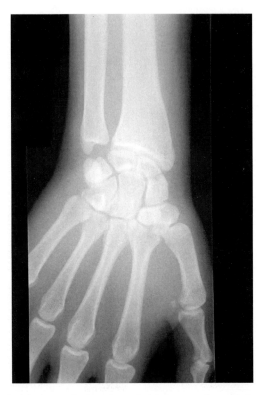

**Fig. 13-16.** A nondisplaced scaphoid fracture through the waist of the bone. This fracture will probably heal with conservative treatment and has less potential for avascular necrosis than a more proximal fracture.

third is known as the waist. Stable fractures are nondisplaced, whereas unstable fractures are defined as those with greater than 1 mm of displacement or a scapholunate angulation of greater than 45° or a lunocapitate angle of greater than 15°, as viewed from a lateral radiograph.

**Clinical presentation.** Scaphoid fractures usually occur in young- and middle-aged patients who have fallen with the outstretched arm and wrist dorsiflexed. Athletes who fall with great force are prone to these fractures. Children typically get a physeal fracture of the radius and older adults fracture the more vulnerable distal radius, although scaphoid fractures do occur in both groups. The history is that of a painful wrist after the fall; typically, the patient will report extreme pain with active motion and trying to grasp objects. On physical examination, the wrist may or may not appear swollen. There is tenderness over the anatomic snuff-box, the distal tuberosity, or the proximal pole distal to Lister's tubercle of the dorsal radius. Pain with wrist dorsiflexion and decreased and painful grip strength are associated with these fractures.[24] Pain with supination against resistance and longitudinal thumb compression pain are reported as other reliable signs.[25] Delayed presentation to the emergency department is common, the patient presuming that the injury is only a sprain.

Children less than 7 years of age rarely get scaphoid fractures because the immature carpus have a cartilaginous covering that resists fracture. The incidence increases with age and the clinical findings are usually similar to adults. Complications such as avascular necrosis and nonunion are very rare in children. Occasionally, these fractures are associated with distal radius fractures.

**Radiographic findings.** Up to 20% of initial wrist radiographs in which scaphoid fractures are present are normal. Only after 10 days to 2 weeks does a resorption line occur demonstrating the fracture. The best radiographic views to diagnose a scaphoid fracture are the posteroanterior (PA), posteroanterior in ulnar deviation (also known as the scaphoid or navicular view), lateral, and oblique views. Figure 13-16 represents a radiograph with a nondisplaced scaphoid fracture. A potentially helpful but nonspecific finding is a navicular fat stripe, which is a radiolucent area next to the scaphoid on its radial aspect. Obliteration of this space is associated with scaphoid fracture but is a relatively rare radiographic finding. As mentioned above, flexion of the scaphoid in the lateral views with increased lunocapitate and scapholunate angles, gives the physician a suspicion of a scaphoid fracture. When hyperflexed, the scaphoid can take on a signet ring appearance in the PA view.

A bone scan can be performed 3 days post-injury and, if normal, essentially rules out occult scaphoid fractures. Tomographic studies are very useful to define whether suspicious areas on the bone are fractures, and can help to elucidate the degree of displacement in unstable fractures.

**Treatment.** Though controversial with respect to methods of immobilization and methods of treatment of unstable fractures, the consensus is that the more complicated and unstable the fracture, the more aggressive the approach. Unstable fractures, as manifested by displacement or associated carpal instabilities and fractures, must be referred to orthopedists for definitive care and possible open reduction and fixation. Stable, nondisplaced fractures without complications can be handled conservatively in the emergency department. A short-arm thumb spica splint or cast in slight volar flexion and radial deviation is the treatment of choice in nondisplaced and occult fractures. Any displaced fracture should be placed in a long-arm thumb spica cast or splint in a position of reduction: wrist flexion and radial deviation. The major complications with this fracture are delayed diagnosis and treatment and nonunion with avascular necrosis.

## Lunate fractures

Lunate fractures are surprisingly uncommon, in view of the bone's central location in the wrist joint. The lunate is interposed between the capitate and radius, though the lunate fossa may actually afford it some protection. Lunate fractures represent only about 2% to 7% of carpal fractures.[26]

**Anatomy and mechanism of injury.** The lunate is located at the midposition of the proximal carpal row. Proximally, it lies in the lunate fossa of the radius; distally, the capitate's proximal convex surface articulates with the concavity of the distal lunate. Ulnarly, the lunate is supported by the triangular fibrocartilage complex, although negative ulnar variance compromises this support. Ligamentous connections to the lunate with the scaphoid and triquetrum create the proximal part of the carpal ring that stabilizes the midcarpal joint laterally and medially. Vascular supply comes from the proximal arcade to its dorsal and volar surfaces.

Dorsiflexion is the most common mechanism of injury to the lunate. As the wrist is dorsiflexed, the capitate is compressed against the volar aspect of the lunar articular surface and the lunate is ulnarly deviated. Ligament attachments can cause either dorsal or volar avulsion fractures. Compressive forces can cause sagittal plane fractures and are facilitated by negative ulnar variance that causes a shearing force over the ulnar aspect of the lunate fossa. Longitudinal compressive force may cause a transverse compression fracture of the bone mass and may be a predisposing cause of avascular necrosis and Kienböck's disease. Fractures of the lunate are extremely rare in children, but do occur and have been reported with greater frequency in older children.

**Classification.** Lunate fractures are usually classified anatomically as dorsal and volar avulsion fractures, transverse and sagittal body fractures, and compression fractures.

**Clinical presentation.** Patients with lunate fractures usually present with a history of a fall on an outstretched arm and complain of middorsal pain. Because early diagnosis is rare, the patient may present days to weeks after a wrist sprain and only at this late stage is the fracture recognized.

**Radiographic findings.** Initial radiographs may be read as negative, just as those of acute scaphoid fractures. When fractured, the cortical defect may be obscured by surrounding carpus and the concavity of the radial lunate fossa. Avulsion fractures dorsally or volarly can be detected in the lateral view, whereas transverse and longitudinal fractures are seen on the anteroposterior views. Negative ulnar variance can be appreciated on this view, and is a clue to mechanism. Late presentation will show evidence of Kienböck's disease with osteosclerosis and collapse of the bone.[8] Figure 13-17 shows the typical radiographic findings of Kienbock's osteosclerosis.

**Treatment.** Nondisplaced fractures can be put in a short-arm cast or splint and referred to orthopedics for close follow-up to assess healing progress. Unstable and displaced fractures should be referred immediately to an orthopedist for possible open reduction and internal or external fixation. Associated carpal instability and potential for nonunion or avascular necrosis makes early follow-up imperative.

## OTHER CARPAL FRACTURES

Most other carpal fractures are rare and sometimes occur in conjunction with other fractures and ligament injuries.[26,27]

### Triquetrial fractures

**Mechanism of injury.** The most common fractures of the triquetrum involve the dorsal aspect and result from an avulsion stress with the wrist in a hyperextended position at the time of a fall or trauma. Fractures of the body of the bone are frequently associated with other carpal fractures and dislocations, specifically perilunate dislocations. Infrequently, compressive transverse or vertical fractures occur secondary to impingement between the hamate and the distal ulna.

**Clinical findings.** A patient with a triquetrial fracture typically presents complaining of dorsoulnar wrist pain after falling on an outstretched arm and hyperextending the wrist. Tenderness can be elicited over the dorsoulnar aspect of the wrist and should make the examiner suspicious of a triquetrial fracture.

**Radiographic findings.** Anteroposterior views of the wrist may be negative unless a body fracture is present. The most common finding is an avulsion fracture seen dorsally on the lateral wrist view. Use of more oblique views may be useful to project the triquetrum above the lunate and make the avulsion fracture more visible. Figure 13-18 shows an avulsion fracture of the dorsum of the triquetrium.

**Treatment.** Undisplaced fractures can be treated with splint immobilization until seen by an orthopedic surgeon unless the fracture is associated with other wrist fractures or dislocations.

### Trapezium fractures

**Mechanism of injury.** The trapezium fracture represents about 5% of all carpal fractures. The most common fracture is a longitudinal fracture with an associated radial dislocation of the first metacarpal. The mechanism is a blow to the thumb with hyperabduction, or a fall on a radially deviated wrist that is also hyperextended, causing the trapezium to be trapped between the base of the first metacarpal and the radial styloid.[27] A trapezial ridge frac-

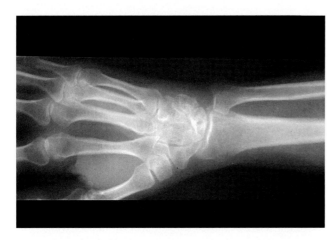

**Fig. 13-17.** The typical radiographic findings of osteosclerosis in Kienböck's disease that represent post-fracture bone changes in the lunate after avascular necrosis has occurred and healed.

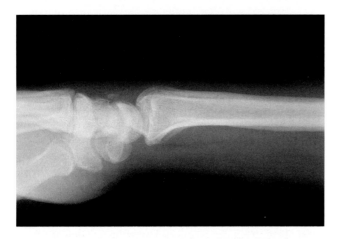

**Fig. 13-18.** An avulsion fracture of the triquetrum seen only in the lateral view just above the dorsal and distal aspect of the lunate.

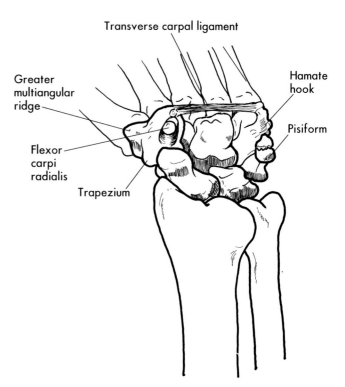

**Fig. 13-19.** A carpal tunnel view can be helpful in appreciating subtle fractures of the carpus. This view can show trapezial ridge fractures as well as fractures of the pisiform and the hook of the hamate.

ture is also common. This fracture results from direct trauma to the ridge area or can occur secondary to an avulsion mechanism produced by traction by the transverse carpal ligament.

**Clinical findings.** Patients with trapezium fractures will present with a history of a fall on the outstretched forearm with wrist in extension. Local tenderness will be present at the base of the thenar eminence and if the wrist is flexed against resistance, pain will result. Occasionally these fractures will have associated carpal tunnel syndrome.

**Radiographic findings.** Longitudinal fractures and associated subluxation of the base of the first metacarpal are seen on plain AP views of the wrist. Trapezial ridge fractures may only be appreciated on a carpal tunnel view (Fig.13-19).

**Treatment.** Displaced fractures of the trapezium with associated metacarpal subluxation require open reduction and pin fixation of the fragments. Trapezial ridge fractures heal poorly, must be treated with a carpal tunnel–release procedure (if this is present), and have had to be excised for

chronic pain problems secondary to poor healing. Simple immobilization of these fractures in a volar splint and referral to an orthopedist will suffice when this fracture is encountered in the emergency setting.

### Trapezoid fractures

Fracture of the trapezoid, the most protected and least-fractured bone of the wrist, is extremely rare and is usually seen with associated with proximal injuries to the second metacarpal.

**Mechanism of injury.** Forces applied longitudinally by the second metacarpal (similar to the mechanism of injury of the trapezium) are postulated as the mechanism for trapezoid fracture. Dorsal dislocation is possible with rupture of the intrinsic ligament connections.

**Clinical findings.** Patients with trapezoid fracture have experienced trauma that causes a longitudinal force on the second metacarpal. Patients present with tenderness over the base of the second metacarpal area, and prominence in that area may represent a dislocation dorsally.

**Treatment.** Unstable fractures and dislocations may require orthopedic referral for ORIF. Nondisplaced fractures should be placed in volar splint and referred for follow-up and final casting.

### Capitate fractures

The literature is variable in reporting capitate fractures as representing 1% to 14% of carpal fractures. Very few capitate fractures have been reported in children.[28] These occur most commonly in association with other carpal injuries, especially scaphoid fractures and perilunate dislocations.

**Mechanism of injury.** Isolated capitate fracture is rarely reported because of its central and relatively protected position between the carpus and the proximal metacarpals. Several mechanisms result in varying degrees of injury. Direct injury to the dorsum of the wrist may injure the capitate solely, whereas a fall on the wrist in dorsiflexion may result in a lesser arc injury and fracture of the scaphoid and capitate without dislocation. More force may cause a perilunate dislocation and fracture through the neck of the bone. A palmar flexion injury may result in associated fracture and displacement of the second and third metacarpals with capitate fracture. Because the blood supply enters at the waist of the capitate, proximal pole fractures can potentially develop avascular necrosis and nonunion. There are four reports of capitate fractures in small children, one of which was in a 10-year-old boy with a hyperextension injury secondary to a fall.[29]

**Clinical findings.** Tenderness over the middorsal wrist and pain on dorsiflexion are the only physical examination clues to capitate fracture. If a scaphoid fracture is present or suspected, the physician should assess for associated capitate fracture.

**Radiographic findings.** Capitate fractures may be diagnosed on plain radiographs, especially in the AP view, but oblique views and tomograms may be necessary to demonstrate more subtle pathology.

**Treatment.** Undisplaced, isolated capitate fractures can be treated initially by short-arm splinting followed several days later by application of a short-arm cast. Displaced fractures require open reduction and internal fixation. Scaphocapitate syndromes will always require open reduction because of rotation of the proximal capitate fragment and associated carpal instability.

### Hamate fractures

Hamate fractures are reported to occur in approximately 1% to 6% of wrist fracture series.[5] The bone is triangular in shape and has a volar hook or hamulus on it, which can be fractured easily.

**Mechanism of injury.** The most common mechanism of injury is that of a fracture to the hook or hamulus that occurs from a direct blow to the palm from an object such as a racquet, golf club, bat, or from a fall on the palmar surface of the hand. The fracture is created by stress transmitted by the volar transverse carpal ligament, the pisohamate ligament, and by force of the blow through the hypothenar eminence. Longitudinal forces, such as a fist against a hard object, along the fifth metacarpal can cause a dorsal fracture-dislocation of the metacarpal with a fragment of the distal hamate. Direct blows can cause body fractures as well as dislocations.

**Clinical findings.** Patients with fractures of the hook of the hamate will present with pain over the hypothenar eminence and will have a history of the pain occurring during racket sports, golf or baseball games, either from just swinging hard and miss-hitting, or from striking the palm during a fall. Body fractures may present with dorsoulnar wrist pain and these patients have a history of striking something with a clenched fist. Difficulty with gripping and pain with wrist rotation may be present. Ulnar nerve impingement has been reported, as well as sensory changes, tendon injuries, and secondary tendinitis.

**Radiographic findings.** Routine radiographic views may show fractures of the body of the hamate but may fail to demonstrate fractures of the hamulus or hook. A special view with the wrist in extreme dorsiflexion and the tube angle at 25° from the plane of the palm shot down the carpal tunnel will show this fracture well. Sometimes special oblique views will demonstrate the fracture, but they are unreliable.

**Treatment.** Fractures of the hook of the hamate should be splinted for comfort and sent to orthopedics for definitive care—which may include excision because of a high incidence of nonunion and chronic pain. Displaced body fractures and associated carpal dislocations require immediate orthopedic referral for open reduction and internal fixation. Nondisplaced fractures require initial splinting and casting after swelling is resolved.

### Pisiform fractures

Again, these fractures are quite uncommon and are usually hard to diagnose initially upon presentation to the emergency department because radiographs may be negative.

**Mechanism of injury.** Almost universally, pisiform fractures result from a fall onto the palm, and because they are contained within the tendon substance of the flexor carpi ulnaris, displacement is uncommon. Fractures are usually avulsion type or are vertical in orientation.

**Clinical findings.** A patient, who has fallen and struck the palmar surface of the hand, complaining of and evidencing hypothenar eminence pain should be suspected of having a pisiform fracture.

**Radiographic findings.** Lateral projections of the wrist or carpal tunnel views will demonstrate these fractures. They are difficult to see on plain films. Avulsion fractures may be seen on the true lateral radiographs. Figure 13-20 demonstrates a fracture through the body of the pisiform in a patient who fell onto his palm during a basketball game.

**Treatment.** Splinting for comfort is initially the treatment of choice. The fracture is stable and immobilization for 3 to 6 weeks in a short-arm cast is recommended. Nonunion and chronic pain are indications for excision similar to the treatment of hamulus fractures.

## DISLOCATIONS AT THE WRIST
### Perilunate and lunate dislocations

These injuries are an extension of lesser-arc injuries through the wrist that first cause carpal instability in the form of scapholunate instability and continue on to cause severe disruption of the midcarpal joint. Formerly, these injuries were divided into two separate entities, but research

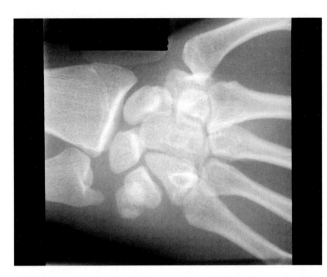

**Fig. 13-20.** A pisiform fracture in a basketball player who had fallen onto his palm during a game. The fracture line is seen on the outer edge of the pisiform and is almost obscured by the triquetrum.

has shown they are a part of a spectrum of injury secondary to extreme forces transmitted through the wrist.

**Mechanism of injury.** Mayfield[30] defined four stages of perilunar instability and ultimate dislocation at the midcarpal joint. The injury occurs in extreme hyperextension, ulnar deviation, and midcarpal joint dorsiflexion. During the first stage, scapholunate instability occurs as the scapholunate interosseous ligaments and the radioscaphoid ligaments are torn. If forces also propagate along the greater arc, this stage can also cause an associated scaphoid fracture (eg, dorsal transscaphoid perilunate dislocation). The second stage, dorsal perilunate dislocation, occurs as the capitate dislocates dorsally from its articulation with the lunate at the midcarpal joint. The third stage occurs when attachments of the lunate and the triquetrum are disrupted as the perilunate dislocation progresses. If greater arc forces are present, an avulsion fracture of the triquetrum occurs; the injury is described as a transtriquetrial perilunate dislocation. This can be with or without an associated fracture of the scaphoid or the capitate (eg, transtriquetrial, transscaphoid perilunate dislocation and the transtriquetrial, scaphocapitate syndrome with perilunate dislocation). The fourth stage is volar dislocation of the lunate. Mayfield views perilunate and lunate dislocations as progressions of the same process and mechanism. With hyperflexion injuries or the reverse mechanism as described previously, both volar perilunate and dorsal lunate dislocations are possible but are very rare.[27] Because of the extreme disruption of the joint, median and ulnar nerve entrapment with carpal and ulnar tunnel symptoms are possible. Tendon entrapment is also possible. These injuries have been reported in children, but are extremely rare.

**Clinical presentation.** Patients with these injuries will have a history of a high-energy mechanism such as a fall from a motorcycle or from a height. Dorsal perilunate

dislocations with or without a lunate dislocation result from landing on the forearm with the wrist in extreme hyperextension. There is visible deformity with a silverfork type configuration similar to a displaced distal radius fracture. The patient holds his or her fingers in slight flexion and experiences extreme pain with attempts to extend them. Paresthesia may be present over either the median nerve distribution or the ulnar distribution. Mechanisms and presentation of volar perilunate dislocations and dorsal lunate dislocations are the opposite. For whatever reason, the patient's wrist is hyperflexed at the time of the injury. The wrist may appear to have shape similar to a Smith fracture (ie, garden-spade deformity). Nerve injury may be less common secondary to their volar position and less tension on the nerves as the deformity progresses. The high-energy nature of these injuries dictates that some will be open fractures with extreme disruption of soft tissues and carpal ligament attachments.

**Radiographic findings.** Radiographic findings with perilunate dislocation are not difficult to recognize as long as the physician is familiar with the normal relations of the carpus. Figure 13-21B shows a radiograph of a dorsal perilunate dislocation. The AP view of the wrist will show what at first may seem like a jumble of bones, as the normal arcs and relationships between the lunate, scaphoid, and capitate have been changed by the dislocation. In volar dislocations, this radiographic finding has been called the crowded carpal sign[31] and represents the distal carpal row overriding the proximal carpal row. The lateral view is more revealing in that the physician can see the capitate's convex proximal surface dorsally or volarly displaced out of the concavity of the distal lunate. The hand distal to the midcarpal joint will be seen displaced entirely dorsal or volar to the axis of the radius. Greater (bony) arc injuries may have associated fractures of the scaphoid and the triquetrum, which can be seen on the AP and lateral respectively.

Lunate dislocations are best seen in the lateral view that will show the lunate to be volarly or dorsally displaced in relation to the lunate fossa of the radius, and not associated with the proximal surface of the capitate. The lunate in this volar position has been described as a spilled teacup.[8] Figure 13-21A is a radiograph showing the volar position and spilled tea-cup description of a lunate dislocation.

**Treatment.** Treatment of perilunate dislocations without associated fracture can be managed by closed reduction through complete muscular relaxation, although a regional block or general anesthesia is required. Because of the complexity of these injuries, orthopedic consultation is a necessity to assure that complications such as other subluxations, fractures, and ligamentous instabilities are identified and treated. Needless to say, open fractures require immediate operative intervention. Perilunate dislocations fall into two large groups: closed dislocations, which autoreduce or are easily reduced, and complicated dislocations, which are open, irreducible, or unstable after initial reduction. Many

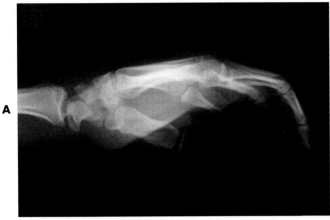

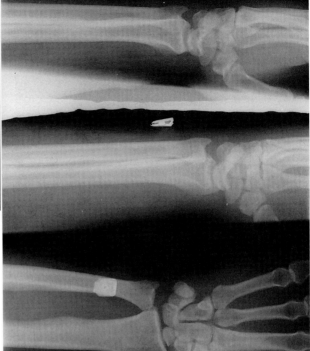

Fig. 13-21. A, Volar lunate dislocation—the spilled tea cup depiction of this type of dislocation. B, A radiograph of a dorsal, perilunate dislocation shows the capitate to be dislocated dorsally above the lunate and the lunate is still in the lunate fossa of the radius. Note that in the lateral view, the hand appears to be normal beyond the articulation of the lunate and capitate.

of these dislocations will also have associated neurovascular compromise. Reports of series of these injuries suggest that the majority of these dislocations, even after what appears to be adequate reduction, will be unstable. The forces required to dislocate the midcarpal joint stretch and tear the supporting ligamentous structures between the scaphoid, lunate, capitate, and triquetrum. Therefore, even with what appears to be a perfect reduction, carpal instability frequently results. Many authors believe immediate open reduction, ligament repair, and pinning of these injuries are the treatments of choice. If attempted in the emergency department, closed reduction is accomplished under adequate relaxation with analgesia and conscious sedation. The wrist is placed in a finger trap apparatus and left for 5 to 10 minutes to allow some muscular relaxation and lengthening. The reduction is performed by dorsiflexing the wrist, applying longitudinal and then volar flexion force to allow the capitate to reduce over the dorsal rim of the lunate and fall into its distal concavity. Obviously, the opposite technique is used to reduce a volar perilunate dislocation. Once the reduction is accomplished, special three-point casting is required to maintain the alignment.

Lunate dislocations represent the extreme of the spectrum of these of injuries. Again, because of the associated disruption of supporting ligaments and the high probability of nerve injury, most of these injuries require orthopedic consultation and open reduction with ligament repair and pin stabilization. Closed reduction can be attempted, but complications of ligamentous instability and residual nerve entrapment syndromes may make surgery inevitable. Closed reduction can be attempted by recreating the peri-

lunate dislocation with dorsiflexion of the wrist when simultaneously applying volar-dorsal force to the lunate to reduce it into the lunate fossa of the radius. Once lunate reduction is accomplished, gradual palmar flexion of the wrist reduces the capitate into the concavity of the distal lunate.

Any associated fracture such as that of the scaphoid, capitate, or triquetrum is tantamount to an unstable situation, and if not dealt with, will invariably result in carpal instability. These injuries, which occur through the greater (bony) arc of force, require open reduction and internal fixation.

### Radiocarpal dislocation

An extreme manifestation of high-energy wrist trauma is complete radiocarpal dislocation, either in the more common dorsal direction or the volar direction. These are rare but potentially devastating injuries that disrupt the ligamentous, stabilizing structures of the wrist and usually have associated fractures of the radius and ulna. This injury may be the extreme manifestation of the progression to a lunate and perilunate dislocation.

### Anatomy and mechanism of injury

The proximal carpal row articulates with the radius and ulna at the scaphoid and lunate fossa and the TFCC complex respectively. The joint is stabilized by strong dorsal and volar ligaments that limit the range of motion at the wrist to approximately 70° in either the dorsal or volar direction. Strong volar ligaments arise from the radius to the scaphoid and lunate whereas the weaker dorsal liga-

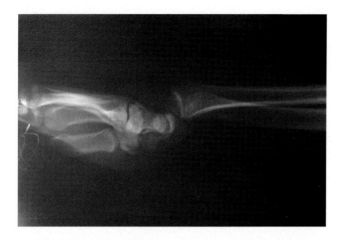

**Fig. 13-22.** A volar radiocarpal dislocation with an associated fracture fragment. The lunate with the rest of the hand attached has been dislocated from the lunate fossa of the radius.

ments go ulnarly from the radius to the triquetrium and prevent radial translocation of the carpus. The ulnocarpal ligament divides into a triquetrial and lunate branch and is an extension of the TFCC. Dorsally, the TFCC is weakly attached to the carpus, and mostly to the triquetrium. Some stabilization is provided by the flexor carpi ulnaris sheath.[2]

The mechanism of injury in this type of dislocation is usually a violent, high-energy force that either places the wrist in extreme dorsiflexion or volarflexion. The dorsal mechanism probably causes a shearing force to be placed by the scaphoid and lunate on the dorsal radius and extreme tension on the volar extrinsic ligaments. With variations in the vector of the force, several things can happen. The Space of Poirer can be opened and enough force can be transmitted to the intrinsic intercarpal ligaments to allow a dorsal perilunate or lunate dislocation. These intercarpal ligaments may remain intact and the entire carpal row will dislocate dorsally over the rim of the radius. There may be associated intercarpal disruption, fracture of the dorsal radius lip or ulnar styloid and rupture of the volar extrinsic ligament system.[32] The most extreme manifestation of the injury involves all of the associated fractures above and intercarpal disruption and volar extrinsic ligament disruption. A similar volar mechanism is described and can have associated radius fractures of the styloid or volar lip, fractures of the ulnar styloid, and intercarpal ligament injuries with associated intercarpal dislocation. Both types of dislocation can have associated median and ulnar nerve injuries; rarely, vascular compromise is possible either secondary to direct injury to the radial or ulnar arteries or because of the extreme swelling.[33]

**Classification.** Patients with radiocarpal dislocation have been classified by Moneim[32] into two therapeutic groups. Type I patients have a radiocarpal dislocation without intercarpal disruption or dislocation. Type II patients have associated intercarpal disruption that Moneim feels is a marker for associated ligament disruption and

ultimate instability and post-reduction complications. Each type of dislocation can have associated fractures of the radius or ulnar styloid and neurovascular complications.

**Clinical presentation.** Radiocarpal dislocation is the result of an extremely high-energy force. These relatively rare injuries are seen in patients with multiple trauma, usually from a fall of some height, a motorcycle accident, or direct crushing-type injury with associated dorsal or volar flexion. The patient complains of severe pain, marked swelling, and possible parethesias in the distribution of the median or ulnar nerves. If the injury is detected early and the swelling is minimal, the dorsal form is similar to Colles fracture with a silverfork appearance. This configuration may be difficult to appreciate if the inevitable massive swelling has occurred. Volar dislocation may resemble a Smith fracture with the typical garden-spade shape. The hand may be swollen and dusky secondary to venous obstruction, or avascular secondary to compromised arterial circulation.

**Radiographic findings.** (Fig. 13-22) The lateral radiograph will be quite revealing, showing the carpus and essentially entire hand either dorsal or volar to the distal radius articulation. The dorsal or volar radial lips may be fractured, but the fracture may be a larger fragment that reminds one of a dorsal or volar Barton fracture. The radial styloid may be fractured and the ulnar styloid is commonly avulsed. The AP radiograph shows ulnar translocation of the carpus with superimposition of the proximal carpal row and the distal radius and ulna. Fractures of the carpus are also possible, so the bones of the proximal carpal row should be scrutinized. Also, carpal instabilities such as scapholunate instability and carpal ring defects causing volar intercalated segment instability (VISI) and dorsal intercalated segment instability (DISI) deformities contribute to the overall morbidity.

**Treatment.** Treatment of type I dislocation is usually closed. The urgency of reduction is in relation to the degree of neurovascular compromise present, but certainly, the sooner reduction is accomplished, the better. Type II dislocations are more complicated, with associated disruption of the carpal relationships, and imply greater ligament injury. Open reduction is therefore considered the treatment of choice, although a type I injury may also require open methods if closed reduction fails. A reasonable approach in the emergency department would be to provide adequate analgesia and conscious sedation and attempt closed reduction under the guidance of an orthopedic surgeon. The reduction can be accomplished with fingertraps and traction or longitudinal traction and manipulation, reversing the deformity and reducing the carpal row back onto the radius. If this is unsuccessful, the patient must go to the operating suite for closed reduction and possible pin fixation. Open reduction and fixation may at this point be necessary. Most of these patients require admission to the hospital to be observed for vascular compromise, and treated for possible associated injuries. After the reduction is accomplished, a long-arm splint or cast is applied.

## Scaphoid dislocation

Isolated scaphoid dislocation is possible but rare.[27] Such injuries may be associated with dislocation of both the scaphoid and lunate as a unit and one report of a transscaphoid-lunate dislocation is in the literature.[27]

**Mechanism of injury.** These injuries may be variants of perilunate- and lunate-type dislocations. Therefore, the postulated mechanism is a fall with high-energy transfer through a dorsiflexed and ulnarly deviated wrist. The scaphoid is forced into the radial styloid and the volar radioscaphoid ligament ruptures with the scaphoid being forced into a volar position. Associated radial styloid fracture is also possible with this injury. Disruption of the blood supply may cause avascular necrosis of the scaphoid, but this is reported as transient; healing usually occurs without residual problems. With severe disruption and volar displacement of the scaphoid, the median nerve may be put under tension in the carpal tunnel. Because the scapholunate and radioscaphoid ligaments are disrupted, scapholunate instability and dissociation occur and residual midcarpal instability ultimately results. Isolated dorsal dislocation is not reported, but is entirely possible.

**Clinical presentation.** Patients with this type of injury will have a history of high-energy injury resulting from a motorcycle accident or fall onto an extended forearm. Patients present with a very swollen, painful wrist and diminished sensation in the distribution of the median nerve (over the thumb and fingers to the radial aspect of the fourth digit).

**Radiographic findings.** Radiographs of the wrist with scaphoid dislocation are abnormal in both the AP and lateral views. An AP view will reveal a space between the radial styloid and scaphoid fossa of the radius and the trapezium, and a vague density of the scaphoid seen behind the capitate's radial border. Even more space and radial translation of the distal carpal row will be seen if the scaphoid and lunate have dislocated as a unit. The lateral radiograph shows a scaphoid that is volar to the capitate and overriding it, resting like a peanut under its volar surface. The scaphocapitate angle will be 0° at this point.

**Treatment.** These complicated injuries should be referred to an orthopedic surgeon as soon as possible. They require early reduction with fixation of pins and ligament repair when necessary to avoid later complications of carpal instability and avascular necrosis. Decompression of the carpal tunnel is also necessary when signs of nerve impingement are present. Closed reduction is accomplished under adequate regional anesthesia or in the operating room under general anesthesia. Longitudinal traction with radial deviation and volar pressure on the subluxed scaphoid reduces it anatomically, but even if normal alignment is present on post-reduction films, residual instability is present and must be addressed.

## Other dislocations of carpal bones

Other carpal bones may be dislocated, but each injury is very rare.[27] The important thing is for the emergency physician to be familiar with the normal anatomy of the wrist and be able to recognize when distortion and displacement of one of the carpus is present. These dislocations are frequently associated with other pathology, specifically with fractures and dislocations of the proximal metacarpals and with fractures of adjacent carpal bones. All of these dislocations and associated fractures require orthopedic consultation and consideration for immediate open reduction and internal fixation.

**Trapezium.** The trapezium can be dislocated both volarly and dorsally, usually as a result of direct trauma to the base of the thumb. Dislocation can occur with simultaneous first metacarpal dislocation or in conjunction with dislocation of the trapezoid and the first and second metacarpal bases. This injury can be reduced closed, but is unstable and usually requires open reduction and internal fixation.

**Trapezoid.** The trapezoid is dislocated after longitudinal force is applied through the second metacarpal; it usually subluxes dorsally. On radiograph, the physician sees misalignment of the base of the second metacarpal and the trapezoid. Dorsal dislocations are reduced closed, whereas a volar dislocation always requires open reduction because of the shape of the bone with its widest portion dorsal to a narrower volar base.

**Hamate.** Hamate dislocation is reported to be rare and occurs mainly in direct trauma and open injuries. Associated injuries include disruption of the hamate and pisiform, along with a dislocation of the fourth and fifth metacarpal bases and with similar disruption including a fracture through the triquetrum (a perihamate, transtriquetrial fracture-dislocation). Open reduction and internal fixation is the treatment of choice for this injury.

**Triquetrial.** Isolated triquetrial dislocation is unusual because of strong ligamentous attachments. When it occurs, the triquetrum dislocates dorsally and can be seen in the lateral or oblique views of the wrist. The treatment goal is stability, particularly on the ulnar aspect of the wrist, which if left unstable due to disruption of the ligamentous connections between the proximal and distal carpal rows, will ultimately result in midcarpal joint collapse into a VISI deformity. These dislocations require open reduction and stabilization with ligament repair.

**Pisiform.** The pisiform is dislocated secondary to longitudinal force along the flexor carpi ulnaris tendon in which it resides. A combination of wrist extension and flexor carpi ulnaris contraction are felt to be the mechanism of most of these injuries. After reduction, recurrent dislocation and chronic pain is very common; definitive treatment is excision.

**Capitate.** Isolated capitate dislocation is extremely rare, but has been reported with an associated open dislocation of the third and fourth metacarpals. Open reduction and internal fixation is the treatment of choice here.

## Carpometacarpal dislocations and fractures excluding the thumb

Acute dislocations of the finger carpometacarpal joints are quite rare and represent less than 1% of hand injuries.[34]

Pure dislocations without associated fracture are even less common. Most dislocations are dorsal as opposed to volar, their orientation determined by the location of the base of the metacarpal in relation to its articulation with the carpal bone. Multiple dislocation is more common than single dislocation. The most common single proximal metacarpal dislocation is the fifth.

**Anatomy and mechanism of injury.** Due to the anatomy of these joints, great force is required to produce these injuries. The second metacarpal articulates with the trapezium radially, the trapezoid centrally, and the capitate ulnarly, with facets that match the surfaces of these carpus.[35] The third metacarpal articulates with the capitate and has a dorsoradial styloid that resists dorsal motion of the joint. Attached by volar and dorsal ligaments and strong transverse intercarpal ligaments, the second and third carpometacarpal joints have minimal motion with a range of 1° to 3° and form a rigid axis about which the first, fourth, and fifth metacarpals rotate when grasping and flattening of the palm occur. The fourth and fifth carpometacarpal joints are more mobile but are strongly attached to the carpus by ligamentous structures. Consequently, these joints are still limited to a range of motion of 25° for the fifth metacarpal and 15° for the fourth.[36] Slight rotation of the fifth carpometacarpal joint is also possible. The fourth metacarpal base articulates with the hamate on a radial facet, and the fifth metacarpal base articulates with the ulnar aspect of the bone. Besides the intrinsic system of intercarpal and dorsal and volar ligaments, the metacarpal bases are stabilized by extrinsic structures. The second metacarpal has insertions for the flexor carpi radialis and the extensor carpi radialis longus. The extensor carpi radialis brevis inserts into the third metacarpal. The fifth metacarpal base is stabilized by the extensor carpi ulnaris and the flexor carpi ulnaris. The exact mechanism of dislocation of the carpometacarpal joints remains obscure, and attempts to consistently reproduce these types of injuries have uniformly failed. Postulated mechanisms for dorsal dislocation include longitudinal force combined with a levering-type vector that disrupts the stabilizing ligaments with or without a fracture of the bone.[36] Another proposed mechanism is that of a dorsally applied force on a flexed wrist that causes a dorsal dislocation. Ironically, the same mechanism has been reported to cause a volar dislocation.[35] The fifth carpometacarpal joint is unique in that it has more mobility and is somewhat less stable than the others. The fifth metacarpal's articulation with the hamate is along a sloping, oblique line and this combined with the pull of the extensor carpi ulnaris, causes dislocations and fractures of the joint to be inherently unstable once the ligamentous structures have been disrupted. The joint is vulnerable not only to the above mentioned forces, but is also more exposed to direct trauma from the ulnar side of the hand. Commonly, the dislocation of the fifth metacarpal base has an associated fracture similar to a Bennett fracture of the thumb metacarpal. Any patient who presents with any metacarpal fracture should be

considered to have an associated adjacent carpometacarpal dislocation until the contrary is proven. Much as the well-known Monteggia and Galleazi fractures of the forearm are produced, fractures of the adjacent metacarpals shorten that segment of the hand and stress and can dislocate the carpometacarpal joint. Carpometacarpal joint (CMC) dislocations are almost always the result of high-energy trauma such as falls from a height, motor vehicle and motorcycle accidents, and machinery injuries that crush and torque the extremity. Kerr[37] reported a hamate fracture and dorsal dislocation of the fourth and fifth CMC joints, the mechanism being a clenched-fisted punch thrown at a brick wall. Other reported causes include karate blows, a lacrosse-stick injury, crushing blows, or a baseball injury.

**Classification.** The only classification system found in the literature is one that addresses the fifth metacarpal base dislocations with associated fourth metacarpal shaft fracture. The class of fracture and therapeutic considerations are dictated by the presence or absence of an associated hamate fracture and by the fracture type.[37] Type Ia lesions have a pure dislocation of the fifth metacarpal at the hamate. Type Ib have a subluxation with a small rim of fracture off of the hamate. Type II injuries have CMC dislocation with associated hamate dorsal rim fracture, and type III lesions have coronal splitting of the hamate.

**Clinical presentation.** The clinical presentation of these injuries varies according to the mechanism of injury and the time of presentation. Usually, unless the injury is quite recent, the patient presents with a markedly swollen hand and quite a bit of pain that is out of proportion to the apparent injury. Shortening of the corresponding finger of the metacarpal involved may be present as well as swelling and tenderness over the CMC joint area. A prominence associated with the dislocated metacarpal base or bases may be palpated, despite the swelling and is appreciated dorsally or volarly, according to the dislocation type. The ulnar nerve can be injured because of this displacement which can then put traction on the nerve, resulting in paresthesias of the ulnar aspect of the fourth digit and of the entire fifth digit. Weakness of the interossei muscles may also be apparent. Median nerve and associated tendon injuries are other reported soft-tissue trauma. Massive hand trauma resulting from motor vehicle accidents, industrial machine accidents, and crush injuries by massive objects may be a clue to these injuries, especially when multiple metacarpals are involved. The patient invariably gives a history of a high-energy mechanism with these dislocations. The most common mechanisms cited include motorcycle accidents, industrial accidents, clenched-fist blows, and falls from a significant height.

**Radiographic findings.** The standard AP, true lateral, and oblique radiographs should be obtained initially. These films will usually reveal the dislocation or will be abnormal enough to arouse suspicion of a significant injury to the carpometacarpal area. The true lateral film will usually show the dislocation, because the involved metacarpal's base will be seen either dorsal or volar to its articulation with the carpal bones. The reference carpal bone is the capitate, which is easily seen in the lateral view and should have a longitudinal axis in direct line with the metacarpal's longitudinal axis and the center of the base. In the lateral view, all metacarpal shafts should be essentially parallel in orientation. Parkinson[1] suggests that angles between the metacarpals in the true lateral view greater than 10°, especially when comparing the second and fifth metacarpals, are diagnostic of CMC dislocation. Figure 13-23 demonstrates this relationship. Figure 13-23 shows three views of a hand with dislocation of the fourth and fifth CMC joints. Fisher[38] described several markers for the radiologic diagnosis of CMC dislocation. The CMC joints as seen in the AP view should all have parallel articular surfaces and the width of the second through fifth joint spaces should be not greater than 1 to 2 mm. The articulation of the CMC joints from the second to the fifth joint describes parallel lines in the shape of the letter M. If these relationships are distorted, CMC dislocation must be ruled out. Finally, apposing surfaces at the articulations in a true AP view do not overlap. Overlapping at these articulations, unless the hand was not perfectly flat on the radiograph cassette, is indicative of CMC pathology and likely dislocation.

**Treatment.** These relatively uncommon injuries are treated in various manners; literature does not absolutely support any one approach. There is no controversy about the fact that closed reduction should be attempted in all cases. This attempt proves one of two things: if the dislocation is reducible and stable, and if percutaneous pin stabilization or open reduction and fixation will be necessary. Initially, the patient should be assessed for complications such as ulnar nerve injury or vascular compromise. If any deficit is present, immediate orthopedic consultation should be obtained. In most cases, these injuries are so potentially complex, consultation is a requirement. Certainly, open fracture dislocations and injuries that dislocate more than one metacarpal are treated by open reduction and internal fixation. Uncomplicated dislocations and fracture dislocations can be managed in the emergency department by closed reduction and if proven to be unstable, by percutaneous pin fixation. The literature suggests that most of these are unstable and will recur if not fixed in some manner, although there have been successful closed reductions followed by casting that have stayed in place. This management approach requires close follow-up.[35]

The reduction is accomplished by creating longitudinal traction with one hand and placing the other fingers over the subluxed metacarpal head. When the traction is being applied, the metacarpal head is then reduced back into its position in the anatomic CMC joint. Reduction may be unsuccessful, due to numerous factors including massive swelling, interposed bone or tendon, and other soft tissue. A splint is placed to hold the reduction until the patient can be evaluated by an orthopedist. Usually, an ulnar gutter splint

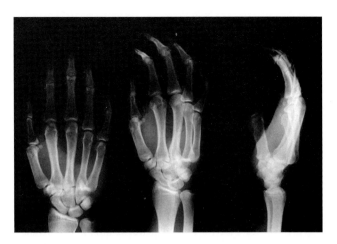

**Fig. 13-23.** Three radiographs showing carpometacarpal dislocation of the fourth and fifth metacarpal bases. Note the angulation between the second and third, and fourth and fifth metacarpals. In a normal hand, the lateral view would show them to be nearly parallel.

or a dorsal-volar splint will suffice until more definitive care can be rendered and until maximal swelling has occurred.

### Ulna dislocations and distal radioulnar joint injuries

Injuries to the ulnar side of the wrist can be as simple as a sprain or as complicated as disruption of the triangular fibrocartilage complex and dislocation of the ulna. There can also be associated carpal fractures, instability of the carpus, and radioulnar joint instability. Patients who complain of pain, either acute or chronic, along the ulnar aspect of the wrist should be evaluated for tears and instability of the joint. These injuries are seen with radius pathology such as Colles- and Smith-type fractures.

**Anatomy and mechanism of injury.** The distal ulna articulates at the sigmoid notch, a groove on the ulnar aspect of the radius' dorsolateral surface. Some movement of the joint is allowed when supination and pronation of the wrist is initiated. This joint (the DRUJ) is stabilized by fibers of the TFCC, a confluence of ligaments that begin on the radius and bridge to the head of the ulna and attach at the base of the ulnar styloid. The ligaments that span the DRUJ form an articular disc that is the main TFCC contribution to the stability of the joint. Fibers sweep from this area along the ulnar styloid to attach to the triquetrum and hamate. Other stabilizing components include the dorsal and volar radioulnar ligaments, the ulnar collateral ligament, and the meniscus homologue on the ulnar aspect of the structure. The extensor carpi ulnaris, as it passes dorsally and radially to the ulnar styloid, also provides support to the joint.

Injury to this area is dependent on the force applied, including its magnitude and vector, and is also a function of the position of the wrist at the time of injury. A fall with the wrist extended is one possible mechanism for dorsal dislocation, whereas the opposite may be true for a volar mechanism, although a direct blow is more likely in this injury. Rotation at the joint is another postulated mechanism. Rotational injuries occur when the hand is fixed and the forearm is acutely rotated about its axis. The force must be sufficient to tear the articular disc area and thus, disrupt the TFCC, to dislocate the ulna. Isolated tears of the dorsal and volar ulnocarpal ligaments is not sufficient to produce the injury.[39] If the ulnar styloid is fractured through its base, a tear of the TFCC is very probable and if displaced, is an indication for operative repair.

**Clinical presentation.** Patients with ulnar dislocations present to the emergency department with a complaint of wrist pain and describe symptoms of a sprain. The wrist is painful and swollen, especially on the ulnar aspect. Supination and pronation are very painful. With dorsal dislocation, the patient holds the wrist in pronation; with volar dislocation, the wrist is held in supination. The history is that of a direct blow over the ulnar wrist, a fall from a significant height on an extended or flexed wrist, or a fall with the wrist fixed in position and the body rotating about it. The classic injury described with this mechanism is a catapulting injury off of a motorcycle with a rotation of the body when the hands continue to grip the handlebars. Point tenderness and fullness in the dorsoulnar aspect of the wrist or on the volar-ulnar aspect of the wrist will be present. Patients presenting with a chronically tender wrist along the ulnar aspect may have had a partial tear of the TFCC that will require follow-up and repair. Many of these are misdiagnosed as simply a sprained wrist and repair is only done months to years later when the patient can stand the pain no longer. Some of these tears are not a result of acute trauma, but are degenerative in nature.

**Radiographic findings.** A true lateral radiograph of the wrist must be obtained to determine dislocation of the ulna. Because of pain, the patient may not be able to supinate or pronate well enough to get this view and diagnosis may depend on history, physical examination, and other imaging techniques. If the true lateral is obtained, the ulna in a dorsal dislocation will be seen as dorsal to the top border of the radius, to which it is usually superimposed on the view. Volar displacement will be obvious as well, in that the ulna will appear to align with the volar border of the radius or may even be inferior to it. CT has been found to be a superior imaging technique to the plain radiograph in demonstrating this injury. CT scan easily shows the wrist in cross-section and demonstrates the volar or dorsal displacement of the ulna from the sigmoid notch of the distal radius. The magnetic resonance imaging (MRI) scan can show the triangular fibrocartilage complex and can demonstrate tears and other pathology without using an invasive method such as arthrography.

**Treatment.** Dorsal dislocations of the ulna can be reduced with supination and can usually be done closed with the patient's arm placed in a long-arm cast in full supination. Volar dislocations are reducible with pronation and manipulation but frequently require open reduction because the ulna is caught under the volar surface of the radius. If reduced in a closed manner, a long-arm cast or splint with the forearm in pronation is applied. Dislocations of the ulna imply a rupture of the triangular fibrocartilage complex; if marked displacement has occurred, it is an indication for open reduction and repair. The repair can also guarantee that the DRUJ is intact and stable. Complications include paresthesia secondary to injury of the ulnar nerve. This sensory change involves the lateral half of the fourth finger and the entire fifth finger. These symptoms are usually not a sign of a permanent injury and resolve with time. The prognosis is good for these injuries, but chronic pain secondary to a nonhealing TFCC occurs.

## OTHER CAUSES OF WRIST PAIN
### Carpal instability

The emergency physician treating a wrist injury should be wary of diagnosing a wrist sprain in any patient with significant tenderness or swelling. In recent years, serious instabilities of the carpal joints have been described with no associated fracture and represent an intermediate but just as devastating injury, especially as it relates to long-term disability. These instabilities have been classified in a very complex system (Table 13-4) that is beyond the scope of this book; however, the important point is that a normal radiograph of a painful wrist does not guarantee that significant injury has been spared. Disruption of the ligaments and the functional relationships of the carpus can cause serious wrist dysfunction if not recognized and treated properly.[30]

**Anatomy and mechanism of injury.** The carpal bones are all connected by strong interosseous ligaments known as the intrinsic ligaments as well as an extensive system of extrinsic ligaments. These connections have enough laxity to permit the carpus to form a dynamic joint but provide enough stability to allow only certain ranges of motion so that other movements of the wrist and fingers can be accomplished in a controlled manner. The carpal bones are arranged in a proximal and distal row that articulate at the midcarpal joint between the lunate and capitate. The connections between the two rows (on the radial side, through the scaphoid; on the ulnar side, through the triquetrum) form a functional ring that, when moved by extrinsic muscle action, allows the midcarpal joint to flex and extend within certain limits. Traumatic injuries that disrupt this system of ligaments allow abnormal motions of the involved carpal bones, which can cause chronic pain with motion and collapse of the joint with motion. Sometimes what appears to be an isolated carpal injury will have an associated carpal instability with a ligament tear, and healing of the fracture does not solve the entire problem. A fracture of the scaphoid can produce such a lesion in that

**Table 13-4.** Classification of carpal instabilities

| Perilunar instability | Midcarpal instability | Proximal carpal instability |
|---|---|---|
| Lesser arc injuries<br>Scapholunate with DISI<br>Triquetrolunate with VISI<br>Complete dorsal or volar<br>Perilunate dislocation<br>Greater arc injuries<br>Unstable scaphoid fx.-DISI<br>Naviculocapitate<br>Perilunate dislocations:<br>  transscaphoid type<br>  transtriquetral type | Midcarpal instability<br>Volar midcarpal joint<br>Dorsal midcarpal joint<br>Displaced distal radius fracture | Dorsal or volar instability at the radiocarpal joint secondary to a Colles or Barton fracture |

the stability of the midcarpal joint is compromised and a deformity of the joint occurs with the lunate becoming volar-flexed and the midcarpal joint collapsing in that direction. This is a VISI deformity. The reverse can also occur with disruption of the supporting ligaments between the triquetrum and its connections with the distal and proximal carpal rows. With this injury, the lunate dorsiflexes and the capitate moves more volarly as the midcarpal joint collapses into a DISI deformity. Another common injury is disruption of the ligaments between the lunate and scaphoid. This is called a *scapholunate dissociation.* Many other less-common instabilities have been described.

**Clinical presentation.** The patient usually presents with a history of wrist trauma, usually secondary to a fall that occurred acutely or a remote injury, and complains of pain in the wrist of some duration. There may or may not be swelling, depending on the timing of the injury. If carefully palpated, tenderness can be elicited over the ligament injured. Injuries to the scapholunate side of the carpal ring usually have tenderness over the anatomic snuff-box and over the area just distal to the Lister tubercle on the radius. Tenderness distal to the ulnar head may indicate disruption of the ring in the triquetrohamate and triquetrolunate areas. If the physician examines the tender area during passive or active motion of the wrist, the bones may be felt to shift with a click or clunking sensation as the unstable carpus reduce to their original unsubluxed position. Tests that can be performed to determine these ligament injuries are termed *shift tests* that may reveal dorsal, volar, medial, or lateral shifts which demonstrate abnormal movements of the carpal rows and relations.

**Radiographic findings.** Wrist radiographs may be within normal limits despite the presence of a carpal instability problem. Scapholunate instability may be seen as a slight, greater than 2-mm widening of the joint between the two bones. A clenched-fist view of the wrist may enhance the radiograph findings of scapholunate instability. The lateral views of the wrist may reveal a VISI that has the lunate

volarflexed and the articulating capitate following it in a more volar direction. The DISI is also seen in these views and is diagnosed by noting the lunate dorsiflexed with its concave articulation and the capitate pointing dorsally. There may be the previously discussed carpal fractures and dislocations that have a high association of carpal instability. This should alert the physician to carefully search for these instabilities when carpal fractures and/or dislocations are present. MRI, with the ability to visualize not only bone but soft tissue, can be extremely useful in identifying these injuries.

**Treatment.** The physician is quite limited in their treatment options in the emergency department setting. Recognition of carpal instability or probable instability is the real challenge. Most of these problems are not acute at presentation and can be managed with early orthopedic follow-up. A volar splint can be applied for comfort until definitive care is arranged.

## DeQuervain tenosynovitis

DeQuervain tenosynovitis is an inflammatory disorder of unknown etiology that involves the extensor pollicis brevis and abductor pollicis longus tendons of the wrist. Suspected etiologies include minor trauma, overuse and repetitive motion type syndromes, and idiopathic causes. It is confused but not associated with arthritic conditions.

**Diagnosis.** The patient complains of pain over the radial aspect of the wrist and relates that it radiates into the hand and up the forearm. Motion of the thumb is extremely painful. Mild erythema and warmth over the involved tendons may be present and passive motion of the thumb will cause the patient's symptoms to recur. Tenderness is universally present over the affected tendons that traverse the radial styloid area; crepitance may be present with palpation. The Finklestein test can be used to confirm the diagnosis. The patient is instructed to squeeze the thumb in the palm with his fingers and ulnarly deviate his wrist. The presenting pain should be recreated with this maneuver.

**Differential diagnosis.** Other disorders that can be confused with DeQuervain disease include arthritis of the first carpometacarpal joint, fracture of the radial styloid, local cellulitis, tenosynovitis of an infectious etiology such as gonococcal, and a soft-tissue contusion. Occult and any arthritic changes will be present on a radiograph. Patients with gonococcal tenosynovitis may have more diffuse involvement, associated fever, and a history of exposure to a sexually transmitted disease. A very specific history of trauma may be soft-tissue contusion as opposed to DeQuervain.

**Treatment.** Conservative treatment consists of immobilization in a thumb spica splint and use of oral nonsteroidal anti-inflammatory drugs (NSAIDs) for 10 days to 2 weeks. If this is not successful, or more immediate relief is required, injection of steroids into the tendon sheaths and surrounding peritendinous areas is very effective. These injections are most effective if done at the point of maximal tenderness and into the surrounding areas to diffuse the drug into the peritendinous areas.

### Other tenosynovitis

Other tendon sheaths can become inflamed and will be evident by pain elicited by motion involving the particular tendon, local erythema of the skin, and crepitance over the affected tendon. After infectious causes are ruled out, these problems can be resolved with immobilization and anti-inflammatory medication.

### Miscellaneous causes of wrist pain

A multitude of other etiologies of wrist pain occurs and a detailed review of each is beyond the scope of this chapter. The reader is referred to the many good reviews on wrist pain available. Some of the other common causes of wrist pain include carpal tunnel syndrome, neuromas and neuropathies, inflammatory conditions such as arthritis, and neoplasms. Ganglion cysts and bone cysts have been known to cause wrist pain as well.

### DISCUSSION

The wrist is anatomically complex and a good working knowledge of the functional anatomy is necessary to properly evaluate and treat wrist injuries. Mechanism of injury is very important in that a history can point the direction to a specific type of injury. The goal in the diagnosis and treatment of wrist injuries is accurate diagnosis and restoration of all anatomic relationships. Knowledge of the rather arbitrary classifications of fractures and dislocations is not as important as assuring that the above principles are followed. Even when no fracture or dislocation is present radiographically, serious injury in the form of ligamentous instability and resulting dysfunction may be present. The physician should always be wary of the perhaps hasty diagnosis of sprained wrist.

### REFERENCES

1. Parkinson RW, Paton RW: Carpometacarpal dislocation: An aid to diagnosis, *Injury* 23: pp. 187–188, 1992.
2. FitzRandolph RL, Hixson ML, Walker CW, Adams BD: Radiographic and orthopedic evaluation of wrist trauma, *Curr Prob Radiol* 1: pp. 3–39, 1991.
3. Palmer AK: The distal radioulnar joint, *Orthop Clin North Am* 15: pp. 321-335, 1984.
4. Mayfield JK, Johnson RP, and Kilcoyne RF: Carpal dislocations: pathomechanics and progressive perilunar instability, *J Hand Surg* 5: 226–241. 1980.
5. Meyer S: Radiographic anatomy of the wrist, *Semin Roentgenol* 26: pp. 300–317, 1991.
6. Melone CP: Unstable fractures of the distal radius. In Lichtman DM, ed: *The wrist and its disorders.* Philadelphia, WB Saunders, 1987, pp. 160–177.
7. Nathan R, Lester B, and Melone CP: The acutely injured wrist: An anatomic basis for operative treatment, *Orthop Rev* 16: pp. 80–95, 1987.
8. Cooney WP, Linscheid RL, and Dobyns JH: Fractures and dislocations of the wrist. In Rockwood CA, Green DP, Bucholz RW: eds: *Fractures in Adults,* vol I. Philadelphia, JB Lippincott, 1991, pp. 372–414, 563–618.
9. Frykman G: Fracture of the distal radius including sequellae-shoulder-hand-finger syndrome, disturbance of the distal radioulnar joint, and impairment of nerve function: A clinical and experimental study, *Acta Orthop Scand* 108 (supp 1): pp. 1–155, 1967.
10. Abbaszadegan H, Jonsson U: Regional anesthesia preferable for Colle's fracture, *Acta Orthop Scand* 61: pp. 348–349, 1990.
11. Kongsholm J, Olerud C: Neurological complications of dynamic reduction of Colle's fractures without anesthesia compared with traditional manipulation after local infiltration, *J Orthop Trauma* 1: pp. 43–47, 1987.
12. Quinton DN: Local anesthetic toxicity of hematoma blocks in manipulation of Colle's fractures, *Injury* 19: pp. 239–240, 1988.
13. Cooney WP, Dobyns JH, and Linscheid RL: Complications of Colle's fractures, *J Bone Joint Surg* 62A: pp. 613–619, 1980.
14. Louis DS: Barton's and Smith's fractures, *Hand Clin* 3: pp. 399–402, 1988.
15. Thomas FB: Reduction of Smith's fracture, *J Bone Joint Surg* 39B: pp. 463–470, 1957.
16. Helm RH, Tomkin MA: The chauffeur's fracture: simple or complex? *J Hand Surg* 17B: pp. 156–159, 1992.
17. Bassett RL: Displaced intra-articular fractures of the distal radius, *Clin Orthop* 214: pp. 148–152, 1987.
18. Markiewitz AD, Andrish JT: Hand and wrist injuries in the preadolescent and adolescent athlete, *Clin Sports Med* 11: pp. 201–225, 1992.
19. Lesko PD, Georgis T, and Slabaugh P: Irreducible Salter type II fracture of the distal radial epiphysis, *J Ped Orthop* 7: pp. 719–721, 1987.
20. Salter RB, Harris WR: Injuries involving the epiphyseal plate, *J Bone Joint Surg* 45A: pp. 586–622, 1963.
21. Campbell RM: Operative treatment of fractures and dislocations of the hand and wrist region in children, *Orthop Clin North Am* 21: pp. 217–243, 1990.
22. O'Brien ET: Fractures of the hand and wrist region. In Rockwood and Green, eds: *Fractures in Children,* vol III. Philadelphia, JB Lippincott, 1991, pp. 372–414.
23. Gumucio CA et al: Management of scaphoid fractures: A review and update, *South Med J* 82: pp. 1377–1388, 1989.
24. Stern JD, Reitman HS: Fractures of the scaphoid bone, *Postgrad Med* 83: pp. 91–96, 1988.
25. Waeckerle JF: A prospective study identifying the sensitivity of radiographic findings and the efficacy of clinical findings in carpal navicular fractures, *Ann Emerg Med* 16: pp. 733–737, 1987.
26. Botte MJ, Gelberman RH: Fractures of the carpus, excluding the scaphoid, *Hand Clin* 3: pp. 149–161, 1987.

27. O'Brian ET: Acute fractures and dislocations of the carpus. In Lichtman DM, ed: *The wrist and its disorders.* Philadelphia, WB Saunders, 1987, pp. 133–135.

28. Light RL: Injury to the immature carpus, *Hand Clin* 4: pp. 415–424, 1988.

29. Young TB: Isolated fracture of the capitate in a 10-year-old boy, *Injury* 17: pp. 133–134, 1986.

30. Mayfield JK: Patterns of injury to carpal ligaments, *Clin Orthop* 187: pp. 36–42, 1984.

31. Klein MB, Webb LX: The crowded carpal sign in volar perlunar dislocation, *J Trauma* 27: pp. 82–84, 1987.

32. Moneim MS, Bolger JT, Omer GE: Radiocarpal dislocation: Classification and rationale for management, *Clin Orthop* 192: pp. 199–209, 1985.

33. Schoenecker PL, Gilula LA, Shively RA, Manske PR: Radiocarpal fracture-dislocation, *Clin Orthop* 197: pp. 237–244, 1985.

34. Mueller JJ: Carpometacarpal dislocations: Report of five cases and review of the literature, *J Hand Surg* 2A: pp. 184–188, 1986.

35. Bloom ML, Stern PJ: Carpometacarpal joints of fingers: Their dislocation and fracture-dislocation, *Orthop Rev* 12: pp. 77–82, 1983.

36. Rawles JG: Dislocations and fracture-dislocations at the carpometacarpal joints of the fingers, *Hand Clin* 4: pp. 103–112, 1988.

37. Cain JE, Shepler TR, and Wilson MR: Hamatometacarpal fracture-dislocation: Classification and treatment, *J Hand Surg* 12A: pp. 762–767, 1987.

38. Fisher MR, Rogers LF, and Hendrix RW: Systematic approach to identifying fourth and fifth carpometacarpal joint dislocations, *Am J Radiol* 140: pp. 319–324, 1983.

39. Aulicino PL, Siegel JL: Acute injuries of the distal radioulnar joint, *Hand Clin* 7: pp. 283–293, 1991.

# The Thumb

*Cheryl D. Adkinson*

The evolution of the opposable thumb is of utmost significance in the human species.[1,2] Although this important development occurred early in primate evolution, this remarkable organ of manipulation has been perfected in modern humans. The thumb has a saddle joint at its base that allows 45° of rotation; it is divergent enough to carry a strong musculature and long enough to allow a precision grip. It is no wonder that the loss of this dominant digit is considered a 40% to 50% disability.[3] Thumb injuries warrant special attention.

This chapter addresses injuries that are unique to the thumb, are of particular importance to the thumb, or are managed differently than apparently similar injuries to the other phalanges. Injuries to the thumb that are not discussed in this chapter can be assumed to be managed the same as similar injuries to other digits, as detailed in Chapters 15 and 16.

Compared with adults, children sustain fewer thumb fractures and tolerate the injuries better. Children heal faster, have less joint stiffness, and show greater remolding of deformities. If improperly treated, however, some thumb fractures may lead to permanent deformity and disability in children.[4] In this chapter, when there are particular points to be made about thumb injuries in children, these are discussed in the section on that injury, under the subheading "Pediatric considerations." When an injury is not addressed specifically in children, the reader may infer that the injury should be evaluated and treated as it is in adults, or that it is seen so rarely in children that there is not sufficient literature on which to base explicit recommendations.

## SENSORY-MOTOR EVALUATION
### Movements

Rather than being aligned with the fingers, the thumb rests with its flexor surface perpendicular to the flexor surfaces of the fingers. Hence, the movements of the thumb are also perpendicular to the movements of the fingers. That is, *flexion* of the thumb moves it across the palm toward the little finger; *extension* moves the thumb away from the little finger in the plane of the palm; *abduction* describes the thumb moving away from the index finger at right angles to the palm; and *adduction* describes the thumb moving back toward the index finger in the plane at right angles to the palm. The unique movement of the thumb, *opposition*, brings the flexor surface of the thumb into contact with the flexor surfaces of the fingers, and requires a combination of flexion, adduction, and internal rotation.[5] These movements are illustrated in Fig. 14-1.

### Functional testing

Functional testing of the thumb should include testing all movements of the thumb. The degree of normal motion, the muscles responsible for various movements, the peripheral nerve supply, and segmental innervation are listed in Table 14-1.

### Sensory supply

Sensory supply to the thumb is by the C-6 dermatome. Both the radial and median nerves supply sensation to the thumb—the radial nerve to the dorsal surface and the median nerve to the palmar surface (Fig. 14-2). The dorsal digital branches of the radial nerve and the volar digital branches of the median nerve supply sensation along the phalanges of the thumb to its tip (Fig. 14-3).

## ANESTHESIA

Anesthesia in the thumb may be achieved by digital block, metacarpal block, or wrist block of the radial and median nerves. Particularly useful for effective anesthesia of the thumb is a median nerve block at the wrist with a radial wheal. These techniques are described in Chapter 3.

## FRACTURES

Fractures of the thumb metacarpal warrant specific discussion because these fractures are distinctly different than fractures of the other metacarpals.

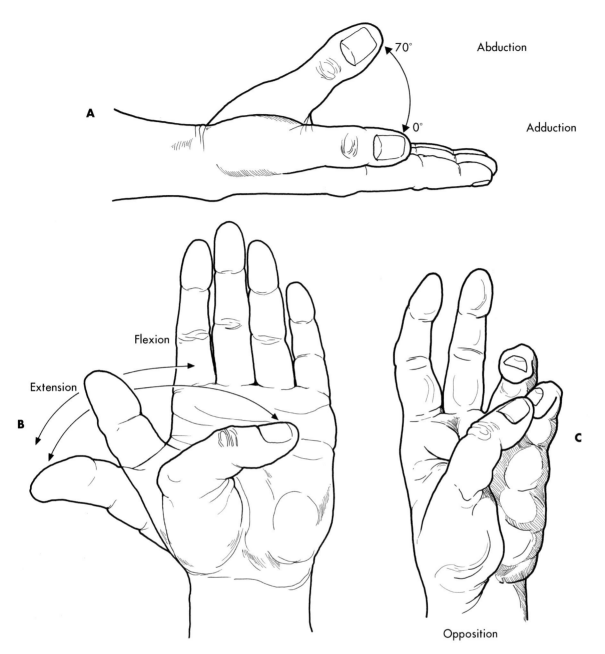

**Fig. 14-1.** Movements of the thumb showing (**A**) abduction/adduction, (**B**) flexion/extension, and (**C**) opposition of the thumb and fifth fingertip.

**Table 14-1.** Functional testing of the movements of the thumb

| | Degrees | Muscle | Nerve | Segmental innervation |
|---|---|---|---|---|
| Metacarpophalangeal joint flexion | 50 | Flexor pollicis brevis | Ulnar, radial | C-6, C-7, C-8 |
| Interphalangeal joint flexion | 90 | Flexor pollicis longus | Median | C-8, T-1 |
| Metacarpophalangeal extension | 0 | Extensor pollicis brevis | Radial | C-7 |
| Interphalangeal joint extension | 20 | Extensor pollicis longus | Radial | C-7 |
| Abduction | 70 | Abductor pollicis brevis | Median | C-6, C-7 |
| | | Abductor pollicis longus | Radial | C-7 |
| Adduction | 0 | Adductor pollicis | Ulnar | C-8 |
| Opposition | NA | Opponens pollicis | Median | C-6, C-7 |
| | | Opponens digiti minimi | Ulnar | C-8 |

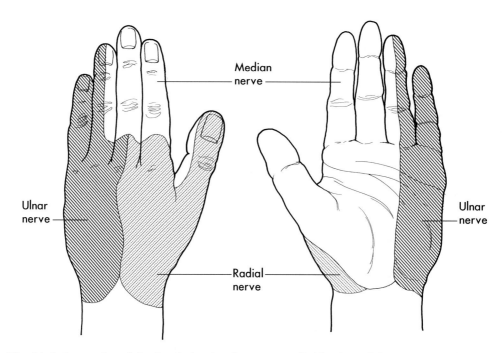

**Fig. 14-2.** Innervation of the thumb showing the areas supplied by the radial nerve and median nerves.

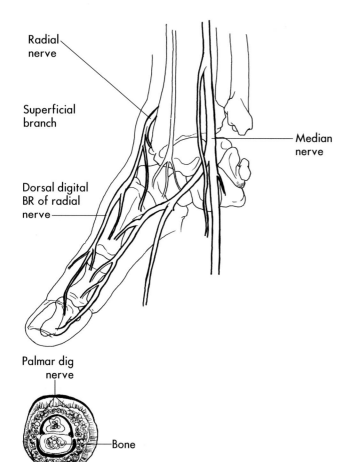

**Fig. 14-3.** Digital nerves of the thumb.

## Metacarpal shaft fractures

Fractures of the shaft of the first metacarpal generally involve the proximal 25% of the bone, and can be seen clearly on routine hand films. The distal fragment is usually adducted and supinated. Treatment involves reducing the fracture by longitudinal traction, with pronation and abduction as needed to correct the angulation. Definitive treatment includes a thumb spica cast for 3 to 4 weeks. Such fractures generally hold their reduction, so operative management is rarely needed. In the emergency setting, a thumb spica splint should be applied and orthopedic follow-up scheduled within a week. Because of the mobility at the carpometacarpal (CMC) joint, some fracture angulation is generally well tolerated.[6]

## Metacarpal base fractures

Most first metacarpal fractures occur at or near the base of the metacarpal. Fracture patterns involving the base of the metacarpal are either intra-articular (Bennett's or Rolando's fractures), extra-articular (transverse or oblique), or, in children, epiphyseal. These four fracture patterns are illustrated in Fig. 14-4. It is imperative to distinguish intra-articular from extra-articular fractures because intra-articular fractures are often unstable and require either pinning after closed reduction or open reduction and internal fixation (ORIF). Extra-articular fractures of the base of the thumb metacarpal are the most common and, fortunately, the easiest to treat. Extra-articular fractures are generally stable after reduction; some angulation is well tolerated.[6]

**Radiologic assessment.** Accurate radiologic assess-

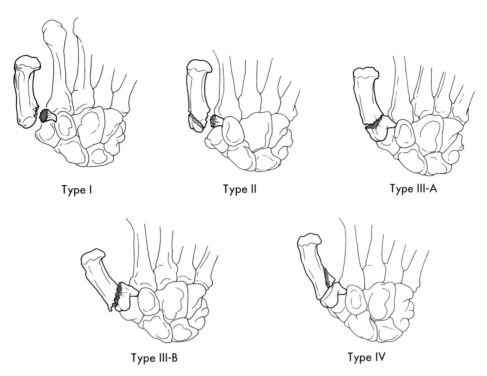

**Fig. 14-4.** Fractures of the base of the thumb occur in four distinct types. Type I (Bennett's fracture-dislocation) and type II (Rolando's fracture) are intra-articular. Type III is extra-articular and may be either (**A**) transverse or (**B**) oblique. Type IV fractures, seen in children, involve injury to the epiphysis.

ment may require a true anteroposterior (AP) and a true lateral view of the metacarpal. Special positioning is necessary to obtain these views. The true AP view (Robert view) is accomplished with the hand in maximal pronation and the dorsal aspect of the metacarpal of the thumb in contact with the x-ray plate. The true lateral view is accomplished by mild hyperpronation of the hand on the x-ray plate (Fig. 14-5). The proper radiographic appearance of these views is also illustrated in Fig. 14-5. Tomograms may be helpful in ascertaining the degree of displacement.[6]

### Intra-articular fractures: Bennett's

*Mechanism.* The usual mechanism for a Bennett's fracture is an axial load to the partially flexed metacarpal. This is a typical position for injuries sustained during fist fights.

*Anatomy.* Bennett's fracture is an intra-articular fracture of the base of the first metacarpal. It is characterized by a small palmar articular fragment that remains in its anatomic position while the metacarpal shaft is displaced in a dorsal-radial direction. The radiographic appearance of a typical Bennett's fracture is illustrated in Fig. 14-6.

*Signs and symptoms/physical findings.* The patient presents with pain, swelling, and limited motion at the base of the thumb metacarpal.

*Radiology.* As noted above, a true AP and a true lateral view may be needed to visualize adequately the Bennett's fracture, and tomograms may be useful as well.

*Definitive treatment.* Many types of splinting, traction, and immobilization have been described to treat this injury. ORIF has become increasingly popular. However, the treatment of choice is attempted closed reduction and percutaneous pinning (Fig. 14-7).[6-8] This is generally accomplished in the operating room with the aid of fluoroscopy, and is followed by immobilization in a short-arm thumb spica cast for 4 to 6 weeks. ORIF is recommended only for cases in which satisfactory closed reduction cannot be achieved.[6-8]

*Emergency management.* Emergency management is prompt orthopedic consultation. If the patient is to be discharged from the emergency department after consultation but before reduction, the fracture should be immobilized in a thumb spica splint.

*Prognosis.* With proper treatment, some limitation of motion may occur, but the incidence of posttraumatic pain is low, and instability is generally not a problem.[7]

### Intra-articular fractures: Rolando's

*Mechanism.* As in Bennett's fracture, the mechanism for the Rolando's fracture is an axial load with the metacarpal in partial flexion.

*Anatomy.* Fortunately, Rolando's fracture (Fig. 14-8) is relatively rare. This fracture, which has numerous variations, is best thought of as a comminuted Bennett's fracture. Its defining characteristic is that, in addition to the small palmar fragment in the Bennett's fracture, there is a large

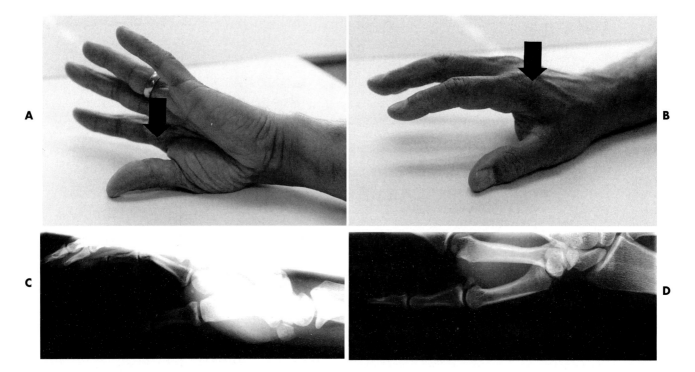

**Fig. 14-5.** Appropriate radiographs for the thumb are the true anteroposterior view (Robert view) and true lateral view. Positions for a true anteroposterior view (**A**) and true lateral view (**B**) are shown. Note that on the true anteroposterior radiograph (**C**) there is no rotation; there is equal concavity on both sides of the phalangeal and metacarpal shafts; and the thumbnail is in the center of the distal thumb. On the true lateral thumb radiograph (**D**), the thumbnail is in profile; the anterior surface of the proximal phalanx is concave; and the phalanges do not appear rotated.

dorsal fragment, creating a T- or Y-shaped fracture at the base of the metacarpal. More typically, the base of the metacarpal is severely comminuted.[7,9]

*Signs and symptoms/physical findings.* The patient with a Rolando's fracture presents with pain, swelling, and limited motion at the base of the first metacarpal.

*Radiology.* As noted above regarding all first metacarpal fractures, a true AP and a true lateral view (Fig. 14-5), may be needed to visualize the Rolando's fracture adequately, and tomograms may be useful as well.

*Definitive treatment.* There are several treatment options for this injury, including closed reduction and immobilization, skeletal traction with early mobilization, soft dressing with early motion, and ORIF. There are no published series comparing outcomes with each of these techniques, but orthopedic texts advise that ORIF is appropriate only for fractures with minimal comminution; more comminuted fractures should be managed closed.[6,7]

*Emergency management.* Because of the variety of treatment options and the poor prognosis of this injury, the emergency physician is advised to obtain prompt orthopedic consultation. If the patient is discharged from the emergency department, the fracture should be immobilized in a thumb spica splint.

*Prognosis.* Prognosis for this injury is poor regardless of method of treatment. Pain, instability, and degenerative arthritis are among the long-term sequelae. Ligament recon-

struction, tendon interposition, and arthrodesis are sometimes used as salvage procedures for chronic problems.[6,7] The patient should be advised of this guarded prognosis.

**Extra-articular fractures**

*Mechanism.* As with intra-articular fractures, an axial load with the metacarpal in partial flexion is the primary mechanism of injury in extra-articular fractures of the thumb metacarpal.

*Anatomy.* Extra-articular fractures of the base of the first metacarpal occur within the joint capsule (Fig. 14-9) but do not involve the articular surface of the joint. It is important to distinguish extra-articular fractures from the intra-articular fractures. Extra-articular fractures are more common and easier to treat. Fractures occurring more distal to the joint capsule are referred to as metacarpal shaft fractures.

*Signs and symptoms/physical findings.* The patient presents with pain and swelling at the base of the thumb metacarpal.

*Radiology.* Extra-articular fractures are either transverse or oblique. It is possible to confuse oblique fractures with intra-articular Bennett's fractures. To avoid this mistake, the radiograph should be inspected carefully to make certain that the fracture does not extend into the joint. Figure 14-10 shows a transverse fracture of the first metacarpal base. If in doubt, true AP and lateral views of the thumb metacarpal should be obtained (Fig. 14-5).

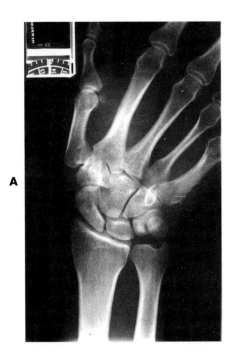

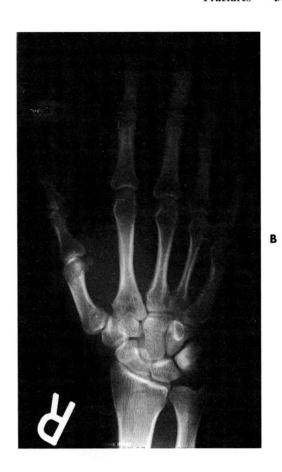

**Fig. 14-6.** Bennett's fracture shown in (**A**) anteroposterior and (**B**) lateral views.

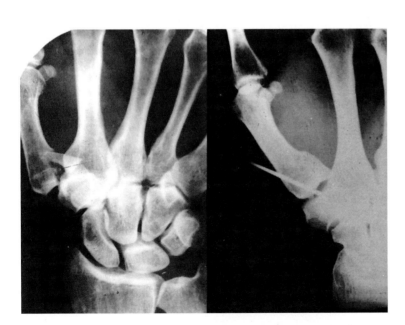

**Fig. 14-7.** Bennett's fracture treated by closed pinning with one Kirschner wire. (From Crenshaw AH, ed. Campbell's Operative Orthopedics, 8th ed. St. Louis: Mosby-Year Book, Inc, 1992.)

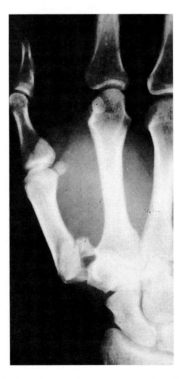

**Fig. 14-8.** Rolando's fracture. (From Crenshaw AH, ed. Campbell's Operative Orthopedics, 8th ed. St. Louis: Mosby-Year Book, Inc, 1992.)

*Definitive treatment.* These fractures generally can be managed by acute closed reduction with the patient under local or regional anesthesia, followed by immobilization in a thumb spica cast for 4 weeks. It is important to avoid hyperextension of the metacarpophalangeal (MP) joint when the plaster is applied. Exact alignment of a transverse fracture need not be achieved. There will be no detectable limitation in range of motion and minimal cosmetic deformity despite 20° to 30° of residual angulation.[7] An oblique fracture that is steeply vertical may be unstable in plaster. If reduction cannot be held in plaster, percutaneous pinning is indicated to secure a closed reduction.[7]

*Emergency management.* Closed reduction with the patient under local or regional anesthesia is appropriate emergency treatment, followed by immobilization in a thumb spica splint. While applying the splint, care should be taken not to hyperextend the thumb at the MP joint. In general, follow-up with an orthopedist is indicated in 1 to 2 weeks. In cases of vertically oriented oblique fractures that may not hold their reduction, and in cases in which alignment after reduction is questionably adequate, orthopedic follow-up should be in 3 to 5 days.

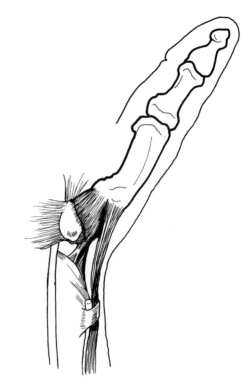

**Fig. 14-9.** Drawing of joint capsule of first metacarpal.

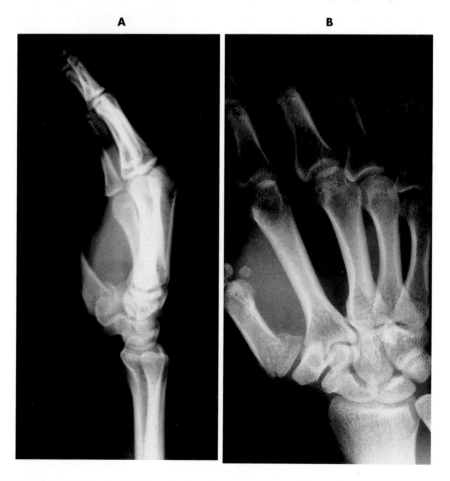

**Fig. 14-10. A,** AP view and, **B,** lateral view of transverse extra-articular fracture of the base of the first metacarpal.

*Prognosis.* Prognosis for this injury is good.

*Pediatric considerations.* The epiphysis of the thumb metacarpal is located at the proximal end of the bone and appears between 24 and 39 months in boys and between 18 and 29 months in girls. Fusion occurs at 16 years in boys and 14 years in girls. A second epiphysis, called a pseudoepiphysis, may appear distally on the metacarpal. This pseudoepiphysis appears earlier than the normal epiphyseal center and often fuses by 6 or 7 years of age. Its only significance is that it must be distinguished from a fracture.[4]

Fractures of the distal portion of the first metacarpal bone are very uncommon in children, whereas fractures of the proximal shaft and metaphysis (base) are quite common. As in adults, they are caused by axial load from a fall or blow. In children, fractures of the proximal end of the first metacarpal bone are classified into four types (Fig. 14-11). Type A is a metaphyseal fracture that is laterally angulated and typically impacted; type B is a Salter-Harris type II fracture that is angulated laterally; type C is a Salter-Harris type II fracture that is angulated medially; and type D is a Salter-Harris type III fracture, which is the pediatric equivalent of a Bennett's fracture.[4]

Type A, B, and C fractures can usually be reduced closed by applying inward pressure at the apex of the angulation and counter-pressure on the metacarpal head. Type C fractures may be more difficult to reduce because the fracture fragment sometimes buttonholes through the periosteum, necessitating open reduction. Once reduced, fracture types A, B, and C should be held in place by a well-molded thumb spica cast.[4]

Type D fractures, the pediatric Bennett's fracture, require surgery for precise reduction. If the fracture is not reduced accurately, the result may be premature closure of the growth plate, with joint deformity and limitation of motion.[4] Orthopedic consultation is advised.

## Phalangeal fractures

Proximal and distal phalangeal fractures of the thumb are evaluated and managed similar to proximal and distal phalangeal fractures of the fingers. The reader is referred to Chapters 15 and 16 for a discussion of these injuries.

## Sesamoid fractures

**Mechanism.** Sesamoid fractures are the result of direct trauma or hyperextension at the MP joint of the thumb. These fractures are rare but should be included in the differential diagnosis of injury to the MP joint of the thumb.[7] Sesamoid bone fractures may be associated with volar plate disruption or with disruption of the accessory collateral ligaments.

**Anatomy.** Sesamoid bones are bones that develop within tendons or ligaments. Almost everyone has two sesamoid bones in the volar plate of the thumb at the MP joint, and most people also have a single sesamoid bone at

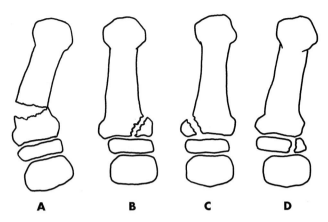

**Fig. 14-11.** Four types of first metacarpal fractures in children. Type A is a metaphyseal fracture; types B and C are Salter-Harris type II physeal fractures with either medial or lateral angulation; type D is a Salter-Harris type III fracture, otherwise known as a pediatric Bennett's fracture.

the interphalangeal (IP) joint of the thumb. The typical radiographic appearance of the sesamoid bones of the thumb is shown in Fig. 14-5. Bipartate sesamoid bones occur in up to 6% of hands. The incidence of bilateral bipartate sesamoid bones of the thumb is unknown.[10] The sesamoids of the MP joint of the thumb are embedded in the fibrous substance of the volar plate. The accessory collateral ligaments insert into the lateral margins of the sesamoids. The tendon of the flexor pollicis brevis inserts into the radial sesamoid and the tendon of the adductor pollicis inserts into the ulnar sesamoid. In the setting of a sesamoid fracture, these muscles separate the fracture fragments by proximal pull.

**Signs and symptoms/physical findings.** Fracture of the sesamoid bones of the thumb is associated with tenderness on the volar aspect of the IP and/or MP joint, with ecchymosis extending into the thenar eminence. Extension, medial stress, and lateral stress at the MP joint may reveal ligamentous instability.[10]

**Radiology.** Fractures of the ulnar sesamoid bone usually may be seen on routine thumb views. To adequately assess the sesamoids, however, radial and ulnar oblique views of the MP joint of the thumb should be obtained. Care should be taken to differentiate fractures from bipartate sesamoid bones. When healthy, these bones have smooth edges, whereas a fractured sesamoid has opposing serrated edges.

**Definitive treatment.** Authors commonly recommend simple immobilization with flexion at the MP joint for 3 to 5 weeks.[7] Surgical repair is reserved for clinical hyperextension instability of the MP joint and open fractures.

**Emergency management.** Care should be taken to assess the integrity of the volar plate and accessory collateral ligaments at the MP joint by stressing these structures. If the joint is stable, the MP should be immobilized in comfortable flexion to approximate the fracture fragments, and orthopedic follow-up in 1 to 2 weeks should be arranged. If the joint is unstable, immediate orthopedic consultation is recommended.

**Prognosis.** The volar plate heals well. Sesamoid fractures generally heal well.

**Pediatric considerations.** Ossification of the sesamoids occurs between 12 and 16 years in boys and 10 and 14 years in girls.[10]

## DISLOCATIONS
### Carpometacarpal dislocations

**Mechanism.** In contrast to the frequent occurrence of fracture-dislocations at the CMC joint of the thumb (eg, Bennett's), pure dislocations at the CMC joint are uncommon. The mechanism of a pure dislocation is the same as that of a fracture-dislocation, ie, a longitudinally directed force applied to the metacarpal in partial flexion. This force levers the base of the metacarpal out of position in a dorsoradial direction. In cases of fracture-dislocations, at least the volar beak of the metacarpal bone breaks off; in the less common pure dislocation, just a tiny fragment of bone may be avulsed off the base of the metacarpal.

**Signs and symptoms/physical findings.** The patient presents with pain, swelling, deformity, and tenderness at the base of the thumb metacarpal.

**Radiology.** This injury is visible on routine films of the hand (Fig. 14-12). If in doubt, true AP and lateral radiographs of the metacarpal should be ordered, as described above and illustrated in Fig. 14-5.

**Definitive treatment.** Treatment of a pure dislocation of the CMC joint of the thumb is surprisingly difficult. There is no agreement on the best approach. Closed reduction is simple but frequently is very unstable. Closed reduction and case immobilization have been successful in cases in which the joint was stable after reduction.[11] Some leading authors recommend closed reduction with the thumb hyperpronated, supplemented by percutaneous Kirschner wires and thumb spica casting for 4 to 6 weeks, followed by cast immobilization for another 4 weeks following wire removal.[7,8] Even with such aggressive management, a good result is not guaranteed.[7] One series

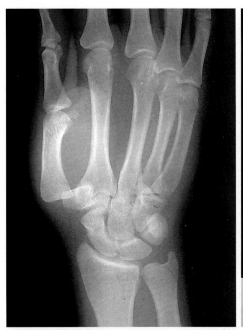
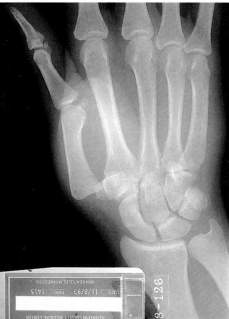
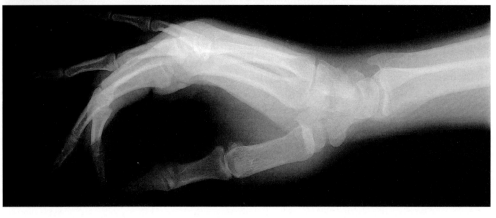

**Fig. 14-12.** Pure dislocation of the carpometacarpal joint of the thumb.

reported the most favorable results when patients were treated on the day of the injury.[11]

**Emergency management.** Appropriate emergency management entails prompt reduction under local or regional anesthesia and splinting in a thumb spica cast. Because percutaneous fixation of this unusual injury is the treatment method preferred by some orthopedists, and because some may wish to accomplish this on the day of injury, consultation should be immediate. Failure to recognize the likely instability of this joint after relocation and to make appropriate arrangements for orthopedic consultation may be associated with a worse-than-necessary outcome. This injury should be considered a high risk for the emergency physician because it *appears* to be easily managed.

**Prognosis.** Prognosis for full recovery is guarded because the joint may sublux or redislocate, despite optimal treatment.

## Metacarpophalangeal dislocations (dorsal)

**Mechanism.** Palmar dislocations are very rare in the thumb MP joint and are not discussed in this chapter. Dorsal dislocations are more common, and are the result of a hyperextension injury that tears the volar plate from its proximal origin. The collateral ligaments usually are not torn, but occasionally one or both may be disrupted.[6]

**Anatomy.** A complex support system around the MP joint makes dislocations at this site uncommon (Fig. 14-13). Most of the stability is due to the two collateral ligaments and the palmar plate. Collateral ligaments are lax in extension and taut in flexion, giving the joint some lateral mobility in extension. The volar plate is thin at its origin on the metacarpal neck and thick at its insertion on the volar base of the proximal phalanx. Hence, when torn, the volar plate tears from its proximal origin.[6]

**Radiology.** Plain films of the hand or thumb will demonstrate this injury.

**Diagnosis.** The most important step in the evaluation of dorsal dislocations is to distinguish between simple and complex dislocations.

In a simple dislocation, nothing is interposed in the joint space and the dislocation can often be reduced closed. A simple dorsal dislocation on standard hand films is illustrated in Fig. 14-14, both pre- and postreduction. A simple dislocation, however, may be converted to a complex dislocation by improper attempts at closed reduction.[6]

In a complex dislocation, the volar plate is entrapped in the joint space between the proximal phalanx and the metacarpal head. Open reduction is required for this injury.

*Clinical examination.* Fortunately, the appearance of the thumb is different in simple and complex dislocations, so it is usually possible to distinguish the two on clinical examination. In simple MP dislocations, the phalanx usually rests on the metacarpal head, so the joint appears to be hyperextended 60° to 90°. In complex dislocations, the proximal phalanx is more nearly parallel to the metacarpal, and only slight hyperextension is noted. Thus, unfortunately, the more serious complex dislocation has a more normal presentation.[6]

*Pathognomonic signs.* There are two pathognomonic signs of complex MP dislocation.[6,7] The first is a simple dimple on the volar aspect of the thenar eminence. The second is visualization of sesamoid bones in the joint space on plain films of the hand (Fig. 14-15). Each of these signs should be sought in the initial evaluation of an MP joint dislocation of the thumb.

**Definitive treatment**

*Simple dislocations.* Closed reduction of simple dislocations generally can be accomplished easily. Proper technique must be employed, however, to avoid converting a simple dislocation into a complex dislocation (Fig. 14-16). Adequate analgesia should be achieved by metacarpal block or median nerve block at the wrist with radial wheal (see Chapter 3 for techniques). To perform closed reduction, the following should be done. The wrist and the IP joint should be flexed to relax the tension on the flexor tendons; the proximal phalanx should then be hyperextended as far as possible on the metacarpal; pressure should then be applied against the dorsal surface of the base of the phalanx until the phalanx is relocated (Fig. 14-17).[6,7]

The physician should be warned that an attempt to reduce the dislocation using the *improper* technique of longitudinal traction and pulling the phalanx back into position may cause either the volar plate to become interposed in the joint[7] or the metacarpal head to buttonhole

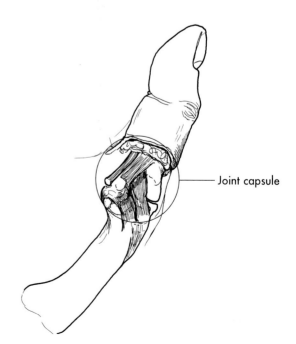

**Fig. 14-13.** Anatomic drawing of metacarpophalangeal joint of the thumb.

Joint capsule

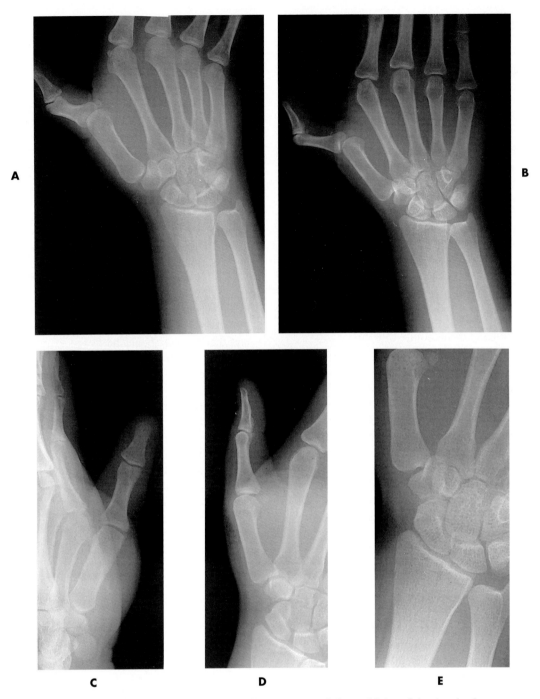

**Fig. 14-14.** Simple dorsal dislocation of the first metacarpophalangeal joint of the thumb, shown pre- (**A** and **B**) and postreduction (**C, D, E**).

between the flexor tendon and lumbrical,[6] thereby converting a simple dislocation into an irreducible complex dislocation.

***Complex dislocations.*** Complex dislocations generally require open reduction. However, a single, gentle attempt at closed reduction is recommended prior to surgery, even when pathognomonic signs of complex dislocation are present.[6,7] The technique for simple dislocations is as described above. If closed manipulation is unsuccessful, an immediate open reduction is indicated.[7]

***Treatment after reduction.*** After reduction, the integrity of the radial and ulnar collateral ligaments must be tested. This is done by applying medial and lateral stress to the joints in extension and flexion. Usually the joint will be stable after closed reduction. If it is, "protected motion" may be started almost immediately.[7] Three to 6 weeks of

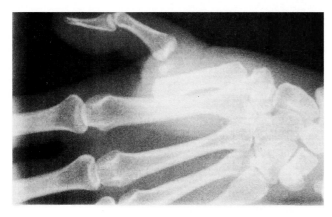

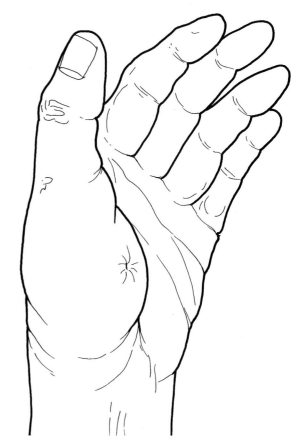

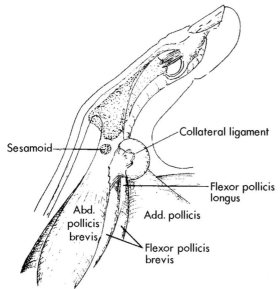

**Fig. 14-15.** X-ray and illustration of complex metacarpopha-langeal dislocation showing sesamoid bones interposed in the joint space, a pathognomonic sign of complex dislocation. (From Beasly RW. Hand Injuries. Philadelphia: WB Saunders, 1981, p 206.)

**Fig. 14-16.** Illustration of complex metacarpophalangeal dislocation showing pathognomonic dimple of the thenar eminence.

protection with a removable thumb spica splint may minimize the soreness that is frequently experienced at the MP joint.[6,7] Satisfactory healing of the volar plate usually occurs with immobilization alone and immediate surgical repair therefore is not recommended.

If the joint is unstable after closed reduction and there is evidence of complete rupture of one of the collateral ligaments, treatment should be the same as that for collateral ligament injuries.

**Emergency management.** Emergency management of simple MP dislocations is closed reduction using the technique outlined above, followed by immobilization in a thumb spica splint, until orthopedic follow-up in 1 week.

Emergency management of complex MP dislocations is a single attempt at closed reduction using the technique outlined above, followed (if successful and stable) by

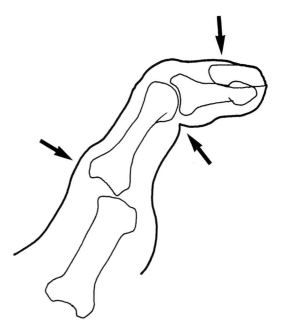

**Fig. 14-17.** Proper technique for reduction of simple dislocation of the metacarpophalangeal joint of the thumb involves *flexing* the wrist and the interphalangeal joint to relax the tension on the flexor tendons, then *hyperextending* the proximal phalanx as far as possible on the metacarpal, then *pushing* against the dorsal surface of the base of the phalanx until the phalanx is relocated.

immobilization in a thumb spica splint with orthopedic follow-up in 1 to 2 weeks. If a gentle attempt at relocation with adequate analgesia is unsuccessful, immediate orthopedic consultation is advised in anticipation of open reduction.

**Prognosis.** Prognosis for this type of injury is generally good. The volar plate usually heals with immobilization alone. In the rare case when improper healing results in chronic pain, instability, or contracture, late reconstruction may be required.[7]

**Pediatric considerations.** The MP joint of the thumb is the most commonly dislocated joint in the hands of children. As in adults, the dislocation is usually directed dorsally, resulting from forced hyperextension, usually when the patient falls and strikes the end of the thumb. Pathophysiology and treatment are the same as in adults.

### Interphalangeal dislocations

**Mechanism.** Pure IP dislocations of the thumb are rare, and result from acute hyperflexion. The more common injury associated with acute hyperflexion is mallet thumb, which is discussed below. When a pure IP dislocation of the thumb does occur, it is almost always dorsal, and is frequently associated with an open wound.[7]

**Signs and symptoms/physical findings.** The patient presents with pain, tenderness, and limited mobility at the IP joint. However, the dislocation may not be apparent on physical examination.

**Radiology.** A true lateral view of the injured digit must be obtained to be certain of identifying this dislocation. The technique for true lateral viewing of the thumb is illustrated in Fig. 14-5.

**Definitive treatment.** Closed reduction is almost always successful if the patient is seen soon after injury. The joint is usually stable after reduction and is splinted in extension for 10 to 12 days. Irreducible dislocations are associated with entrapment of the volar plate in the soft tissue of the joint, and require open reduction. Dislocations present for more that 2 to 3 weeks usually require open reduction, which is technically difficult in this setting and frequently results in poor joint mobility.[7]

**Emergency management.** After digital block, the dislocation should be reduced by gentle hyperextension and longitudinal traction while applying volar-directed pressure over the dorsal surface of the base of the distal phalanx. Radial, ulnar, dorsal, and volar stability should be checked explicitly following reduction. The reduced dislocation should be splinted in extension and the patient followed up with an orthopedist in 1 to 2 weeks. If attempted reduction fails, there may be associated entrapment of the volar plate in the joint space. Orthopedic consultation should be sought for open reduction.

Open IP dislocations should be managed like other open-joint injuries, with prompt surgical débridement, irrigation, and closure in the operating room.

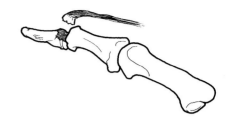

**Fig. 14-18.** Mallet thumb.

**Prognosis.** If treated acutely, these injuries heal well.

## TENDON AND LIGAMENT INJURIES
### Open tendon injuries

Open tendon injuries of the thumb should be managed as described in the section on open tendon injuries in Chapter 16.

### Closed tendon injuries

#### Mallet thumb

*Mechanism.* The mechanism of injury is a blow to the tip of the thumb, resulting in acute hyperflexion at the IP joint.[12] Mallet thumb is more common than pure dislocation of the thumb at the IP joint[7] (Fig. 14-18).

*Anatomy.* In this injury, the extensor pollicis longus is avulsed from its insertion into the base of the distal phalanx. There is often a small dorsal bone fragment off the distal phalanx.

*Signs and symptoms/physical findings.* Mallet thumb is evidenced clinically by a closed flexion deformity at the IP joint, similar to that of mallet finger. The distal phalanx is subluxed volarly.

*Radiology.* A routine hand or thumb film should be adequate for diagnosing this injury, which is similar to the mallet finger.

*Definitive treatment.* Either splinting or operative repair is appropriate for this injury, depending on the patient's specific circumstances.[7] In the largest series available,[13] the authors reserved recommendation for operative repair for cases of open injuries of the tendon; otherwise, they recommended closed management. For successful closed management, the IP joint must be maintained continuously in full extension for 6 to 8 weeks. Finger casts, plaster splints, and prefab finger splints such as stack splints are all appropriate (Fig. 14-19). The patient must be diligent about care of the skin under these splints, and must also avoid flexing the joint during splint changes.

*Emergency management.* Acute injuries should be splinted carefully with the IP joint in extension and the patient should be referred within 3 to 5 days to an orthopedist.

*Prognosis.* Prognosis for normal joint function is good in compliant patients.

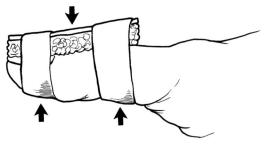

Dorsal padded aluminum splint

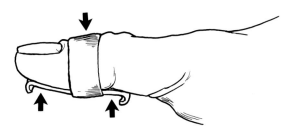

Volar unpadded plastic or aluminum splint

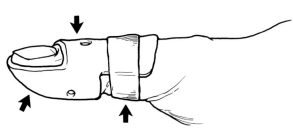

Stack splint

**Fig. 14-19.** Numerous methods of splinting the interphalangeal joint in extension.

### Trigger thumb

*Mechanism.* Trigger thumb (Fig. 14-20) is a common injury.[14] An isolated traumatic event is rarely identified as its cause. Women are more frequently affected than men, and the dominant hand is more likely to be affected than the nondominant hand.[15]

*Anatomy.* The painful snapping of the trigger thumb is caused by the flexor tendon passing through its too-tight tendon sheath. This relative constriction almost always occurs at the metacarpal head, and may be caused by a nodule on the flexor tendon that catches on the tendon sheath.[5,15]

*Signs and symptoms/physical findings.* The patient presents with complaints of painful snapping of the thumb on flexion and extension. On examination, a palpable or audible snapping can be appreciated as the patient flexes and extends the thumb. Triggering may be confused with a locked MP joint, subluxation of the MP joint, a tendon

tumor, or partial tendon laceration, so care should be taken to assess the problem with an eye to these alternative diagnoses.[15]

*Radiology.* Radiography is not helpful in the diagnosis of trigger thumb.

*Definitive treatment.* Steroid injection with or without immobilization of the IP and MP joints in 15° of flexion resolves trigger thumb in most cases.[15] Surgical release is another option.

*Emergency management.* The emergency physician may reassure the patient by explaining the pathology involved, and he or she may offer interim treatment with a nonsteroidal analgesic. Steroids can weaken tendons and result in tendon rupture, so the emergency physician should refer patients for steroid injection to a physician who can provide close follow-up.

*Prognosis.* Although conservative treatment is effective in most cases, it is less likely to be effective in patients with diabetes or rheumatoid arthritis, or in patients in whom the injury involves multiple digits. Surgical release is generally, but not always, successful and can result in painful scarring.[15]

### Ulnar collateral ligament injuries

*Mechanism.* Injury to the ulnar collateral ligament of the thumb is 8 to 10 times more frequent than injury to the radial collateral ligament of the thumb.[16,17] Laxity of the ulnar collateral ligament of the MP joint of the thumb is commonly referred to as "gamekeeper's thumb." Although technically inaccurate, this term has come to be applied to both acute and chronic laxity. The original description by Campbell[18] referred to the chronic laxity noted in Scottish gamekeepers, who sustained this injury by repetitively breaking the necks of wounded hares. Another term applied to the same injury is "skier's thumb," due to the association of this injury with skiing.[19,20] In skiers, ulnar collateral ligament injury is second in incidence only to trauma of the medial collateral ligament of the knee.[20]

In skiers, injury to the ulnar collateral ligament occurs because the pole strap or hand grip inhibits release of the pole at the moment of impact, forcibly abducting and extending the thumb.[21] Modifications in hand grips on ski poles have accomplished little in reducing the incidence of this injury.[20] Although skiing accounts for a high percentage of cases of this injury, the injury is seen in other sports, particularly football.[17]

Sudden abduction stress at the MP joint of the thumb, combined most likely with hyperextension, results in partial or complete disruption of the ulnar collateral ligament of the thumb. This ligament can be torn distally, proximally, or along its course.[20] A totally transected distal ulnar collateral ligament can become entrapped in the intact adductor aponeurosis of the dorsal expansion at the MP joint. This soft tissue interposition, or so-called "Stener" lesion, is reported to occur in 14% to 66% of patients with MP instability (see Fig. 14-21).[20]

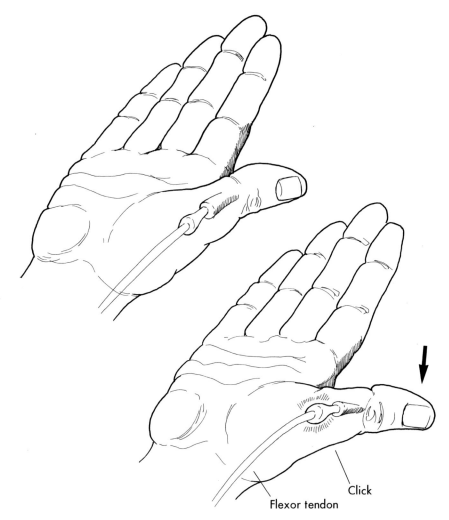

**Fig. 14-20.** Trigger thumb.

*Anatomy.* The ulnar collateral ligament is a 4 mm × 8 mm × 12 mm band that originates from the metacarpal head and inserts on the lateral tubercle of the proximal phalanx volar to its origin. The ulnar collateral ligament is tight in flexion and lax in extension.[20]

*Signs and symptoms/physical findings.* The acutely traumatized patient complains of a swollen, painful MP thumb joint. Frequently, the point of maximum tenderness can be localized to the ulnar aspect of the joint. In the presence of a normal plain radiograph and an appropriate history, a diagnosis of ulnar collateral ligament injury can be made on this finding alone.

*Radiology.* Fractures can occur in association with injury to the ulnar collateral ligament. Hence, the affected joint should be radiographed prior to any manipulation that might displace a nondisplaced fracture. The presence of a nondisplaced fracture does not rule out a complete ligamentous avulsion or complete tear.[20] Furthermore, plain films may be normal in severe ulnar collateral ligament injury.

*Diagnosis.* A diagnosis of ulnar collateral ligament injury is made on the basis of appropriate history and findings of tenderness over the ulnar collateral ligament and pain with stress of the ligament. The goals of further examination and studies are to differentiate a partial from a complete tear of the ulnar collateral ligament, and to determine the presence or absence of soft tissue entrapment (Stener lesion) of a completely torn ulnar collateral ligament. This is not as easy as it sounds.

If plain films are normal, laxity is assessed clinically by determining the extent to which the joint "opens up" or is radially deviated with abduction stress at the MP joint (Fig. 14-22). The test should be done with the MP both in full flexion and in extension. Flexion isolates the ulnar collateral ligament; rotation of the proximal phalanx should be avoided.[20] Instability in extension implies injury to the volar plate and accessory collateral ligaments, as well as injury to the ulnar collateral ligament.[22] The uninvolved thumb should be used as a comparison.[23,24] Unless the joint is grossly unstable, stress testing should be performed

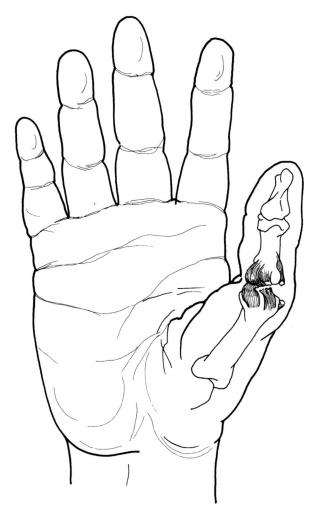

**Fig. 14-21.** Stener's lesion, showing the torn ulnar collateral ligament caught in the adductor aponeurosis of the metacarpophalangeal joint of the thumb.

under adequate analgesia because pain and muscle spasm may give a false impression of stability. Analgesia can be achieved by local infiltration or by regional block of the radial and median nerves at the wrist.[7] A goniometer should be used in judging laxity, and the measured degree of laxity documented. Unfortunately, the criteria for laxity are controversial, varying from 10° to 45° greater than the unaffected side, with some authors recommending an absolute value of greater than 35°.[8,20,25]

When the diagnosis of complete rupture remains questionable, many authors recommend the addition of stress radiography to characterize the injury.[20] Adequate analgesia is necessary to obtain useful stress radiographs. Unfortunately, there is little agreement as to how to perform and assess stress radiographs.[20,25] Therefore, the emergency physician probably should not order stress films unless requested to do so by the consulting orthopedist, in which

case they should be done in the manner favored by the consultant.

Arthrography has been recommended as an adjunctive diagnostic procedure, and may distinguish complete tear with entrapment from complete tear without entrapment; however, the sensitivity and specificity of this test have not been established.[20] This test has no role in the emergency management of ulnar collateral ligament injuries.

***Definitive treatment.*** There is general agreement that partial tears (sprains) of the ulnar collateral ligament are best treated by immobilization in a thumb spica cast for 3 to 6 weeks.

Most authors prefer surgical repair of acute complete tears of the ulnar collateral ligament. This preference is based on the belief that a high percentage of complete tears are associated with soft tissue interposition of the torn ulnar collateral ligament in the adductor aponeurosis, although actual figures vary from 14% to 66%.[20] Most authors think that the results of acute surgical repair are better than those of delayed reconstruction and favor repair "as soon as feasible." Delay of more than 3 weeks has been associated with an increased incidence of pinch weakness.[26]

***Emergency management.*** After making the best assessment possible, partial ulnar collateral ligament injuries should be immobilized in a thumb spica splint. The MP joint should be splinted in slight flexion (eg, up to 30°); hyperextension must be avoided; and the patient followed up with an orthopedist in 1 to 2 weeks.

Injuries known or suspected to be complete tears of the ulnar collateral ligament, as well as injuries of the ulnar collateral ligament associated with fractures, should be immobilized in a thumb spica splint with the MP joint in slight flexion. Follow-up with an orthopedist should be within 3 to 5 days, so that surgery, if needed, can be performed acutely.

***Prognosis.*** With prompt recognition and treatment, symptomatic and functional outcome for ulnar collateral ligament injuries is generally good. Unrecognized and untreated injuries of this ligament result in a weak and painful pinch, and a joint prone to arthritis.[20]

***Pediatric considerations.*** Relatively little attention has been focused on ulnar collateral ligament injuries in the pediatric population. Forced abduction stress at the child's MP joint may result in any one of four injuries (Fig. 14-23). The ulnar collateral ligament may be sprained or ruptured; there may be a simple Salter Harris type I or II fracture of the proximal physis; or there may be a Salter Harris type III avulsion fracture of the ulnar ¼ to ⅓ of the epiphysis of the proximal phalanx. The latter injury is referred to as a "pseudogamekeeper's thumb" because there is the appearance of joint instability on examination, yet the injury is entirely bony. These injuries usually occur in adolescents or preadolescents. The most common childhood gamekeeper's thumb is the Salter Harris type

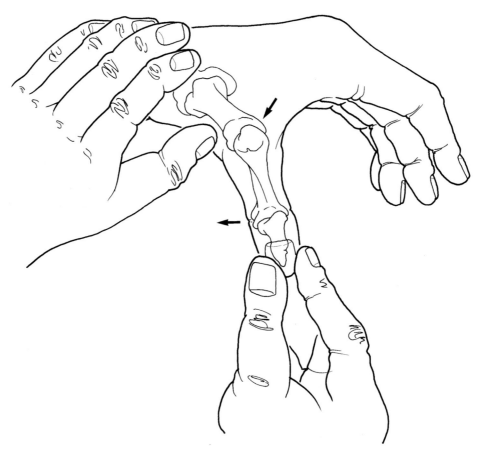

**Fig. 14-22.** Abduction stress of the metacarpophalangeal joint of the thumb shows widening of the metacarpophalangeal joint space in an ulnar collateral ligament tear.

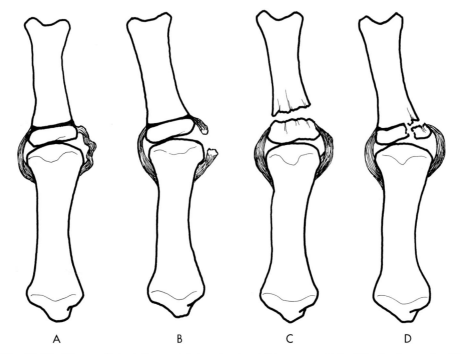

**Fig. 14-23.** Ulnar collateral ligament injury in the child may result in (**A**) simple sprain; (**B**) rupture of the ligament; (**C**) "pseudogamekeeper's thumb" due to a Salter-Harris type I or II fracture of the proximal phalanx; or (**D**) a Salter-Harris type III avulsion fracture.

III. This injury has been coined the "breakdancer's thumb."

The examination findings and radiologic evaluation of these injuries in the child is the same as in the adult. Treatment consists of cast immobilization for the sprained ulnar collateral ligament, surgical repair for the complete ulnar collateral ligament tear, reduction and cast immobilization for the Salter Harris type I or II injury of the proximal physis, and surgical repair for the Salter Harris type III injury.[4]

**Radial collateral ligament injury.** Because radial collateral ligament injury of the MP joint of the thumb is much rarer than other thumb injuries, it will be covered briefly.

*Mechanism.* The injury occurs as a result of lateral stress during hyperextension of the thumb.

*Anatomy.* There is no abductor aponeurosis in which the torn radial collateral ligament can get caught, so entrapment, as seen in the Stener lesion with ulnar collateral ligaments, cannot occur.

*Signs and symptoms/physical findings.* Patients usually present late and complain of pain with such movements as unscrewing jars and opening car doors. Tenderness is noted at the MP joint on the radial side, and stress of the radial ligament elicits pain. The radial aspect of the metacarpal head may appear prominent.[7]

*Definitive treatment.* There is little literature regarding the acute management of this injury. One respected text recommends immobilization in a thumb spica cast for 3 to 4 weeks.[7]

*Emergency management.* The emergency physician is advised to splint the acute injury in a thumb spica splint and arrange for prompt follow-up with an orthopedist. A patient with a chronically unstable radial collateral ligament at the time of initial presentation should be referred to an orthopedic surgeon for elective reconstruction. No acute intervention is needed.

## SOFT TISSUE INJURIES
### Soft tissue injuries to tip and nailbed

Soft tissue injuries to the tip of the thumb and nailbed are managed like soft tissue injuries of the fingertips. The reader is referred to Chapter 15, for a discussion of these injuries.

### Amputations

The thumb is the most important digit of the hand. Therefore, thumb amputation is a potentially debilitating injury. The care rendered by the emergency physician is extremely important in determining the functional outcome of this injury.[3,27]

A *complete amputation* is total separation of the digit or a segment of the digit from the remaining hand. A *partial* or *incomplete* amputation has some bridging tissue, however minor, between the severed part and its base. Complete amputations, in popular terminology, may be *replanted;* partial amputations, *revascularized.* The distinction is arbitrary and has little to do with prognosis (Fig. 14-24).

**Mechanism.** Local crush injury is the most common mechanism of thumb amputation, and guillotine injury the least common.[3] Total amputations occur with the same frequency as partial amputations.[28] Lawn mowers and power saws are commonly involved.[27] In farm accidents, the classic injury is a total avulsion of the thumb resulting from catching a winter glove in the power take-off of a tractor.[25]

Thumb amputation is at least four times more common in males than in females.[3,25,29] It occurs most frequently during the productive years of the 20s to 40s,[3,25,29] and affects the dominant hand three fourths of the time.[25]

**Anatomy.** Bones, soft tissue, tendons, vessels, and nerves are all involved in this type of injury. The extent of damage to the vascular bundle often is not apparent at the time of initial inspection.

**Radiology.** Radiographs should include the joint above the level of apparent injury.

**Definitive treatment**

*Rationale for attempted replantation.* The first successful thumb replantation was performed in 1968.[30] Since then, improvements in surgical technique, optics, and surgical equipment have made replantation a common and very successful procedure, and improvements continue to evolve. In replantation centers, large series have reported successful thumb replantation rates of 70% to 90%.[3,29]

Not all amputations are equally amenable to replantation. Guillotine amputations are associated with greater success than crush or avulsion injuries.[3,25,27,29,31] A narrow zone of injury is more favorable than a wide zone of injury.[29] Young patients fare somewhat better than old patients, and children have the best final outcomes if the replantation is successful, even though survival of the digit itself is slightly lower in children than in adults.[29] Healthy patients fare better than those with underlying disease, and clean amputations fare better than grossly contaminated ones. A remarkably high success rate of 68% has been achieved, however, even in *unselected* thumb amputations, and a success rate of 46% has been achieved even in *unselected* total avulsion injuries.[29]

Because the thumb is so essential to the function of the hand, attempted replantation is almost always indicated.[25,27,29,31] A successful replantation is far superior functionally and cosmetically to any available alternative treatment, including simple debridement and closure, pollicization of another digit, or transfer of a toe to the hand.[27,29] The functional gain from thumb replantation exceeds that of any other digit reattatchment.[21] Total loss of the thumb is associated with a 40% to 50% disability.[3] Total medical costs for thumb amputation with replantation, including settlement and temporary disability, are one-fourth of the total costs for amputation without replantation.

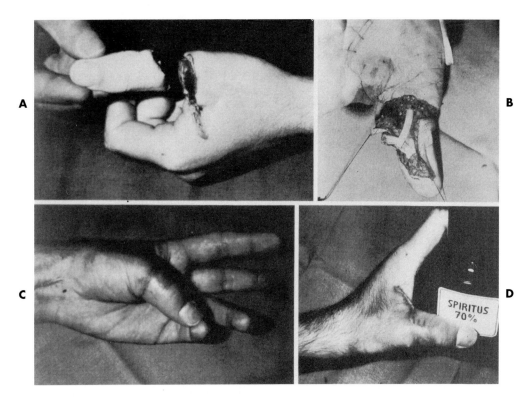

**Fig. 14-24.** Of all digits, the thumb is given highest priority in considering reattachment. **A,** Thumb amputated at the metacarpophalangeal joint level. **B,** The essential pulley mechanism of the flexor pollicis longus tendon was destroyed, precluding function by primary tendon repair. The vital pulley system is reconstructed from tendon over a pliable silicone rod to maintain space for secondary replacement of the flexor tendon with a graft. **C and D,** Useful functional recovery despite restricted motion at the metacarpophalangeal and interphalangeal joint levels. (Courtesy of Dr. Viktor Meyer.) (From Beasly RW. Hand Injuries. Philadelphia: WB Saunders, 1981, p 333.)

This does not include additional costs to society resulting from the fact that only 10% of patients not undergoing replantation return to work.[32]

*Contraindications.* There are few contraindications to attempted thumb replantation. Foremost among the contraindications are associated life-threatening injuries, the inability to safely undergo prolonged surgery, and severely mangled or crushed parts.[21,32] Consideration must be given to the presence of advanced vessel disease and to severe mental instability that would preclude rehabilitation.[27] Total ischemia time must also be considered, but the limits are not clear. The likelihood of successful replantation decreases with a warm ischemia time greater than 6 to 8 hours,[27,33] but when the digit is cooled properly, 12 to 24 hours and even up to 33 hours of ischemia may be tolerated.[3]

*The replantation procedure.* Replantation is performed by a microvascular surgeon and often involves a team of surgeons. Specialized instruments and microscopes are needed for this procedure, which is usually available only at major centers.

The procedure involves the following sequence: identification and tagging of neurovascular structures, cleaning and débridement, bone fixation and shortening, extensor tendon repair, flexor tendon repair, arterial anastomoses, nerve repair, venous anastomoses, and skin coverage.[27] The procedure lasts approximately 5 hours.[25] Intraoperative complications include the usual anesthetic risks. Immediate postoperative complications include vascular thrombosis, hemorrhage, and infection. Patients may return emergently to the operating room one or more times to reestablish adequate blood flow in the first several days following the operation.[3]

**Emergency management: evaluation and treatment.** Unless higher priority injuries exist, the emergency physician should consider all thumb amputations to be candidates for replantation, treat the patient and the amputated part accordingly, and promptly arrange transfer of the patient and amputated part to a replantation center. The physician should, of course, be aware of the limitations of replantation, and be careful to avoid encouraging unrealistic expectations for the patient or family. Both goals are well served by explaining to the

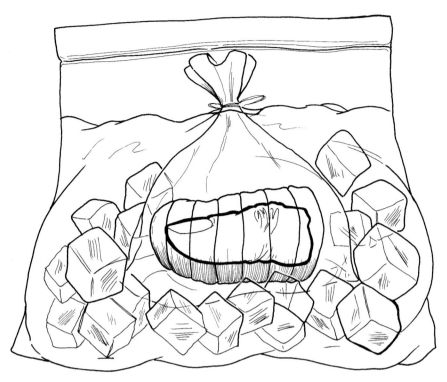

**Fig. 14-25.** The amputated digit should be wrapped in saline-soaked gauze and placed in a sealed plastic container, which is then immersed in a solution of ice and water.

family that the purpose of transfer for more specialized evaluation is to render whatever care is necessary to give the best possible outcome, whether that be replantation or otherwise.[3,27]

*The patient and stump.* After evaluating injuries that are potentially more serious, the physician should turn his or her attention to the site of the amputation to assess the degree of associated injury and the level of the injury. Hemorrhage should be controlled with direct pressure; clamps and tourniquets should not be used. The wound should be irrigated with normal saline; antiseptics should be avoided because of potential damage to viable tissue. Handling of the injured part should be minimized and no débridement undertaken. The neurovascular status should be ascertained, and motor and tendon function determined. The stump should then be dressed with sterile, saline-soaked gauze, splinted for protection, and elevated. The patient should be given tetanus if due, a systemic broad-spectrum antibiotic (eg, cephalosporin), and systemic analgesia as needed.[3] Preoperative laboratory studies should be ordered to expedite operative management.

*The amputated part.* The amputated part should be inspected gently to determine tissue loss, the degree of crush, and contamination. Handling should be minimized.

Normal saline irrigation is indicated; antiseptics and débridement are avoided. The part should then be wrapped in saline-moistened gauze and placed in a water-tight plastic bag or container, which is immersed in a container of ice and water (Fig. 14-25). It is important to cool the part as soon as possible, and it is imperative to avoid freezing any portion of it through direct contact with ice. The container should be labeled properly. Even severely crushed amputated parts not likely to be used for replantation are treated in this manner, because portions of the tissue may be valuable for closure or reconstruction.[3]

*Incomplete amputations.* Care of incomplete amputations is the same as for complete amputations, with the exception that the splint is applied to protect both the stump and the partially amputated digit. Tissue bridges should never be severed. After splinting, ice should be applied over the dressing and the hand should be elevated.[3]

*Documentation.* Written documentation should be made of the following: the mechanism of injury, the exact time of injury, the time the amputated part was cooled, all treatments rendered (irrigation, tetanus, antibiotics, analgesics, splinting, elevation), neurovascular and motor function at the time of evaluation, the patient's past medical and surgical history, prior injuries to the affected thumb, handedness, allergies, medications, tetanus status, habits, vocation, and avocations.[3] The originals or copies of radiographs should be sent with the patient.

**Prognosis and complications.** As noted above, successful replantation rates as high as 70% to 90% have been achieved for the thumb. To be deemed a success, the replanted thumb must have sensation, motion, and stability, and must be relatively pain-free and cosmetically acceptable to the patient. Replantations of the thumb have generally met these criteria.[3,25,27,29,31] Cold intolerance is a common problem after replantation, but this largely resolves after 1 to 2 years.[27] Decreased two-point discrimination is common despite nerve repair, but protective sensibility or better is the usual outcome.[27,31] Range of motion at the IP and MP joints may be decreased, but mobility at the CMC joint is generally sufficient to give a total active range of motion close to 80% or normal.[25]

If a replantation is to fail, it usually does so within 7 postoperative days. The average number of additional procedures per patient undergoing attempted replantation is 1.8.[29] Patients frequently return to work in 7 to 12 weeks, but some may require prolonged rehabilitation. Potential complications in the viable replantation include delayed bony union, bony nonunion, tendon adhesions, neuroma, and scar contracture.[29]

## DISCUSSION

The thumb is the most important digit of the hand. Hence, every thumb injury should be evaluated carefully. The following points warrant emphasis.

Radiologic evaluation of the thumb frequently requires true AP and true lateral views, so the treating physician should be aware of the technique for achieving these views.

It is important to distinguish intra-articular from extra-articular fractures of the base of the first metacarpal, because intra-articular fractures are frequently unstable and require surgical intervention, whereas extra-articular fractures are amenable to closed reduction and splint immobilization.

Sesamoid fractures should be considered in the differential diagnosis of pain at the volar crease of the first MP joint, as well as disruption of the volar plate and collateral ligaments.

Reduction of a pure dislocation of the CMC joint is easy, but the joint is frequently unstable after reduction, so care should be taken in postreduction evaluation. Orthopedic consultation is advised for this injury.

Dorsal dislocation of the MP joint is common. Care is necessary to distinguish simple from complex dislocations. The complex dislocation involves entrapment of the volar plate in the joint space and generally requires open reduction. The simple dislocation is amendable to closed reduction. Proper technique for closed reduction is important in order to avoid conversion of a simple dislocation into a complex dislocation.

Ligamentous integrity at the MP and IP joints should be assessed for all thumb injuries. The initial goal in evaluating ulnar collateral ligament injury is to distinguish the nonoperative partial tear from the complete tear requiring timely surgical intervention.

Replantation should be considered for all thumb amputations. The initial care rendered by the emergency physician is of paramount importance in the functional outcome of these injuries. Surgical consultation should be sought promptly.

Although the majority of thumb injuries can be managed properly by the emergency physician, the thumb is so important to the function of the hand that prompt orthopedic consultation is advised for any thumb injury for which the proper management is not clear to the examining physician.

## REFERENCES

1. Campbell BG: *Human evolution,* ed 2, Chicago, 1966, Aldine Publishing Company.
2. Jones S, Martin R, and Pilbeam D: The Cambridge encyclopedia of human evolution, Cambridge, UK, 1992, Cambridge Press.
3. Dalsey W: Management of amputated parts. In Roberts JR, Hedges JR, eds: *Clinical procedures in emergency medicine,* Philadelphia, 1985, WB Saunders.
4. O'Brien ET: Fractures of the hand and wrist region. In Rockwood CA, Wilkins KE, and King RE, eds: *Fractures in children,* Philadelphia, 1991, JB Lippincott.
5. Hollinshead WH: *Textbook of anatomy,* ed 3, Hagerstown, MD, 1974, Harper & Row.
6. Ashkenaze DM, Ruby LK: Metacarpal fractures and dislocations, *Orthop Clin North Am* 23:19-33, 1992.
7. Green DP, Rowland SA: Fractures and dislocations of the hand. In Rockwood CA, Green DP, and Bucholz RW, eds: *Rockwood and Green's fractures in adults,* Philadelphia, 1991, JB Lippincott.
8. Isani A: Small joint injuries requiring surgical treatment, *Orthop Clin North Am* 17:407-419, 1986.
9. Green DP, O'Brien ET: Fractures of the thumb metacarpal, *South Med J* 65:807, 1972.
10. Patel MR, Pearlman HS, Bassini L, and Ravich S: Fractures of the sesamoid bones of the thumb, *J Hand Surg* 15-A:776-781, 1990.
11. Watt N, Hooper G: Dislocation of the trapeziometacarpal joint, *J Hand Surg,* 12-B:242-245, 1987.
12. Blair WF, Steyers CM: Extensor tendon injuries, *Orthop Clin North Am* 23:141-148, 1992.
13. Miura T, Nakamura R, and Torii S: Conservative treatment for a ruptured extensor tendon on the dorsum of the proximal phalanges of the thumb (mallet thumb), *J Hand Surg,* 11-A:229-233, 1986.
14. Hoppenfeld S: *Physical examination of the spine and extremities,* New York, 1976, Appleton-Century-Crofts.
15. Thorson E, Szabo RM: Common tendonitis problems in the hand and forearm, *Orthop Clin North Am* 23:65-74, 1992.
16. Moberg E: Fractures and ligamentous injuries of the thumb and fingers, *Surg Clin North Am* 40:297-309, 1960.
17. Osterman AL, Hayken GD, Bora WM: A quantitative evaluation of thumb function after ulnar collateral repair and reconstruction, *J Trauma* 21:854-860, 1981.
18. Campbell CS: Gamekeeper's thumb, *J Bone Joint Surg* 37-B:148-149, 1955.
19. Gerber C, Semm E, and Matter P: Skier's thumb, surgical treatment of recent injuries to the ulnar collateral ligament of the thumb's metacarpophalangeal joint, *Am J Sports Med* 9:171-177, 1981.
20. Newland CC: Gamekeeper's thumb, *Orthop Clin North Am* 23:41-48, 1992.
21. Engkvist O, Balkier B, and Lindsjo U: Thumb injuries in downhill skiing, *Int J Sports Med* 3:50-55, 1982.

22. Kahler DM, McCue FC: Metacarpophalangeal and proximal interphalangeal joint injuries of the hand, including the thumb, *Clin Sports Med* 11:57-76, 1992.

23. Bowers WH, Hurst LC: Gamekeeper's thumb: evaluation by arthrography and stress roentgenography, *J Bone Joint Surg* 59-A:519-524, 1977.

24. Burton RI, Eaton RG: Common hand injuries in the athlete, *Orthop Clin North Am* 4:809-838, 1973.

25. Bowen CVA, et al: Rotating shaft avulsion amputations of the thumb, *J Hand Surg* 16-A:117-121, 1991.

26. Helm RH: Hand function after injuries to the collateral ligaments of the metacarpophalangeal joint of the thumb, *J Hand Surg* 12-B:252-255, 1987.

27. Gaul JS, Nunley JA: Digital replantation. In Nyhus LM, ed: *Surgery,* Norwalk, CT, 1989, Appleton & Lange.

28. Kleinert HE, et al: Digital replantation: selection technique and results, *Orthop Clin North Am* 8:309-318, 1977.

29. Ward WA, Tsai TM, and Breidenback W: Per primam thumb replantation for all patients with traumatic amputations, *Clin Orthop* 266:90-95, 1991.

30. Komatsu S, Tamai S: Successful replantation of a completely cut off thumb: case report, *Plast Reconstr Surg* 42:374-377, 1968.

31. Bieber EJ, et al: Thumb avulsion: results of replantation/revascularization, *J Hand Surg* 12-A:786-790, 1987.

32. Chase RA: Costs, risks and benefits of hand surgery, *J Hand Surg* 8:644, 1983.

33. Berger A, et al: Replantation and revascularization of amputated parts of extremities: a three-year report from the Viennese replantation team, *Clin Orthop* 133:212-214, 1978.

34. Harris JH, Harris WH: *The radiology of emergency medicine,* ed 2, Baltimore, 1981, Williams & Wilkins.

35. Stener B: Displacement of the ruptured ulnar collateral ligament of the metacarpophalangeal joint of the thumb: a clinical and anatomical study, *J Bone Joint Surg* 44-B:869-879, 1962.

36. Stener B: Skeletal injuries associated with rupture of the ulnar collateral ligament of the metacarphalangeal joint of the thumb: a clinical and anatomical study, *Acta Chir Scand* 125:583-586, 1963.

37. Stevenson TR: Fingertip and nailbed injuries, *Orthop Clin North Am* 23:149-159, 1992.

# Examination of the Hand and Management of Fingertip Injuries

*Robert A. Rusnak*

The earliest fossil evidence of primates dates to approximately 55 million years ago.[1] From that time, the hand has evolved as the premier biomechanic instrument. Guided by the mind, the human hand fashioned tools and ultimately built the machines that have, in turn, created the world in which we live. Care of the injured hand should well be given with an understanding of and respect for its evolutionary history and importance. Moreover, for the particular patient involved, the functional result and ultimate outcome of treatment is often determined by the initial treating physician.

This chapter presents an approach to the examination of the hand, emphasizing those aspects most important to emergency physicians, rather than detailed descriptions of structure and function that are more appropriately covered in textbooks on anatomy or surgery of the hand.

## HISTORIC FACTORS

Vital information regarding any patient with a hand complaint includes the following: 1) right- or left-handedness; 2) patient occupation; 3) hobbies that require fine motor control (eg, playing a musical instrument); 4) previous injuries or infections; 5) medical problems (eg, diabetes mellitus, scleroderma, chronic arthritis, peripheral vascular disease); 6) congenital abnormalities that may directly affect the functional result of any hand injury or infection; 7) medications; 8) possible allergies; and 9) patient tetanus immunization status.

After obtaining this information, a detailed history of the mechanism of injury, or the sequence of signs and symptoms that brought the patient to the emergency department should be obtained. For example, in cases of injury with lacerations, the patient should be asked if the hand was injured in flexion or extension. In the case of a finger injury, if the finger was being actively flexed at the time of injury, retraction of an injured tendon may be present if the hand is examined in extension. Because nerves and blood vessels are closely linked in the hand, bleeding that is not easily controlled with pressure may imply a vascular injury as well as a possible nerve or tendon injury. Injuries that occur during an assault (ie, a fight strike) can lead to lacerations by incisor teeth of the extensor tendons or penetration of the dorsal joint capsule or synovium of the metacarpophalangeal joints (MCPJ). Human or animal bites not only injure soft tissue but may also injure bone or cause serious infections.

During history taking, it is also imperative to assess the need for immediate operative treatment or immediate referral to an orthopedic or plastic surgeon or a tertiary care center. Such injuries include but are not limited to the following: 1) extensive mangling; 2) degloving injuries; 3) massive contamination with dirt, gravel, or barnyard detritus; 4) high-pressure injection injuries; 5) amputations or partial amputations proximal to the distal interphalangeal

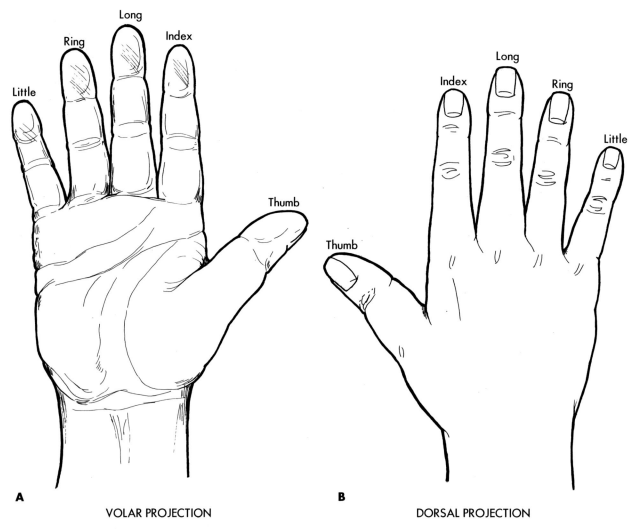

**Fig. 15-1. A** and **B,** Surface anatomy of the hand.

joint; 6) deep space or tendon sheath infections; and 7) open fractures proximal to the distal interphalangeal joint. In such cases, emergency department care is limited to: 1) careful physical examination to determine the structures injured; 2) the institution of prophylactic intravenous antibiotics; 3) control of bleeding; 4) splinting in a functional position; and 5) appropriate measures to conserve amputated segments. These measures include wrapping the amputated segment in sterile gauze moistened with sterile normal saline, placing this wrapped segment in a sterile specimen cup, and placing the cup on ice.

## ANATOMY

The surface anatomy of the palm is illustrated in Fig. 15-1. The bones and joints are illustrated in Figs. 15-2 and 15-3 in both volar and dorsal projections; the bones include fourteen phalanges and five metacarpals. The vascular anatomy of the hand is listed in Fig. 15-4. It is important to note that the apex of the superficial palmar arch lies just proximal to the proximal transverse palmar skin crease—

that is, proximal to a line drawn transversely across the palm at the level of the thenar web space—as indicated in Fig. 15-4. All fingers have both a radial and ulnar digital artery with accompanying ulnar and radial digital nerves. See Table 15-1 for the nerve supply of commonly tested hand muscles.

The extension of the index finger is accomplished by two extensor tendons, the extensor digitorum, and the extensor indicis proprius. Extension of the middle, ring, and little fingers is done by a single-extensor digitorum tendon inserted into the base of the distal phalanx. The flexor digitorum profundus tendon is inserted into the volar base of the distal phalanx, producing flexion of the distal interphalangeal joint and MCPJ; the flexor digitorum superficialis tendon is inserted into the proximal base of the middle phalanx, producing flexion of the proximal interphalangeal joint (PIPJ). See Fig. 15-5 for a diagram of the anatomy of the flexor superficialis and profundus tendons.

The ulnar nerve supplies all the intrinsic muscles of the hand except for five muscles controlled by the median

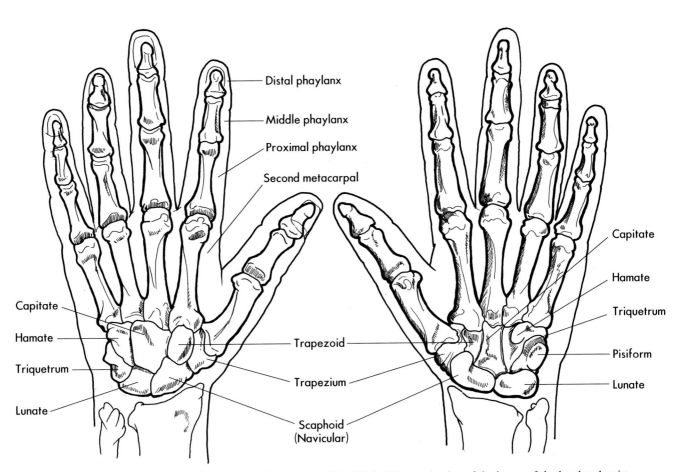

**Fig. 15-2.** Dorsal projection of the bones of the hand and wrist.

**Fig. 15-3.** Volar projection of the bones of the hand and wrist.

nerve. The muscles supplied by the ulnar nerve include: 1) the three hypothenar muscles (the abductor digiti quinti, the flexor digiti quinti, and the opponens digiti quinti); 2) the seven interosseus muscles; 3) the ulnar two lumbrical muscles; and 4) the adductor pollicis. The median nerve supplies the flexor carpi radialis, the flexor digitorum profundus (also supplied by the ulnar nerve), the flexor pollicis longus, the abductor pollicis brevis, and the opponens pollicis. The radial nerve supplies all the post-axial hand muscles.

One of the key elements in understanding tendon structure in the hand is the presence of synovial sheaths that surround the flexor tendons in the fingers and the palms. The extent of these tendon sheaths is illustrated in Fig. 15-6. These have important implications for the spread of infection along the digits and into the palmar and carpal spaces. Tenosynovitis from a puncture wound or cut on the finger can extend proximally along these tendon sheaths to cause localized collections of pus in the palm or wrist. Tenosynovitis is diagnosed by tenderness along the tendon sheath proximal or distal to a puncture wound or healing laceration and pain on active and especially passive motion. Tenosynovitis of the flexor tendons or infection of the flexor sheath in the palm or wrist requires hospitalization and intravenous antibiotics.

## JOINTS

There are five carpometacarpal joints, five metacarpophalangeal, and nine interphalangeal joints; all of these are true synovial joints. See Fig. 15-7 for a diagram of a proximal interphalangeal joint that includes its supporting structures, the radial and ulnar collateral ligaments, the anterior fibrocartilagenous volar plate, and the flexor tendons immediately anterior to the volar plate.

## PHYSICAL EXAMINATION

Preparation for the physical examination should include the following: 1) exposure of the entire extremity; 2) a comfortably seated or supine patient; 3) appropriate lighting; 4) a tourniquet (either a 1-inch Penrose drain secured by a hemostat, a blood pressure cuff inflated to 250 mm Hg, or a pneumatic tourniquet), to allow examination of selected lacerations for the presence of tendon or joint involvement; 5) appropriate instruments for exploration, including skin hooks; 6) appropriate wound-care techniques and materials such as sterile gloves, protective eye wear, and mask; 7) a comfortably seated physician, and 8) most importantly, uninterrupted time.

Before proceeding with the actual details of the physical examination, a discussion of terms is in order. The fingers should be named thumb, index, middle, ring, and little

(Fig. 15-1). Descriptions of injury or swelling should be described as ulnar or radial rather than medial or lateral, to avoid confusion between the supinated and pronated hand. The rotational axis of the hand includes the middle finger, its metacarpal, the capitate, the lunate, and the distal radius; pronation, supination, and interossei function occur around this axis (Figs. 15-8, 15-9, and 15-10).

A systematic approach to any hand complaint is mandatory. The physician should inspect the hand, making note of its color and the appearance of the digits distal to an injury or

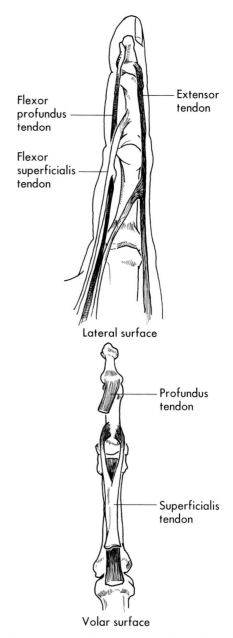

**Fig. 15-5.** Anatomy of the flexor superficialis, and profundus tendons of the digit, volar and lateral projections.

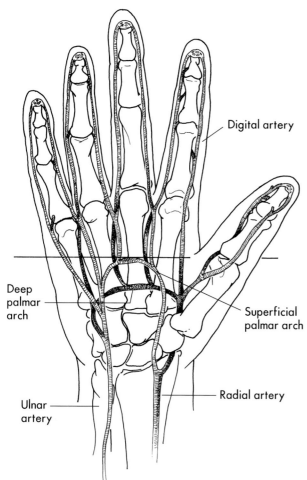

**Fig. 15-4.** Vascular anatomy of the hand, volar projection.

**Table 15-1.** The nerve supply of commonly tested hand tendons

| Median nerve | Ulnar | Radial nerve |
|---|---|---|
| Flexor carpi radialis | Flexor carpi ulnaris | Extensor digitorum |
| Flexor digitorum superficialis | *Flexor digitorum profundus | Extensor indicis proprius |
| Flexor digitorum profundus | Adductor pollicis | Extensor carpi radialis longus/brevis |
| *Flexor pollicis longus | Flexor pollicis brevis | Extensor pollicis longus |
| Abductor pollicis brevis | Hypothenar muscles | Extensor pollicis brevis |
| Opponens pollicis | Interossei | Abductor pollicis longus |
| | | Extensor digiti minimi |

*also innervated by the ulnar nerve

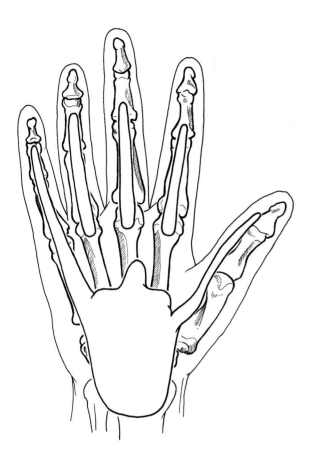

**Fig. 15-6.** The most common arrangement of flexor tendon sheaths in the hand.

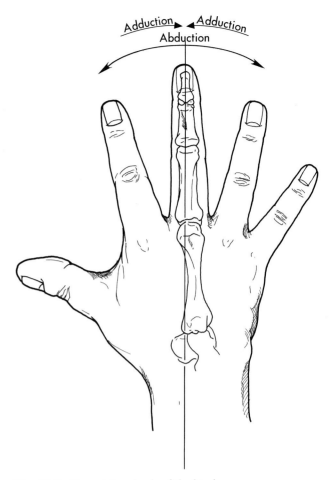

**Fig. 15-8.** The rotational axis of the hand.

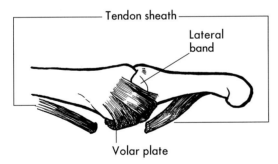

**Fig. 15-7.** The proximal interphalangeal joint.

laceration; the position of the hand relative to the uninjured extremity; and the presence of edema, abrasions, bruises, deformities, or puncture wounds. A good screen for injury is a test of the patient's grip strength; following this ask the patient to draw all the fingers into a cone starting from a position of full extension (to perform this maneuver, the radial, medial, and ulnar nerves must be intact; Fig. 15-11). Next, each digit should be examined for tendon function, fingertip two-point sensory discrimination, and capillary refill. Lastly, wrist flexion, extension, and ulnar and radial deviation should be checked, passively and actively and against resistance (Figs. 15-9 and 15-10).

Next, the joints should be examined for active and passive range of motion, and to determine the presence of any synovial swelling, erythema, or tenderness. Synovial thickening is assessed by palpating the distal and proximal surfaces along the dorsal or volar side of the hand joint. A velvety thickening above the bony surfaces (ie, the inability to clearly palpate the bony joint surfaces) as compared with the other hand is good evidence of its presence. Appreciation of this sign takes practice.

The digital nerves to the fingers contain sensory, motor, and autonomic function. Because the fingers and palm are liberally supplied with sweat glands, a complete injury of both digital nerves or of the radial, medial, or ulnar nerves causes loss of sweating to the affected sensory areas. This can be best appreciated by observing the digits through the positive 20 diopter objective of an ophthalmoscope to look for beads of sweat on the distal finger (these appear as tiny silvery-white dots on the skin surface). In small children unable to adequately cooperate for testing, this can be determined by immersing the injured hand in warm water for several minutes, then examining the injured hand for wrinkling on the skin of the fingertip. Loss of wrinkling indicates a nerve injury.

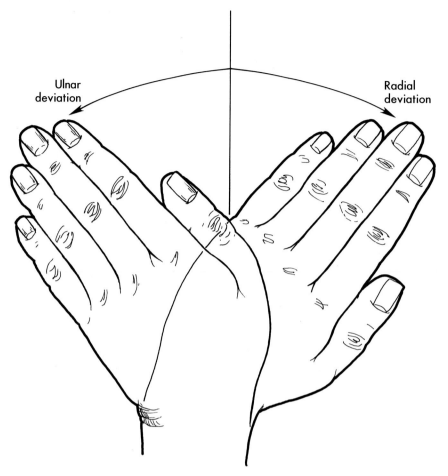

**Fig. 15-9.** Standard nomenclature for hand movements (ulnar and radial deviation).

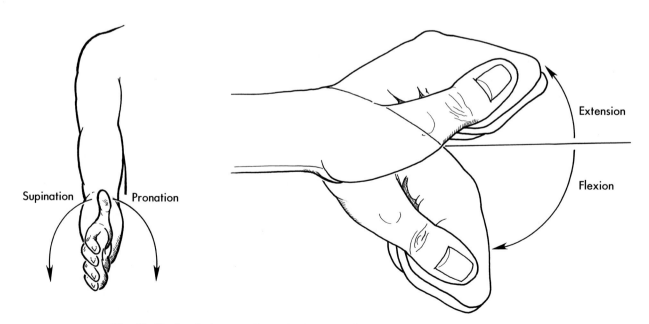

**Fig. 15-10.** Standard nomenclature for hand movements (supination, pronation, extension, flexion).

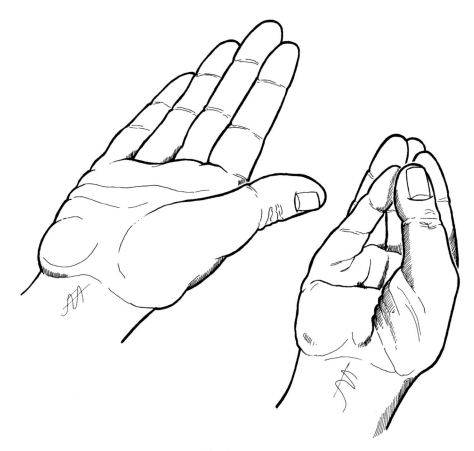

**Fig. 15-11.** Demonstration of coning of the fingers.

When checking for tendon function, the full range of motion and strength should be assessed. In the presence of a partial laceration, the patient may be able to move the joint through a full range of motion, but experience pain radiating either proximally or distally along the course of the tendon when the injured tendon is tested against resistance. The standard method for testing flexor digitorum superficialis function is to hold the fingers not being tested in extension when the patient attempts to maximally flex the finger being tested at the MCPJ and the PIPJ (Fig. 15-12). If limited flexion of the little finger is present (at least 45° of flexion at the MCPJ and PIPJ should normally be present), then modified testing is required. In the modified test described by Stein et al[2] for testing the function of the flexor digitorum superficialis to the little finger when flexion seems limited during standard testing, the index and middle fingers are held in extension and the patient is instructed to flex the ring and little fingers maximally at the MCPJ and PIPJ (Fig. 15-13). Using this modified technique, the authors demonstrated that 77% (154 patients) of patients had full flexor superficialis function of the little finger, 19% (38 patients) had incomplete function, and 8 of 200 hands demonstrated absence of the flexor superficialis in the little finger (in three of these patients, this finding was bilateral and in one, unilateral). Therefore, whenever the integrity of the flexor digitorum superficialis tendon to

the little finger is in question, this modified test should be performed. Patients with an unequivocal flexor tendon laceration should be referred to a specialist; those who demonstrate incomplete tendon function or pain radiating proximally or distally along the course of the tendon when the tendon is stress-tested (a sign of a partial laceration) should have a careful wound exploration to rule out a partial tendon laceration, or should be referred to a specialist.

The flexor digitorum profundus tendons are tested by fully extending the finger, stabilizing the MCPJ and PIPJ in full extension, and asking the patient to flex the fingertip at the distal interphalangeal joint and hold flexion against resistance (Fig. 15-14).

## MUSCLE AND NERVE TESTING

Table 15-1 lists commonly tested tendons of the hand and their innervation. These movements may be demonstrated to the patient by the examiner prior to each tendon or nerve test.

### Median nerve

The flexor pollicis longus tendon is tested by stabilizing the thumb at the MCPJ and asking the patient to flex the tip of the thumb; the examiner's other hand provides resistance against the flexion (Fig. 15-15). The flexor digitorum superficialis tendon is tested by holding the digits not being

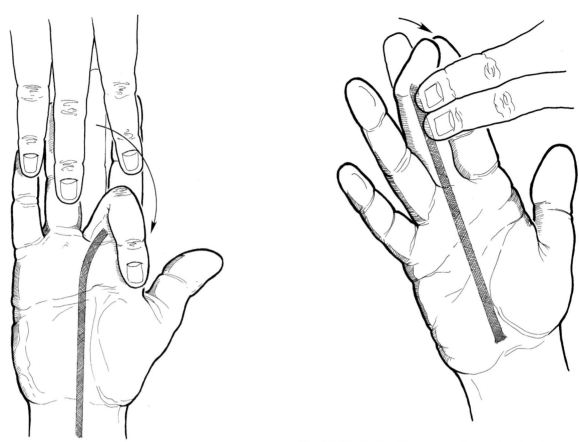

**Fig. 15-12.** Testing for flexor digitorum superficialis tendon function.

**Fig. 15-14.** Testing flexor profundus tendon function.

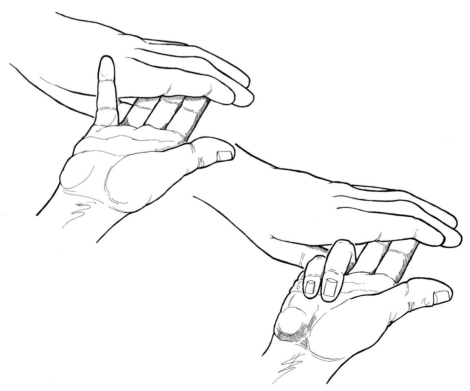

**Fig. 15-13.** Modified testing of flexor digitorum superficialis function to the little finger.

tested in full extension and asking the patient to flex the finger being tested onto the palm (Fig. 15-12); resistance is supplied by the examiner's free hand. Each digit is tested in turn. The opponens pollicis muscle is tested by asking the patient to make a loop with the thumb and the little finger, with the nail parallel to the palm (Fig. 15-16). The strength of the muscle is then tested by inserting a finger into the loop and trying to break the loop when the patient exerts force between the tip of the thumb and the tip of the little finger. The abductor pollicis brevis tendon is tested by asking the patient to raise the thumb above the surface of the palm as if it were a flag pole (ie, at a 90° angle) (Fig. 15-17). Strength is tested by attempting to push the thumb into the axis of the index finger, and confirmed by palpation of the thenar eminence to detect muscle contraction. The flexor carpi radialis tendon is tested by asking the patient to flex the hand at the wrist and palpating the tendon, which inserts into the volar surface of the trapezoid and capitate bones (Fig. 15-18).

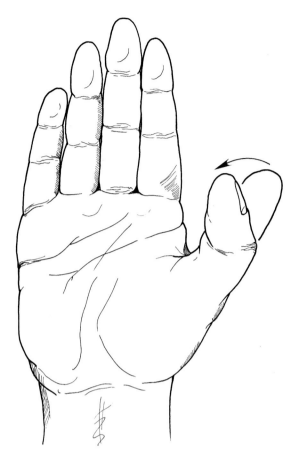

**Fig. 15-15.** Testing flexor pollicis longus tendon function.

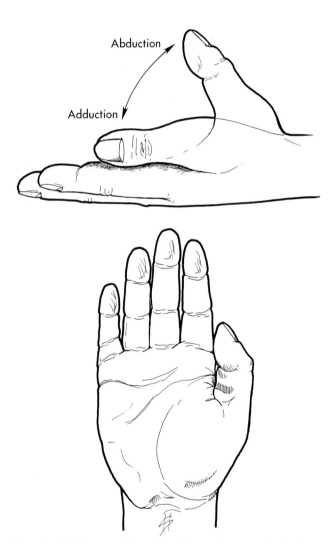

**Fig. 15-17.** Testing abductor pollicis brevis muscle function. Thumb abduction and adduction occur in a plane perpendicular to the extended index finger.

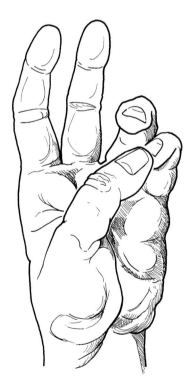

**Fig. 15-16.** Testing opponens pollicis muscle tendon function.

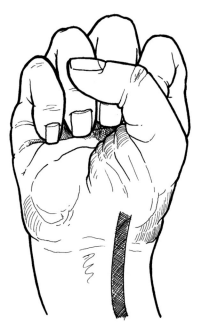

**Fig. 15-18.** Testing flexor carpi radialis tendon function.

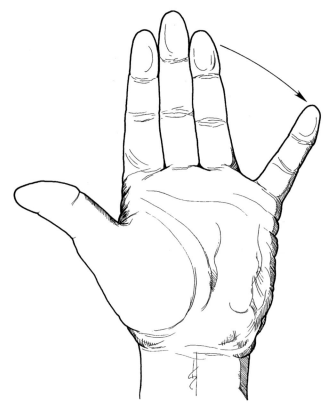

**Fig. 15-19.** Testing muscles of the hypothenar compartment.

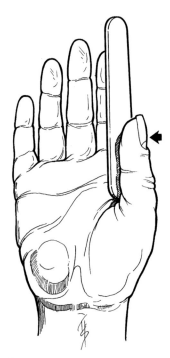

**Fig. 15-20.** Testing for muscle strength of the adductor pollicis muscle.

## Ulnar nerve

The flexor digitorum profundus tendon is tested by stabilizing the PIPJ in full extension, and asking the patient to bend the tip of the finger against resistance (Fig. 15-14). Interosseus muscle function is tested by asking the patient to spread the fingers apart (the fingers should abduct away from the middle finger; Fig. 15-8). The examiner should test for strength by pushing the fingers together against resistance. The muscles of the hypothenar compartment (ie, the abductor digiti minimi, the flexor digiti minimi, and the opponens digiti minimi) are tested by asking the patient to fully extend all the fingers and then move the little finger away from the other fingers (Fig. 15-19). Strength is tested by resistance against the examiner's free hand. The adductor pollicis muscle is tested by asking the patient to hold a piece of paper or a tongue blade between the thumb and the volar surface of the index finger. Strength is assessed by noting how difficult it is to remove this object (Fig. 15-20). The flexor carpi ulnaris tendon is tested by asking the patient to flex the hand at the wrist, palpating the tendon that inserts into the pisiform bone, and attempting to extend the hand when the patient supplies resistance (Fig. 15-21).

## Radial nerve

The tendons of the extensor pollicis brevis and the abductor pollicis longus are tested by asking the patient to move the thumb away from the hand as if the patient were hitchhiking (Fig. 15-22) (note: thumb extension occurs in the plane of the palm). The strength of these tendons is assessed by active resistance against this motion. The extensor carpi radialis longus and brevis tendons are tested by asking the

patient to make a fist and extend the hand at the wrist (Fig. 15-23). The extensor pollicis longus tendon is tested by asking the patient to place the hand on a flat surface and lift the thumb away from that surface (Fig. 15-24). The extensor indicus proprius tendon is tested by asking the patient to

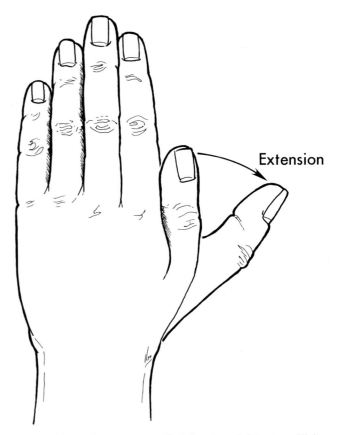

**Fig. 15-22.** Testing extensor pollicis brevis and abductor pollicis longus muscle and tendon function. Thumb extension occurs in the plane of the palm.

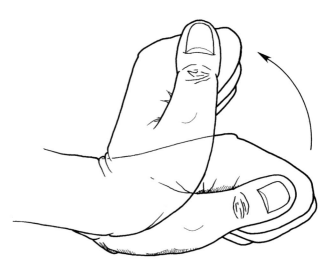

**Fig. 15-23.** Testing extensor carpi radialis longus and brevis tendon function.

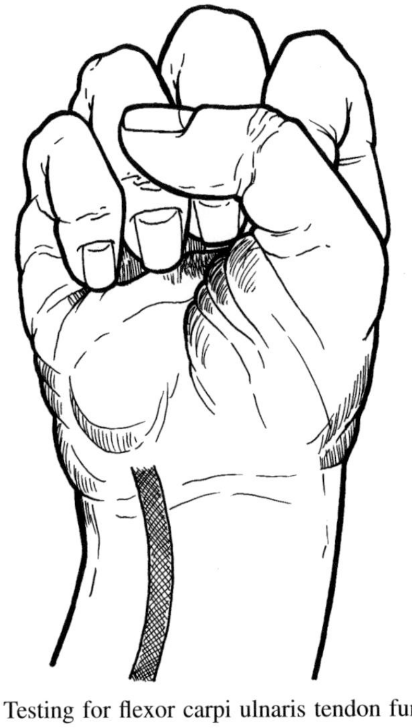

**Fig. 15-21.** Testing for flexor carpi ulnaris tendon function.

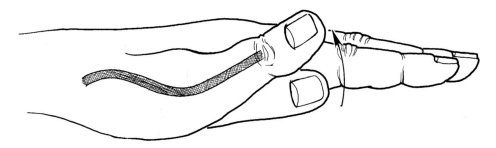

**Fig. 15-24.** Testing extensor pollicis longus muscle and tendon function.

make a fist and extend the index finger (Fig. 15-25). The extensor digitorum tendons are tested by asking the patient to extend the digits at the MCPJ and checking the strength of extension against resistance in each of the fingers (Fig. 15-26). The extensor digiti minimi is similarly tested by asking the patient to make a fist and then extend only the little finger at the MCPJ (Fig. 15-27). Strength is tested against resistance. The extensor carpi ulnaris tendon that inserts into the dorsal ulnar surface of the little finger metacarpal is tested by asking the patient to extend the hand at the wrist and bend the hand toward the ulna against resistance (Fig. 15-28).

### Nerve sensory branches

The sensory branches of each of the nerves are indicated in Fig. 15-29. The most specific area of radial nerve sensation is over the skin of the first dorsal interosseus muscle. The most specific area of median nerve function is the skin over the volar tip of the index finger, and the most specific area of ulnar nerve sensation is the skin over the volar tip of the little finger.

Sensory testing is the most unreliable component of the entire neurologic examination; however, a simple paper clip can be used in an objective means of evaluation. Sensation should be tested by uncoiling the paper clip, rolling it into a two-point discriminator (Fig. 15-30) with the two points roughly 5 mm apart (the upper limit of two-point sensation in normal patients), asking the patient to avert or close his or her eyes, and touching either one or two points to the digit being tested. Widened two-point sensation implies a nerve injury. For lacerations distal to the proximal palmar skin crease, each digit should be tested over the radial and ulnar side of the volar skin pad, as this cutaneous landmark defines the point at which the palmar digital nerves divide into the radial and ulnar branches.

### SOFT TISSUES

All wounds should be examined thoroughly to determine the extent of injury, the involvement of deeper structures (eg, tendons, nerves, and joint capsules), and the possible presence of a foreign body. Because blood vessels and nerves are closely approximated in the hand, the presence

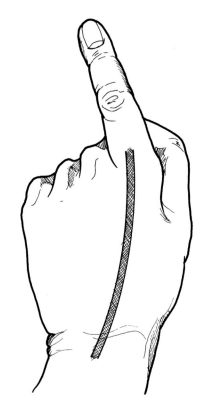

**Fig. 15-25.** Testing extensor indicis proprius muscle and tendon function.

of bleeding that does not easily respond to direct pressure and elevation should heighten suspicion of a nerve injury. It is also important to note: 1) if the injury is a cut or a crush; 2) if it is clean or contaminated; 3) if there is skin loss; and 4) if there is an amputated or partially amputated segment. A white, partially amputated segment implies arterial ischemia; a cyanotic or violaceous tip or flap is indicative of poor venous return. If there is any question about the viability of a distal partially amputated segment or flap, surgical consultation is advisable, because maintaining length of the finger is one of the primary goals of treatment. Digital nerve injuries, especially of the thumb and index fingers, flexor tendon injuries (complete or partial), and injuries of the radial or ulnar artery should be referred to a specialist in hand or plastic surgery.

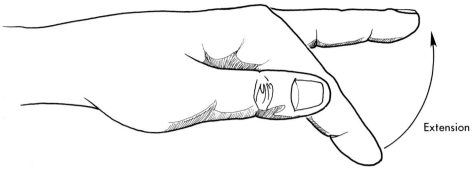

**Fig. 15-26.** Testing extension of the fingers (testing extensor digitorum function).

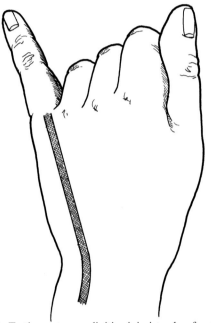

**Fig. 15-27.** Testing extensor digiti minimi tendon function.

## DISCUSSION

The human hand has had a long and successful evolutionary history. The ultimate success of any initial hand injury or infection often depends on the steps taken by the initial treating physician. These steps demand a careful examination that includes appropriate light anesthesia, hemostasis, instrumentation, infection control measures, and uninterrupted time. Other steps include the use of appropriate and standard nomenclature in charting and when describing cases to consultants. Extensive injuries should be expeditiously referred to specialists after a brief initial examination, splinting, and intravenous antibiotics.

## FINGERTIP AMPUTATION AND FINGER PAD TISSUE LOSS

The fingertip is the most commonly injured part of the hand.[3] Two common presentations include sharp injuries such as the loss of a portion of one of the fingertips while

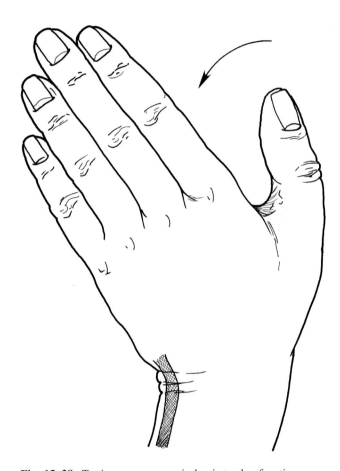

**Fig. 15-28.** Testing extensor carpi ulnaris tendon function.

slicing food or from a cut on broken glass, or a crush-type injury such as when the finger is caught in a door and part of the tip is amputated. Although these injuries may seem trivial, they can result in a surprisingly high degree of disability and time lost from work. The average healing time in three studies was 21 to 27.3 days.[4-6] Conservative treatment has been studied for both sharp and crush injuries,[5] and seems especially applicable in cases of crush injury when the viability of the surrounding soft tissues is in question. Conservative treatment of fingertip injuries has been studied in both children and adults in lesions that vary

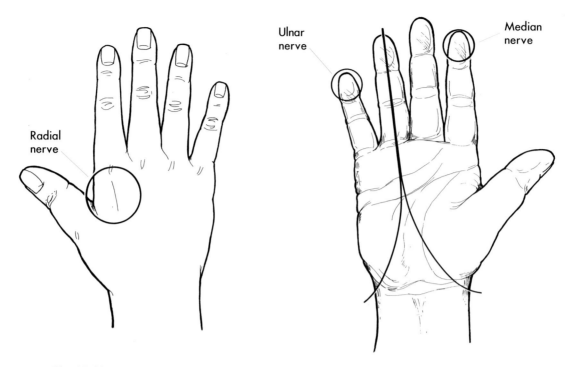

**Fig. 15-29.** Sensory distribution of radial, median, and ulnar nerves. Circle indicates area of most specific sensory function.

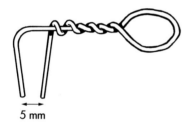

**Fig. 15-30.** Easily constructed device, made from a standard paper clip, for checking two-point discrimination.

from 0.5 cm² or larger (in children) to 6.25 cm² (in adults); and involve the terminal phalanx without injury to tendons or joints.⁴,⁷ These studies excluded injury proximal to the nail or nail bed.

The principles of treatment advocated by most authors⁴⁻¹⁵ include the following: thorough cleaning with sterile solutions with or without prior soaking; nipping protruding bone with a bone rongeur to a level 3 to 5 mm below that of the surrounding soft tissue; sterile dressings with antibiotic ointment over the amputated part covered by vaseline gauze and a tube gauze dressing (three studies used silver sulfadiazene occlusion dressings over the amputated fingertip⁶,¹⁴,¹⁵); leaving the nail and nail bed untouched (if uninjured) or careful repair of the nail matrix; dressing changes daily or every other day to remove crusts from the healing amputation; referral to occupational therapy or physical therapy for stump skin toughening exercises after complete epithelialization; and the use of dry dressings once firm granulation tissue is present.

Complications of both conservative and surgical treatment include intolerance to cold, numbness, tenderness, and increased two-point discrimination.⁴,⁵ Fingernail deformity is more likely to occur when greater than two-thirds of the nail is involved or when the amputation is at or proximal to the lunula of the nail.⁵ Surgical treatment has additional complications including prolonged pain and joint stiffness (secondary to prolonged immobilization after grafting), postoperative infection, and graft failure.⁴,⁵,¹³,¹⁶ Proposed surgical treatments for fingertip amputations include split-thickness skin grafting, a variety of flaps, numerous plastic surgical closures, and primary closure with or without trimming of soft tissue or bone.¹⁶⁻¹⁸ Several articles have reported that conservative treatment is equal to or better than surgical treatment, and that it avoids the problems inherent in surgical treatment such as joint stiffness, postoperative infection, and graft failure.⁴⁻¹⁵ On balance, I prefer conservative treatment of fingertip injuries to the distal phalanx because of their excellent cosmetic results, decreased infection rate, and simplicity of treatment. Conservative treatment is especially useful when crush injuries have caused the amputation. However, surgical treatment might have advantages in cases in which there is a high likelihood of fingernail deformity (when more than two-thirds of the nail is lost) that is unacceptable to the patient, and in cases in which preservation of digit length is a high priority (eg, in injuries to the dominant thumb). Amputation injuries that involve the joint or tendons or are proximal to the insertions of the extensor and flexor tendons in the distal phalanx, or those that occur proximal to the lunula (where the likelihood of nail deformity is high) will require surgical consultation. Also, extensive volar angulation of the amputation segment has a less favorable outcome when treated conservatively.

## SUBUNGUAL HEMATOMA

A subungual hematoma is defined as blood between the nail and nail matrix. Two issues bear on the treatment of a subungual hematoma; the first is the possibility of an underlying laceration of the nail matrix and the second is the possibility of an underlying fracture of the distal phalanx. In one study of 47 patients with subungual hematomas,[19] radiographs were obtained in each patient after fingertip injuries. The nail was removed and the nail matrix inspected for a laceration beneath the hematoma. If the laceration was less than 2 to 3 mm in length, the nail was replaced over the nail bed, tucked into the nail fold, and the patient discharged; if a laceration needed repair, it was closed with fine (6-0) sutures and the nail was replaced in its previous anatomic position to prevent adhesions from forming between the nail matrix and the nail fold. In this study, 95% of patients with a fracture of the distal phalanx had a reparable laceration of the nail matrix. Furthermore, in 60% of patients with a subungual hematoma that involved more than 50% of the nail surface, the laceration was reparable. In patients with a subungual hematoma covering more than 50% of the nail surface area, or a subungual hematoma associated with a tuft fracture, these authors recommended that the nail be removed and the nail matrix be explored to search for a reparable laceration. This study stands in contrast to another study that involved patients ranging in age from 3 to 60 years with or without an associated fracture of the distal phalanx.[20] Inclusion criteria in this study were a closed hematoma, an intact nail, and no laceration of the skinfold or disruption of the nail. In this study, there was no correlation between the size of the hematoma and fracture. The procedure used in this study to treat subungual hematoma was simple trephination. There were no soft tissue infections, osteomyelitis, or permanent nail deformities.

Usual methods for draining a subungual hematoma include the following: a hot paper clip, disposable cautery, or use of a nail drill. In the hot paper clip technique, a standard paper clip is uncoiled and held in the jaws of a hemostat; the tip is heated with an alcohol lamp or cigarette lighter until the tip glows. The tip is then placed over the nail plate that overlies the area of hematoma. Pressure is applied until the nail is melted away and the paper clip enters the pool of the hematoma. Several cycles of heating the paper clip and applying pressure to the area of the nail generally are required before the hematoma is entered. Disposable cautery is a direct method of releasing a subungual hematoma. The cautery unit is turned on and the glowing tip is pressed to the nail surface until the tip melts through the nail and enters the pool of the hematoma. The nail drill is a battery-powered, hand-held device that uses

sterile disposable bits to bore small holes in the nail. After trephination of any sort, approximately 4 months generally are required for a new nail to replace the damaged one. Important principles in the treatment of subungual hematoma include adequate anesthesia prior to the procedure using a digital block and the use of multiple holes (or one large 3 to 4-mm hole).

Before treating a subungual hematoma, it is important to document the sensory examination to two-point discrimination over the fingertip and to document the presence of extensor tendon function since injuries that produce a subungual hematoma may sometimes avulse the extensor tendon.

We support the conservative treatment of uncomplicated subungual hematomas. Uncomplicated patients include those with a closed hematoma, an intact nail, and no associated laceration of the skinfold or disruption of the nail.[20] Patients who have significant crush injuries, fingertip lacerations that involve the nail itself, and injuries that avulse, split, or disrupt the nail should have the nail removed and the nail matrix inspected. If a suturable laceration is found, it should be repaired (Fig. 15-31) and the untrimmed nail replaced in its anatomic position between the nail fold and nail matrix. The nail should then be sutured into place laterally to prevent adhesions from forming between the nail matrix and the nail fold. A band-aid is a sufficient dressing after treatment of an uncomplicated subungual hematoma not associated with fracture. A tube gauze dressing is the ideal dressing for those patients who required removal of the nail, suture of an underlying laceration in the nail matrix, and replacement of the nail between the nail matrix and nail fold. A follow-up wound check 2 days posttreatment is recommended for patients who have had suturing of the nail matrix or an open wound of the fingertip.

All patients with subungual hematomas do not require radiography. Those with obvious deformity, pain on palpation over the volar pad, or pain with longitudinal compression of the digit, or those whose hands are intrinsic to their profession (eg, musicians, typists, computer chip assembly workers) are likely to benefit from an x-ray. In these patients, the diagnosis of a fracture may modify their ability to work or may form the basis of a disability based on worker compensation rules. Fractures should be reduced appropriately and splinted in extension using a metal or plastic splint for a period of 2 to 3 weeks. One study[13] does not recommend antibiotics for subungual hematomas after trephination, even in the presence of a fracture. I support this view.

Lacerations of the nail matrix are generally repaired to prevent a deformed nail matrix because the nail matrix is a mold over which the new nail grows. If this mold is deformed, as new nail grows, this deformity will result in a new nail that is cosmetically unacceptable; will catch on objects in the environment during daily living activities; and is difficult to correct following initial mistreatment.

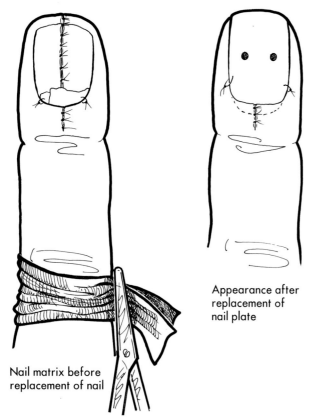

Nail matrix before
replacement of nail

Appearance after
replacement of
nail plate

**Fig. 15-31.** Repair of laceration to nail matrix. Figure on right shows damaged nail replaced by a stent to prevent adhesions from forming between nail matrix and proximal nail fold.

Generally accepted treatment guidelines for suturing a lacerated nail matrix include[3,17,21-24] gentle débridement; cleaning and removal of all foreign bodies; saving even the smallest fragment of *viable* nail matrix (to prevent a defect in this tissue); retaining the nail plate to be used as a subsequent dressing; meticulous repair of the nail matrix laceration using a fine absorbable suture (eg, 6-0 suture); reinsertion of the nail plate or a substitute (generally vaseline gauze) between the nail matrix and the nail fold after laceration repair to prevent adhesions between these parts until the new nail forms in 2 to 3 weeks (the nail is usually held in place by sutures placed laterally rather than directly proximal so that they do not enter the germinal matrix of the nail); applying a sterile nonadherent dressing (generally vaseline gauze with antibiotic ointment); and the appropriate reduction/splinting of any fractures of the distal phalanx (Fig. 15-31). As the new nail plate forms, the reinserted nail plate (or its substitute) is dislodged and will fall away.

## FINGERTIP INJURIES

Fingertip injuries include amputations, traumatically avulsed nails, crush injuries, and nail bed lacerations. Simple fingertip injuries should not involve tendons, amputations at or proximal to the distal interphalangeal joint, or the potential use of grafts or flaps; these can be treated by most emergency department physicians. Principles of treatment for these injuries include maximizing digit length; stump coverage with adequate nontender soft tissue (ensuring that sensitivity is as good as possible); minimizing joint stiffness; and limiting employment disability.[6] In questionable cases, especially those that involve the dominant hand, it is advisable to seek subspecialty consultation. Wounds with excessive loss of volar tissue (less dorsally) no longer have adequate palmar pulp tissue to support the nail adequately. Consequently, 20% to 25% of these patients will develop a hooked nail (ie, nail growth over the end of the finger).[18] Another instance when early consultation may be appropriate is when amputations are associated with a severe crushing component because of the possibility in these cases of tissue necrosis.[17] Common amputation injuries include: losses after slicing injuries while cooking or cleaning or those in which the fingertip is crushed after being caught in a door. In these cases, there may be an associated avulsion of the proximal nail (because the nail beneath the lunula and nail root is not as firmly adherent to the nail matrix as it is more distally). Treatment in these cases involves[3,17,21-23] careful examination of flexor/extensor function; checking two-point discrimination over both the radial and ulnar sides of the distal tip; radiography to rule out a fracture; a digital block using a long-acting anesthetic; hemostasis during repair using a finger tourniquet (a 1-inch Penrose drain placed just above the metacarpophalangeal joint and secured by a hemostat); thorough cleaning and minimal débridement of the nail bed and germinal matrix; meticulous reapproximation of the nail bed matrix (if a laceration is present) using fine absorbable sutures (6-0 suture); preservation of the skinfold around the nail by careful reapproximation of the edges; prevention of adhesions between the nail fold and the nail matrix by replacing the avulsed nail (or gauze-packing if the avulsed nail is too badly damaged) between these parts and suturing it in place with laterally placed sutures (so that the sutures do not enter the germinal matrix of the nail) (Fig. 15-31); and the appropriate reduction and splinting of fractures.

The procedure for removing a nail after a partial avulsion or searching for a laceration is surprisingly simple. The key element is dense fingertip anesthesia using a digital block. The nail itself is easily removed by opening the jaws of Mayo scissors and passing the blunt rounded tip (with the smooth side toward the nail matrix) between the nail plate and matrix from the distal portion of the nail to the proximal portion just under the nail fold. Several passes may be necessary to loosen the entire nail; the tip of the nail then may be grasped by a hemostat and pulled directly out longitudinally. Nail elevation may also be accomplished using a specific instrument, a Freer elevator, although this instrument is not commonly available in most emergency departments. After removal, the nail should be washed but not trimmed. After the nail bed has been repaired, the avulsed nail should be replaced in its anatomic position or vaseline or adaptic gauze placed between the nail fold and nail matrix to prevent adhesions. Both the replaced nail and the gauze should be held in place by sutures placed laterally on the ulnar and radial side of the nail to prevent suturing into the germinal nail matrix (Fig. 15-31). Thereafter, a nonadherent dressing (vaseline or adaptic gauze followed by antibiotic ointment) should be placed over the injury followed by tube gauze dressing. Patients with fractures should be fitted with an alumofoam splint or the equivalent and should be scheduled for a wound check 2 days postinjury. Controlled studies of the use of antibiotics after such injuries have not been done. One paper suggests that antibiotics are not helpful even in the presence of a tuft fracture.[13] In immunocompromised patients (those with AIDS, diabetes mellitus, peripheral vascular disease, or Raynaud's phenomena), administering 3 days of penicillin V potassium, 500 mg four times daily, or a first-generation cephalosporin seems prudent. Controlled studies in this setting are lacking, however.

## FOREIGN BODIES

Wood, metal, and glass are the most commonly found foreign bodies in the hand.[24] One study found that 37.5% of foreign bodies in the hand are missed by the first examining physician.[24] Therefore, a high level of suspicion and knowledge of the mechanism of injury are important factors when considering the presence of a foreign body. The most common hand injury is a puncture wound;[25] these appear innocent but may hide significant foreign bodies.[26,27] Because the path of migration of a foreign body cannot be predicted,[25] it is important to examine *all* areas of the hand, wrist, and forearm during examination, not just the immediate area beneath the wound. Foreign bodies can migrate into the forearm following a puncture wound in the web space, and have been reported to migrate from the wrist to the digit.[27,28] Plain radiography can detect 80% of all foreign bodies when at least two views are obtained.[29] The principle of trauma radiology is that the joints both above and below the wound site or injury should be radiographed. Several studies[24,30,31] found that radiography detected 100% of metal foreign bodies, 95% of glass foreign bodies, and 15% of wooden foreign bodies. Most glass foreign bodies are visible on plain radiographs; in fact, fragments as small as 0.5 mm will appear on plain films if not obscured by bone, and fragments as small as 2 mm will be visible in the presence of overlying bone.[31] A study of glass, gravel, wood, and plastic embedded into cadaver hands revealed that all glass was readily identified by CT.[32] If gravel was highly suspected and not visible on plain radiographs, then CT scanning readily detected it.[32] In the same study,[32] plastic (the density of which is similar to that of soft tissue) was not readily detected by CT scanning, and MRI was recommended as the diagnostic method of choice to detect plastic foreign bodies. This same study[32] also revealed that xeroradiography was no more helpful than plain radiography in identifying foreign bodies. Several

studies recommended CT scanning if a wooden foreign body was not seen on plain radiographs.[33-35] Ultrasound is useful in detecting nonradio opaque foreign bodies in the hand.[29,36-40] Visualizing foreign bodies using ultrasound depends on the differences in acoustic impedance between the foreign body and the surrounding soft tissues, not on the density of the foreign body. The detection of foreign bodies by ultrasound is contingent on the experience of the ultrasonographer, the size of the foreign body (3 to 4 mm being the reported lower limit of resolution), and the use of a linear array transducer (rather than the more commonly available pieshape).[29,36-40] See Figure 15-32 for a flow diagram useful in the diagnostic approach to foreign body detection in the emergency department.

Undiagnosed or unsuspected foreign bodies can lodge in tendons[41,42] cause tendon rupture,[42,43] lead to tenosynovitis,[28] be the nidus for unusual infections[44] or synovitis;[45] present as nodules;[46] cause osteolytic lesions of bones[47] or osteomyelitis and septic arthritis,[48,49] and cause delayed lacerations of major nerves.[50,51] Criteria for the removal of foreign bodies in the hand have been proposed by several authors[26,52] and include the following: foreign bodies located in the fingers; those likely to provoke significant tissue inflammation (wood stained with analine dyes or coated with creosote, or wood having a high resin or oil content); thorns, cactus spines, and plant parts,[53,54] those heavily contaminated with cloth or soil,[55] those associated with a fracture or infection[52,56] located near or producing a functional abnormality of vessels, joints, nerves or tendons; if the patient has an allergy to the foreign body; and patients who will be taken to the operating room for débridement of other associated hand injuries. One author[25] recommends that if a glass foreign body has penetrated the fascia of the palm, then a formal exploration in the operating room of the deep structures of the hand is in order because injury to tendon, nerves, and vessels are difficult to detect clinically. Removal of a foreign body requires adequate anesthesia; hemostasis using a 1-inch Penrose drain secured with a hemostat or use of a pneumatic tourniquet; adequate exposure; bright lights; patient cooperation; and most importantly, uninterrupted time. Should any one of these elements be lacking, the emergency room physician should seek subspecialty assistance. When removing wood splinters, it is appropriate to open the entire track under local anesthesia and tourniquet control. If there is doubt about the removal of a wooden foreign body, the patient should be scheduled for repeat examination in 5 to 7 days.[57] If signs of infection are present at the time of repeat examination, the wound should be explored or the patient should have a CT scan of the wound to look for an occult foreign body. In cases of subungual wood splinters, one author[25] recommends removal of the nail overlying the foreign body; this ensures direct access and complete removal. Open wound management techniques are appropriate when a patient with a known retained foreign body is discharged from the emergency department to be definitively treated by a subspecial-

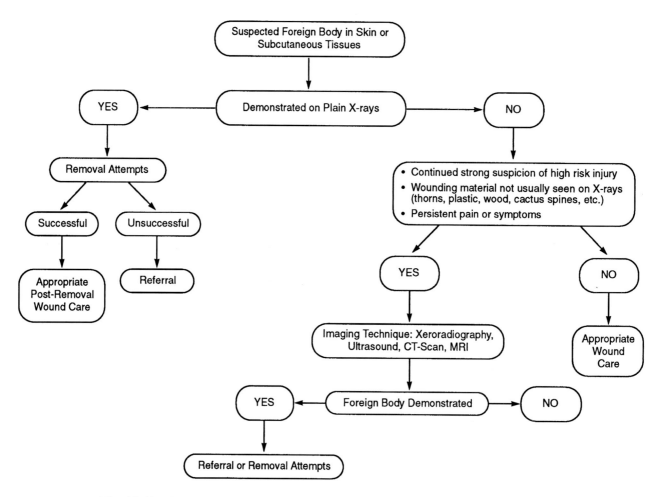

**Fig. 15-32.** Flow diagram useful in the diagnostic approach to foreign body detection in the emergency department. (Reproduced from Schwartz GR, Cayten CG, Mangelsen MA, et al: *Principles and practice of emergency medicine*, ed. 3, Baltimore, Md, 1992, Lea & Febiger. Reproduced with permission.)

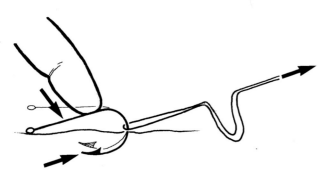

**Fig. 15-33.** Removal of a fishhook with a piece of string.

ist. In such patients, the emergency department physician should explain in unequivocal terms that the patient does, in fact, have a retained foreign body, the reason for its nonremoval in the emergency department (physician inexperience, depth of penetration, location near vital structures, lack of uninterrupted time), and the absolute need for appropriate and timely subspecialty referral. This conversa-

tion should be documented in the medical record. Because of implications for employment and in order to maximize functional results, emergency department physicians should attempt to remove only superficial foreign bodies in the digits, hand, or wrist.

**Embedded fishhooks**

Patients occasionally present to the emergency room for removal of a fishhook embedded in the soft tissues of the skin. There is a simple technique to remove an embedded hook without anesthesia if only a single hook is involved.[58,59] This method is also effective if a single barb of a treble hook is embedded, but other barbs should be safely covered first with cloth tape to prevent further puncture wounds. Safety glasses should also be worn by the physician during this maneuver.

A piece of string or a twill tape approximately 36 inches long should be tied in a circle. This is then placed around the curved portion of the fishhook at skin level. One finger is used to place pressure on the shank of the hook perpendicular to the site of skin entry to unlock the barb. The other hand provides an aggressive, brisk pull (along the axis of the shank) on the string encircling the curved portion of the hook while perpendicular unlocking pressure is applied to the shank. The motion of this brisk pull is initiated with 75% slack in the encircling string, and the force is continued throughout the full arm swing. This must be done with confidence in the pull as the encircling string is snapped (Fig. 15-33).

The hook frequently will fly across the room, so bystanders should not stand in line with your pull. This method is very successful as long as perpendicular pressure is applied to unlock the barb. Patients should be assured this is a painless procedure and is commonly used by experienced fishermen. Patients are often amazed when the hook is removed without them knowing. This method is not recommended for hooks embedded near neurovascular structures or tendons.

## Gunshot wounds

**Nail gun and high pressure injection injuries.**[63] Gunshot wounds can cause extensive injury to vascular structures and muscles. Nail gun injuries can produce injuries just as destructive as those from high-powered handguns.[60] The innocent-appearing puncture wound caused by a high-pressure injector can mask significant disabling injuries of tendon sheaths, neurovascular structures, and muscle.[61,62] In the presence of a high-pressure injection injury, there should be no preoperative infiltration of local anesthesia in the injured hand because local infiltration into tissues already distended with injectate may lead to further tissue distension, with secondary vascular spasm and consequent increased ischemia and tissue destruction.[52] All patients with gunshot wounds to the hand, nail gun injuries, and wounds caused by high-pressure injectors should be admitted to the hospital. Only after consultation and with the consent of an orthopedic or hand surgeon should any of these patients be discharged from the emergency department. In such cases a note in the hospital chart should document the conversation, the name of the consultant, and the disposition agreed to by the specialist.

## REFERENCES

1. Martin RD: Primate origins: Plugging the gaps. *Nature* 363: 223-234, 1993.
2. Stein A, Lemos M, and Stein S: Clinical evaluation of flexor tendon function in the small finger. *Ann Emerg Med* 19: 991-993, 1990.
3. Hart RC, Kleinert HE. Fingertip and nailbed injuries, *Emerg Med Clin North Am* 11:755-765, 1993.
4. Ipsen T, Frandsen PA, and Barfred T: Conservative treatment of fingertip injuries, *Injury* 18:203-205, 1987.
5. Chow SP, Ho E: Open treatment of fingertip injuries in adults, *J Hand Surg* 7(A):470-476, 1982.
6. Arbel R, Goodwin DRA, and Otremski I: Treatment of fingertip injuries with silver sulfadiazine occlusion dressing, *Injury* 20:161-163, 1989.
7. Rosenthal LJ, Reiner MA, and Bleicher MA: Nonoperative management of distal fingertip amputations in children, *Pediatrics* 64:1-3, 1979.
8. Bossley CJ: Conservative treatment of digit amputations, *NZ Med J* 82:379-380, 1975.
9. Das SK, Brown HG: Management of lost fingertips in children, *Hand* 10:16-27, 1978.
10. Douglas BS: Conservative management of guillotine amputation of the finger in children, *Aust Paediatr J* 8:86-89, 1972.
11. Illingworth CM: Trapped fingers and amputated fingertips in children, *J Pediatr Surg* 9:853-858, 1974.
12. Louis D, Palmer A, and Burney R: Open treatment of digital tip injuries, *JAMA* 244:697-698, 1980.
13. Lamon RP, Cicero JJ, Frascone RJ, Hass WF: Open treatment of fingertip amputations, *Ann Emerg Med* 12:358-360, 1983.
14. Fox JW, Golden GT, Rodeheaver G, et al.: Non-operative management of fingertip pulp amputation by occlusive dressings, *Am J Surg* 133:255-256, 1977.
15. deBoer P, Collinson PO: The use of silver sulfadiazine occlusive dressings for fingertip injuries, *J Bone Joint Surg* 63-B:545-547, 1981.
16. Russell RC, Casas LA: Management of fingertip injuries, *Clin Plast Surg* 16:405-425, 1989.
17. Zook EG, Doermann A: Management of fingertip trauma, *Postgrad Med* 83:163-176, 1988.
18. Burkhalter WE: Fingertip injuries, *Emerg Med Clin North Am* 3:245-253, 1985.
19. Simon RA, Wolgin M: Subungual hematoma: association with occult laceration requiring repair, *Am J Emerg Med* 5:302-304, 1987.
20. Seaberg DC, Angelos WJ, and Parris PM: Treatment of subungual hematomas with nail trephination: a prospective study, *Am J Emerg Med* 9:209-210, 1991.
21. Kleinert HE: Fingertip injuries and their management, *Am Surg* 25:41-51, 1959.
22. Melone CP, Grad JB: Primary care of fingernail injuries, *Emerg Med Clinic North Am* 3:255-261, 1985.
23. Rosenthal EA: Treatment of fingertip nailbed injuries, *Orthop Clin North Am* 14:675-697, 1983.
24. Anderson MA, Newmeyer WH III, and Kilgore ES: Diagnosis and treatment of retained foreign bodies in the hand, *Am J Surg* 144:63-67, 1982.
25. Stein F: Foreign body injuries of the hand, *Emerg Med Clinic North Am* 3:383-390, 1985.
26. Marquis GP: Radiolucent foreign bodies in the hand: case report, *J Trauma* 29:403-404, 1989.
27. Chow J: Foreign body migration in the hand (letter), *J Hand Surg* 13(A):462, 1993.
28. Merrell JC, Russell RC, and Zook EG: Non-suppurative tenosynovitis secondary to foreign body migration, *J Hand Surg* 8:340-341, 1983.
29. Donaldson JS: Radiographic imaging of foreign bodies in the hand, *Hand Clin* 7:125-134, 1991.
30. Morgan WJ, Leopold T, and Evans R: Foreign bodies in the hand, *J Hand Surg* 9-B:194-196, 1983.
31. Tandberg D: Glass in the hand and foot: will an x-ray film show it? *JAMA* 1872-1874, 1982.
32. Russell RC, Williamson DA, Sullivan JW, Suchy H: Detection of foreign bodies in the hand, *J Hand Surg* 16-A:2-11, 1991.
33. Rhoades CE, Soye I, Levine E, Reckling FW: Detection of a wood foreign body in the hand using computed tomography: case report, *J Hand Surg* 7:306-307, 1982.
34. Firooznia H, Bjorkengren A, Hofstetter SR et al.: Computed tomographic localization of foreign bodies lodged in the extremities, *Comput Radiol* 8:237-239, 1984.
35. Bodne D, Quinn SF, and Cochran CF: Imaging foreign glass and wooden bodies of the extremity with CT and MR, *J Comput Assist Tomogr* 12:608-611, 1988.
36. Lejeune A: Detection of foreign bodies in hand, *J Hand Surg* 18-A:166-168, 1993.
37. Fornage BD, Schernberg FL: Sonographic preoperative localization of a foreign body in the hand, *J Ultrasound Med* 6:217-219, 1987.
38. Hansson G, Beebe AC, Carroll NC, Donaldson JS: A piece of wood in the hand diagnosed by ultrasonography, *Acta Orthop Scand* 59:459-460, 1988.

39. Gooding GAW, Hardiman T, Sumers M, et al.: Sonography of the hand and foot in foreign body detection, *J Ultrasound Med* 6:441-447, 1987.

40. Fornage BD, Schernberg FL, and Rifkin MD: Ultrasound examination of the hand, *Radiology* 155:785-788, 1985.

41. Arbel R, Kaplin O, and Goodwin DRA: The disappearing needle, *J Hand Surg* 12-B:127-128, 1987.

42. Jozsa L, Reffy A, Demel S, Balint JB: Foreign bodies in tendons, *J Hand Surg* 14-B:84-85, 1989.

43. Jablon M, Rabin SI: Late flexor pollicis longus tendon rupture due to retained glass fragments, *J Hand Surg* 13-A:713-716, 1988.

44. Fayman M, Braun S: A foreign body related actinomycosis of a finger, *J Hand Surg* 10-A:411-412, 1985.

45. Klein B, McGahan JP: Thorn synovitis: CT diagnosis, *J Comput Assist Tomogr* 9:1135-1136, 1985.

46. Wong RC: Embedded foreign body presenting as an umbilicated dermal nodule, *Int J Dermatol* 27:254-255, 1988.

47. Merrell JC, Petro JA, and Miller SH: Osseous foreign body reaction in the hand, *Ann Plast Surg* 4:154-157, 1980.

48. Greene WB: Unrecognized foreign body as a focus for delayed *Serratia marcesens* osteomyelitis and septic arthritis, *J Bone Joint Surg* 71-A:754-757, 1989.

49. Vincent K, Szabo RM: *Enterobacter agglomerans* osteomyelitis of the hand from a rose thorn: a case report, *Orthopedics* 11:465-467, 1988.

50. Craig EV: Delayed laceration of ulnar nerve following hand trauma, *JAMA* 253:1014, 1985.

51. Browett JP, Fiddian NJ: Delayed median nerve injury due to retained glass fragments: a report of two cases, *J Bone Joint Surg* 67-B:382-384, 1985.

52. Smoot EC, Robson MC: Acute management of foreign body injuries of the hand, *Ann Emerg Med* 12:434-437, 1983.

53. Lindsey D, Lindsey WE: Cactus spine injuries, *Am J Emerg Med* 6:362-369, 1988.

54. Lammers RL: Soft tissue foreign bodies, *Ann Emerg Med* 17:1336-1377, 1988.

55. Haury BB, Rodeheaver GT, Pettry D, et al.: Inhibition of non-specific defenses by soil infection potentiating factors, *Surg Gynecol Obsetet* 144:19-24, 1977.

56. Edlich RF, Rodeheaver GT, Morgan RF et al.: Principles of emergency wound management, *Ann Emerg Med* 17:1284-1302, 1988.

57. Rand C: Cocktail stick injuries: delayed diagnosis of a retained foreign body, *BMJ* 295:1658, 1987.

58. Danesh J, Donoghue M, and Dixon G: Fishhook injuries: wound anglers and string theory (letter), *NZ Med J* 105:136, 1992.

59. David SS: Fishhook removal, *Lancet* 338:1463-1464, 1991.

60. Edlich RF, Silloway KA, Rodeheaver GT et al.: Industrial nail gun injuries, *Comp Ther* 12:42-46, 1986.

61. Herrick RT, Godsil RD, and Widener JH: High pressure injection injuries to the hand, *South Med J* 73:896–898, 1980.

62. Fialkov JA, Freiberg A: High pressure injection injuries: an overview, *J Emerg Med* 9:367-371, 1991.

63. Curka PA, Chisholm CD: High pressure water injection injury to the hand, *Am J Emerg Med* 7:165-167, 1989.

# Hand Injuries and Infections

*Stephen W. Smith*

In this chapter, relevant diagnostic issues are covered. Issues necessary for choosing either surgical or non-surgical treatment are discussed, as is the urgency of surgical referral. Management of conditions that do not require surgery by a specialist and thus can be undertaken by the emergency physician are discussed in detail. Operative techniques employed by the specialist are beyond the scope of this chapter.

Most importantly, it is imperative to refer all but the most trivial hand injuries for follow-up with a hand surgeon.

# FRACTURES: GENERAL OVERVIEW

Fracture of the proximal phalanx results in the greatest degree of disability, followed by the middle phalanx, the metacarpal bones, and lastly, the distal phalanx. Injuries up to 6 weeks old may still be amenable to reduction without osteotomy.

## Indications for reduction

Fractures that are displaced, rotated, or angulated should be slated for reduction.

## Indications for surgery

Injuries requiring surgery are categorized as follows:
1) Unstable reductions (the reduction must not depend on the splint for its stability). The possible exception is in the use of the Burkhalter-Reyes method of dynamic splinting for unstable proximal phalangeal fractures described below.
2) Some open fractures.
3) Involvement of the joint and fragment > 20% of the joint surface and displaced.
4) Persistent soft-tissue interposition after closed reduction (rare in the hand)
5) Other specific injuries detailed below.

## Follow-up and duration of immobilization

Follow-up within 1 week is necessary to assure continued alignment of all of phalangeal fractures. The most common mistake in treating these injuries is to overtreat by immobilizing for too long a period of time. It is rarely necessary to immobilize even unstable closed phalangeal fractures for longer than 3 weeks.[1] Clinical healing (resolution of swelling and tenderness) requires 3 to 4 weeks, and it is at this time that range of motion should begin. The physician should not wait for radiographic healing, which usually takes much longer—averaging 5 months with a range of 1 to 17 months.[2] Tenderness is a good indicator of the need for continued immobilization.[3] After this time, buddy taping may be used for stability, allowing motion and preventing further stiffness. Physical therapy should be started and continued until stiffness is resolved.

## Complications

Complications of fractures include malfunction from excessive residual angulation, nonunion, malrotation, joint stiffness (often from excessive or inappropriate splinting), degenerative joints (when the articular surface is involved), and adhesions of the flexor and extensor mechanisms to the fracture site, especially in fractures with much soft-tissue injury.

Complications can best be avoided by careful examination to identify pathology and providing early follow-up with a hand surgeon regardless of the emergency department management.

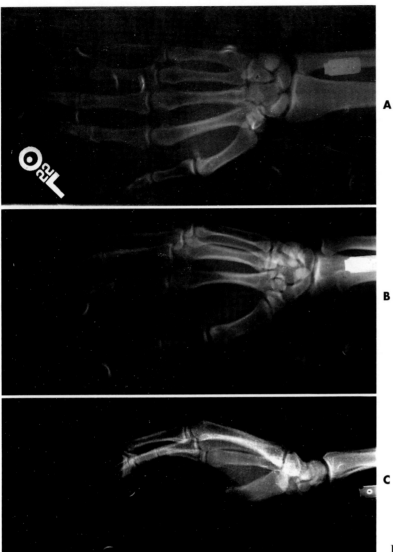

**Fig. 16-1. A,** Normal AP, **B,** oblique, and **C,** lateral of the hand for comparison.

## Radiography (see Fig. 16-1 for normal hand)

**Indications for radiography.** For many hand injuries, significant fracture may be ruled out by clinical exam, saving the patient both time and money. The more experienced and knowledgeable physician will be better able to determine which injuries may harbor significant fractures. It is helpful to remember that soft-tissue injury is tender to palpation, as are fractures, but only with fractures may tenderness be elicited by stressing the bone at a distant site, or by palpating where there is no overlying soft-tissue tenderness. If the physician is in doubt, or inexperienced with a particular injury, it is safest to order a radiograph of the injury.

**Pitfalls in radiography.** When viewing the anteroposterior (AP) film it is a common pitfall for the physician to miss angulation and sometimes even displacement of fractures, especially those of the base of the proximal phalanx.[4] Therefore, a minimum of three views is necessary to assure correct diagnosis: AP, lateral, and at least one oblique. Even so, the base of the proximal phalanx can be very difficult to

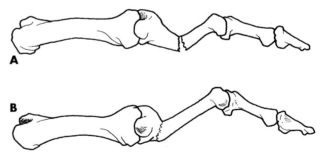

**Fig. 16-2. A,** Sketch of a midshaft proximal phalanx fracture with apex volar angulation. This creates an obvious deformity on radiographs whereas, in **B,** the same degree of angulation at the base results in a subtle but functionally significant deformity. These base fractures are commonly overlooked on radiographs.

visualize because of superimposition of the other phalanges, especially after reduction when the film detail is also obscured by the splint. In addition, for the same amount of angulation, a base fracture remains clinically unrecognized more often than a shaft fracture (Fig. 16-2). Fractures at the

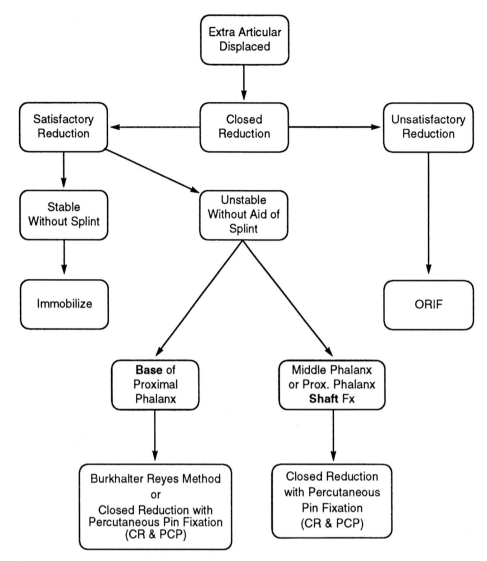

**Fig. 16-3.** Algorithm for treatment of proximal or middle phalangeal fractures.

bases of the metacarpals are notoriously difficult to visualize on radiograph. Rotation is also very difficult to detect radiographically; it must be assessed clinically.

### Stable, nondisplaced fractures

There are occasions when it is sufficient to simply tape the injured finger to an adjacent one (ie, buddy tape) and allow active motion, otherwise known as *dynamic splinting.* This allows for early motion, reducing joint stiffness and promoting earlier return of function. This therapy applies only to unquestionably stable fractures; that is, fractures that are transverse and impacted. Displacement, rotation, or angulation in any plane demands more aggressive therapy. If dynamic splinting is undertaken early (ie, within 1 week), follow-up is mandatory to detect any subsequent displacement or angulation, and to remedy such instability before healing occurs.

### Anesthesia

Reduction is best carried out under wrist anesthesia (eg,

ulnar or median nerve block). Metacarpal head blocks and digital blocks may be acceptable for phalangeal fractures.

### PHALANGEAL FRACTURES
### Proximal and middle phalanges (Fig. 16-3)

**Recognition of rotation.** Rotation of phalangeal fractures is both common and commonly missed. Permanent disability can only be avoided by careful attention to detail. Rotation should always be checked on physical exam, and should be suspected especially with oblique and spiral fractures. First, with the digits in the semiflexed position, the hand should be examined; the nails of the four digits should be coplanar (Fig. 16-4). It is helpful to compare the examined hand with the opposite hand. Second, the hand should be examined with the digits in as much flexion as possible. All four digits should point to the region of the scaphoid bone (Fig. 16-5). When the fracture is rotated, that digit will point askew (Fig. 16-6). As little as 10° of rotation can be disabling.

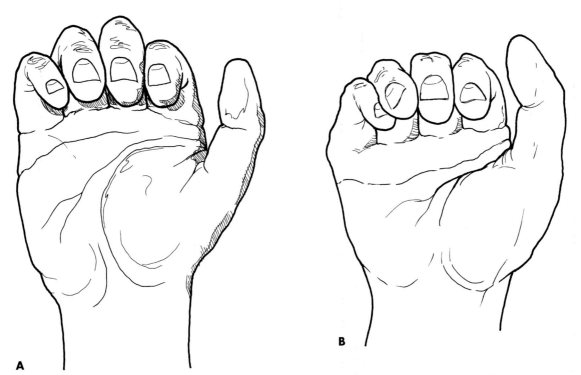

**A**    **B**

**Fig. 16-4.** Sketch of **A,** coplanar and **B,** rotated fingernails. It is helpful to compare with the opposite hand.

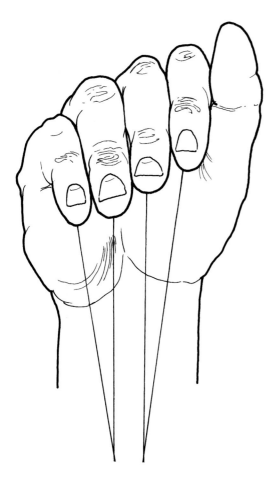

**Fig. 16-5.** Sketch of normal hand with all flexed fingers pointing to the scaphoid bone.

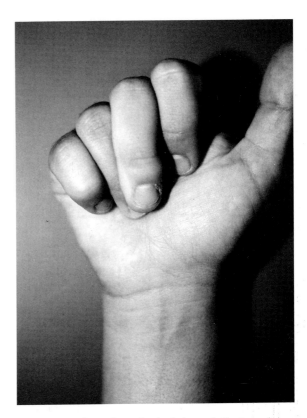

**Fig. 16-6.** Rotation of proximal phalangeal fractures becomes evident when the PIP joint is flexed and the finger points askew.

**Management of rotation**

*Proximal phalanx.* Grossly unstable rotation must be fixed operatively. Stable rotatory reductions of proximal phalangeal fractures can be controlled by splinting in flexion at the proximal interphalangeal (PIP) joint. However, great care must be taken to frequently flex and extend the PIP joint through range of motion. Stiffness of the PIP joint is a potential complication if it is left in flexion for as little as 1 week.[5] It is easier to control rotational alignment if an adjacent finger is incorporated into the cast or splint. The Burkhalter-Reyes dynamic splinting method described below is the best splinting method for stable rotatory reductions: digits are all flexed in unison at the PIP joint, adjacent fingers preventing the fractured one from rotating out of alignment. This method avoids the complication of PIP joint stiffness.

*Middle phalanx.* The majority of reductions of rotated middle phalangeal fractures will be unstable. These must be referred for closed reduction and percutaneous pin fixation.

**Fractures that are stable after closed reduction**

Closed reduction and splinting are sufficient if the fracture is stable after reduction without the aid of a splint. If postreduction radiographs show good alignment, the splint is placed. The splint will be used to ensure the stability of the reduction, not to hold in place an unstable reduction. Many fractures will not fall into this category and will need operative fixation. Spiral oblique fractures, for example, will almost always shorten without fixation as will other fractures in which the muscle-tendon forces resist stable reduction.

**Splinting of stable reductions.** Volar angulation has important implications for splinting. The preferred position for immobilization of the hand is the James[5] position—the metacarpal phalangeal (MP) joints in at least 70° of flexion and the interphalangeal (IP) joints ideally in full extension. Joint stiffness is minimized because the ligaments are thus immobilized in the position of maximum length. However, in order to help maintain reduction of proximal phalangeal fractures, preventing volar angulation, the IP joints need to be in some degree of flexion: no more than 15° to 20° for the PIP, and no more than 5° to 10° for the distal interphalangeal (DIP) joint. Immobilization of the injured digit alone suffices except in the situation of rotational malalignment.

Splinting can be done with an ulnar or radial gutter (Fig. 16-7), depending on which digit is affected, or with an outrigger splint, which is a short arm cast with an aluminum extension for the affected finger.

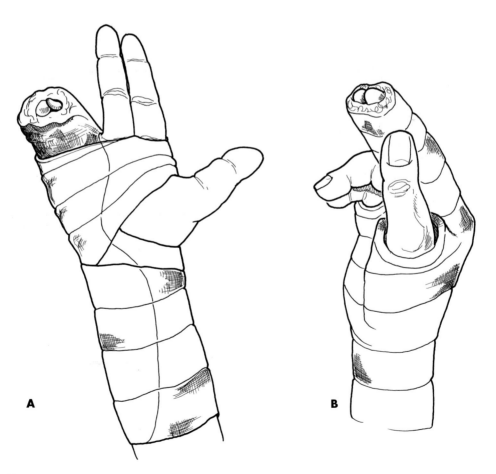

**Fig. 16-7. A,** An ulnar gutter splint immobilizes the fourth and fifth fingers, leaving second and third free. **B,** A radial gutter splint performs the reverse.

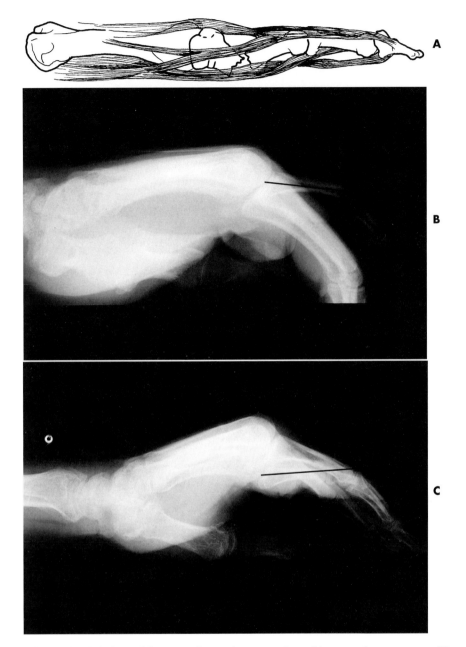

**Fig. 16-8.** Proximal phalangeal fractures almost always angulate with apex volar recurvatum. The interossei insert volarly at the base of the proximal phalanx, flexing the MP joint; the attachment of the middle phalanx tends to extend the distal fragment. The geometry of the fracture in **A** demonstrates the subtlety of recognition. A lateral view, **B,** is essential to making the diagnosis and even then, **C,** it can be difficult. (See also Fig. 16-2).

The Burkhalter-Reyes method described below in the management of unstable fractures can also be used in stable fractures to prevent PIP stiffness from developing during immobilization.

## Proximal phalangeal fractures

Proximal phalangeal fractures almost always angulate with apex volar recurvatum (Figs. 16-2 and 16-8). (Apex volar means the apex of the angulation is volar and the distal fragment is angulated in the dorsal direction.) The in-

terossei insert volarly at the base of the proximal phalanx, flexing the MP joint, and the attachment of the central slip to the dorsal base of the middle phalanx tends to extend the distal fragment. It is difficult to appreciate angulation of fractures of the base,[4] but if recognized, they have a low incidence of complications when treated closed as long as the residual angulation is not greater than 20°.

If the fracture heals with excessive angulation, the extensor hood over the PIP joint shortens and slips volar to the PIP axis, preventing full PIP extension, and the fracture apex interferes with the flexor tendons, limiting flexion. Furthermore, there may be adhesions of the flexor tendons to the fracture site.[4] More than 25° (30° in children) of apex volar angulation can result in loss of both flexion and extension of the PIP joint.[4] Apex volar angulation up to 20° is acceptable.[3]

**Unstable fractures.** If the fracture reduction does not hold, closed reduction with percutaneous pin fixation is the most common management. However, Burkhalter and Reyes[6,7] describe a technique of splinting for midshaft and base fractures that Green and Rowland[8] list as their preferred method of treatment for fractures of the base of the proximal phalanx. Burkhalter and Reyes describe success using this technique with unstable base *and* shaft fractures. This method helps to prevent joint stiffness through early active motion.

*Closed reduction: the Burkhalter-Reyes method.* Unstable fractures of the proximal phalanx have been preferably treated surgically, but at a cost of prolonged immobilization and stiffness of the PIP joint. Stiffness after fractures in the hand is a greater problem than it is in other parts of the body. Immediate or early motion is important to avoid hand stiffness. It is also important to remember that "absolute anatomical restoration of extra-articular fractures is not necessary in order to achieve union with excellent function, nor is rigid fixation of the skeleton necessary in order to achieve union or to begin early motion."[6]

After reduction, a short arm cast is applied with the wrist in 30° of extension and the metacarpal joints hyperflexed to 90° (Fig. 16-9). On the volar side, the cast extends to the proximal palmar crease, allowing full flexion of MP and IP joints. Dorsally, the cast extends to the level of the PIP joint. The dorsal compression at the PIP joint keeps the MP joint in full flexion and simultaneously prevents recurvatum. This management allows early active motion. The patient is encouraged to flex simultaneously all PIP and DIP joints actively. Such active flexion rotates the incorrectly rotated fracture back into its correct plane. Full flexion of the PIP joint is regained within a few days; full extension requires more time to recover, and may be aided with a rubber extension band, especially if more than 40° of extension is lost. Bone healing and recovery of motion are achieved simultaneously, resulting in less stiffness than surgical treatment. "Clinical alignment is far more important than radiographic alignment. This fracture will not be reduced anatomically, and there may be some shortening and displacement. If the digits are well aligned with simultaneous distal flexion and the lateral view shows no persisting dorsiflexion instability, the reduction is satisfactory."[6] Immobilization is continued for about 4 weeks or until local tenderness is absent. As always, early follow-up is essential to ensure no loss of reduction.

In summary, the most common method of treatment of unstable proximal phalangeal fractures remains surgical. Fractures at the base of the phalanx have a low incidence of

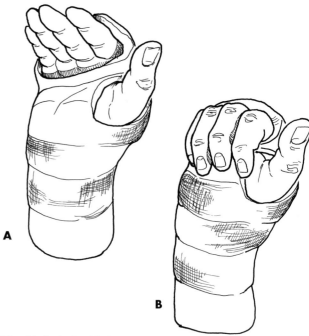

**Fig. 16-9. A,** Burkhalter-Reyes splinting method. A dorsal hood to the PIP joint, compressing the proximal phalanges, keeps the MP joint in full flexion and prevents recurvatum. **B,** The patient is encouraged to flex simultaneously all PIP and DIP joints actively.

complications if they are treated closed, thus Green and Rowland prefer the Burkhalter method for base fractures. Burkhalter and Reyes use this method for shaft fractures as well. Burkhalter emphasizes that "the method requires great attention to detail on the part of the surgeon to achieve a reduction and requires enough maturity to be able to abandon the method if failure is likely."[6] If the reduction is unacceptable after 1 to 2 weeks, the method may be abandoned for surgical repair.

**Neck fractures (distal to the shaft of proximal phalanx).** This fracture usually angulates 60° to 90° (Fig. 16-10) apex volar and reduction is very difficult to maintain. It should be referred for surgery.

### Middle phalangeal fractures

Middle phalangeal fractures tend to angulate apex dorsal if the fracture is proximal to the insertion of the flexor superficialis and volar if the fracture is distal (Fig. 16-11). If the closed reduction holds well (more the exception than the rule), these fractures can be simply splinted across both IP joints, the joints in full extension. Immobilization need not cross the MP joint, but active MP flexion must be emphasized. Any instability requires percutaneous pin fixation. Rotation is difficult to detect clinically, and should be looked for on the lateral radiograph, which will show a double shadow of the two condyles of the head (Fig. 16-12). Rotation must be treated surgically, usually with pin fixation.

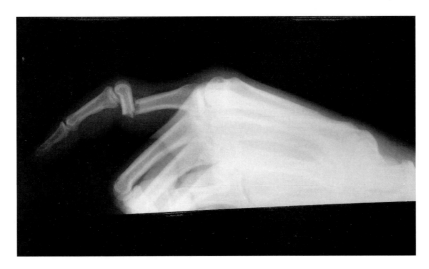

**Fig. 16-10.** Proximal phalangeal neck fracture. These often are severely angulated because of the pull of the extensor tendons. Because reduction is very difficult to maintain, these fractures require surgery.

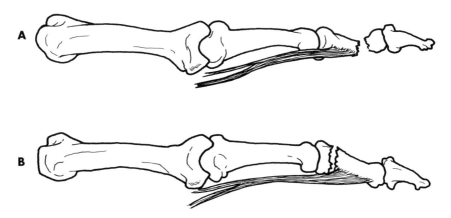

**Fig. 16-11.** The action of the superficialis tendon on middle phalanx fractures is to cause apex volar angulation (**A**) if the fracture is distal and apex dorsal angulation (**B**) if the fracture is proximal.

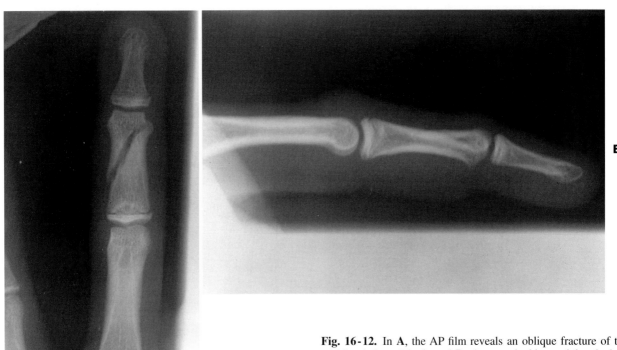

**Fig. 16-12.** In **A**, the AP film reveals an oblique fracture of the middle phalanx. The lateral **B**, shows a double condylar shadow, revealing unsuspected rotation, which may be difficult to detect clinically.

### Comminuted fractures (Fig. 16-13)

These fractures must be referred for open reduction internal fixation (ORIF) or pin fixation. They are usually the result of penetrating, crush, or rotatory injuries.

### Condylar fractures (Fig. 16-14)

These are always displaced and require ORIF, whether in children or adults.

### Intra-articular fractures (Fig. 16-15)

These are usually avulsion fractures, which are discussed below. Intra-articular fractures, which are not avulsions, are almost always the result of a great deal of axial impaction trauma and require ORIF to restore the joint surface.

### Avulsion fractures (see also joint injuries—dislocations and ligamentous injuries)

Nondisplaced fractures can be treated with dynamic splinting (ie, buddy taping) and require early range of motion exercise to prevent joint adhesions.

### Avulsion fractures at the base of the proximal phalanx

These are usually lateral at the insertion of the collateral ligaments. Most are nondisplaced or minimal fractures not affecting the joint surface and may be managed by buddy taping (Fig. 16-16). "If the x-ray film shows wide displacement of a tiny avulsion chip (greater than 2 to 3 mm) or if the fragment involves more than 20% of the articular surface and is displaced or rotated, we believe that primary operative treatment is indicated"[9] (Figs. 16-15 and 16-17). In children, the analogous injury is a Salter III fracture of the epiphyseal base (discussed in the section *Hand Fractures in Children*).

### Avulsion fractures at the base of the middle phalanx

**Dorsal chip.** A dorsal avulsion fracture may create a Boutonniere deformity that will often not be apparent during initial physical exam. Boutonniere deformities are discussed in the section on blunt tendon injuries. Because of the potential bad outcome, a displaced dorsal avulsion fracture should be referred for possible ORIF unless it is a minimally displaced fragment. If not displaced, the treatment is identical to blunt central slip tendon rupture as discussed: splinting the PIP joint alone in extension, emphasizing active DIP flexion. (See also *Volar PIP Fracture-Dislocation* and Fig. 16-18.)

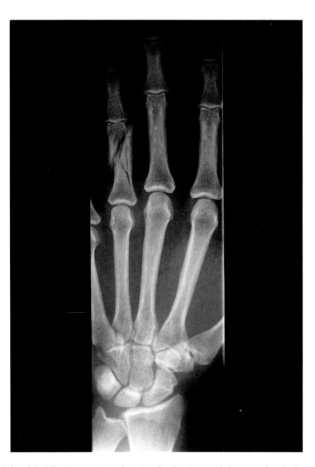

**Fig. 16-13.** Comminuted butterfly fracture of the proximal phalanx. These require ORIF or pin fixation as treatment.

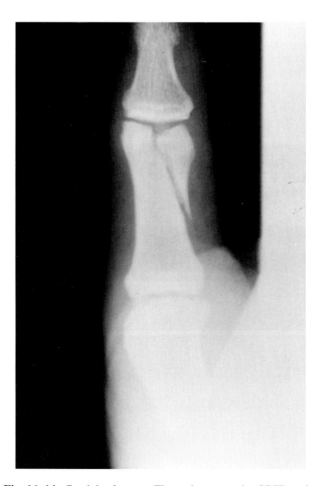

**Fig. 16-14.** Condylar fracture. These always require ORIF or pin fixation as treatment.

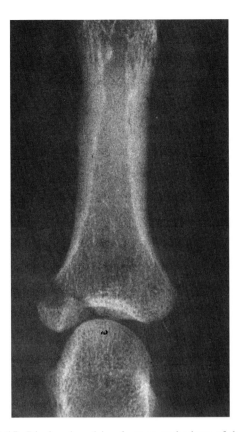

**Fig. 16-15.** Displaced avulsion fracture at the base of the proximal phalanx. It is displaced less than 2 to 3 mm, but it involves more than 20% of the articular surface. It therefore requires ORIF. (From Rockwood CA, Green DP, Bucholz RW, eds.: *Fractures in Adults.* ed 3, Philadelphia, 1991, JB Lippincott, p 477.)

**Volar chip.** Tiny chip fractures with minimal displacement are treated identically to hyperextension volar plate injuries (see *Injuries of the PIP Joint*). Dorsal extension block splinting at 15° to 20° flexion followed by buddy taping or 3 to 6 weeks of buddy taping alone allows early active motion. Obviously, hyperextension is to be avoided.

Larger volar chip fractures are usually associated with dorsal dislocation of the middle phalanx on the proximal phalanx. These injuries are discussed in detail in the section on *Injuries of the PIP Joint*.

**Lateral chip.** Tiny chip fractures with minimal (< 2 to 3 mm) displacement are treated with simple immobilization (of the PIP joint only), if the joint is stable. If unstable, it should be treated as for collateral ligament rupture. Unstable PIP injuries are discussed in the section *Injuries of the PIP Joint*. Larger fractures or those with more displacement (> 2 to 3 mm) must be evaluated on the basis of the continuity of the articular surface: if greater than 20% of the joint surface, the fracture should be referred for ORIF.

### Distal phalangeal fractures

Distal phalangeal fractures (Fig. 16-19) include crush injuries resulting in the tuft fracture—the less common transverse shaft fractures and avulsion fractures caused by the flexor and extensor tendons. Also included in this group are longitudinal fractures and base fractures. The thumb is the most frequently injured digit followed by the index and

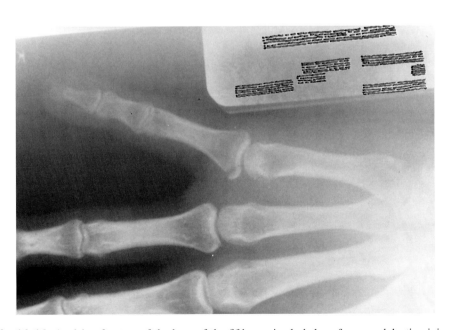

**Fig. 16-16.** Avulsion fracture of the base of the fifth proximal phalanx from an abduction injury. The joint surface is well maintained because the fragment is less than 20% and is displaced less than 2 to 3 mm. This injury is best managed by buddy taping alone.

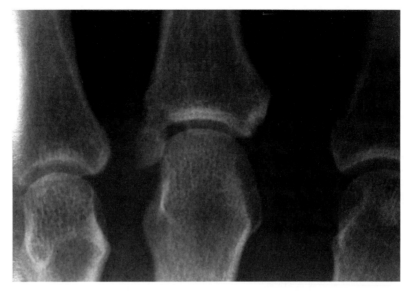

**Fig. 16-17.** If MP joint disruption involves a significantly displaced (2 to 3 mm) avulsion fracture at the base of the proximal phalanx, surgical fixation is indicated. (From Rockwood CA, Green DP, Bucholz RW, eds: *Fractures in Adults.* ed 3, Philadelphia, 1991, JB Lippincott, p 519.)

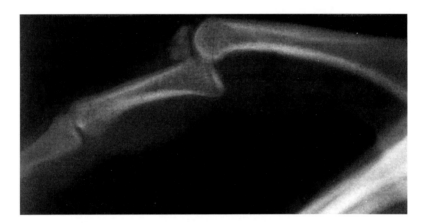

**Fig. 16-18.** Volar fracture-dislocation of the PIP joint. After reduction, if the joint is congruous and the fragment is reduced in full extension of the PIP joint, only the PIP joint should be splinted in full extension and active and passive DIP motion encouraged. (From Rockwood CA, Green DP, Bucholz RW, eds: *Fractures in Adults.* ed 3, Philadelphia, 1991, JB Lippincott, p 509.)

middle fingers, and the nondominant side is the most frequently affected.[10]

In the case of crush injuries, attention is to be focused primarily on concomitant soft-tissue injury: subungual hematomas and burst lacerations. The bone need not be splinted except to cushion the finger from the pain of further external trauma. The splint may be discontinued when tenderness is resolved. Management of soft-tissue injuries and subungual hematomas is discussed in the chapter on *Nailbed Injuries.* Splinting too tightly will cause severe pain. The splint should not involve the PIP joint. It should be removed daily to allow for range of motion exercises. Any further radiographs should be avoided, as they are not needed and, because radiographic healing is slower than clinical, they only serve to disappoint the patient.

Displaced or angulated shaft fractures require reduction and either splinting or Kirschner wire fixation (Fig. 16-20).

The patient should always be examined for the presence of a mallet finger with any distal phalangeal injury.

**Prognosis.** The prognosis for distal phalanx fractures is dependent on the degree of soft-tissue injury and is generally very good, with functional recovery in 3 to 4 weeks.

However, in DaCruz' study[10] of distal phalangeal fractures, a large proportion of patients, especially those with fractures of the tuft and shaft (as opposed to longitudinal or base) had numbness, disabling cold hypersensitivity, and hyperesthesia of the fingertip lasting 6 months or longer.[11] Many patients had difficulty with fine functions of the fingertip. Only one-third of patients were fully recovered at 6 months. Comminuted tuft fractures fared the worst, with a high incidence of nonunion and osteolysis thought to be caused by disuse. Longitudinal fractures fared well.

Extensor tendon avulsion fractures result in a mallet fracture. Depending on the amount of displacement and of articular surface involved, there are proponents of ORIF. Nevertheless, splinting alone gives as good or better results for all of these fractures except many of those with volar subluxation of the distal on the middle phalanx. This topic is discussed in greater detail in the section on *Tendon Injuries-Mallet Finger.*

Flexor Digitorum Profundus (FDP) tendon avulsions (Fig. 16-21) occur with forced extension of the DIP joint with simultaneous attempted flexion, as happens when a football player catches his finger on the jersey of another. It occurs almost exclusively in the ring finger. The tendon and fracture chip virtually always retract far proximally up the finger, usually hanging up on the split in the superficialis tendon at the PIP joint, but may retract farther proximally in the hand. These need referral and operative repair. This injury is often missed on initial exam and if unrecognized there is a greater likelihood of scarring with resultant difficulty retrieving the tendon and bone fragment.

## METACARPAL FRACTURES (METACARPALS II THROUGH V)

The metacarpal bones can be anatomically divided into base (at the proximal end), shaft, head, and neck. The metacarpal bones of the index (second) and long (third) fingers are rigidly fixed to the distal carpal row; the second is fixed to the trapezium and trapezoid, and the third to the capitate. The metacarpals of the ring (fourth) and little

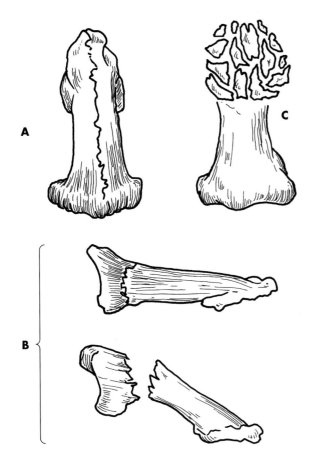

**Fig. 16-19.** The distal phalanx may be fractured longitudinally (**A**), usually without displacement; it may be fractured transversely (**B**), often with angulation (which can be reduced and splinted closed, although it sometimes requires pin fixation); or (**C**), the tuft can be crushed (the most common distal phalanx fracture).

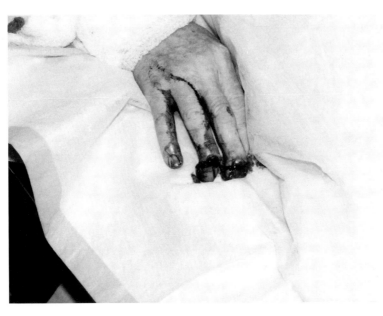

**Fig. 16-20.** Near amputation of distal phalanges 3 and 4, with open fractures of the distal phalanx. The nail matrix and blood supply were still intact, and this was treated with thorough irrigation, intravenous antibiotics, reduction, suturing, and splinting. The reduction was adequate and stable so that pin fixation was not needed. In other cases, pin fixation may be required.

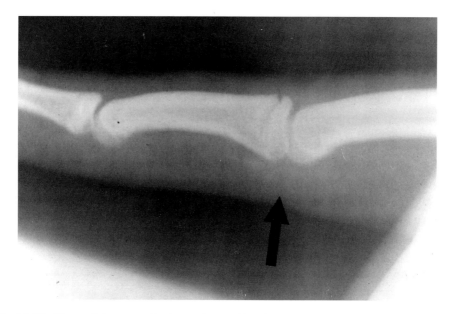

**Fig. 16-21.** Flexor digitorum profundus tendon avulsion fracture. These are easily missed and may cause significant disability if not recognized and repaired. The bone fragment anterior to the base of the middle phalanx is very subtle and difficult to visualize, but note the hyperextension of the distal phalanx. The patient with this type of avulsion will be unable to flex the distal phalanx.

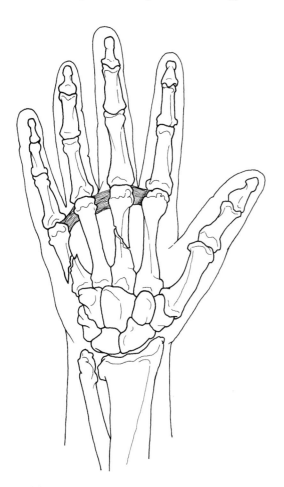

**Fig. 16-22.** The MC heads are linked by the transmetacarpal ligament. Thus, oblique fractures of the shaft of the third and fourth MCs are relatively stable, whereas fractures of the shaft of the second and fifth are more prone to shortening.

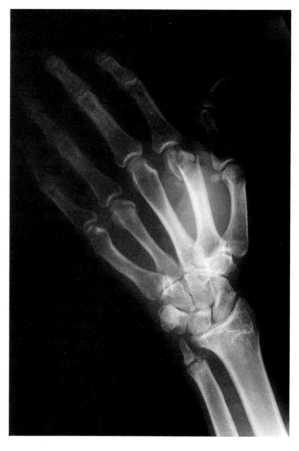

**Fig. 16-23.** The second (index) metacarpal is fractured through both the neck and the head. The joint surface is relatively well maintained and if a neck fracture was not also present, conservative therapy would be adequate. However, the neck fracture needs operative stabilization.

(fifth) finger are able to flex and extend up to 30° because of a mobile articulation with the hamate bone. Because of this mobility, the fourth and fifth metacarpals are better able to compensate for fracture angulation.

The metacarpal heads are linked by the transmetacarpal ligament. Thus, oblique fractures of the shaft of the third and fourth metacarpals are relatively stable, whereas fractures of the shaft of the second and fifth are more prone to shortening (Fig. 16-22).

### Metacarpal head fractures (Fig. 16-23)

These are always intra-articular fractures. If nondisplaced, these may be managed with splinting alone. Comminuted fractures must be referred for surgical fixation, although if severely comminuted, these will often not be surgically correctable and a hand surgeon may choose to treat conservatively. If conservative therapy is chosen, the defects will fill in with fibrocartilage and often result in good function despite poor radiographic appearance.

All simple displaced fractures involving the joint require operative fixation. These fractures should be splinted for comfort and referred for surgery within 3 days.

### Metacarpal neck fractures

**Fracture of the neck of the fifth metacarpal (Boxer's fracture) (Fig. 16-24).** The Boxer's fracture is the most common hand fracture. It is the result of axial impact of the head of the fifth metacarpal against an unyielding surface (whether a wall or a face), and is very difficult to hold in reduction. The interossei, as with all metacarpal fractures, exert an apex dorsal deforming force (*apex dorsal* means the distal end is angulated in the volar direction). This force, combined with the often-seen comminution of the volar cortex, tends to make reduction of these fractures very unstable. Furthermore, it is impossible to create a splint that supports the reduction with the requisite three-point fixation unless the metacarpal joint is immobilized in extension, which if left for longer than 10 days results in complications much worse than dorsal angulation. Fortunately, reduction is rarely necessary.

An unequivocal indication for reduction is to correct significant rotational deformity or lateral angulation. These deformities must be reduced and either splinted or fixed with Kirschner wire, or managed by ORIF.

Apex dorsal angulation (measured as the total angulation, this includes the natural 15° of angulation at the metacarpal neck) alone has been treated by many methods, including closed reduction and immobilization, Kirschner wires, ORIF, and simple symptomatic care without any reduction. Simple splinting for comfort with early mobilization, or even no splinting at all and immediate mobilization,[12] gives excellent functional results because the mobil-

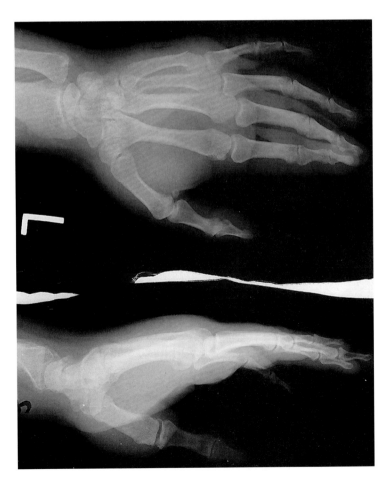

**Fig. 16-24.** Lateral and oblique views of a Boxer's fracture with 30° to 35° of angulation. If there is no rotation, this fracture may be treated symptomatically, with no reduction necessary.

ity of the fifth metacarpal compensates for angulation. Loss of knuckle prominence and a dorsal hump may cause an unacceptable cosmetic deformity that can only be corrected by surgery, at a cost of significantly longer rehabilitation.[13] In a study by Arafa,[14] immediate mobilization of all Boxer's fractures, regardless of the degree of angulation, resulted in excellent function with a short period of disability. Thirty-four percent of patients (all of whom were manual workers) returned to work within 2 weeks, and 82% returned within 4 weeks. Fourteen percent of patients lacked greater than 15° of extension, but without functional impairment, only 5% had an obvious cosmetic deformity, and only 10% had measurable weakness detected by grip-strength meter, none of whom had noticed subjective weakness. Similar results were obtained by McKerrell,[12] and as in other series, patients who underwent closed reduction lost the reduction at follow-up. McKerrell's operative group did not return to work for an average of 58 days. No author reported difficulties with a palmar prominence.

Closed reduction has been advocated and is widely practiced. Studies recommending closed reduction comment on the difficulty in maintaining the reduction, yet recommend the treatment based on successful results obtained. The results were no doubt successful only because no treatment is necessary in the first place (any treatment works well). In a study of police and fire fighters whose fractures were manipulated only if angulation was greater than 40°, even those with residual angulation of greater than 60° returned to work fully functional within 4 weeks.[15]

Closed reduction can be more harmful than helpful. Splinting of the metacarpal joint in less than 70° of flexion for longer than 10 days can lead to permanent and disabling stiffness. Despite valiant attempts to splint the metacarpal in flexion, these efforts nearly universally fail (Fig. 16-25). The only way to hold the Boxer's fracture in reduction and retain the metacarpal joint in flexion is the 90°-90° method used by Jahss,[16] in which both the MP and PIP joints are splinted at 90°—but this method is only mentioned to condemn it. This method may be used for reduction, but never for immobilization because it often leads to skin necrosis over the PIP joint and permanent disabling flexion contracture of the PIP joint.

Hunter,[15] Arafa,[14] and Ford[12] all achieved successful results without reducing even fractures greater than 40°. Pseudoclawing (Fig. 16-26) is a complication of a greatly angulated neck fracture (usually > 40°). MP extension results in PIP flexion because the volarly angulated metacarpal head is pulling on the flexor tendons. Pseudoclawing on initial exam is an indication for attempted reduction. Because of the mounting evidence and their own experience, Green and Rowland[17] have changed their preferred method of treatment, abandoning closed reduction unless the angulation is greater than 40°.

### Management of Boxer's fractures

1) Simple, less than 40° (including the natural metacarpal neck angle) fractures, without significant rotation or angulation, without pseudoclawing; the patient does not insist on perfect cosmesis—these fractures should be treated without reduction, a removable splint used for comfort only. Mobilization should be encouraged as soon as pain allows (usually within a few days). Patient should be referred to a hand surgeon within 1 week.

2) Simple fractures as above, but cosmesis is a major concern (unusual)—these fractures should be splinted for comfort and referred for surgical fixation

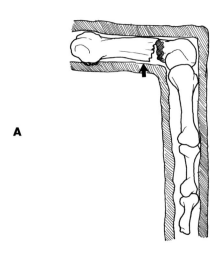

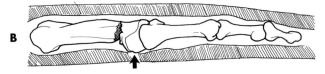

**Fig. 16-25. A,** The reason a splint cannot maintain reduction of a Boxer's fracture if the MP joint is flexed. For maintenance of reduction, it is necessary to have three-point fixation with one point of fixation on the head of the MC. However, if the joint is in flexion, the proximal phalanx is anterior (volar) to the MC head, preventing the splint from finding purchase on this point. **B,** How splinting in extension can hold the reduction; however, the MP joint cannot be held extended for longer than 7 to 10 days without disabling stiffness resulting.

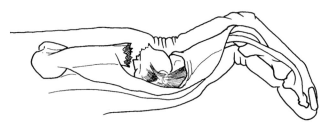

**Fig. 16-26.** Sketch illustrating pseudoclawing, which results from large angulation of an MC neck fracture. The angulated fragment pulls on the PIP flexor tendon, causing PIP flexion especially during MP extension.

within 5 days. The drawbacks are a long rehabilitation (average 2 months) and risk of infection.

3) Rotation, lateral angulation, dorsal angulation greater than 40°, especially if pseudoclawing is present—these fractures can be treated by attempting closed reduction and ulnar gutter splinting.

*Method of reduction.* After ulnar or hematoma block, with plaster ready to be immediately applied, the proximal phalanx can be used to push the metacarpal head posteriorly and the flexed middle phalanx can be used as a lever to crank the fracture into rotatory reduction. The wrist should be splinted in 30° of extension. The only way to hold this reduction is to leave the MP joint in full extension (Fig. 16-25B), which must only be attempted in reliable patients who will return for followup within 7 days to be resplinted with the MP joint in at least 70° of flexion; this is critical to avoid permanent disabling joint stiffness. The IP joints should be left in near full extension. It is common for the reduction to be lost, so follow-up within 5 days is essential to reassess the need for surgical correction.

**Fourth metacarpal neck fracture.** Like the fifth metacarpal, the fourth is quite mobile and the hand will not have functional deficits despite significant volar angulation. Because of the transverse metacarpal ligament, rotation and lateral angulation are limited in the third and fourth metacarpal neck fractures,[18] and even volar angulation is less than that in the fifth metacarpal neck fracture. All of the treatment considerations for fifth metacarpal neck fractures apply here, except that no more than 30° of volar angulation should be accepted. Rotation must be corrected.

**Second and third metacarpal neck fracture.** Very little fracture angulation can be tolerated in the immobile second and third metacarpals; therefore, all of these fractures should be referred for closed reduction and percutaneous Kirschner-wire fixation or ORIF within 5 days.

## Metacarpal shaft fractures

Metacarpal shaft fractures may rotate, shorten, or angulate. They may be transverse, oblique, or comminuted. As with neck fractures, the force of the interossei muscles tend to cause apex dorsal angulation. As in metacarpal neck fractures, angulation is poorly tolerated in the second and third metacarpals. In shaft fractures as compared with neck fractures, for any given angulation the cosmetic defect is more pronounced and the incidence of clawing is greater (Fig. 16-27). Therefore, less angulation can be tolerated in shaft fractures of the fourth and fifth metacarpals than in neck fractures. Fortunately, there usually is greater purchase for three-point fixation in the case of shaft fractures and they are more amenable to closed reduction and splinting. Shortening is acceptable up to 5 mm[19] in metacarpal fractures, except in the case of the subcapital spiral oblique fracture (Fig. 16-28), which may shorten and impinge on the metacarpal joint.

**Rotation of metacarpal fractures.** Correction and maintenance of rotational deformity is the most critical aspect of the care of metacarpal fractures. In a normal hand, with the metacarpal joints in extension, the fingers are free to ad- and abduct, but when the metacarpal joints are flexed, the fingers press tightly into each other and become laterally fixed. A very small amount of metacarpal rotation will disrupt this fine mechanism and cause the fingers to cross when the MP joints are flexed.

Fortunately, as described by Burkhalter,[6] this can be used to advantage when correcting the rotation. With the MP joints blocked in full 90° flexion by a well-padded plaster hood over the PIP joints, the adjacent fingers will correct the rotation. The fingers may be free to flex and extend fully at the PIP and DIP joints, but the patient must be instructed to flex and extend the fingers simultaneously to prevent overlap. Leaving the fingers free and encouraging early motion prevents stiffness and promotes early function.

**Transverse metacarpal shaft fractures (Fig. 16-29).** Transverse metacarpal fractures usually occur as the result of a direct blow.[20] Single, closed transverse fractures may be reduced and splinted in the emergency department. After appropriate anesthesia, rotational and angular deformities, and displacement should be corrected and a dorsal-volar splint applied. As stated above under *Metacarpal Shaft Fractures,* the more proximal the fracture, the less angulation may be tolerated. To hold rotation, the splint should include the finger and at least one adjacent normal finger. The Burkhalter method described above gives good rotational stability and early motion. Shortening is seldom a problem in transverse fractures. Because of the trauma to soft tissues from a direct blow, swelling may make splinting or casting ineffective or impractical, necessitating pin fixation. Early follow-up is essential to ensure no loss of reduction. The fracture should be immobilized until swelling and tenderness is gone, which should be no longer than 4 weeks.

Indications for referral and possible surgery are open fractures, inability to reduce or to maintain reduction, and multiple (more than one) fractures with displacement or angulation.

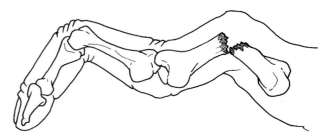

**Fig. 16-27.** An identical degree of angulation in a midshaft fracture causes more pseudoclawing that in a neck fracture. Therefore, less angulation is tolerated for midshaft than for neck fractures.

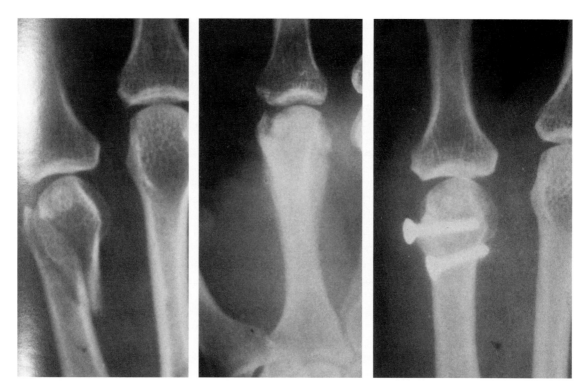

**Fig. 16-28.** Subcapital spiral oblique fracture. Any shortening, even if less than 5 mm, is an indication for surgical fixation because the fracture fragment may impinge on the joint. (From Rockwood CA, Green DP, Bucholz RW, eds: *Fractures in Adults.* ed 3, Philadelphia, 1991, JB Lippincott, p 493.)

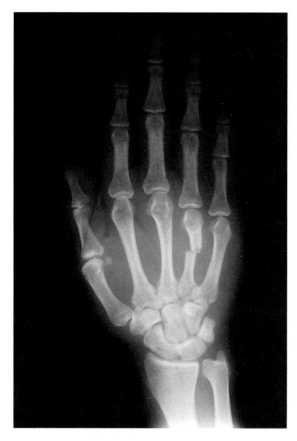

**Fig. 16-29.** Transverse fourth metacarpal shaft fracture. This fracture may be easily reduced, closed, and splinted.

**Oblique metacarpal shaft fractures (Fig. 16-30).** "Spiral oblique fractures of the metacarpal shaft result from a torque force with the finger acting as a long lever."[20] These fractures tend to shorten and rotate more than angulate. Correction of rotation (see discussion on evaluation of rotation) may be difficult to hold with external immobilization and often require surgical treatment. If there is no rotation and less than 5 mm of shortening, such fractures may be treated by immobilization and referral within 1 week to assure no change. Angulation may be reduced as in transverse fractures.

Rotation that persists despite reduction attempt, or shortening greater than 5 mm are indications for very early referral for closed reduction and wire fixation, or for ORIF. Open or multiple fractures should also be referred for surgery. Subcapital spiral oblique fractures require fixation to prevent impingement on the joint (Fig. 16-28).

**Comminuted metacarpal shaft fractures.**[20] Comminuted fractures are usually caused by severe trauma such as gunshot wounds or crush injuries. There are usually severe open soft-tissue injuries that may only rarely be treated with simple external immobilization. After appropriate emergency care of soft tissue, these patients usually require immediate consultation. For comminuted fractures with less severe soft-tissue injuries, management follows the principles of care outlined for oblique metacarpal fractures.

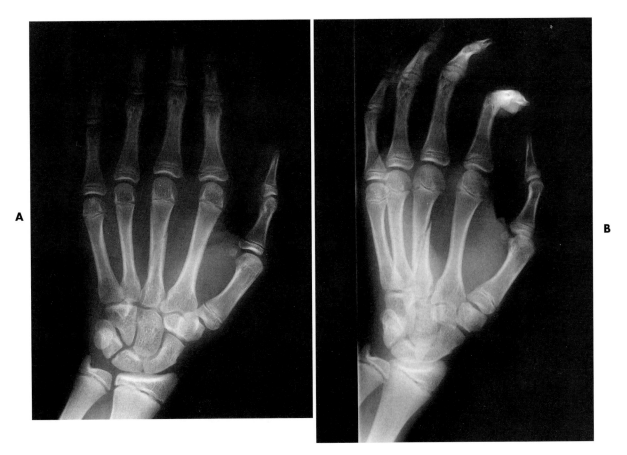

**Fig. 16-30.** Oblique shaft fracture of the third metacarpal, AP and oblique views. There is very little shortening (< 5 mm), and as long as there is no rotation on clinical exam, this fracture may be treated without manipulation by splinting alone.

## Metacarpal base fractures

Metacarpal base fractures are serious injuries and are often missed by the emergency physician and radiologist. The most common causes of metacarpal base fractures are punching and falling on an outstretched hand. There may be associated carpal bone fractures, especially of the hamate.

Fractures at the bases of the second and third metacarpal are rarely displaced and usually only require splinting for comfort. These are usually intra-articular but cause little disability because of the immobility of the second and third carpometacarpal (CMC) joint. These fractures should be splinted with the wrist in 30° extension and the metacarpal joints free.

The fourth metacarpal base fracture is more often associated with displacement or CMC dislocation than the second and third, and the fifth is nearly always associated with dislocation or instability (see carpometacarpal dislocations in *The Wrist*). Early diagnosis of CMC dislocations is essential to prevent chronically impaired wrist function.[21] Injuries around the CMC joint are easily missed on radiograph. In one study[22] of CMC dislocations, the injury was overlooked in 15 of 21 patients that presented to the emergency department, with delay in diagnosis of up to 8 weeks.

In the instance of fracture-dislocations of the second through fourth metacarpal base, closed reduction and splinting under regional anaesthesia is acceptable, but requires early follow-up to assure maintenance of reduction. Rotatory alignment is critical (Fig. 16-31).

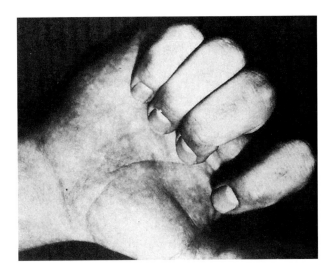

**Fig. 16-31.** Result of inadequately treated rotated fractures of the bases of metacarpals 3, 4, and 5. (From Rockwood CA, Green DP, Bucholz RW, eds: *Fractures in Adults*. ed 3, Philadelphia, 1991, JB Lippincott, p. 494.)

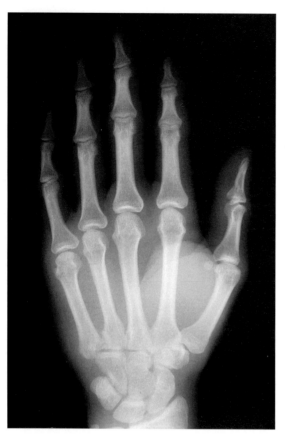

**Fig. 16-32.** Fracture dislocation of the base of the fifth metacarpal. These are nearly always unstable and require pin fixation. (See also Fig. 16-33.)

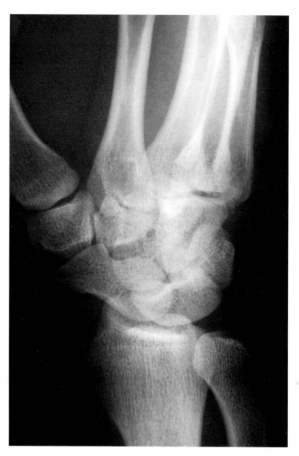

**Fig. 16-33.** Fifth MC base dislocation. Recognition of metacarpal base fracture-dislocations and simple dislocations may be very difficult. This oblique view (compared with normal hand in Fig. 16-1) demonstrates that: 1) the fourth and fifth MCs are not parallel; and 2) the fifth MC is not flush with the hamate bone. On the contrary, there is a step-off.

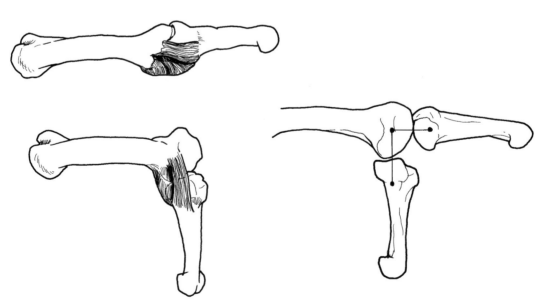

**Fig. 16-34.** Sketch that shows that the radius of the head of the MC is longer in the dorsal-volar than in the longitudinal direction. Therefore, when the joint is flexed, the collateral ligaments are stretched taut and will not shorten if splinted in this position. If splinted in extension, they are relatively lax and will shorten, causing disabling joint stiffness.

The fifth metacarpal base is different (Figs. 16-32 and 16-33); the base is not stabilized on both sides, the extensor carpi ulnaris inserts and pulls at the base of the fifth metacarpal, and the fifth CMC joint is important for mobility. Thus, they nearly always displace or dislocate. These fractures will nearly always require closed reduction with pin fixation.

**Splinting of metacarpal base fractures.** As always, splints must be applied with the MP joint in at least 70° of flexion to prevent disabling contracture of the collateral ligaments (Fig. 16-34). IP joints should not be included in the splint.

## HAND FRACTURES IN CHILDREN

Most fractures of the hand in children do well with closed reduction and splinting; however, there are some that require operative fixation. Some specific injuries are discussed below; those injuries that are not discussed are managed as adult fractures.

Malalignment and angulation of fractures in young children are often corrected by remodeling. Remodeling will not correct angulation of the phalangeal neck, where there is no physis, because remodeling only readily occurs near a physis. The physes are proximal in the phalanges and distal in the metacarpals. Remodeling will neither correct rotation nor correct displaced intra-articular fractures or medial-lateral angulation of the middle phalanx, although it will correct up to 15° of medial-lateral angulation at the base of the proximal phalanx.

A convenient splint for the young child is called a *boxing-glove cast.* No conventional splint will withstand the activity of a young child. Therefore, it is usually necessary to cover the splint in gauze and then add an outer layer of plaster to protect the entire casing. Alternatively, the splinted arm can be firmly wrapped against the body to prevent any trauma to the splint.

### Proximal phalanx

The most common hand fracture in children is a Salter-Harris type II (Salter II) at the base of the proximal phalanx (Fig. 16-35), usually of the little finger, with abduction deformity. This is best treated by hyperflexing the MP joint and forcing the finger into adduction. Rotational deformity must of course also be corrected. Remodeling will correct any residual angulation that is less than 15° in any plane, but will not correct rotation (the middle phalanx, in contrast, will only remodel in the flexion-extension plane). Residual angulation greater than 15° or residual rotation will require operative fixation. An adjacent finger should be incorporated into the splint with the MP joints in flexion.

Salter I fractures (Fig. 16-36) should be reduced if displaced and splinted with the MP joints in flexion.

Shaft fractures are treated as in adults, but residual fracture angulation less than 15° is acceptable in any plane in the proximal phalanx, although rotation is not.

Neck fractures may occur in young children who catch a finger in a door and withdraw it quickly. The head rolls

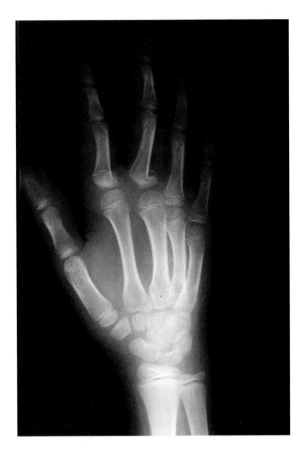

**Fig. 16-35.** Salter II fracture of the proximal phalanx. These are readily managed with closed reduction and splinting.

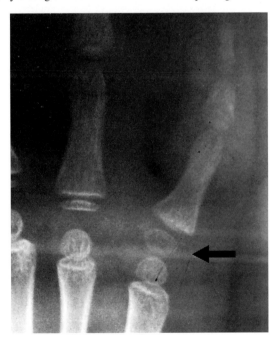

**Fig. 16-36.** A 3-year-boy was seen for a swollen fifth finger and metacarpophalangeal joint. Radiograph reveals a round appearance of the epiphysis of the base of the proximal phalanx (*arrow*) because the physis has fractured (Salter I) and the epiphysis has dislocated and rotated onto its end. This injury was not appreciated and resulted in very poor function. (From Rockwood, Wilkins, and King, eds: *Fractures in Children.* 3rd ed, Philadelphia, 1991: JB Lippincott, p 330.)

with apex volar angulation of 60° or more, so that the joint surface points dorsally. This deformity will obviously severely limit flexion. It must be treated operatively, usually with closed reduction and percutaneous pin fixation. Unfortunately, this fracture is often overlooked as it requires a high-quality lateral radiograph to be detected. If missed, new bone will fill in the volar defect, making correction very difficult. These usually will not remodel because they sit at the phalanx distal end, which has no physis.

## Middle phalanx

In children, middle phalangeal fractures usually occur at the base and are of the Salter III type. These require operative fixation whenever the fragment is displaced, just as in an

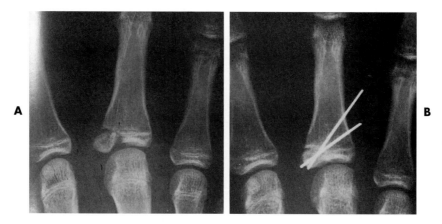

**Fig. 16-37. A,** A 15-year-old boy sustained this avulsion fracture at the base of proximal phalanx that is displaced more than 1.5 to 2.0 mm and also involves a large portion of the articular surface; it therefore required surgical treatment. **B,** Appearance 1 month after open reduction and Kirschner wire fixation. (From Rockwood, Wilkins, and King, eds: *Fractures in Children.* 3rd ed, Philadelphia, 1991, JB Lippincott, p 333.)

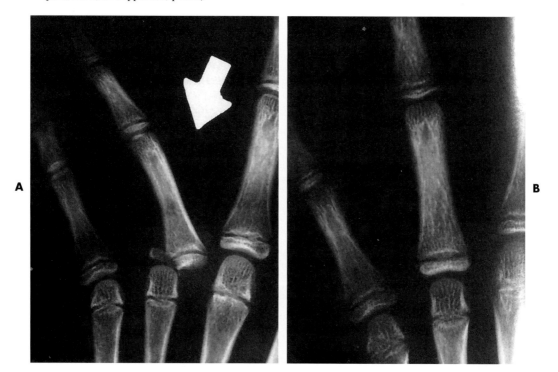

**Fig. 16-38. A,** A 9-year-old girl sustained this radial fracture-dislocation of the middle finger in a fall on the stairs. After reduction, the epiphyseal fragment was in near anatomic reduction because it was held in place by the ligament. Therefore, no pinning was necessary. **B,** Six weeks after closed reduction and immobilization in a radial gutter splint for 3 weeks, there was full motion and normal stability. (From Rockwood, Wilkins, and King, eds: *Fractures in Children.* 3rd ed, Philadelphia, 1991, JB Lippincott, p 360.)

adult. A displaced avulsion fracture of significant size (>20% of joint surface) would be surgically treated. Shaft and neck fractures are treated as in an adult.

### Avulsion fractures of the proximal and middle phalanges

Treatment is the same as in adults. These fractures appear different because they are usually Salter III fractures in which a piece of the epiphysis attached to the ligament breaks off.

"If the fragment involves a significant portion of the articular surface and is displaced more than 1.5 to 2 mm, then exact open reduction and Kirschner-wire fixation is indicated"[23] (Fig. 16-37). Figure 16-38 demonstrates an exception. In this Salter III fracture-dislocation of the proximal phalanx, the avulsion fracture was held in position by the ligament. After treatment, closed reduction alignment and splinting alone produced satisfactory results.

### Distal phalanx

There are two injuries in children that must be specifically addressed: the open Salter I fracture of the epiphysis (Fig. 16-39), and the Salter III mallet fracture.

The Salter I fracture usually happens as a result of a finger catching in a door. There is a transverse fracture through the physis and the epiphysis remains undisplaced, but the remainder of the phalanx is angulated in the volar direction (apex dorsal) and the metaphysis slides out from under the eponychium and is exposed (it is an open fracture). This injury results in a significant incidence of osteomyelitis and should therefore be treated with prophylactic IV antibiotics and thorough irrigation and debridement; flexion of the nail will lift the fracture out of the nail fold and expose it for irrigation.

Reduction is accomplished by hyperextension and placement of the nail back into the fold. The nail should be left

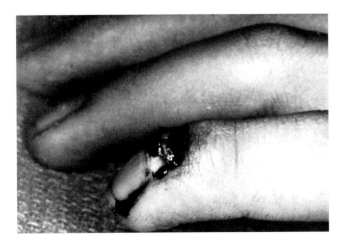

**Fig. 16-39.** Photograph of an open Salter I fracture of the epiphysis of the distal phalanx. (From Rockwood, Wilkins, and King, eds: *Fractures in Children.* 3rd ed. Philadelphia, 1991, JB Lippincott, p 325.)

in place to maintain stability of the reduction. If the nail is nearly completely avulsed, it must be removed, but this is usually not the case. Entrapment of the nailbed in the fracture site should be suspected and, if it is not extracted, nonunion will result. To help identify this problem, post-reduction radiographs should be scrutinized for widening of the fracture site. The finger is splinted as for a mallet finger and prophylactic oral antibiotics should be administered. Persistent displacement requires early referral, usually within 3 days. Otherwise, follow-up should be initiated in 2 weeks.

According to Campbell,[24] even a small amount of blood around the epinychium indicates an (possibly already reduced) open fracture that requires full irrigation and debridement to avoid complicating osteomyelitis. This is a minority viewpoint and it would be aggressive to further open and irrigate such a fracture on this assumption alone; however, it is prudent to treat with antibiotics.

Management of the Salter III mallet fracture, which is displaced and involves greater than one-third of the joint surface, is controversial and should be referred to a hand surgeon for possible operative therapy. In the interim, reduction and splinting, as in a mallet fracture, should be attempted.

### Metacarpal fractures

Shaft fractures are treated as in adults. Neck fractures have less tendency to displace because of a thick periosteal sleeve. Management is also the same as in adults. Head fractures are also treated as in adults—displaced fractures require ORIF to restore the articular surface. Nondisplaced fractures may be splinted with the MP joint in 30° of flexion. It is important to look for joint space widening associated with these fractures; this indicates possible hemarthrosis that should be drained to help prevent avascular necrosis of the metacarpal head.

## SOFT-TISSUE INJURIES: HAND INFECTIONS

Infections of the hand can be divided into those that can be incised and drained in the emergency department, treated as an outpatient, and those that require drainage by a hand surgeon in the operating suite or required admission to the hospital. Hand infections are usually initiated by trauma and very often require some form of surgical drainage; they should be considered a surgical disease.

In the history and physical examination the physician should always inquire about instigating trauma and possible retained foreign body, premorbid illness, especially diabetes or vascular disease, previous antibiotic therapy, tetanus immunization, and previous infection or surgery of the hand (including minor surgery such as laceration repair). Joint spaces, deep spaces, and tendon sheaths, all being closed spaces with poor blood flow, are especially vulnerable and must be examined with particular attention. Also vulnerable, of course, are contaminated or fractured bones and wounds with retained foreign bodies

---

### Hand infections

*High-risk injuries*

   Closed fist injuries
   Bites
   Punctures
   Involvement of tendon, joint, deep space, bone, muscle
   Aquatic injuries *(Aeromonas)*
   Wounds presenting late (especially after 12 hours)

*Patients with:*

   Vascular disease
   Immune compromise

*Pitfalls*

   Retained foreign bodies
   Lack of adequate drainage and debridement

*Indications for immediate consultation*

   Infection of tendon, joint, deep space, or bone
   (Usually) uninfected wounds with gross contamination
      of tendon, joint, deep space, or bone
   Deep foreign bodies
   Systemically ill
   Too busy to perform appropriate surgical care for
      superficial infections which could otherwise be done
      in the ED

*General therapy for all hand infections*

   Incision and drainage
   Debridement
   Splinting
   Elevation

*Aids to examination of hand wounds**

   Create a bloodless field by exsanguinating the distal
      extremity and applying a tourniquet
   Use regional blocks for anaesthesia. However, a Bier
      block is relatively contraindicated for an infected
      extremity

*Never use blind clamping in the hand to stop bleeding: pressure or a temporary tourniquet will almost always suffice. There are too many small and important structures in the hand that are vulnerable to blind clamping. Small nerves run with every artery.

---

(see box on this page). For serious infections antibiotics should always be immediately administered by the intravenous route, as adequate tissue levels are reached higher and faster (Table 16-1).[25]

### Antibiotic therapy

**Prophylactic antibiotics.**[26] In low-risk, nonbite wounds of the hand, prophylactic antibiotics have been shown to be ineffective.[27-29] Prophylactic antibiotics have only been proven effective in elective surgery when the antibiotic is given prior to skin disruption. The maximal acceptable delay for antibiotic delivery to wounds is estimated at 3 hours.[24]

Wound-tissue levels of antibiotic are much higher and reached much earlier with intravenous administration than with oral or intramuscular injection.[24] Immediate intravenous antibiotic prophylaxis has not been studied, but may be effective by quickly delivering antibiotic into the wound. Outpatient oral antibiotics are not in the patient's hands until after emergency department discharge. Early administration of prophylactic intravenous antibiotics is recommended for high-risk wounds only (see the box on this page). Simple bite wounds to the hand should receive at least oral prophylaxis (see discussion below). Antibiotic coverage should be continued orally for 3 days only.

**Organisms and antibiotics.**   Skin infections in the normal host that are caused by trauma in the home are almost always caused by *Staphylococcus aureus* (50% to 80%) or Group A beta-hemolytic *Streptococcus* because these organisms so frequently colonize the skin. Staphylococcus infections tend to develop over several days and to abscess, whereas *Streptococcus* causes a rapidly progressive cellulitis or lymphangitis that can be accompanied by systemic symptoms and extensive tissue damage.

Most routine infections will be adequately treated with an antistaphylococcal antibiotic such as a semisynthetic penicillin (eg, dicloxacillin) or a first-generation cephalosporin (eg, cephalexin). For patients with penicillin allergy, a cephalosporin is recommended unless the reaction to penicillin is severe. For this type of penicillin allergy, erythromycin is recommended. Vancomycin is very effective, but is also very expensive and must be administered intravenously; it should be reserved for severe infections or infections with methicillin-resistant *Staphylococcus*.

**Serious and severe infections.**   An intravenous first-generation cephalosporin or semisynthetic penicillin (eg, cefazolin or nafcillin) suffices for deep-hand infections without special contamination and without sepsis. Severe infections with fever and sepsis, immunosuppression, or special contamination should be treated with broad-spectrum intravenous antibiotics. Single-agent therapy is convenient in the emergency department and can be accomplished with ampicillin-sulbactam (AM/SB), with the more expensive ticarcillin-clavulanate (TC/CL), or with the most broad-spectrum but also most expensive, imipenem.

Other infectious etiologies must be considered, depending on the circumstances of the trauma—bites (eg, human, cat, dog), intravenous drug users, diabetics, farm contamination, fresh or sea water contamination.

**Bites.**[26] Bites of the hand are wounds that may be particularly prone to infection because of the high concentration of bacteria in oral flora. Human, cat, and dog bites are individually discussed below, but there are general considerations in dealing with bites. First, the issue of rabies must be dealt with. Second, even in the wound that is not infected, aggressive exploration, debridement, and irrigation are required to prevent infection. Involvement of deep spaces, tendon, joint, or bone require intravenous antibiotic prophylaxis and often irrigation and debridement by a hand surgeon in the operating suite. Third, the

**Table 16-1.** Antibiotics for hand infections in the emergency department*

| Infection | Organism | Antibiotic |
|---|---|---|
| Routine | *Staphylococcus* and *Streptococcus* | Antistaph antibiotic: semisynthetic penicillin or first generation cephalosporin<br>Serious infection†: intravenous cefazolin |
| Human bite–prophylaxis in hand bites indicated | *Staphylococcus, Streptococcus, Eikenella,* anaerobes | Penicillin plus first generation cephalosporin or second generation cephalosporin (eg, cefuroxime) (also AM/CL)<br>**Serious infection:**† AM/SB, TC/CL, or Imipenem |
| Cat bite–prophylaxis indicated | *Staphylococcus, Streptococcus, Pasteurella,* anaerobes | See Human bite |
| Dog bite–prophylaxis indicated | *Staphylococcus, Streptococcus,* anaerobes, *Pasteurella* (infrequent) | Dicloxacillin or first generation cephalosporin†<br>**Serious infection:** see Human bite |
| Diabetic–rule out gas gangrene and necrotizing fasciitis | **Mild infection:** *Staphylococcus, Streptococcus*<br>**Serious infection:** add *enterococcus,* anaerobes, gram negatives including *Pseudomonas* | **Mild infection:** first generation cephalosporin or diclox<br>**Moderate (oral regimen) infection:** clindamycin plus ciprofloxacin<br>**Serious infection:**† same as #2<br>**Gas gangrene infection:** add penicillin G to intravenous regimen |
| Farm injury | **Mild infection:** *Staphylococcus, Streptococcus*<br>**Serious infection:** gram negatives, anaerobes, gas gangrene | See Diabetic |
| Intravenous drug use | **Mild infection:** *Staphylococcus, Streptococcus* | Same as for Dog bite |
| Fresh water | *Aeromonas* | Norfloxacin (second choice: TMP sulfa) |
| Sea water or seafood handlers | If bullous lesions present–*Vibrio vulnificus* | Doxycycline plus an aminoglycoside |
| High-pressure injection injury | Gram positive, gram negative, anaerobes | Always a serious infection (TC/CL or AM/SB or imipenem) |

*Severe infections involving fever and sepsis should always be treated with broader spectrum antibiotics. Single agent therapy is convenient in the ED and can be accomplished with ampicillin/sulbactam (AM/SB), with the more expensive ticarcillin/clavulanate (TC/CL), or with the most broad spectrum but also most expensive imipenem/cilastatin.

†Serious infections include involvement of tendon or sheath, joint, bone, and deep space, include those with retained foreign body, and include those with systemic signs or symptoms. Outpatient treatment is only instituted after adequate drainage and debridement.

AM/SB = ampicillin/sulbactam

TC/CL = ticarcillin/clavulanate

AM/CL = amoxicillin/clavulanate

physician might be tempted to close primarily superficial bite wounds of the hand, but with the possible exception of dog bites, this should be avoided. Though it is not proven that simple cutaneous bite wounds have a higher incidence of infection than routine wounds, cosmesis of the hand is not usually important enough to risk primary closure. Moreover, hand wounds that heal by secondary intention typically have a good cosmetic result.

All of the literature on bites is based on small studies with many variables. There are no conclusive trials of antibiotics for either prophylaxis or treatment. Recommendations for treatment are based mostly on culture and sensitivity results and may have very little relationship to clinical efficacy. In short, very little is known for certain about antibiotic efficacy. On the other hand, the benefits of appropriate surgical care are well known.

**Human bites.** Human bite–wound infections are polymicrobic in 50% of patients.[30] *Staphylococcus aureus* has been found in up to 80% of human or animal bite infections[31]; therefore antibiotics must be penicillinase resistant. Aerobic *Streptococcus* are very prevalent in hand infections and anaerobes of all kinds are also common.[32,33] *Eikenella corrodens,* an anaerobic gram-negative rod, is isolated from approximately 25% to 30% of human bite wounds.[34-37] It is resistant *in vitro* to penicillinase resistant synthetic penicillins (eg, nafcillin, dicloxacillin), most aminoglycosides, and clindamycin,[33] and is usually sensitive to penicillin G. Twenty percent resistance to penicillin was found in one study.[38] The relationship between *in vitro* sensitivities and clinical efficacy is not fully known. In human bites to the hand, to cover for both *Staphylococcus* and *Eikenella,* penicillin plus either dicloxacillin or a first-generation cephalosporin should be administered, both prophylactically and therapeutically.

Based on its antimicrobial activity, amoxicillin-clavulanate (AM/CL) has been heavily marketed as an effective single-agent for bite wounds. However, it has only been studied once[39] in a very small number of patients, and though in this small study it was as effective as penicillin +/− dicloxacillin, it also resulted in a 30% incidence of loose stools. Nevertheless, *in vitro* it is active against *Staphylococcus*, *Streptococcus*, *Eikenella*, and other anaerobes and is commonly used and probably effective.

Despite the common recommendation that all patients with infected human bite wounds to the hand and all patients with new bite wounds involving deep structures be admitted to the hospital, Dreyfuss[34] has demonstrated that the critical element is the surgical care received. His patients fared very well as outpatients—only 6% required admission. Closed-fist injuries are discussed below under surgical management of hand infections.

In a very nice prospective study[40] of uninfected human bite wounds less than 24 hours old and not involving joint or tendon, 48 patients were randomized to either placebo, an oral second-generation cephalosporin, or intravenous cefazolin and penicillin. Seven of 15 patients receiving placebo and zero of 33 receiving antibiotics developed infection. Uninfected human bite wounds of the hand should be treated as is customary with at least 3 days of prophylactic antibiotics. Until further research is available, a first- or second-generation cephalosporin +/− penicillin is recommended.

**Cat bites.** Cat bites are particularly dangerous because their sharp pointed teeth create puncture wounds that may be avascular and cannot be irrigated. *Pasteurella multocida,* a facultative anaerobic coccobacillus, is found in a majority of wounds caused by cat bites and also in wounds caused by dog bites.[41-44] *Staphylococcus* and *Streptococcus* are, of course, also found. Whereas penicillin alone is not adequate coverage for *Staphylococcus*, dicloxacillin or a first-generation cephalosporin may not be ideal coverage for *Pasteurella*. This diclox or cephalexin alone may not be adequate therapy. Penicillin plus an antistaphylococcal antibiotic is recommended. Patients with fresh cat bites should receive prophylactic coverage with the above regimen.

Amoxicillin-clavulanate is often recommended because, as a single agent, compliance is better; it may be effective, but is not proven to be superior, is more expensive and has more side effects (especially diarrhea).

**Dog bites.** Callaham concludes[26,45,46] from his own data that simple dog-bite wounds are comparatively safe except in high-risk situations such as hand bites. Cummings' recent meta-analysis[47] of all randomized studies of antibiotic prophylaxis for dog-bite wounds showed a protective effect (seven infections prevented per 100 patients treated), which appears to be greater in hand wounds. Therefore, prophylactic antibiotics should be given for dog-bite wounds to the hand. Unless any of the high-risk factors above are present, loose suturing of simple wounds is probably safe after thorough irrigation and debridement.

*Staphylococcus*, *Streptococcus*, anaerobes, and, rarely, *Pasteurella* are cultured from infected dog-bite wounds. Despite the occasional presence of *Pasteurella*, dog-bite infections may be treated without penicillin, unless cultures dictate otherwise. Dicloxacillin or a first-generation cephalosporin alone are adequate, unlike cat or human bites, for both prophylaxis and treatment.

**Intravenous drug users.** Intravenous drug users who present with infections[48] may mix nonsterile drug powder with tap water, wash the skin with saliva, and inject into the hand or fingers with a used needle. The injections may be part or all subcutaneous and are exacerbated by inflammatory fillers added to the drug. Abscesses may be concealed by subcutaneous fibrosis resulting from chronic lymphedema. Veins are often used near the PIP joint, where infections may result in pressure necrosis or infection of the very superficial joint or tendon sheath. Infections are often severe and these infections require antibiotics to cover *Staphylococcus*, *Streptococcus*, anaerobes and gram negatives. Necrotizing fasciitis is commonly initiated by intravenous drug use. Ampicillin-sulbactam (AM/SB), ticarcillin-clavulanic acid (TC/CL), or imipenem are excellent single agents.

**Other bacterial infections.** Serious hand infections in diabetics[49,50] carry a high morbidity, with amputation often necessary. Gram negatives are cultured in up to 60% of patients. Those who also have renal transplants have a 100% amputation rate caused by immunosuppressive drugs and to poor perfusion distal to an unused AV fistula.

Gram-negative coliforms are found in wounds on the farm. *Aeromonas hydrophila* is associated with injuries occurring in fresh water. *Vibrio vulnificus* is associated with sea-water contamination including fish and seafood handlers, presents with hemorrhagic bullous lesions, occurs especially in patients with liver disease, and carries a very high mortality.[51]

### Minor infections

**Paronychia.**[52] Paronychia is an infection of the nail fold (ie, eponychium). When it develops a collection of pus, the pus is between the nail and the fold, not in the subcutaneous tissue as is an abscess. The infection may uncommonly spread to the subungual area, but only if left untreated. Instigating factors include trauma to the nail fold, nail biting and finger sucking. In patients exposed to chronic soaking of hands, as in dishwashers, the infection is often chronic and fungal (ie, candidal) and may involve more than one digit. Paronychias are very painful, but do not spread rapidly or cause systemic toxicity. If untreated, they may develop into a felon, osteomyelitis, flexor tenosynovitis, or chronic candidal infections.

Paronychia must be drained if a pus collection develops under the nail fold. Often what appears to be simple cellulitis without purulence does indeed harbor a small pocket of pus that must be drained; when in doubt, drainage should be attempted. If no abscess is present, the patient can be treated with antibiotics (see below) and soaks. Soaks should be in water that is as hot as the patient can tolerate, four times daily for 10 minutes.

*Drainage.* Because the collection of pus is between the nail and fold (Fig. 16-40), standard skin incision used for subcutaneous abscess is contraindicated. Instead, drainage is easily accomplished by inserting an 11-blade up under the eponychium along the surface of the nail and parallel to its plane, to separate the nail and eponychium (Fig. 16-41). Unless it is a very small collection of pus, the physician should assure drainage by spreading under the eponychium with a curved mosquito clamp (Fig. 16-42). Longitudinal incision parallel to the nail should be avoided because it is unnecessary and creates a skin bridge that may necrose. For a small paronychia, the procedure is so quick that it may be merciful to proceed without anesthesia, sparing the patient the discomfort of a digital block.

Larger paronychias must be treated under a block (see chapter on anesthesia). A small amount of iodoform gauze may be left in place, or alternatively zinc oxide can be thickly applied to keep the wound open and draining, as Kilgore and colleagues[53] recommend. If the infection has

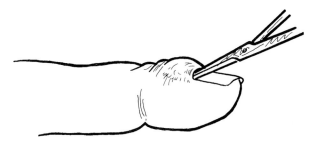

**Fig. 16-42.** Unless it is a very small collection of pus, the physician should assure drainage by spreading under the eponychium with a curved mosquito clamp.

spread under the nail, whole or partial nail removal is required. If there is surrounding cellulitis or induration, antibiotics may be helpful (see below) and warm soaks four times daily should be prescribed.

*Antibiotics.* Paronychia is usually a mixed-aerobic and anaerobic infection, remarkably similar to human-bite infections with occasional *E. corrodens* cultured. Antibiotic sensitivities are varied and there are no clinical trials to provide guidance for antibiotic therapy. As with all pus collections, drainage is the treatment and antibiotics may offer nothing. Routine wound cultures are not warranted. Penicillin, erythromycin, first-generation cephalosporins, amoxicillin-clavulanate, clindamycin, and semisynthetic penicillins are all possibly effective, but it is not clear which is best. The vast majority of patients do well as long as the surgical care is adequate.

*Prognosis.* Patients should be free of pain within 5 to 7 days of adequate drainage. If trouble persists, a foreign body, an unusual organism, or a complicated infection should be suspected and the patient referred to a specialist. Such patients may have any of the complications listed below, or may have herpetic whitlow.

*Complications*
1) felon
2) osteomyelitis
3) flexor tenosynovitis
4) chronic paronychia (ie, *Candida albicans*)

Herpetic whitlow may have a similar appearance to paronychia. However, whitlow should be distinguished by vesicles and should be suspected if the patient is a health-care worker or a young child. The incidence of this infection has diminished with the widespread use of gloves in health care. It is important to distinguish whitlow because it should not be incised and because the health-care worker must be aware of the infectivity of his or her wound. The only treatment is analgesia and protective bandaging. Whitlow resolves in 3 to 4 weeks.

*Felons.*[53,54] A felon is an infection of the closed-space fatpad of the distal finger. It presents as a very painful and throbbing swelling. There is often a history of some penetrating trauma to the digit which at the time seemed trivial to the patient. The infection is enclosed with no

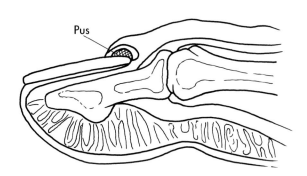

**Fig. 16-40.** Paronychia. Sketch of sagittal view of pus beneath the eponychial fold.

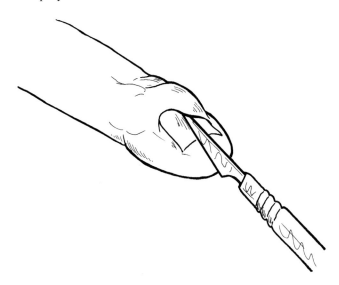

**Fig. 16-41.** Paronychia drainage procedure. An 11-blade should be inserted up under the eponychium along the surface of the nail and parallel to its plane, to separate the nail and eponychium.

---

*Complications of felons*

Cellulitis and lymphangitis
Osteomyelitis
Septic arthritis
Flexor tenosynovitis

*Complications of drainage of felons:*

Septic arthritis and flexor tenosynovitis
Lateral incision: unstable finger pad, neuromas, partial or
    complete loss of fingertip sensation
Volar longitudinal incision: scar on sensitive volar pad

---

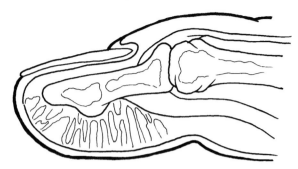

**Fig. 16-43.** Fibrous connections from bone to skin give the fingertip its stability.

outlet, and if left untreated will cause pressure necrosis of the adjacent bone and skin. Skin slough and osteomyelitis are common sequelae if the felon is not drained. *Staphylococcus* is the most common etiologic agent. Antibiotics are no substitute for drainage, although they may arrest a very early infection before it abscesses. Radiographs to diagnose osteomyelitis are only necessary if presentation has been delayed. Complications of felons are listed in the box above.

Fibrous connections from bone to skin give the fingertip its stability (Fig. 16-43). According to Kilgore,[53] these are multiple fibrous strands that radiate from the periosteum, and not septae that divide the fingertip into compartments, as most authors write. Kilgore states that because the fingertip is not divided into multiple compartments, drainage procedures need not divide all the fibrous connections, as is often recommended. He states that they are least concentrated in the center of the fatpad; hence, the center of the fatpad is the most distensible area and pus will localize there (Fig. 16-44). It is these arguments that he uses to support the midline volar longitudinal incision as adequate for drainage and least destructive to the fingertip (Fig. 16-45).

*Drainage.* Drainage must be performed under regional anesthesia. The fish mouth incision (Fig. 16-46C) is mentioned only to condemn it. By disrupting the fibrous strands, this incision leaves the fingertip unstable. The so-called hockey stick incision (Fig. 16-46D) may also leave the fingertip unstable. Transverse incisions across the pad may sever nerves and lead to a totally anesthetic fingertip. Similarly, lateral through and through incisions have also severed nerves, causing an anesthetic fingertip.

A longitudinal midline volar incision or a high unilateral incision is recommended (Fig. 16-46). The longitudinal volar incision into the pad is particularly effective for felons that are well localized in the center of the pad, especially if they are pointing. The longitudinal incision is the method least likely to injure nerves and is therefore the least likely to cause pain and fibrosis. However, the most dreaded complication of drainage of a felon is tenosynovitis from entry of the flexor sheath by the knife, and this complication is most common when the longitudinal volar incision is

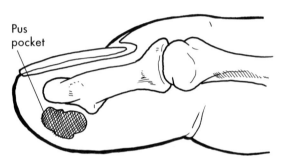

**Fig. 16-44.** The center of the fatpad is the most distensible area of the finger and pus will localize there.

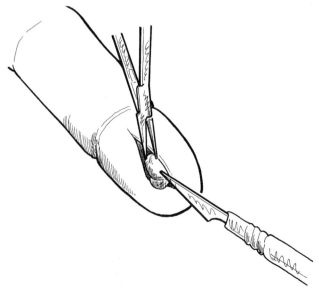

**Fig. 16-45.** The drainage technique using a midline volar longitudinal incision. Spread with scissors or with a clamp to open the entire abscess cavity.

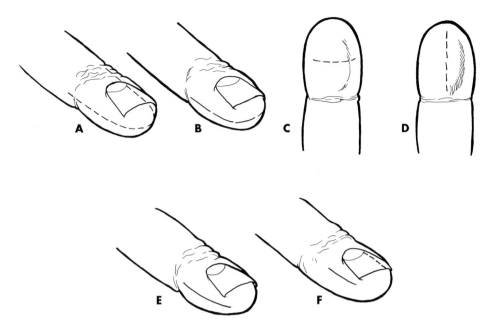

**Fig. 16-46.** Incisions used for drainage of felons. **A,** This fish mouth incision should not be used. **B,** This hockey stick incision should not be used. **C,** Transverse volar incision is not as effective as the longitudinal volar incision, **D, E,** The high-lateral incision, is recommended, but do not go through and through as in **F.**

extended too proximally. The other minor disadvantage is that of a scar on the important sensory surface of the finger. The high lateral incision may be more effective for felons that diffusely infect the entire pad. However, it has a higher incidence of nerve injury with subsequent hypoaesthesia or pain. Do not incise across the DIP joint or flexion contracture will result. The incision should not come close to the joint and tendon structures, which may extend up to 1 cm beyond the joint crease.

Using a longitudinal midline volar incision under regional anesthesia, the point of maximal tenderness is incised the length of the abscess by an 11-blade. Again, the physician must be exceedingly careful not to carry the incision too proximal into the flexor tendon sheath. A mosquito clamp should be spread in the cavity to assure drainage. The wound can then be packed loosely with gauze. To keep the wound draining, Kilgore and colleagues[53] prefer to apply a thick coat of zinc oxide instead of packing the wound.

In a high lateral incision under regional anesthesia, the incision is carried to the bone and then volar to the bone, proceeding past the midline. It must be high lateral, just below the nail margin, to avoid the neurovascular bundle and to avoid dividing the fibrous strands of the volar fatpad, which must remain a single unit to ensure fingertip stability. It is not necessary to carry the incision all the way through and out the opposite side, as is sometimes practiced, and this may result in an anesthetic fingertip.

For both types of incisions, the proximal end of the incision should be about 1 cm distal to the flexion crease. Care must be taken to not probe or cut proximally where

the flexor tendon sheath or the DIP joint may be violated, leading to tenosynovitis or septic arthritis. A mosquito clamp should be spread in the abscess cavity to assure drainage. To keep the wound draining, Kilgore and colleagues[53] prefer to apply a thick coat of zinc oxide instead of packing the wound.

After drainage and loose packing, the hand must be splinted and elevated and oral antistaphylococcal antibiotics prescribed.

### Deep hand infections[55]

**Recognition of deep hand infections.** Most crucial for the emergency physician is determining when a hand infection involves deep spaces, bone, joint, or tendon sheath. A swollen, red, and painful hand must always be assumed to harbor deep infection. There are five major spaces in the hand: 1) the deep palmar space; 2) the thenar space; 3) the dorsal subaponeurotic space; 4) the hypothenar space; and 5) the subfascial web space. Infections in any of these spaces must be suspected if there is swelling of the hand, if the pain is more generalized than a local abscess, and if hand function causes pain. All deep-space infections and flexor tenosynovitis require immediate drainage in the operating room by an experienced hand surgeon.

Radiographs of the seriously infected hand are essential to look for gas, fracture, and osteomyelitis.

The deep palmar (midpalmar) space is bordered radially by the septum from the third metacarpal to the profundus tendon of the long finger, ulnarly by the septum from the fifth metacarpal to the sublimis of the little finger, palmarly by the flexor tendons and dorsally by the metacarpals (Fig.

16-47). Infection may enter via direct trauma, from the flexor tendon sheaths, or least commonly by hematogenous spread. Infection here will cause palmar swelling, often massive, and severe pain with movement of the flexor tendons. It often penetrates dorsally, and leads to dorsal swelling (eg, collar button abscess). Drainage will usually be by a deep transverse palmar incision.

The thenar space (Fig. 16-47) is bordered ulnarly by the septum from the third metacarpal to the profundus tendon

of the long finger. It is bordered by the adductor pollicis dorsally and the index finger flexors volarly. Infection here will first present as swelling of the web space on the volar aspect and of the thenar eminence. It may penetrate to the dorsal side next to the first dorsal interosseous muscle. The position of greatest volume of the thenar space, and therefore of greatest comfort, is the abducted position. Passive adduction of the thumb increases pain. Besides direct trauma, it may become infected via the flexor sheath of the

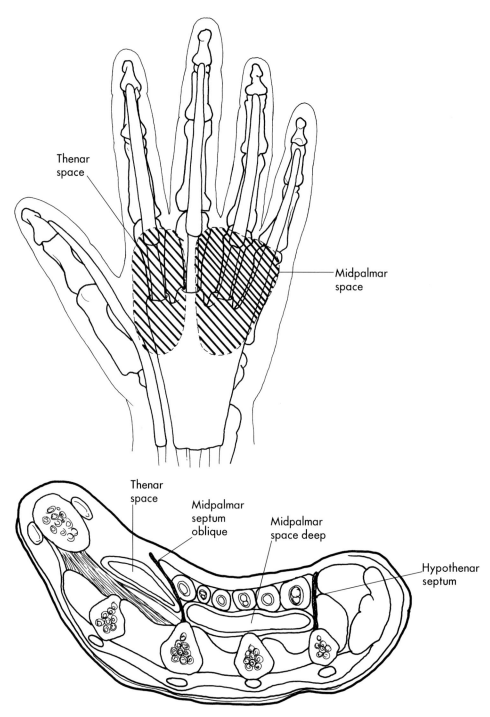

**Fig. 16-47.** AP and cross-section sketches of the deep palmar spaces.

index finger. Drainage will usually be by a curvilinear incision around the border of the thenar eminence. If there is dorsal extension, further drainage by incision of the dorsal web space is necessary.

The dorsal subaponeurotic space lies deep to the extensor tendons on the dorsum of the hand. It is easy to underdiagnose infection of this space as a simple subcutaneous abscess. It is drained usually by two longitudinal incisions over the second and fifth metacarpals.

The subfascial web space is the subfascial space between the fingers. It becomes infected when an infected palmar blister penetrates the skin and also the closely adherent underlying fascia. It can easily be misdiagnosed as a superficial infection, but should be distinguished by the resting abducted position of the digits.

The hypothenar space (Fig. 16-47) lies ulnar to the midpalmar deep space and infection here is recognized by swelling and tenderness of the hypothenar eminence.

Collar button infections (Fig. 16-48) are a result of a palmar infection producing sufficient pressure to break through between the metacarpals to the dorsal subcutaneous area, resulting in an abscess that points both dorsally and volarly. Drainage must be by both palmar and dorsal incisions of the web space.

### Tenosynovitis

The flexor tendons are enclosed in lubricating synovial sheaths that allow tendon glide. The tendons and sheaths have poor blood supply. When seeded with bacteria, they readily become infected. The purulence and inflammation of infection increase the pressure in the sheath and propagate a vicious circle of ischemia and infection. The sheaths lie beneath the subcutaneous tissue except at the finger flexion creases where they are directly subcutaneous and relatively constricted. Infection will progress proximally up the sheaths, relieving pressure, and may be slowed at these flexion creases, but will inexorably progress without treatment. The sheaths of the thumb and little finger are continuous with the wrist tenosynovium (Fig. 16-49) and infections will easily and rapidly decompress and progress toward the wrist. The tenosynovium of the middle three fingers ends in the midpalm. Therefore infection of these sheaths is contained and a greater degree of pressure may build, until the infection bursts through its containing sheath into the midpalmar space or thenar space.

Extensor tendons do not lie in sheaths but do become infected. Contamination of the flexor tendon and sheath is much more likely to lead to infection than a wound that contaminates the extensor tendon. Wounds of any tendon require thorough irrigation and prophylactic antibiotics.

Kanavel[56] described the four cardinal signs of flexor tenosynovitis, and these can be generalized to extensor as well:
1) tenderness over the tendon sheath
2) symmetric swelling of the finger
3) pain on passive extension (flexion for extensor tenosynovitis)
4) flexed resting position of the finger

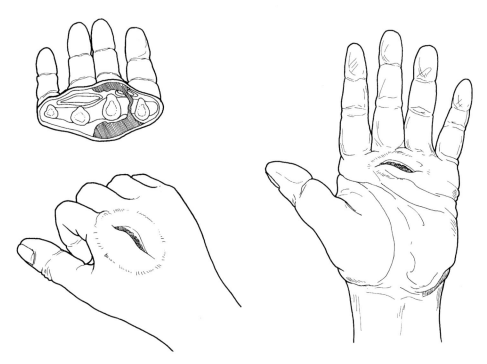

**Fig. 16-48.** Collar button abscess is a result of a palmar infection producing sufficient pressure to break through between the metacarpals to the dorsal subcutaneous area, resulting in an abscess that points both dorsally and volarly. Drainage should be performed from both sides as shown.

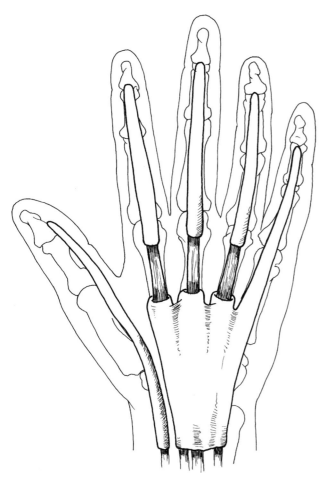

**Fig. 16-49.** The sheaths of the thumb and little finger are continuous with the wrist tenosynovium and infections will easily and rapidly decompress and progress toward the wrist. Because the tenosynovium of the middle three fingers ends in the midpalm, infection of these three sheaths may burst into the palmar spaces.

Infection of the tendon sheath is usually by direct trauma and the infecting organism is most commonly *S. aureus,* but many other pathogens may be present; therefore, broad-spectrum antibiotics are preferred because of the seriousness of the infection. Unfavorable sequelae range from scarring of the tendon onto its sheath with subsequent loss of flexor function to deep space infection of the hand or wrist with possible systemic sepsis. Nearly all flexor tenosynovitis requires immediate drainage in the operating room by an experienced surgeon. Very early pyogenic flexor tenosynovitis may respond to splinting, elevation, heat, and intravenous antibiotics, which should be administered immediately in the emergency department. These infections will require drainage if not significantly improved in 12 to 24 hours.

Extensor tenosynovitis also requires immediate consultation and intravenous antibiotics, but can often be managed conservatively with elevation and splinting as an inpatient.

All patients with tenosynovitis need admission and immediate consultation.

### Septic arthritis and joint penetration

Both septic arthritis and wounds with joint penetration are orthopedic emergencies. The joints of the hand, like all others, are relatively avascular and thus very susceptible to infection if contaminated. Any penetrating injury to a joint may cause septic arthritis and must be treated aggressively with intravenous antibiotics and debridement and irrigation in the operating room.

The physician must always assume that a wound overlying a joint may have penetrated into the joint until proven otherwise. Any wound over the MP joint should be considered a closed or clenched-fist injury (CFI) until proven

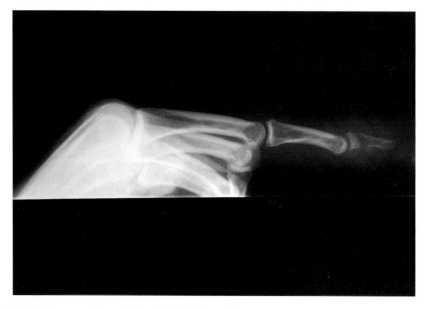

**Fig. 16-50.** Osteomyelitis of the distal phalanx after an open transverse fracture. Note the nonunion, the moth-eaten appearance, the periosteal calcification, and the dorsal subluxation. Osteomyelitis may also be the result of any of the soft-tissue infections, including felon and paronychia.

otherwise. The fist-to-mouth mechanism will usually be denied by the patient. Wound exploration is critical to this determination.

In the hand, septic arthritis is most often encountered as the sequela of a penetrating joint injury, especially CFI (see below), but may occur without apparent trauma as well. Clinical findings include swelling, redness, warmth, and tenderness of the joint. The sine qua non of septic arthritis is pain with joint movement, and if this finding occurs in conjunction with any of the above findings, septic arthritis must be seriously suspected. Radiographs may show air in the joint, fracture, joint-space narrowing, or joint destruction. In the setting of trauma, the diagnosis may be clinical, without the need for arthrocentesis. Gout may mimic septic arthritis. Septic arthritis must be treated with intravenous antibiotics and immediate drainage in the operating room.

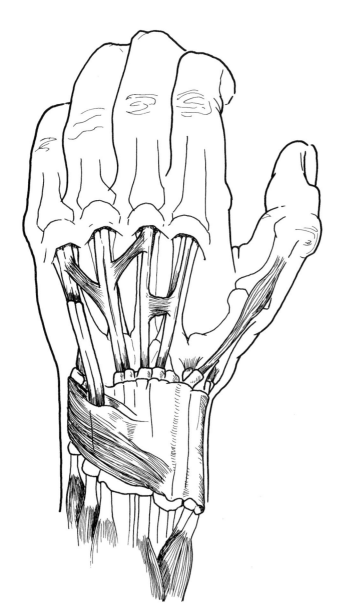

**Fig. 16-51.** Sketch of the extensor tendons, compartments, and juncturae tendinum.

**Closed-fist injury.** Closed-fist injury occurs when the flexed MC joint of a fist strikes a tooth. All too often the extensor tendon and the joint are penetrated and inoculated. CFI accounts for much of the morbidity associated with human bites. Patients often do not present until infection has set in, and too often when they do present in a timely manner, the seriousness of the injury goes unrecognized. Because the MC joint is in full flexion at the time of extensor tendon and of joint penetration, the depth of the wound may be easily concealed. It is necessary to examine the patient in the position of injury (ie, with the MC joints flexed). If the hand is examined with the MC joint extended, the lacerated area of the tendon will be proximal to the wound, and an intact section of tendon will cover the entrance wound to the joint. Radiographs may show air in the joint and fractures or indentations of the articular bone. All wounds in the area of the MC joints should be considered CFI until proven otherwise. It is safest to obtain immediate consultation.

### Osteomyelitis

Osteomyelitis should be suspected in any indolent infection near a bone and should be looked for on any radiograph of an infected hand. Treatment often requires admission for intravenous antibiotics and surgery to remove infected bone. Consultation is essential, although depending on the acuity of the infection, may not need to be immediate (Fig. 16-50).

### Atypical infections

Indolent infections may be mycoses such as blastomycosis or coccidiomycosis, tuberculosis or infection with atypical mycobacteria, or some cutaneous malignancies.

Trauma from contact with vegetation (eg, wood or thorn bushes) is an occupational hazard of farmers, gardeners, florists, timber workers, and others and may result in sporotrichosis, an infection with the fungus *Sporothrix schenkii*. A lesion on the hand may be followed by subcutaneous nodules and lymphadenopathy spreading over days to weeks up the arm and unresponsive to antibiotic therapy.

### SOFT-TISSUE INJURY: TENDON
### Anatomy

Tendon anatomy is discussed in the previous chapter on *Evaluation of Hand Injuries.* Further aids to anatomy will be found in Fig. 16-51, showing the six tendon compartments of the wrist; in Fig. 16-52, showing finger tendon anatomy; and in Figs. 16-53 and 16-54 illustrating the two tendon zone classifications.

**Indications for possible emergency department management**

1) extensor tendon over metacarpals (Zone III) > 50% lacerated
2) any amount of laceration of extensor apparatus over the finger, and over the MP or PIP joints
3) blunt distal phalanx extensor tendon rupture (mallet finger)
4) blunt PIP lateral band rupture (Boutonniere deformity)

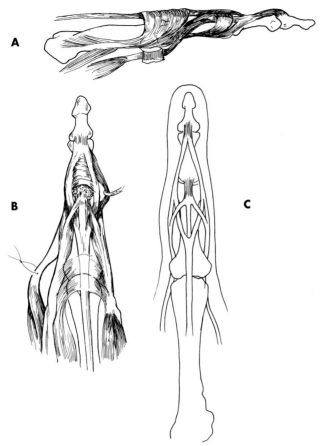

**Fig. 16-52.** Sketch of finger extensor apparatus (**A** and **B**), with schematic (**C**).

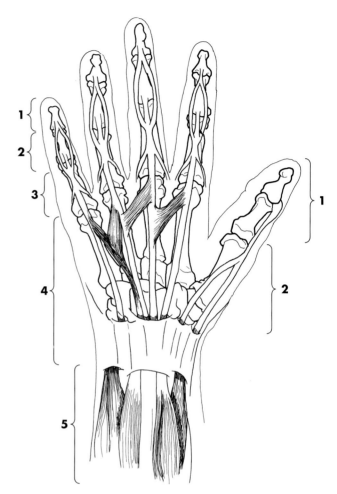

**Fig. 16-53.** Sketch of traditional tendon zones.

The following injuries may be done by a confident and experienced emergency physician, although some hand surgeons advise against it:
1) open mallet finger (laceration)
2) open central slip rupture (laceration)

**Indications for repair by consultant**
1) any flexor tendon, as well as partial lacerations
2) most long extensors at the wrist level
3) contaminated, inaccessible, or untidy lacerations, poor visualization, uncooperative or intoxicated patient
4) lack of experience, confidence, or time

**Referral.** Injuries indicating need for a referral include any tendon laceration that requires repair, but cannot be done by the emergency department physician. This category may include anything except for simple less than 50% lacerations of long extensor tendons. All repairs will of course require follow-up by a consultant.

**Timeliness of referral.** Repairing tendons in the emergency department is a difficult undertaking because it requires a period of uninterrupted concentration. In a busy department, it is usually best to call a consultant who can devote his or her undivided attention to the task.

However, if you have the time or if there is no consultant readily available, your patient will benefit from the conve-nience of immediate rather than delayed primary repair. If no consultant is available and your department is busy, delayed primary repair is very acceptable and should be performed before the healing process of the tendon begins, preferably within 5 days. If the delay is longer than 5 days wound healing may be well underway and this secondary repair is significantly more difficult. Additionally, with extensor tendons, the longer the wait, the greater the retraction and difficulty of retrieval. Obviously, immediate repair should never be attempted if the time or confidence is lacking.

If the patient is referred to a hand surgeon for immediate repair, the patient may be prepared for surgery in consultation with the specialist. In addition to standard preoperative care, a second-generation cephalosporin or semisynthetic penicillin effective against *Staphylococcus* and *Streptococcus* should be administered, and if there is a delay before the patient can go to the operating suite, the wound should be irrigated thoroughly before a bandage is applied.

If the patient is referred to a hand surgeon for delayed primary repair of the tendon, the wound should be thoroughly irrigated under local anesthesia, the skin approxi-

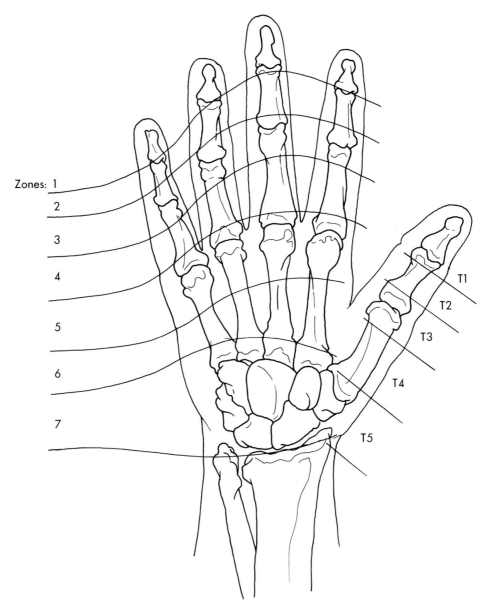

Zones: 1
2
3
4
5
6
7

T1
T2
T3
T4
T5

**Fig. 16-54.** Sketch of Verdan zone classification.

mated loosely with simple nylon sutures, and prophylactic antibiotics with *Staphylococcus* and *Streptococcus* coverage should be prescribed. If the mechanism of injury implicates contamination with other pathogens, appropriate prophylactic antibiotic therapy should be instituted.

**Flexor tendon lacerations**

Diagnosing flexor tendon laceration may be difficult—the flexor tendons are usually cut with the fingers flexed as in grabbing a knife. Because the wound is examined with the fingers extended, the shorn tendon end will be pulled distal to the laceration. A lacerated sheath with intact flexion is a clue that the tendon is partially lacerated but is now pulled distally out of view by the extended finger.

Flexor tendons in the hand and wrist should only be repaired by expert hand surgeons because of the difficulty

and the high incidence of complications. When injured tendons heal, they form adhesions that inhibit glide. If this happens to tendons with long excursions, it will result in motion limitation and poor function. Flexor tendons have a very long excursion—up to 7 cm in the hand—and run in relatively immobile synovial sheaths to which they readily form adhesions. Thus, flexor tendon repairs often heal poorly even when performed by the most experienced hand surgeons.

If only the sheath is violated but the tendon unharmed, the sheath may be closed by the emergency physician after copious irrigation. If the sheath is lacerated, however, the tendon is usually at least partially lacerated somewhere within the sheath and this must first be ruled out.

Partial lacerations require repair if, during active motion (usually under regional anesthesia), there is a block or clicking sound. Most partial lacerations do not require repair. If there is no block or click (ie, no tendon repair is required), the involved finger should be splinted with 30° of wrist flexion and 90° of MCP flexion. The splint should then allow active IP extension. A rubber band secured through a hole in the fingernail of the involved finger should be used to passively maintain the finger in the flexed position. The patient should be referred within 1 week to a hand surgeon and should return for a pop or snap, indicating complete rupture of the tendon. Splinting for 3 weeks will be required.

If delayed primary repair will be undertaken, the wrist should be splinted in 30° of flexion and the MCP joint at 70° to 90° after appropriate wound care.

### Extensor tendon lacerations

Extensor tendons have only about 2 cm of excursion over the metacarpals, where the structures they may adhere to are loose and will not fix the tendon; thus extensor tendons may, with some exceptions, be repaired in the emergency department if conditions are suitable.

Extensor tendon lacerations of the wrist are one exception. At the wrist, the tendons have about 4 cm of excursion and the extensor retinaculum has a fixed synovial sheath. Extensor tendon lacerations at this level may lead to adhesions that unacceptably limit glide. Therefore, these should be referred to a hand surgeon for immediate or delayed primary repair. After prophylactic antibiotics and loose skin closure, the wrist should be splinted in 40° of extension, with the metacarpophalangeal (MCP or MP) joints in 30° of flexion and the IP joints in full extension.

### Extensor tendon repair

**Accessibility.** Extensor tendon repair requires accessibility. Tendons must not be retracted, or, if they are retracted, they must be easily retrievable without damaging vital structures. Fortunately, juncturae tendinum crosslink the extensor digitorum communis (this does not include the extensor pollicis longus). If the laceration is distal to the juncturae, the proximal end will be attached to adjacent tendons, preventing excessive retraction. In fact, to facilitate apposition of the two ends for repair, the proximal end of the tendon can be pulled into apposition with the distal end by the juncturae if the adjacent fingers are flexed (Fig. 16-55). The longer the time from injury, the more retraction will occur. Blind grasping for a tendon should never be attempted.

The wound must be easily extendable, if extension is necessary for accessibility. Wound extension for any purpose must never cross a natural hand crease perpendicularly, especially on the flexor surface, and care must be taken not to extend the wound across important neurovascular structures, especially the cutaneous branches of the radial and ulnar nerves. Extensions should be along the crease lines.

**Tidiness.** Tendon repair also requires tidiness. There must be no contamination of the tendon. It must be sharply lacerated, without any crush injury. Retrieval of the tendon ends must be done delicately to avoid any further trauma. The wound itself must be clean such that primary closure is possible.

**Visualization.** Repair requires excellent visualization. The tendon ends must be brought into a well-lighted and

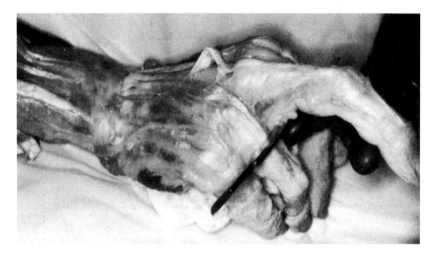

**Fig. 16-55.** Photo of cadaver demonstrating the action of the juncturae tendinum (the cross connections between the tendons of the extensor communis). When the adjacent fingers 2 and 4 are flexed, the attached juncturae pull the proximal part of the middle tendon distally. This has two practical uses if the tendon is lacerated distal to the insertion of the juncturae. First, when trying to locate the proximal end of the transected tendon, it may be brought into view by flexing the adjacent fingers. Second, after tendon repair, tension may be taken off of the repair by splinting adjacent fingers in flexion. The laceration may not be recognized when it is proximal to the juncturae because the adjacent tendons will be able to extend the involved digit through the juncturae. (From Beasley RW: *Hand Injuries.* Philadelphia, 1981, WB Saunders, p 254, with permission.)

bloodless field. A Bier block may be necessary, as simple tourniquets become too painful for the patient after 15 to 20 minutes.

Lastly, repair requires a cooperative and sober patient who will remain motionless during the procedure and understand the importance of postoperative care.

**Partial tendon laceration.** Partial tendon lacerations are diagnosed by direct visualization upon wound exploration, but should be strongly suspected if tendon tension against resistance produces pain. Laceration of the extensor communis proximal to the juncturae tendinum may go unrecognized because the pull of the juncturae from adjacent tendons will result in weak extension of the involved finger.

Over the metacarpals, tendons with less than 50% laceration need not be repaired, but should be splinted. However, partial lacerations over the joints (ie, MP, PIP, or DIP) can cause serious functional problems unless repaired. All partial tendon lacerations, even if not repaired, require splinting.

**Technique of repair.** First, crushed edges of the tendon must be sharply debrided, saving as much tissue as possible. If adjacent tendons are injured and are to be repaired, they will tend to cross-heal and adhere to one another (Fig. 16-56). To avoid this problem, differential debridement can be undertaken so that the repair is at different levels. Tendons must be minimally handled.

Suture should be nonabsorbable, preferably braided polyester. Nylon or prolene are also acceptable. Simple sutures are inadequate because they will rip through the longitudinal fibers of the tendon. The modified Kessler suture (Fig. 16-57) holds nicely. A figure 8 may be used for flat tendons such as extensor hood and lateral bands. Some authors recommend two independent sutures for added assurance. When placing and tightening the suture, bunching of the tendon should be avoided. Avoid strangulation of the tendon vascular supply and minimize exposed knots and suture. Lastly, if one is particularly skilled and at leisure, exposure of raw surfaces of tendons, which have a propensity to adhesions, can be minimized by finishing with a fine monofilament running suture of the edges (Fig. 16-58). I have found this to be impractical for flat extensor tendons.

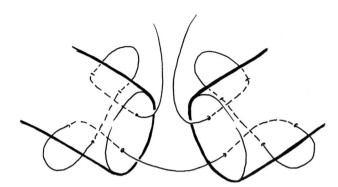

**Fig. 16-57.** The modified Kessler suture.

**Splinting.** Splinting of extensor tendon repairs is designed to release the tension on the tendon when also allowing the joints to be immobilized in the manner that best preserves their mobility. Generally, this means that the wrist should be extended to approximately 30°, the IP joints extended, and the MP joints in 15° of flexion.[58] For a severed single extensor communis, immobilizing adjacent fingers in more flexion than the affected one helps to release tension (Fig. 16-59).

One author recommends MP extension,[59] but given the propensity for permanent extension contracture at the MP joint that James[5] highlights in an excellent article, I would try to avoid this and only splint the MP joints in full extension for a maximum of 7 to 10 days and then only in a very reliable patient. The MCP joints should not be splinted in anything but full flexion, unless, as in the case of extensor tendon repair (or maintenance of reduction of Boxer's fractures), it is unavoidable.

Finger extensors should be immobilized for 3[58] to 4[59] weeks, at which time the extension splint is removed six to eight times daily for gentle active flexion and extension. The patient must always be warned against forced flexion of the involved digit or wrist.

Wrist extensors must be splinted at least 4 weeks[59] and as much as 6 weeks[58] followed by rehabilitation. There are dynamic splinting techniques in which immediate ROM is initiated. Rehabilitation of extensor tendon injuries is be-

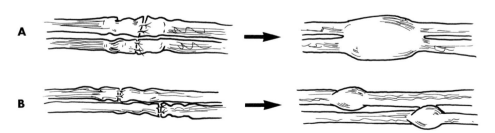

**Fig. 16-56. A,** Adjacent severed tendons may heal together. This may be avoided if, **B,** the tendons can be repaired at different levels such that the adjacent tendon surface is undamaged and less likely to scar together.

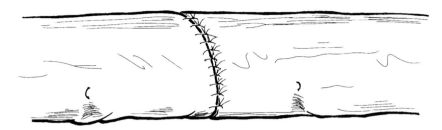

**Fig. 16-58.** Though impractical in most instances, raw surfaces at the repair site may be cleaned up with a fine monofilament suture. This procedure helps to minimize scarring.

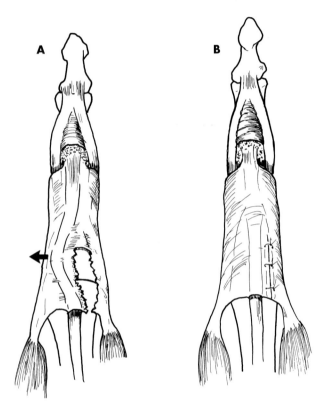

**Fig. 16-59.** Sketch of torn sagittal band with lateral slippage. Repair is essential to maintain the position of the extensor tendon over the MP joint.

yond the scope of this text. I refer you to an excellent review.[59]

**Metacarpal phalangeal joint (zone III injuries or Verdan zone V).** At the MP joint, the fascia is intimate with the tendons and there is no sheath. This extensor apparatus consists of the extensor tendon and sagittal bands that stabilize the long extensor tendon over the MP joint. Partial laceration of a sagittal band may be difficult to appreciate because of the intimacy with the fascia, but it can lead to slippage of the tendon and finger drift to one side (Fig. 16-59). Thus, any tendon laceration at the MP joint must be repaired. This may be accomplished with a figure 8 stitch using 3-0 or 4-0 braided polyester, nylon, or prolene. Also, keep in mind that any laceration over the

metacarpals is likely to be caused by a fist-mouth injury and thus be unacceptably contaminated. As always, if there is any doubt about the extent of the injury, it should be referred to a hand surgeon for immediate or delayed primary repair within 5 days. In any case, the patient must be followed-up by a hand surgeon. Splinting should be with the wrist in 30° extension, the MP joint in 15° flexion, and the IP joints in slight flexion.

**Proximal interphalangeal joint (zone II and Verdan zone III).** At the PIP joint, any amount of tendon laceration may weaken the lateral band or the central slip, with the potential to develop over weeks into a Boutonniere deformity, even if the patient has full function on initial exam. If there is any lack of function on initial exam, the central slip may be completely lacerated (see discussion on central slip rupture below). If the injury is well defined and all lacerated tissue is clearly exposed to view, it may be repaired by a confident and experienced emergency physician and referred for follow-up. The consequences of a poor repair are rather grave, with possible resultant Boutonniere deformity. If there is any doubt, the patient should be referred to a hand surgeon for immediate or delayed primary repair.

In any case, immediate intravenous antibiotics should be given, and the wound well irrigated. If immediate emergency department repair is chosen, all lacerated tendon should be repaired. The central slip may be approximated using a horizontal mattress suture. A nonabsorbable suture should be used (eg, nylon, prolene, or braided polyester), as with all tendon repairs. Splinting should be as for a central-slip rupture, with the PIP joint in extension and the MP and DIP joints free to actively flex and extend. In any case, the patient should be referred within 3 to 5 days to assure stability of the repair.

**Distal interphalangeal joint (zone I and Verdan zone I).** At the DIP joint, extensor laceration may result in a mallet finger. If uncomplicated, a confident emergency physician may suture this laceration using a horizontal mattress. After closure, the finger should be splinted as with a blunt mallet finger. Lacerations may involve other supporting structures and may require both repair and pinning by a hand surgeon.[58] In any case, the patient should be referred for early follow-up (3 to 5 days) to assure stability of the repair.

### Blunt injuries

**Mallet finger (of tendon origin and of bony origin).** "Mallet finger" refers to the loss of active extension of the DIP joint as a result of rupture of the extensor tendon or avulsion of the proximal dorsal bone of the distal phalanx where the tendon inserts. The injury results from forced passive flexion against a taut tendon, such as when a football or basketball strikes the extended finger. When the avulsion is of one third of more of the articular surface, it is referred to as a mallet fracture, or mallet finger of bony origin. Avulsion fractures of smaller size are treated identically to those of pure tendon origin.[60] There is much written on mallet finger and much controversy, because all treatments result in some cosmetic or functional loss. However, only rarely are there severe complications or limitations of function after any method or even after no treatment at all. Surgical repair has never proven superior to conservative therapy (ie, splinting), and has often resulted in more complications.[61,62] All authors agree that simple closed ruptures or avulsions that involve less than one-third of the articular surface, without joint dislocation or instability, should be treated conservatively.

*Splinting of mallet finger.* The DIP joint should be continuously splinted in mild (0° to 5°) of hyperextension for 6 to 8 weeks, followed by 2 to 4 weeks of night splinting. The DIP joint should never for even a moment drop out of extension during this time. The degree of hyperextension should never cause pain or blanching of the skin over the DIP joint, as this may lead to skin necrosis. When the splint is removed, some extension may be lost over the first few weeks, but usually is regained by scar contracture over the ensuing 6 months.

Splinting has complications, the worst being skin necrosis or maceration. The dorsal DIP alumafoam splint leaves the patients finger pad free and may enable him or her to continue working, but this splint is associated with a high incidence of skin complications[61] and one must be very vigilant with its use. If this splint is used, a layer of absorptive padding must be applied. The most commonly used and recommended splint during the first few weeks is the Stack splint[63] (Fig. 16-60 C) because it causes less pressure over the initially tender and swollen DIP joint. The Stack splint, however, often does not hold the DIP joint in completely full extension and one must be sure the tip of the finger is in contact with the end of the splint to maintain adequate extension.[64] Another popular splint, the Abouna splint (Fig. 16-60 D), made of rubber coated wire, was compared with the Stack splint.[65] The two splints were equally effective, with cure or significant improvement in 50%. However, the Stack splint was found to be superior with respect to patient satisfaction and hygiene. Any splint must be removed periodically for skin care and this procedure must be done with assistance so that the DIP is not allowed to flex.

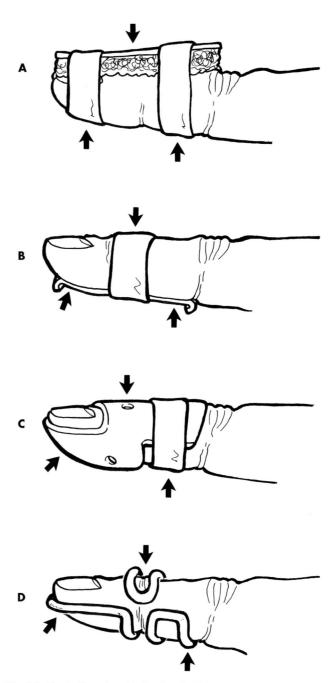

**Fig. 16-60. A,** Dorsal padded splint. **B,** Volar unpadded splint. **C,** Stack splint (recommended). **D,** Abouna splint.

Early referral to a hand surgeon for DIP pinning is appropriate for patients, such as surgeons or dentists, who must continue to use their fingers.

Late mallet finger refers to deformities seen at least 3 to 4 weeks after the injury. Even up to 6 weeks after injury, these respond to splinting. Beyond 6 weeks, mallet finger can be left untreated if there is no loss of function, or can be treated with prolonged splinting or pinning.

*Splinting the proximal interphalangeal joint in flexion.* Many authors have recommended immobilizing the PIP joint in 45° to 60° of flexion to relax the lateral bands and allow closer approximation of disrupted elements, and thus faster healing. Permanent, disabling PIP flexion contracture is a potential complication. PIP flexion has variously been accomplished by plaster casts, internal wires, or splints, and may allow a shorter period of splinting. In 1988 Evans and Weightman[66] described a two-part pipflex splint (Fig. 16-61) that combines a DIP immobilization splint and a dynamic spring splint that holds the PIP joint in flexion, but allows the joint to be extended at intervals only under close supervision. The PIP joint must be extended passively at least once a week to prevent crippling contracture.

Most authors agree that only the DIP joint need be immobilized in simple mallet finger. However, there is an exception—if there is concomitant PIP hyperextension or volar plate injury, the PIP joint must be splinted in slight flexion to prevent swan neck deformity (see discussion below).

***Prognosis and complications.*** Most patients will have some permanent extension limitation, averaging about 10° (range 0° to 30°) and flexion limitation averaging about 15° (range 0° to 40°). Extension limitation is greatest in those with greater degrees of flexion deformity on initial exam. Also associated with worse prognosis are age over 60 years, delay in treatment more than 4 weeks, and short stubby fingers.[67] There may also be limitation of PIP ROM.[61,68] Function limitation is greatest for those with mallet fractures. A dorsal bump with minor aching and cold intolerance[68] are common chronic problems.

Swan neck deformity (Figs. 16-62 B and 16-63) is the most debilitating complication of mallet finger. It is a chronic condition of PIP hyperextension and persistent DIP flexion deformity that is difficult to correct surgically. Swan neck deformity occurs most commonly in association with: 1) a large amount of flexion deformity; 2) PIP hyperextension; or 3) PIP volar plate injury at initial exam. It may be prevented if PIP hyperextension or volar plate injury are present at initial exam; the PIP joint should then be splinted in slight flexion.[69]

Complications already mentioned were those associated with splinting.

Open mallet finger caused by a laceration at the DIP joint is discussed above in the section on *Extensor Tendon Repair–DIP joint.*

**Mallet fractures.** When an avulsion fracture is greater than one-third of the joint surface (Fig. 16-64), it is called a

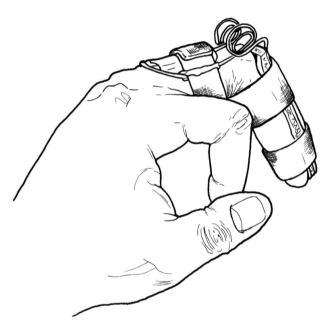

**Fig. 16-61.** Sketch of Pipflex splint, which holds the DIP extended and loosens the lateral bands by flexing the PIP joint with a spring, allowing the PIP joint to be extended at intervals under close supervision. If the PIP joint is not regularly extended, crippling contracture will result.

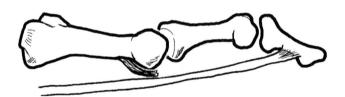

**Fig. 16-63.** Type II hyperextension injuries involve laxity or rupture of the volar plate. If not splinted properly, a hyperextension deformity may persist along with a flexion deformity of the DIP joint caused by the pull of the flexor tendon.

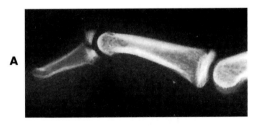
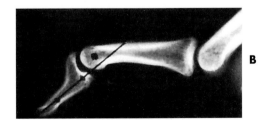

**Fig. 16-62. A,** An adolescent presenting with a mallet fracture that was treated with a splint with questionable compliance. **B,** On late follow-up, a reasonable joint surface has formed, but the distal phalanx is in volar subluxation and a swan neck deformity is present. (From Campbell RM: Operative therapy of fractures and dislocation of the hand and wrist region in children, *Orthop Clin North Am* 21(2):222, 1990.)

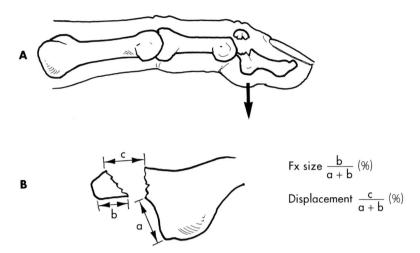

**Fig. 16-64. A,** Sketch of mallet fracture with subluxation. **B,** Method of determining fracture size and displacement.

$$\text{Fx size } \frac{b}{a+b} \text{ (\%)}$$

$$\text{Displacement } \frac{c}{a+b} \text{ (\%)}$$

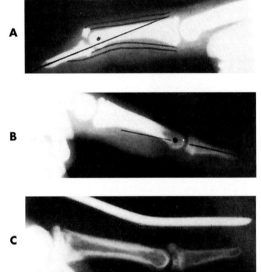

**Fig. 16-65. A,** Mallet fracture involving one-third of the articular surface of the joint. The dorsal displacement of the fracture fragment is obvious, but the volar subluxation of the remaining distal phalanx by the profundus tendon is subtle. Comparison with **B,** the normal side, reveals the subluxation. **C,** Splinting in slight extension holds the subluxation reduced. (From Campbell RM: Operative therapy of fractures and dislocation of the hand and wrist region in children. *Orthop Clin North Am* 21(2):222, 1990.)

*mallet fracture.* In this case, the joint may be unstable because "the major portions of both collateral ligaments remain attached to the . . . fragment."[69] The distal phalanx will sublux in the volar direction because of the volar force exerted by the flexor profundus. However, the physician must be very careful in evaluating this volar subluxation because it may be very subtle and easily missed and may determine treatment. When in doubt, comparison films of the other hand should be ordered (Fig. 16-65). It is also helpful to draw a line through the axis of the distal and middle phalanx as in Fig. 16-65.

There is no universal agreement regarding treatment for mallet fractures, especially those with greater than 2 to 3 mm displacement. Most authors recommend ORIF, but without strong data to support this view. Their are no randomized series to answer this question, and only one large series[70] in which many such fractures were treated with splinting alone. The results in this series were identical to those achieved by surgery. Green and Rowland[71] leave mallet fracture with volar subluxation (Fig. 16-66 B) of the distal phalanx as their only indication for ORIF. However, even when subluxation is present, some hand surgeons prefer to treat with splinting alone, as long as the splint easily maintains reduction.

Figure 16-66 A illustrates a large mallet fracture, but without subluxation; it should therefore be treated identically to simple mallet finger, with splinting alone. Figure 16-62 demonstrates the results of an inadequately treated mallet fracture.

***Referral.*** As with all hand injuries, timely follow-up with a hand surgeon is essential to ensure good progress and compliance. The patient with mallet finger should be

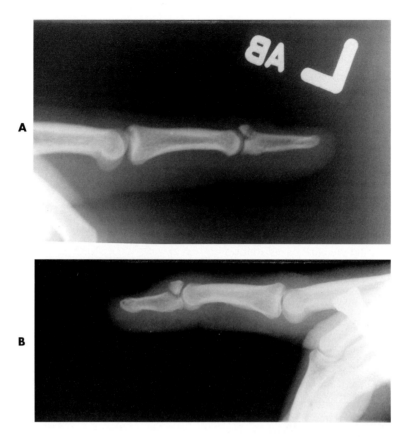

**Fig. 16-66. A,** Mallet fracture with greater than one-third of the joint surface affected, but without any volar subluxation. This may be treated as a simple mallet finger by splinting alone. Compare with **B,** in which there is subtle volar subluxation that often requires pin fixation. This fracture-subluxation may be treated with reduction and splinting if the splint succeeds in easily maintaining the reduction and the patient is very reliable and followed closely. Also note the beginnings of a swan neck deformity with PIP hyperextension and DIP flexion. This necessitates splinting of the PIP joint as well, in a minimum of flexion.

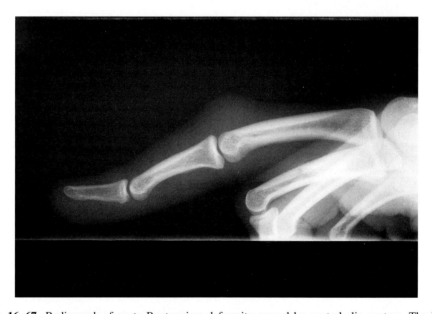

**Fig. 16-67.** Radiograph of acute Boutonniere deformity caused by central slip rupture. The PIP joint is in extension, but only because the DIP joint is hyperextended by the taut lateral bands. Notice the post–rupture soft-tissue swelling of the dorsal PIP joint.

seen within 1 to 2 weeks. Mallet fractures should be seen within 1 week, and fractures with subluxation must be referred immediately for possible ORIF.

**Central slip rupture and boutonniere deformity.** Boutonniere deformity (Fig. 16-67) refers to the deformity that chronically develops after rupture of the central slip or avulsion of the proximal dorsal lip of the middle phalanx. It is a chronic condition in which the PIP joint is flexed and unable to be extended and the DIP joint is hyperextended (Fig. 16-68). Emergency physicians commonly miss the central slip rupture that leads to this very disabling problem.

*Proximal interphalangeal joint anatomy and central slip rupture.* The extensor hood at the PIP joint is very complicated (Fig. 16-52). Normal function is as follows: the extensor hood is acted upon by the lumbricals to extend both the PIP and DIP joints (the long extensors extend the MP joints). The extensor hood extends the PIP joint via the central slip, the hood attachment to the dorsal base of the middle phalanx (Fig. 16-52). The extensor hood extends the DIP joint via the lateral bands that run on either side of the central slip and attach distally at the dorsal base of the distal phalanx. These two joints are always extended in unison under normal conditions. The DIP joint cannot be actively fully extended without full extension of the PIP joint, and vice versa. Lumbrical contracture pulls the entire extensor hood proximally, exerting pull on both the central slip and lateral bands.

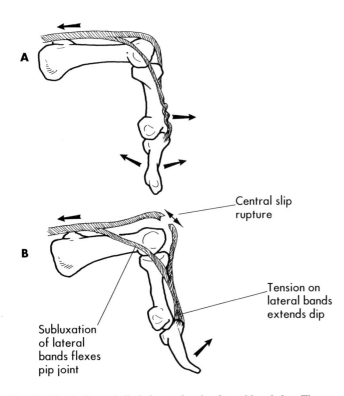

**Fig. 16-68. A,** Central slip is intact, leaving lateral bands lax. The DIP joint is not tethered. **B,** After central slip rupture, the proximal extensor mechanism has slipped proximally, tightening the lateral bands, thus extending the DIP joint.

When the central slip ruptures, the extensor hood mechanism is no longer tethered distally to the middle phalanx; rather, it is allowed to be pulled proximally by the resting tension of the lumbricals without extending the PIP joint (its connection to the PIP joint disrupted). The lateral bands are naturally pulled taut as well, extending the DIP joint even though the PIP joint can no longer be extended (Fig. 16-68). If the triangular ligament, which holds the lateral bands dorsal and close to the midline, also ruptures, or if it simply weakens over time, the lateral bands will sublux to a position volar to the axis of the PIP joint so that in their taut state they will flex the PIP joint as well as extending the DIP joint. With central slip rupture alone, the resulting tension on the lateral bands over time usually causes volar subluxation even without direct injury. Thus, central slip rupture alone will develop into a boutonniere deformity over a period of weeks. With rupture of the triangular ligament alone leaving the central slip intact, the PIP joint will still be able to be extended, the extensor hood mechanism will not be pulled proximally, and the DIP joint will not be extended (pathologically) at rest (ie, boutonniere deformity will not develop).

*Diagnosis of central slip rupture.* Immediately following injury, the lateral bands have not yet subluxed, unless there was concomitant triangular ligament rupture. Therefore, there will be no boutonniere deformity; that is, there will be no pathologic PIP flexion, but there will be DIP extension from lateral band tension. Lack of boutonniere deformity acutely does not rule out central slip rupture and, indeed, boutonniere deformity may develop later. Closed injuries to the central slip are often missed by the emergency physician, with often disabling results.

The patient usually presents with a painful, swollen PIP joint. On closer examination, maximal tenderness will be dorsal rather than lateral. Elson[72] describes a method for functionally diagnosing this injury (Fig. 16-68): the patient flexes the PIP joint 90° over the edge of a table, then attempts to extend the PIP joint. If the central slip is ruptured, the taut lateral bands will hyperextend the DIP joint first and any PIP extension that occurs will be the result of this extending force on the distal phalanx. PIP extension will be weak, but may be present. If pain limits this maneuver, it should be performed under digital or metacarpal head block. Pain and intact function may represent a partial rupture. Radiographs should of course always be taken, because of the frequency of avulsion fracture at the dorsal base of the middle phalanx, an injury which results in the same functional examination at the time of injury but may require different management (Fig. 16-69).

*Treatment of central slip rupture (prevention of chronic boutonniere deformity).* Most of the literature on boutonniere deformity is devoted to the very difficult task of surgical repair of the chronic condition. There is scant literature on the initial management of central slip rupture or acute boutonniere deformity. However, if recognized, this disabling problem can be prevented.

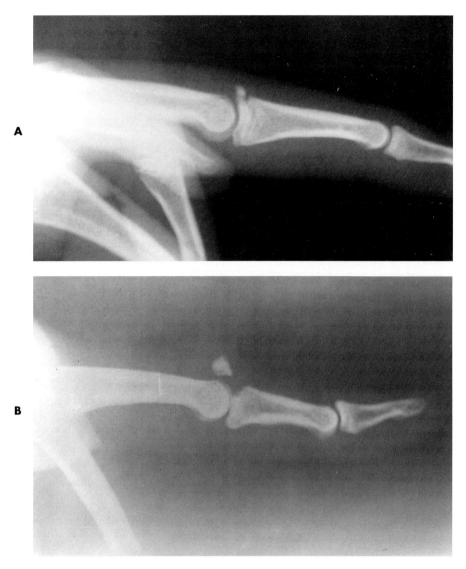

**Fig. 16-69. A,** Small avulsion fracture without loss of central slip function (notice the PIP joint is extended whereas the DIP joint is not hyperextended). This injury should be splinted with the PIP joint in extension and the DIP free to flex. **B,** Large central slip avulsion fracture with loss of independent PIP extension. The PIP joint is in extension, but only because the DIP joint is hyperextended by the taut lateral bands. This requires surgical reduction and fixation.

Without avulsion fracture present, the PIP joint should be splinted in full extension, leaving the MP and DIP joints free. Active DIP flexion should be encouraged as it is essential for central slip healing (Fig. 16-70). By flexing the DIP joint, the lateral bands are pulled distally, pulling the PIP extensor hood mechanism distally, allowing the two ends of the ruptured central slip to approximate. Splinting should be prescribed for approximately 6 weeks and "treatment should not be considered complete until active flexion of the distal joint is equal to that in the opposite normal finger."[73] The reason for this is that until the PIP extensor mechanism is tethered to the middle phalanx by the healed central slip, the lateral bands will not be lax enough to permit full flexion of the DIP joint.

With avulsion fracture (Fig. 16-69) present, "A bouton-

niere injury with a displaced avulsion fracture of significant size demands open reduction and internal fixation."[73]

Open injury is discussed in the section *Extensor Tendon Repair–PIP Joint.*

## SOFT-TISSUE INJURIES (DISLOCATIONS AND LIGAMENTOUS INJURIES)

Dislocations of joints of the hand are very commonly seen in the emergency department. Whether the injury will ultimately require surgery or not, the dislocation should be reduced if possible.

Radiography should always be performed after joint reduction. It is not always necessary to radiograph an obviously dislocated joint prior to relocation if it is clear by

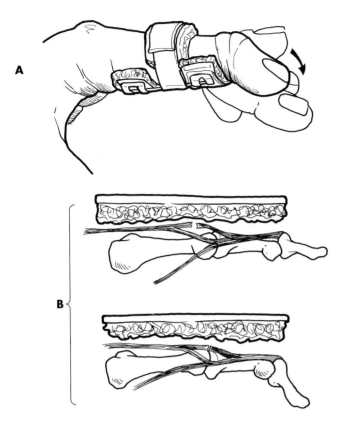

**Fig. 16-70. A,** Method of splinting the PIP joint only, so that the DIP can go through ROM and **B,** the underlying anatomic rationale for this method.

physical examination that there are no complicating fractures that will suffer further damage from the manipulation.

### Indications for nerve block before reduction

Most authors recommend nerve block before reduction of closed dislocations. In my experience and that of many emergency physicians, if reduction is swift, it may be performed without nerve block with no greater overall discomfort to the patient. However, there are two other disadvantages to reducing without nerve block: first, if no anesthesia is used, it may be difficult after reduction is complete to thoroughly assess the stability (ie, integrity of the collateral ligaments and volar plate) and the function (ie, active flexion and extension) of the joint; if these are not assessed in the emergency department, the patient will require earlier follow-up with a hand specialist for evaluation when the swelling and pain have subsided. Second, if the reduction cannot be accomplished swiftly, nerve block will be required anyway.

### General indications for surgery of joint injuries

1) irreducible dislocations
2) unstable fracture-dislocations
3) disruption of the collateral ligaments and volar plate
4) many articular fractures with incongruency of the joint surface

### Injuries of the distal interphalangeal joint

Dislocations of the DIP joint are very uncommon and virtually always dorsal. Volar subluxation occurs in the context of mallet fracture and requires operative fixation. Mallet fracture is discussed in detail in the section on tendon injuries.

Dorsal DIP dislocations are often open. These must of course be treated, after digital or wrist block, with irrigation of the wound and joint and with prophylactic antibiotics, which should be administered intravenously and early. Reduction is accomplished with gentle longitudinal traction and volar pressure. Closure of the skin should be performed loosely.

**Dorsal distal interphalangeal joint fracture–dislocations.** Avulsion fracture of the volar plate (Fig. 16-71) may occasionally complicate a dorsal dislocation. Because the flexor digitorum profundus (FDP) tendon inserts into this fragment, a complete disruption with fragment dislocation always requires surgery. If active DIP flexion is absent, complete disruption should be suspected.

If the fracture fragment is greater than one-third the articular surface, the reduction is likely to be unstable and the FDP tendon is likely to be involved. If after reduction there is no residual subluxation of the distal on the middle phalanx and the fracture fragment is in near anatomic reduction, closed therapy with splinting is appropriate. However, if there is either subluxation of the distal phalanx or dislocation of the fragment, surgery is necessary.

Recently, Hamer and Quinton described satisfactory results with conservative therapy of 22% to 47% avulsion-subluxations using a dorsal extension block splint.

The PIP joint was (splinted) in 15° to 30° of (flexion), and the injured joint flexed to a position that maintained reduction (between 30° and 60°). The MCP joints were not immobilized if at all possible. The splint was held on with adhesive tape at the level of the middle and proximal phalanx, but the terminal phalanx was not taped so that the affected joint could be flexed but not extended.[74]

The splint is then extended 10° each week and serial radiographs are taken to assess joint congruity and maintenance of reduction. Failure to maintain the reduction is an indication for internal fixation.

Despite the recommendations of this paper concerning treatment of DIP fracture subluxation, most hand surgeons recommend very early referral for surgical repair. Splinting in 60° of flexion may lead to severe flexion contracture of the joint. If the subluxation can be held by a dorsal extension block splint in the emergency department, closed reduction and splinting may be attempted if the patient is referred within 3 days to a hand surgeon for evaluation and possible surgery. Radiographs after splinting are essential to ascertain maintenance of reduction and joint congruity. Additionally, surgical repair is required if the fracture fragment remains displaced more than 2 mm after reduction (Fig. 16-71 B).

Irreducible dislocations of the DIP joint occur when the volar plate, the FDP tendon, or a bone fragment lodge in the joint. These require ORIF.

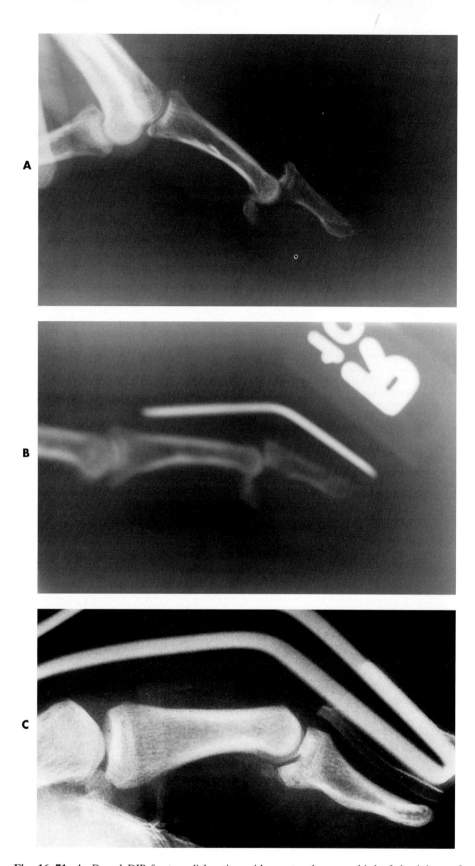

**Fig. 16-71. A,** Dorsal DIP fracture-dislocation with greater than one-third of the joint surface affected. Most surgeons recommend ORIF for treatment. **B,** Dorsal splinting was attempted in lieu of surgery, but the distal phalanx remains subluxed. Although this may be corrected by splinting in a greater degree of flexion, severe flexion contracture may result. Additionally, the fracture fragment is much too far displaced for conservative treatment. **C,** Adequate reduction of a DIP dorsal fracture dislocation by 30° of extension block splinting. The fragment is not displaced and there is no residual subluxation. There is very little residual joint incongruity or V sign (see Fig. 16-72). Surgery may still be necessary and the patient should be referred within 3 days. (Part C From Hamer DW, Quinton DN: *J Hand Surg [Br]* 17B(5), 1992, with permission.)

With delayed presentation from 2 to 4 weeks, the soft tissues may be contracted to the point that closed reduction is impossible. Reduction may still be attempted in the emergency department, but if unsuccessful the patient must be immediately referred to a hand surgeon for possible ORIF. Longer delays make ORIF impossible because of degeneration of the articular cartilage and severe periarticular soft-tissue contraction.[69] These usually require arthrodesis.

**Volar distal interphalangeal joint dislocations.** Volar DIP dislocations and fracture-dislocations are rarely complete. After reduction, they are managed as mallet finger and mallet fracture.

### Injuries of the proximal interphalangeal joint

The PIP joint is the most frequently injured joint in the hand, and is most frequently injured by being struck by a ball in sports. It is the most important joint for hand function, partly because of its large normal ROM of from 105° to 120°. It is a hinged joint and, unlike the MP joint, it has no mediolateral laxity.

Unfortunately, the PIP joint is also very susceptible to stiffness from injury, splinting in any amount of flexion, or surgery. Rowland and Green state "It is unusual to obtain full ROM after any procedure on the PIP joint."[75] When treating injuries of other parts of the hand, the PIP joint must not be immobilized in flexion. Stiffness results from shortening of the volar plate.

It is very important to ascertain whether PIP injury involves the volar, lateral, or dorsal structures. If a dislocation was reduced prior to presentation, it must be determined if it was dorsal (volar plate injury), volar (central slip injury), or lateral (collateral ligament injury). On examination, the dislocation may be tender or lax on the volar aspect (volar plate), laterally (collateral ligaments), or dorsally (central slip). If it is tender dorsally, it must be examined to ensure that the PIP extension is fully intact (see *PIP Anatomy and Central Slip Rupture* in the section on *Tendon Injuries*). If central slip rupture is inadvertently treated as a volar plate injury by splinting in slight flexion, the central slip will not heal and debilitating boutonniere deformity will result.

**Radiography.** "More errors are made in the diagnosis of PIP joint injuries because of failure to obtain lateral view radiographs than any other single reason."[76]

**Hyperextension injury and dorsal dislocation (volar plate injury).** Hyperextension is the most common mechanism for PIP joint injury, causing volar plate injury. The volar plate may completely tear without dislocation. The physician must be sure that there is no subluxation of the joint when treatment is concluded. Lateral radiographs (Fig. 16-73) are critical for evaluation of presence or absence of the V sign (Fig. 16-72), indicating joint incongruity (subluxation). Any apparent subluxation must be corrected by splinting in more flexion or by surgery. Liss and Green[77] have classified hyperextension injury as follows:

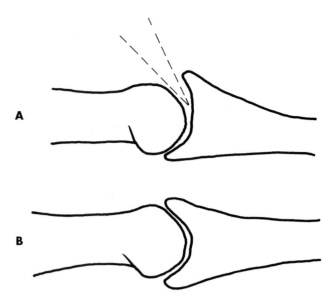

**Fig. 16-72. A,** The V sign indicating joint subluxation. **B,** The joint is congruous and there is no V sign.

Type I injury—first-degree sprain of volar plate. There should be no prehospital history of dislocation-relocation with this injury. There is pain on the volar aspect of the PIP joint. Radiograph results are normal. On examination, there may be ecchymosis and volar tenderness and the joint may have no hyperextension laxity to passive stress. Treatment consists of buddy taping or splinting in slight flexion for comfort until pain subsides—usually no more than 1 week—followed by active ROM exercises. The patient's return to sports should be possible within 2 weeks, although "buddy taping the injured finger to an adjacent one is advisable for several weeks."[77]

Type II injury—second- or third-degree sprain with hyperextension laxity on examination under nerve block, but no subluxation or dislocation. This injury should be treated with splinting in 15° of flexion for 7 to 14 days. If there is persistent laxity after this period, an additional 2 weeks of splinting is necessary. Flexion contracture is common and rehabilitation is critical; maximum improvement may take as long as 18 months and residual joint enlargement is permanent.

Type III injury–subluxation (joint incongruity or V sign) (Fig. 16-73) on lateral radiograph but no dislocation. Subluxation is reduced by flexing the joint and maintaining it with an extension block splint. Fifteen degrees flexion is usually sufficient; more flexion can be detrimental, but reduction should be ascertained by radiograph results. Persistent joint incongruity requires immobilization in a greater degree of flexion.

Type IV injury–dorsal dislocation (Fig. 16-74), in which there is always disruption of the fibrocartilaginous volar plate, usually at its relatively weak distal aspect near the insertion in the middle phalanx. There is always longitudinal disruption of the accessory collateral ligaments, but the

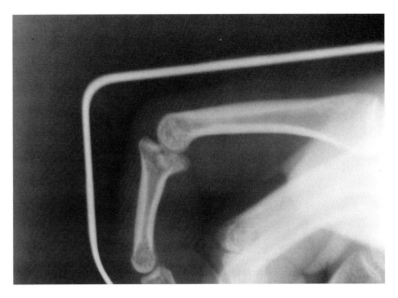

**Fig. 16-73.** Reduced PIP dorsal fracture-dislocation. Joint congruity has not been achieved despite greater than 60° of flexion. Notice the pronounced V sign made by the dorsal opposing joint surfaces. Surgical repair is necessary.

collateral ligaments themselves may be left intact (Fig. 16-75). There may also be a small avulsion chip fracture at the base of the middle phalanx. A larger fracture (greater than 20% to 30% of the joint surface) at the volar base of the middle phalanx is a fracture-dislocation (Fig. 16-76) and is a much more serious injury.

***Treatment of dorsal dislocation.*** Dorsal dislocations are often reduced before the time of presentation. If the joint remains dislocated, it may be reduced before radiography if by physical examination the physician is certain of no significant fractures. "Reduction is accomplished by accentuating the deformity and then applying traction to the finger while flexing it to reduce the joint."[78] Nerve block is standard but not always necessary, as long as examination for stability and function can be subsequently carried out without it. Full extension and passive stress of the volar plate should be avoided.

Concomitant collateral ligament injury (mediolateral instability on stress exam) requires operative repair. If the joint has lateral stability, active post–reduction ROM from 20° to 90° will also be stable. If lateral stability is in question, the joint can be compared with the opposite side.

Most dorsal dislocations do not manifest mediolateral instability and can be treated conservatively. As in Type III injuries, simple dorsal splinting or extension block splinting (Figs. 16-77 and 16-78) may then be initiated at no more than 15° to 20° of flexion and reduced over 2 to 4 weeks followed by buddy taping until full painless motion is restored. Post–reduction radiographs are necessary to assure joint congruity and also to rule out fracture-dislocation, a more serious injury. If the joint remains incongruous, splinting in a greater degree of flexion is necessary.

**General treatment of all volar plate injuries.** Green and Rowland[79] prefer to treat all volar plate injuries, including dislocations, with 3 to 6 weeks of buddy taping only, if radiographs reveal no joint incongruity. Complications of volar plate injury are listed in the box on this page.

***Open dislocations of the proximal interphalangeal joint.*** Stern and Lee[80] conclude that parenteral antibiotics are necessary and that open debridement and reduction with operative repair of the volar plate is indicated in the treatment of open dorsal PIP dislocations. Liss and Green[77] argue in response that it is unnecessary to repair the volar plate and that it leads to a higher rate of residual stiffness. The decision of operative fixation may best be made in consultation with the hand surgeon. Should conservative therapy be decided, parenteral antibiotics must be administered and the wound and joint must be thoroughly irrigated and debrided before loose skin closure. Splinting is as for closed dislocations.

---

*Complications of volar plate injury*

  Persistent instability

  Swan neck deformity from persistent hyperextension
    laxity

  "Pseudoboutonniere deformity"[78] after injury involving
    avulsion of the proximal attachment of the volar
    plate and subsequent scarring and contracture such
    that there is PIP flexion contracture and lateral
    band contracture with DIP extension.

  Limitation of ROM

  Pain and swelling of the joint, may be chronic

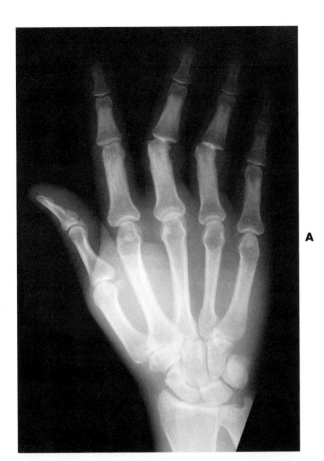

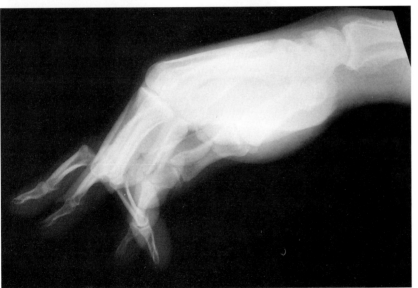

**Fig. 16-74. A,** AP and **B,** lateral views of third and fourth PIP dorsal dislocations. It is preferable to order finger radiographs rather than hand radiographs to prevent other fingers from obscuring the view.

**Dorsal fracture–dislocations.** The dorsal fracture-dislocation (Fig. 16-76) is the result of the base of the middle phalanx being driven into the head of the proximal phalanx during dislocation, fracturing off the volar aspect of the base of the middle phalanx, usually with comminution of the fragment. The articular surface may be disrupted and, if the fragment is more than 30% of the joint surface, the collateral ligaments are usually attached to it, resulting in instability and subluxation.[77] This is a far more serious injury than dislocation alone.

**Treatment.** Fragment sizes less than 30% of the joint surface "are easily reduced and predictably maintained by flexion splinting."[81] After closed reduction, if radiographs reveal congruity of the articular surfaces (ie, there is no V sign as described by Light[82]) (Figs. 16-72 and 16-73) and no subluxation of the middle phalanx on the proximal phalanx (Fig. 16-79), and exam reveals collateral ligament stability, this injury may be treated by the McElfresh[83] method of extension block splinting at 15° to 20°.

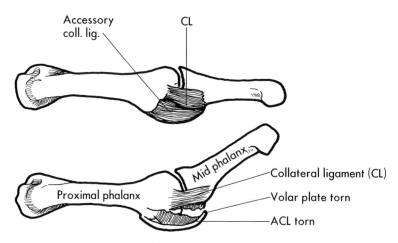

**Fig. 16-75.** Ligamentous rupture with PIP dislocation. The volar plate ruptures distally and a tear develops between the collateral ligaments and the accessory collateral ligaments. The collateral ligaments themselves usually remain intact. If they are ruptured, as evidenced by mediolateral instability, surgery is indicated.

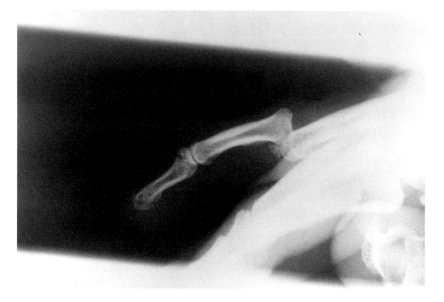

**Fig. 16-76.** PIP dorsal fracture-dislocation, approximately 30%. Treatment with dorsal extension block splinting should be undertaken, with the PIP joint flexed to 60°. Post–splinting radiograph must demonstrate no residual subluxation of the middle on the proximal phalanx.

With fragment sizes greater than 30% of the joint surface, or joint incongruity and subluxation, some authors recommend surgery,[77,78] but both McElfresh[83] and Hamer and Quinton[74] have demonstrated that the method of extension block splinting should be attempted. The reduction is maintained by holding the joint at 60° in an extension block splint. If radiographs reveal persistent subluxation, more flexion may be necessary. If this fails, surgery is indicated (Fig. 16-73). If it succeeds, follow-up within 1 week is essential to ensure maintenance of reduction and to begin the weekly gradual extension of the splint.

Unlike DIP fracture-dislocations in which the FDP tendon attaches to the fragment, the bone fragment need not be anatomically reduced. As long as there is no joint subluxation, the joint surface will adequately remodel.

Surgical treatment should be reserved for injuries in which the joint is unstable or remains subluxed despite conservative therapy, usually when the fragment is larger than 50%, although Rowland and Green "have been able to use it effectively in some patients with up to 70% involvement."[84] Hamer and Quinton had good to excellent results in seven of 12 patients with 50% to 70% involvement. The other five patients had severe comminution or a depressed central fragment, both of which portend a poor prognosis by any treatment. Various methods of pin fixation have been described to treat dorsal fracture-dislocation. Pin fixation is difficult because of the comminution of the fragment and the resulting stiffness associated with surgery. For fragments larger than 50%, consultation with a hand surgeon is recom-

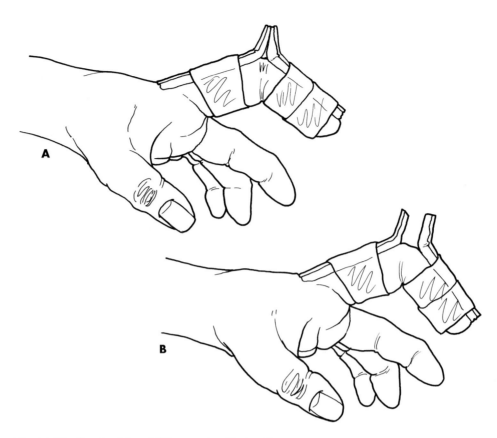

**Fig. 16-77.** Sketch of dorsal PIP extension block splint.

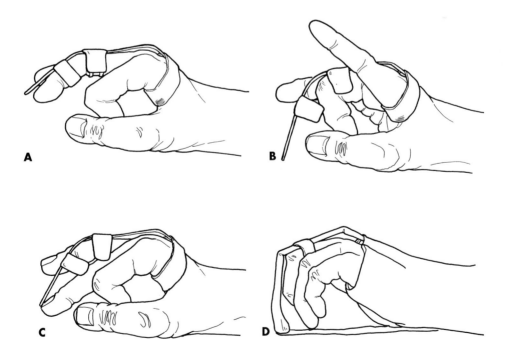

**Fig. 16-78. A,** Aluminum dorsal extension block splint. **B,** Demonstration of allowable PIP flexion in the extension block splint. **C,** If the proximal phalanx is not well secured to the splint, MP joint flexion is possible, allowing the PIP joint to be extended too far. **D,** Malleable outrigger secured to plaster short arm cast. The outrigger is prevented from bending (ie, extending too far) by an attachment to the cast.

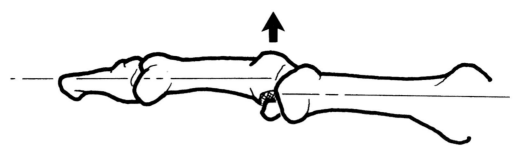

**Fig. 16-79.** To assess subluxation at the PIP joint, determine whether the long axes of the phalanges align.

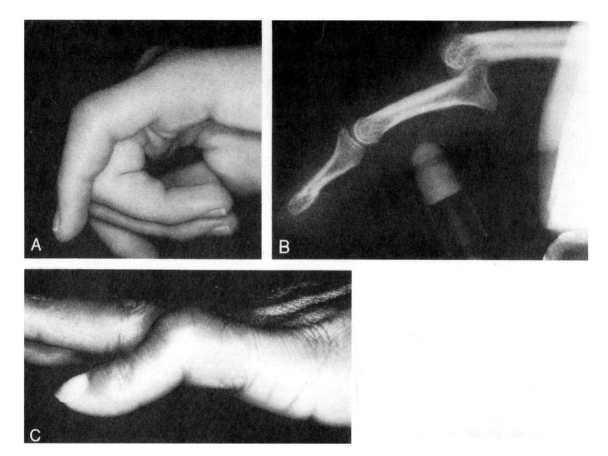

**Fig. 16-80. A,** A patient presents with a painful PIP joint which superficially does not appear to be dislocated. **B,** Radiograph is surprising, showing a rare PIP volar dislocation. **C,** Boutonniere deformity resulting from an untreated volar dislocation. (From Melone CP: Joint Injuries of the Fingers and Thumb, *Emer Med Clin North Am* 3(2):326, 1985.)

mended; all of these patients should be referred for very early follow-up (ie, 1 to 3 days).

***Extension block splinting.*** Extension block splinting is a means of dynamic splinting, allowing ROM of the affected joint to help prevent stiffness, but limiting full extension that may further damage or prevent healing of the volar plate. There are two methods of extension block splinting. Strong's method[85] (Fig. 16-77) is simpler but should only be used in very reliable, compliant patients. The traditional method (Fig. 16-78) is best employed using a plaster short arm cast with a malleable outrigger. As always, it is essential to keep the MP joint in at least 70° of

flexion. It is also essential that the proximal phalanx be taped to the splint; otherwise MP flexion will allow PIP extension. The end of the malleable outrigger should be secured to the cast to prevent its extension. The patient is encouraged to actively and passively flex the finger, extension being prevented by the splint.

***Irreducible dislocations.*** These occur as a result of entrapment of the volar plate or flexor tendons and require ORIF.

**Volar dislocation.** This is a rare injury and there is very little literature about it. It may be very subtle on physical examination (Fig. 16-80). The injured element is primarily

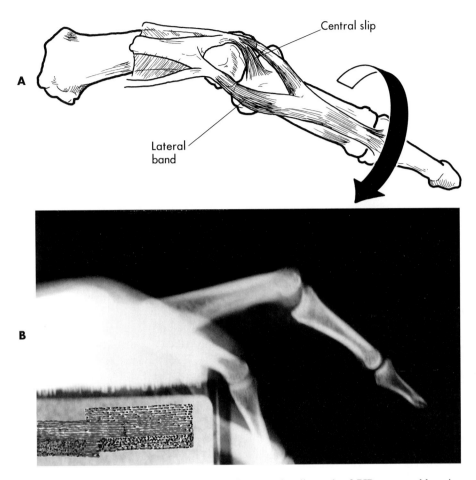

**Fig. 16-81. A,** Schematic of rotary subluxation. **B,** Lateral radiograph of PIP rotary subluxation showing oblique view of proximal phalanx (both condyles of the head are visible instead of overlapping) and simultaneous true lateral view of the middle phalanx.

the central slip of the extensor mechanism because the thin dorsal capsule provides little stability. "Dorsal joint stability is primarily dependent on the integrity of the central extensor tendon (central slip) and its insertion into the dorsal base of the middle phalanx. Secondary stability is provided by the extensor expansion, the lateral bands, and the transverse retinacular ligaments."[77] There may also be collateral ligament rupture.

There is disagreement over whether open or closed treatment is indicated. Green and Rowland[86] favor closed treatment identical to the treatment of blunt central slip rupture, even if there is an avulsion of the dorsal base of the middle phalanx, unless the fragment is displaced and does not reduce in full extension. Treatment is by splinting only the PIP joint in full extension and encouraging active and passive DIP flexion (see *Central Slip Rupture* in the section on *Tendon Injuries*). If the fragment is displaced, pin fixation may be necessary. With concomitant collateral ligament rupture, the patient should be referred for ORIF.

**Rotary proximal interphalangeal subluxation (Fig. 16-81).** Rotary subluxation is an uncommon injury. It has some of the clinical and radiologic features of volar dislo-

cation, but it is different. Pathognomonic is the lateral radiograph, which reveals a true lateral profile of the proximal phalanx and an oblique view of the middle phalanx (Fig. 16-81 B). Green and Rowland previously believed that this was an irreducible dislocation but have since had success and describe the procedure as follows:

Under digital-block anesthesia, gentle traction is applied to the finger with both the MP and PIP joints flexed at 90°. This maneuver relaxes the volarly displaced lateral band and allows the band to be disengaged and slip dorsally when a gentle rotary and traction force is applied. Further relaxation of the extensor mechanism can be achieved by dorsiflexion of the wrist. A small pop may be felt as the lateral band reduces to its dorsal position. Successful reduction is followed by full active and passive motion of the PIP joint and . . . must . . . be confirmed by . . . a true lateral view. If the joint has been successfully reduced, no immobilization is required and early active motion can be started immediately with buddy-taping.

Failure of closed reduction is an indication for open reduction.[87]

**Collateral ligament injury and lateral dislocation.** Collateral ligament injury, or the jammed finger, is the most common finger injury in sports. The injury may be an isolated partial tear, unassociated with dislocation or volar plate injury, or a complete tear with or without dislocation; according to Eaton,[88] if it is a dislocation, there will always be volar plate injury. Collateral ligament rupture usually happens at the proximal attachment. If the joint is not dislocated and there is no laxity, or laxity with a good endpoint at less than 20° on stress radiograph, it is a partial tear. Angulation of greater than 20° on stress radiograph is diagnostic of significant complete rupture.[89] Joint incongruity on radiograph suggests soft-tissue interposition and is an indication for ORIF.

Partial tear (second-degree sprain) or first-degree sprain may be treated only by buddy taping to the finger adjacent to the injured ligament until full painless motion is restored. If not possible because of excessive pain, splint in slight flexion followed by buddy taping when the pain has subsided.

Treatment for complete rupture (unstable with or without having been dislocated) engenders some controversy. Surgery leads to greater joint stability but of course at a cost of limited ROM. For complete rupture of the radial collateral ligament of the index finger stability is most important and there is little disagreement that operative fixation is the treatment of choice. For other PIP collateral ligament injuries, splinting in slight flexion followed by buddy taping or simply buddy taping for 6 weeks is sufficient. The finger adjacent to the injured ligament should be buddy taped against it. Chronic complications include instability and often painful swelling, and patients should be warned that they will have painful swelling for many months.

For athletes, McCue[78] recommends surgical repair of all collateral ligament tears, but his opinion is not unopposed. Green[90] successfully used buddy taping for 2 months on a basketball player who continued playing.

### Injuries of the metacarpophalangeal joint

The MP joint, unlike the PIP joint, is not hinged. Rather, the metacarpal head is a convex surface articulating with the concave surface of the base of the proximal phalanx, allowing both flexion-extension, abduction-adduction, and circumduction. In full flexion, abduction-adduction is limited by the collateral ligaments, which are stretched taut to their full length because the distance from the axis of motion to the volar surface of the MC head is longer than to its distal surface (Fig. 16-34). Thus, the physical examination for collateral ligament laxity should be performed with the joint in full flexion.

Joint stability is provided primarily by the collateral and accessory collateral ligaments.[91] The fibrocartilaginous volar plate, which is laterally continuous with the transmetacarpal ligament, prevents hyperextension and dorsal dislocation when the joint is in extension.

**Metacarpophalangeal dislocation.** Dislocation is almost exclusively dorsal, with rupture of the volar plate at its proximal attachment to the metacarpal. It happens more often to the index and little fingers because they are more exposed to trauma and they are continuous with the transmetacarpal ligament on only one side. The mechanism of injury is hyperextension.

Dislocations may be classified as simple (reducible) and complex (irreducible). Complex dislocations involve entrapment of the volar plate (Fig. 16-82), whereas simple do not. Simple dislocations are, in fact, subluxations because the joint surfaces remain intact. Care must be taken during reduction not to convert a simple to a complex dislocation.

On examination, the two types of dislocations can be distinguished: simple dislocations present with a dramatic hyperextension deformity of 60° to 90°, whereas in complex dislocations, the proximal phalanx and metacarpal are nearly parallel. Complex dislocations of the index finger exhibit in the distal palm "a bony hard prominence that is the head of the second metacarpal, and on either side of it, the palmar skin is puckered."[92] In complex dislocations, the flexor tendons deviate to the ulnar side, manifesting on examination as ulnar deviation of the affected finger. Finally, a sesamoid bone in the joint on radiograph is pathognomonic of complex dislocation. "The surgeon should not have to resort to multiple unsuccessful attempts at closed reduction to conclude that he or she is dealing with an irreducible dislocation."[93]

To reduce a simple dislocation, simple longitudinal traction should not be applied because it may lead to entrapment of the volar plate and conversion to a complex dislocation. If not reduced under wrist block, pain may make the joint irreducible and deceive the physician into

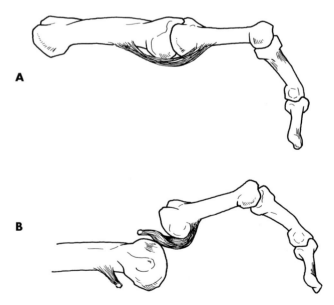

**Fig. 16-82.** Sketch of interposition of volar plate, which often complicates a metacarpophalangeal dislocation and may make it impossible to reduce closed.

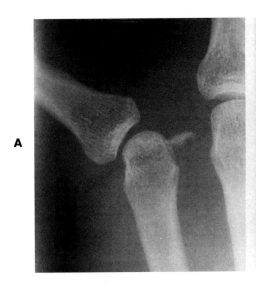 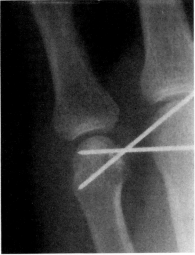

**Fig. 16-83. A,** If disruption of the MP joint involves a displaced avulsion fracture off the head of the metacarpal, surgical fixation, **B,** is indicated. (From Rockwood CA, Green DP, Bucholz RW, eds: Fractures in Adults. ed 3, Philadelphia, 1991, JB Lippincott, p 519.)

believing the dislocation to be complex. The joint should be reduced as follows:[78,92,93] 1) the wrist and PIP joint should be flexed to loosen the flexor tendons; 2) the hyperextension deformity should be exaggerated to 90° when holding the joint surfaces in contact to prevent interposition of the volar plate; and 3) the proximal phalanx is then advanced distally and volarly into flexion with continued contact between the joint surfaces maintained. Reduction should be easy and accompanied by, according to Rowland and Green, "a palpable and audible clunk."[94]

The joint may then be alternatively splinted in 70° for 7 to 10 days or buddy taped. The prognosis is very good, with rare complications or recurrences.

Complex dislocations are difficult to reduce primarily because of interposition of the volar plate and the subsequent chinese finger trap which tightens around the MC head when reduction is attempted. Campbell[95] states that, nevertheless, 50% can be reduced closed, and Rowland and Green[96] state that one attempt at gentle closed reduction should be attempted. The same technique should be used as for simple dislocations. If unsuccessful, open reduction should be immediately undertaken.

**Metacarpophalangeal collateral ligament injuries and lateral instability.** Collateral ligament sprains and disruptions are uncommon because the joint is protected from lateral stress. They most commonly occur with a sudden deviation of the finger in an ulnar direction, particularly when the MP joint is in flexion and the ligament taut. These injuries present as pain at the MP joint, swelling in the depression between MC heads, and pain with ligament stress, even with lateral deviation when the ligaments are relaxed in extension. The act of joint flexion alone is painful because it tenses the injured collateral ligament. MP

joint instability (eg, collateral ligament rupture) is best detected by stressing the joint in the flexed position because in extension the ligament is normally lax.

Incomplete MP collateral ligament tears may be treated with buddy taping and continued until symptoms have resolved.

Collateral ligament disruptions of the interior fingers can usually be treated with splinting in 50° or less of flexion or even buddy taping.[97] If splinted in full flexion the ligament may heal in the stretched position and be too lax.

Complete disruption of the radial collateral MP ligament of the little finger with subsequent ulnar deviation may require open repair.[97] A hand surgeon should be consulted or the patient sent for early follow-up.

Avulsion fractures, whether off the lateral base of the proximal phalanx or off the metacarpal head, require operative fixation "if the x-ray film shows wide displacement of a tiny avulsion chip (greater than 2 to 3 mm) or if the fragment involves more than 20% of the articular surface and is displaced or rotated"[98] (Figs. 16-17 and 16-83).

*Carpometacarpal Injuries* are discussed in the chapter on *Wrist Injuries.*

### REFERENCES

1. Rockwood CA, Green DP, Bucholz RW, eds: *Fractures in Adults,* 3rd ed, Philadelphia, JB Lippincott, 1991, p 479.
2. Green DP, Rowland SA: Fractures and dislocations in the hand, In *Fractures in Adults* 3rd ed. Rockwood CA, Green DP, Bucholz RW, eds: Philadelphia, JB Lippincott, p. 479.
3. Watson FM: Fractures in the hand: Metacarpals and phalanges, *Emerg Med Clin North Am* 3(2): 295, 1985.
4. Coonrad R, Pohlman M: Impacted fracture in the proximal phalanx of the finger. *J Bone Joint Surg* 51(A):1291-1296, 1969.
5. James JIP: Common, Simple Errors in the Management of Hand Injuries. *Proc Royal Soc Med* 63:70, 1970.

6. Burkhalter WE, Reyes FA: Closed treatment of fractures of the hand, *Bull Hosp Jt Dis* 44(2):145-162, 1984.

7. Reyes, FA, Latta, LL: Conservative management of difficult phalangeal fractures, *Clin Orthop* 214:23-30, 1987.

8. Green DP, Rowland RA. In Rockwood CA, Green DP, Bucholz RW, eds: *Fractures in Adults,* 3rd ed, Philadelphia, 1991, JB Lippincott, 474.

9. Rockwood CA, Green DP, Bucholz RW, eds: *Fractures in Adults,* 3rd ed, Philadelphia, 1991, JB Lippincott, p. 519.

10. DaCruz DJ, Slade RJ, Malone W: Fractures of the distal phalanges, *J Hand Surg* 13B(3):351, 1988.

11. DaCruz DJ, Slade RJ, Malone W: Fractures of the distal phalanges, *J Hand Surg* 11A:351, 1986.

12. Ford DJ, Ali MS, Steel WM. Fractures of the fifth metacarpal neck: is reduction or immobilization necessary? *J Hand Surg* [Br] 14B(2):165-167, 1989.

13. McKerrell J, Bowen V, Johnston G, Zondervan J: Boxer's fractures—Conservative or operative management? *J Trauma* 27(5):486-490, 1987.

14. Arafa M, Haines J, Noble J, Carden D: Immediate mobilization of fractures of the neck of the fifth metacarpal, *Injury* 17:277-78, 1986.

15. Hunter JM, Cowen NJ: Fifth metacarpal fractures in a compensation clinic population. A report on 133 cases, *J Bone Joint Surg* 52A:1159-1165, 1970.

16. Jahss SA: Fractures of the metacarpals: A new method of reduction and immobilization, *J Bone Joint Surg* 20:178-186, 1938.

17. Green DP, Rowland SA: Fractures and Dislocations in the Hand In Rockwood CA, Green DP, Bucholz RW (eds): *Fractures in Adults,* 3rd ed., Philadelphia, 1991, JP Lippincott, p 488.

18. Royle SG: Rotational deformity following metacarpal fracture, *J Hand Surg* 15B(1):124-5, 1990.

19. Bloem JJAM: The treatment and prognosis of uncomplicated dislocated fractures of the metacarpals and phalanges, *Arch Chir Neerl* 23:55-65, 1971.

20. Rockwood CA, Green DP, Bucholz RW (eds): *Fractures in Adults,* 3rd ed, Philadelphia, 1991, JB Lippincott, pp. 490, 491.

21. Fisher MR, Rogers LF, Hendrix RW: Systematic approach to identifying fourth and fifth carpometacarpal joint dislocations, *AM J Roentgenology* 140:319-324, 1983.

22. Henderson JJ, Arafa MAM: Carpometacarpal dislocation: An easily missed diagnosis, *J Bone Joint Surg* 69-B, (2):212-214, 1987.

23. Rockwood CA, Wilkins KE, King RE, eds: *Fractures in Children,* 3rd ed, Philadelphia, 1991, JB Lippincott, p 329.

24. Campbell RM: Operative treatment of fractures and dislocations of the hand and wrist region in children, *Orth Clin N Am* 21(2):220, 1990.

25. Alexander JW, Alexander SE: Influence of route of administration on wound fluid concentrations of prophylactic antibiotics, *J Trauma* 16:488-495, 1976.

26. Callaham M: Controversies in antibiotic choices for bite wounds, *Ann Emerg Med* 17(12):1321-1330, 1988.

27. Grossman JAI, Adams JP, Kurec J: Prophylactic antibiotics in simple hand lacerations, *JAMA* 245:1055-1056, 1981.

28. Haughey RE, Lammers RL, Wagner DK: Use of antibiotics in initial management of soft tissue hand wounds, *Ann Emerg Med* 10:187-192, 1981.

29. Worlock P, Boland P, Darrell J, et al: The role of prophylactic antibiotics following hand injuries, *Br J Clin Pract* 34:290-292, 1980.

30. Hausman MR, Lisser SP: Hand infections, *Orthop Clin North Am* 23(1):171, 1992.

31. Chuinard RG, D'Ambrosia RD: Human bite infections of the hand, *J Bone Joint Surg* 59A(3):416-418, 1977.

32. Brook I: Microbiology of human and animal bite wounds in children, *Pediatr Infect Dis Journal* 6(1):29-32, 1987.

33. Goldstein EJC, et al: *Eikenella corrodens* in hand infections, *J Hand Surg* 8(5):563-567, 1983.

34. Dreyfuss UY, Singer M: Human bites of the hand: A study of one hundred six patients, *J Hand Surgery* 10A:884-889, 1985.

35. Faciszewski T, Coleman DA: Human bite wounds, *Hand Clinics* 5:561-569, 1989.

36. Snyder CC: Animal bite wounds, *Hand Clinics* 5:571-590, 1989.

37. Bilos ZJ, Kucharchuk A, Metzger W: *Eikenella corrodens* in human bites, *Clin Orthop* 134:320-324, 1978.

38. Rayan GM, et al: *Eikenella corrodens* in human mouth flora, *J Hand Surg* 13A(6):953-956, 1988.

39. Goldstein EJC, Reinhardt JF, Murray PM, Finegold SM: Outpatient therapy of bite wounds. Demographic data, bacteriology, and a prospective, randomized trial of amoxicillin/clavulanic acid versus penicillin +/− dicloxacillin, *Int J Dermatol* 26(2):123-127, 1987.

40. Zubowicz VN, Gravier M: Management of early human bites of the hand: A prospective study, *Plast Reconstr Surg* 88(1):111-114, 1991.

41. Arons MS, Fernando L, et al: *Pasteurella multocida*—The major cause of hand infections following domestic animal bites, *J Hand Surg* 7A:47-52, 1982.

42. Goldstein EJ, Citron DM, et al: Bacteriology of human and animal bite wounds, *J Clin Microbiol* 8:667-672, 1978.

43. Lucas GL, Bartlett DH: *Pasteurella multocida* infection in the hand. *Plast Reconstr Surg* 67:49-53, 1981.

44. Phipps AR, Blanshard J: A review of in-patient hand infections, *Arch Emerg Med* 9:299-305, 1992.

45. Callaham M: Prophylactic antibiotics in common dog bite wounds: A controlled study, *Ann Emerg Med* 9:410-414, 1980.

46. Callaham M: Treatment of common dog bites: Infection risk factors, *JACEP* 7:83-87, 1978.

47. Cummings P: Antibiotics to prevent infection in patients with dog bite wounds: A meta-analysis of randomized trials, *Ann Emerg Med* 23(3):535-540, 1994.

48. Reyes FA: Infections secondary to intravenous drug abuse, *Hand Clin* 5(4):629-633, 1989.

49. Mann RJ, Peacock JM: Hand infections in patients with diabetes mellitus, *J Trauma* 17(5):376-380, 1977.

50. Francel TJ, Marshall KA, Savage RC: Hand infections in the diabetic and the diabetic renal transplant recipient, *Ann Plast Surg* 24(4):304-309, 1990.

51. Morse Jr GJ, Black RE: Cholera and other vibrioses in the US, *NEJM,* 312:343-350, 1985.

52. Roberts JA: The clinical approach to paronychia, *Emerg Med News* 15(4):4, 1993.

53. Kilgore, et al: Treatment of felons, *Am J Surg* 130:194-198, 1975.

54. Canales FL, Newmeyer WL III, Kilgore ES: The treatment of felons and paronychias, *Hand Clin* 5(4):515-523, 1989.

55. Nevasier RJ: Infections, in Green DP, ed: *Operative Hand Surgery.* New York, 1988, Churchill Livingstone, pp. 1027-1047.

56. Kanavel AB: *Infections of the Hand,* ed 6, Philadelphia, 1933, Lea & Febiger.

57. Patzakis MJ, Wilkins J, Bassett RL: Surgical findings in closed fist injuries, *Clin Orthop* 220:237-240, 1987.

58. Herndon JH: Tendon injuries—extensor surface, *Emerg Med Clin North Am* 3(2):333, 1985.

59. Lovett WL, McCalla MA: Management and rehabilitation of extensor tendon injuries, *Orthop Clin North Am* 14(4):819, 1983.

60. Rockwood CA, Green DP, Bucholz RW, eds: *Fractures in Adults,* 3rd ed, Philadelphia, 1991, JB Lippincott, p 446, 1991.

61. Stern PJ, Kastrup JJ: Complications and prognosis of treatment of mallet finger, *J Hand Surg* 13A:341-6, 1988.

62. Robb WAT: The results of treatment of mallet finger, *J Bone Jt Surg* 41B:546-549, 1959.

63. Stack HG: A modified splint for mallet finger, *J Hand Surg* [Br] 11(2):263, 1986.

64. Rockwood CA, Green DP, Bucholz RW, eds: *Fractures in Adults,* ed 3, Philadelphia, 1991, JB Lippincott, p 449.

65. Warren RA, Norris SH, Ferguson DG: Mallet finger: A trial of two splints, *J Hand Surg* 13B(2):151-153, 1988.

66. Evans D, Weightman B: The Pipflex splint for treatment of mallet finger, *J Hand Surg* 13B(2):156-8, 1988.

67. Abouna JM, Brown H: The treatment of mallet finger. The results in a series of 148 consecutive cases and a review of the literature, *Br J Surg* 55(9):653-667, 1968.

68. Clement R, Wray RC: Operative and nonoperative treatment of mallet finger, *Ann Plast Surg* 16(2):138, 1986.

69. Lenzo SR: Distal joint injuries of the thumb and fingers, *Hand Clin* 8(4):772, 1992.

70. Wehbe MA, Schneider LH: Mallet fractures. *J Bone Joint Surg* 66A(5):658-669, 1984.

71. Green DP, Rowland SA: Fractures and Dislocations in the Hand, In Rockwood CA, Green DP, Bucholz RW, eds: *Fractures in Adults,* ed 3, Philadelphia, 1991, JB Lippincott, p 453.

72. Elson RA: Rupture of the central slip of the extensor hood of the fingers, *J Bone Joint Surg* 68B(2):229, 1986.

73. Rockwood CA, Green DP, Bucholz RW, eds: *Fractures in Adults,* ed 3, Philadelphia, 1991, JB Lippincott, p. 478.

74. Hamer DW, Quinton DN: Dorsal fracture subluxation of the distal interphalangeal joint of the finger and the interphalangeal joint of the thumb treated by extension block splintage. *J Hand Surg [Br]* 17B(5):591, 1992.

75. Rockwood CA, Green DP, Bucholz RW, eds: *Fractures in Adults,* ed 3, Philadelphia, 1991, JB Lippincott, p. 505.

76. Rockwood CA, Green DP, Bucholz RW, eds: *Fractures in Adults,* ed 3, Philadelphia, 1991, JB Lippincott, p. 503.

77. Liss FE, Green SM: Capsular injuries of the proximal interphalangeal joint, *Hand Clin* 8(4):758, 1992.

78. Kahler DM, McCue FC III: Metacarpophalangeal and proximal interphalangeal joint injuries of the hand, including the thumb, *Clin Sports Med* 11(1):63, 1992.

79. Rockwood CA, Green DP, Bucholz RW, eds: *Fractures in Adults,* ed 3, Philadelphia, 1991, JB Lippincott, p. 507.

80. Stern PJ, Lee AF: Open dorsal dislocations of the proximal interphalangeal joint. *J Hand Surg* 10A:364-370, 1985.

81. Hastings H II, Carroll C IV: Treatment of closed articular fractures of the metacarpophalangeal and proximal interphalangeal joints, *Hand Clin* 4(3):517, 1988.

82. Light TR: Buttress pinning techniques, *Orthop Rev* 10:49-55, 1981.

83. McElfresh E, Dobyns J, O'Brien E: Management of fracture disloca-

tion of the proximal interphalangeal joints by extension block splinting. *J Bone Joint Srg (Am)* 54:1705, 1972.

84. Rockwood CA, Green DP, Bucholz RW, eds: *Fractures in Adults,* ed 3, Philadelphia, 1991, JB Lippincott, p 513.

85. Strong ML: A new method of extension-block splinting for the proximal interphalangeal joint—preliminary report. *J Hand Surg* 5:606-607, 1980.

86. Green DP, Rowland SA: Fractures and dislocations in the hand, In Rockwood CA, Green DP, Bucholz RW, eds: *Fractures in Adults,* ed 3, Philadelphia, 1991, JB Lippincott, p 508.

87. Green DP, Rowland SA: Fractures and dislocations in the hand, In Rockwood CA, Green DP, Bucholz RW, eds: *Fractures in Adults,* ed 3, Philadelphia, 1991, JB Lippincott, p 510.

88. Eaton RG: *Joint Injuries of the Hand,* Springfield, IL, 1971, Charles C. Thomas, pp 9-34.

89. Kiefhaber TR, Stern PJ, Grood ES: Lateral stability of the proximal interphalangeal joint, *J Hand Surg* 11A:661, 1986.

90. Rockwood CA, Green DP, Bucholz RW, eds: *Fractures in Adults, 3* ed, Philadelphia, 1991, JB Lippincott, p 504.

91. Minami A, An KA, Cooney WP, et al: Ligament stability of the metacarpophalangeal joint: A biomechanical study, *J Hand Surg* 10A:255, 1985.

92. Zemel NP: Metacarpophalangeal joint injuries in fingers, *Hand Clinics* 8(4):747, 1992.

93. Rockwood CA, Green DP, Bucholz RW, eds: *Fractures in adults,* ed 3, Philadelphia, 1991, JB Lippincott, p 520.

94. Rockwood CA, Green DP, Bucholz RW, eds: *Fractures in Adults,* ed 3, Philadelphia, 1991, JB Lippincott, p 521.

95. Chrenshaw AH, ed: Campbell's Operative Orthopedics, ed 8, St. Louis, 1992, Mosby-Year Book, Inc, 3076.

96. Green DP, Rowland SA: Fractures and dislocations in the hand, In Rockwood CA, Green DP, Bucholz RW, eds: *Fractures in Adults,* ed 3, Philadelphia, 1991, JB Lippincott, p 522.

97. Isani A: Small joint injuries requiring surgical treatment, *Orthop Clin North Am* 17(3):414, 1986.

98. Rockwood CA, Green DP, Bucholz RW, eds: *Fractures in Adults,* ed 3, Philadelphia, 1991, JB Lippincott, p 519.

# CHAPTER 17

# The Hip

*Joel S. Holger*

Hip pain is a common presenting symptom in emergency medicine. The hip has a primary role in weight-bearing and gait, and a painful joint is often the result of traumatic or inflammatory processes. Clinical findings are often nonspecific, pain may be referred in other areas of the body, and abnormalities may manifest themselves in an abnormal gait. There is a wide range of differential diagnoses to consider when presented with a patient with hip pain.

For patients with a clear history of trauma and hip pain, the evaluation focuses on the history and examination. A more organized process of evaluation is required for patients without such a history, for those with insidious onset, or for those with gait and weight-bearing abnormalities. Because the hip joint has L-3 innervation, pain is commonly referred to the thigh and knee, especially the medial aspect. Pain originating in the lumbosacral spine may radiate to the hip area, as can pain referred from the abdominal and retroperitoneal areas.

Physical examination includes adequate exposure, inspection, palpation, and range-of-motion testing, followed by radiologic evaluation. Neurologic function and vascular status is documented. Palpation is performed over the hip joint at one to two fingerbreadths below the midpoint of the inguinal ligament. Palpation should be completed over the greater trochanter and adjacent prominences of the pelvis. Leg shortening and rotation are noted. Manual distraction of the extremity in an axial direction followed by axial compression may help elicit pain in an occult fracture. The extremities are examined for symmetry and passive range of motion. Normal passive range of motion is as follows: flexion, 140°; external rotation, 45°; internal rotation, 45°;

abduction, 45°; adduction, 25°; and extension, 25°. One gait abnormality often encountered is the "antalgic" gait, which is a short-stance phase on the affected extremity, since these patients do not want to stand for long on a painful extremity.

## ANATOMY AND BLOOD SUPPLY

The hip is a ball-and-socket joint surrounded by synovium with a rounded femoral head that articulates with the acetabulum; each of these is covered by articulating cartilage. The femoral head has a central defect, the fovea centralis, where the ligamentum teres arises from the acetabular notch and attaches to the femoral head. The cartilage of the femoral head is thickest at the superior portion over the weight-bearing surface, absent over the fovea, and thinnest at its termination at the femoral neck. The acetabular cartilage is horseshoe-shaped and arches around the acetabular fossa. A fibrocartilaginous labrum attaches to the margins of the acetabulum, widening the socket and adding stability. The hip capsule arises from the rim of the acetabulum and attaches to the intertrochanteric crest anteriorly and the midportion of the femoral neck posteriorly, covering about two thirds of the neck in this area. Three major ligaments strengthen the capsule: the iliofemoral, the ischiofemoral, and the pubofemoral.

The blood supply to the femoral head comes primarily through the circumflex branches of the profunda femoris artery; these branches form an extracapsular ring at the base of the femoral neck. Smaller retinacular branches arise from this ring, penetrate the capsule and course posteriorly along the neck, and enter the femoral head at its surgical neck (Fig. 17-1). A small and probably insignificant contribution comes from the foveal artery, which passes through the ligamentum teres. Venous drainage passes through the medullary space of the femoral neck before entering the metaphysis via the subtrochanteric veins. This retinacular blood supply is especially vulnerable in displaced and impacted fractures of the femoral neck and is significantly compromised during dislocations of the joint, thereby accounting for the complication of avascular necrosis as a result of injury.

## RADIOLOGIC EVALUATION OF THE HIP

Hip disorders are routinely evaluated using an anteroposterior (AP) radiologic view of the full pelvis with both hips in neutral position, and a conedown AP and cross-table lateral view of the affected hip (Fig. 17-2). The full-pelvis view allows for comparison with the contralateral side. In the conedown view, the beam is centered over the proximal femur and offers a slight change in radiologic appearance. Radiographs should be carefully examined for evidence of shortening of the femoral neck, disruption of

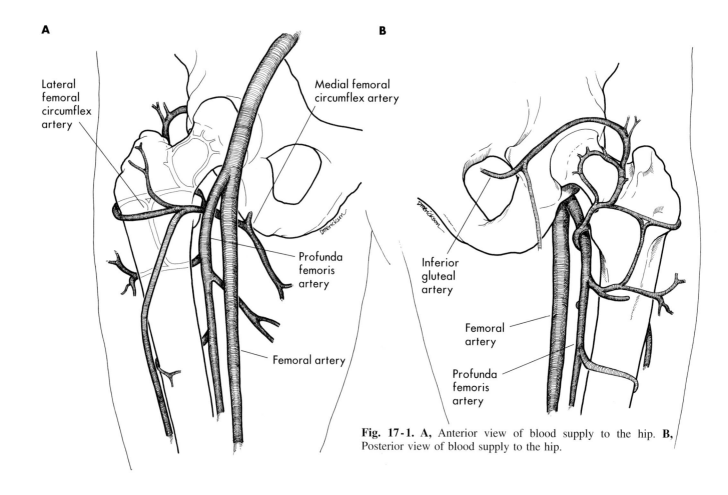

**A,** Lateral femoral circumflex artery; Medial femoral circumflex artery; Profunda femoris artery; Femoral artery

**B,** Inferior gluteal artery; Femoral artery; Profunda femoris artery

Fig. 17-1. **A,** Anterior view of blood supply to the hip. **B,** Posterior view of blood supply to the hip.

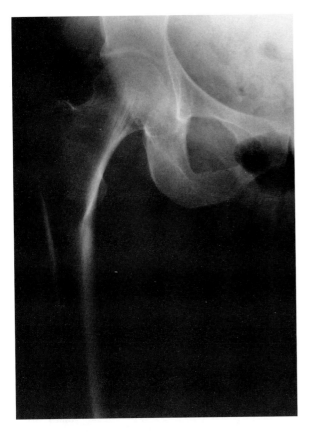

**Fig. 17-2.** Normal anteroposterior view of the hip.

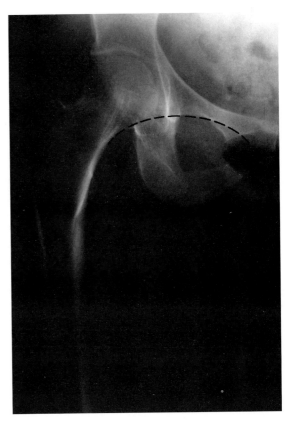

**Fig. 17-3.** An interruption of Shenton's line is suspicious for fracture of the hip.

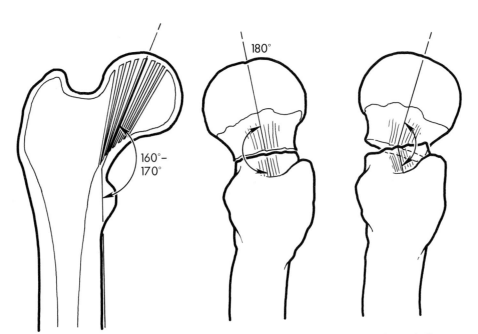

**Fig. 17-4.** Normal angles of trabecular lines from the femur to femoral head. A change indicates an acute fracture or chronic deformity.

the cortical line on the superior or inferior margins of the neck, and any interruptions in Shenton's line (Fig. 17-3).

The normal relationship of the femoral shaft to the femoral neck is an angle of 120° to 130° on the AP view. More important, however, is the measurement of the angle of trabecular lines from the medial femur to the head on the AP view, normally 160° to 170°. These lines form a straight line of 180° on the lateral view (Fig. 17-4). Changes in these relationships suggest acute fracture or a chronic deformity.

Ultrasonography, bone scanning, computed tomography (CT), and magnetic resonance imaging (MRI) add valuable information to the plain radiograph. Ultrasonography is used in evaluating displacement of the hip in the neonate and the infant up to 6 months of age. Other uses include needle guidance during arthrocentesis and periosteal fluid aspiration.

Bone scanning is valuable in visualizing stress or occult fractures of the femoral neck and in diagnosing avascular necrosis. The limitations of this technique are its lack of specificity (arthritis and synovitis may mimic fractures) and the time interval between the traumatic event and the appearance of an abnormal bone scan. Maximal sensitivity does not develop until 24 to 72 hours post fracture especially in older patients who need more time for osteoblasts to incorporate isotope (Fig. 17-5).

Computed tomography is often the next imaging procedure following radiography used to evaluate hip trauma. It is helpful in identifying stress fractures, in imaging the joint after reduction of dislocations and associated pelvic fractures, and in evaluating both benign and malignant tumors as well as other hip diseases.[1] Its disadvantages are cost, gonadal radiation exposure, and its inability to visualize cartilaginous fragments.

Magnetic resonance imaging offers high sensitivity in diagnosing stress fractures and is more sensitive than CT with regard to viewing the soft tissues and avascular necrosis.[2] Its main disadvantage is cost, but it offers the advantage of no ionizing radiation.

A patient who has suffered a traumatic event may have normal radiographs, and significant hip pain with weight-bearing (or may refuse to bear weight). Occult fracture in these patients is a real possibility, especially fracture of the femoral neck or acetabulum, and the emergency physician should formulate a plan, often in communication with the patient's primary physician or orthopedist, regarding further imaging of the hip and follow-up examinations. Bone scanning, CT, and MRI are highly valuable in these situations.[3,4]

## HIP FRACTURES

Fractures of the hip are associated with the physiologic changes of aging. Osteoporosis is seen in patients with both femoral neck and intertrochanteric fractures. Eighty percent of these fracture patients are women, in whom there are higher rates of osteoporosis. The incidence of hip fracture

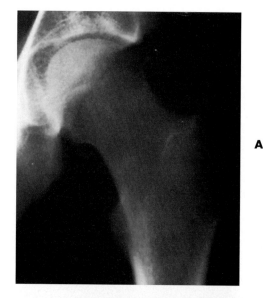

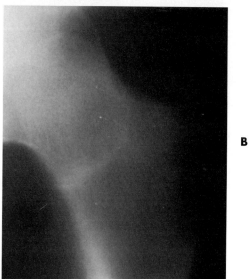

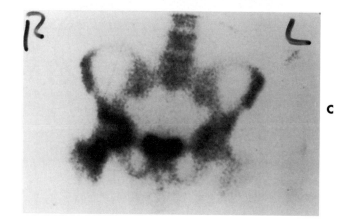

**Fig. 17-5.** Stress fracture of the femoral neck. **A,** Radiograph suggesting inferior femoral neck fracture. **B,** Computed tomogram showing compression in this area. **C,** Bone scan showing increased uptake in the area of the fracture. (From Crenshaw AH, ed: Campbells Operative Orthopaedics, St. Louis, 1992, Mosby Year Book p. 1143.)

doubles every 5 years after the age of 50 years, and the average fracture occurs sometime during the seventh and eighth decades of life.[5] Falls occur with higher frequency in the aging population, and this, in conjunction with decreased bone mass, is the most common etiology of hip fractures. Between 15% and 20% of patients die as a result of these fractures. Medical problems such as infection and sepsis, anemia, heart failure, and medication side effects may predispose to the event. These problems should be checked for during the evaluation of hip fracture patients.

Patients presenting with hip fractures may not have a history of trauma. Likewise, elderly patients may fracture the femoral neck while walking, suggesting that postural instability causes torsional forces above the neck that may fracture osteoporotic bone.[6]

Fractures in patients younger than 50 years of age are generally related to high-energy trauma, which is often associated with other, more severe injuries. These fractures tend to be more highly displaced. Fractures of the femoral shaft may be present with both intertrochanteric and femoral neck fractures. Patients sustaining high-energy injury or multiple trauma should be evaluated for these fractures. Stress or "fatigue" fractures of the femoral neck may be seen in young patients, most notably males in military training and athletics, but these may also be seen in the elderly. This type of fracture is thought to occur from repetitive stress to bone that may be weakened by increased bone resorption, until the cumulative stress overcomes the structural strength of the bone.

## FEMORAL NECK FRACTURES

Fractures of the femoral neck are also called *subcapital* or *intracapsular fractures.* The femoral neck lies within the joint capsule of the hip and has no or a minimal periosteal layer, with a very precarious blood supply to the femoral head. These conditions predispose to the most common problems in healing, nonunion, and avascular necrosis of the femoral head. As noted earlier, the blood supply to the femoral head comes primarily from an extracapsular arterial ring, which ascends in anterior, posterior, medial, and lateral groups around the neck, which then form an intra-articular ring near the femoral head. The lateral group that supplies the lateral weight-bearing portion of the femoral head is at risk during fracture and from subsequent intracapsular hematoma formation, influencing treatment decisions because of an increased incidence of avascular necrosis.

### Clinical presentation

The patient presenting with a femoral neck fracture often has a history of trauma, most commonly a fall. Pain is located in the groin, proximal thigh, and may be referred to the mid- or distal femur, especially with attempts at manipulation of the hip. The involved extremity lies in external rotation and is shortened if there is displacement of the fracture. Pain is accentuated with any movement of the

hip, and the majority of patients are unable to tolerate any hip flexion. Neurovascular status of the extremity distal to the injury is usually always intact; if it is unclear, a separate or associated injury should be sought. Potential predisposing medical conditions to the fall should be evaluated at this time and may be initially clinically occult.

### Classification

Structurally, there are three types of femoral neck fractures: impacted, nondisplaced, and displaced. Garden's classification[7] is most commonly used (Fig. 17-6).

### Stage I impacted fractures

Impacted fractures are crush injuries of the femoral neck, with the trabeculae and cortex pushed into the femoral head. There is some abduction, and the inferior cortex is intact. These are the most stable femoral neck fractures, and for treatment reasons it is important to distinguish them from other fracture types. Despite the relative stability, 16% of patients eventually disimpact.[4] Current recommendations are that all patients undergo internal fixation, which is accomplished by inserting multiple threaded screws or Knowles pins for fixation (Fig. 17-7). Commonly, three to five screws or pins are placed from the lateral aspect of the greater trochanter into the femoral head. There is minimal perioperative morbidity, union rates are high, and the possibility of disimpaction is eliminated.

### Stage II nondisplaced femoral neck fractures

In nondisplaced femoral neck fractures, the fracture line extends across the femoral neck but is not displaced. These fractures are complete, have no impaction, are unstable, and eventually become displaced if they are not stabilized. Internal fixation is required to obtain high union rates. Surgical treatment for stage II fractures is similar to that for stage I fractures, with multiple screw fixation used most commonly. In unusual circumstances, some surgeons prefer to use primary prosthetic replacement (see section on surgical repair of stage III and stage IV fractures).

### Stage III and stage IV fractures

Both stage III and IV fractures are displaced; the difference between the two types is the degree of displacement. In stage III injuries, the femoral head is abducted relative to the pelvis. In stage IV, the head is adducted relative to the pelvis and represents full displacement. In stage III, the fracture fragments are in contact with each other, while in stage IV they are completely separated. In each of these injuries, there is a much higher incidence of disruption of the blood supply and avascular necrosis. Treatment options and prognosis are similar. For these reasons, the injuries are often discussed together.

### Surgical repair of stage III and stage IV fractures

Treatment options for displaced femoral neck fractures include internal fixation, following open or closed reduction,

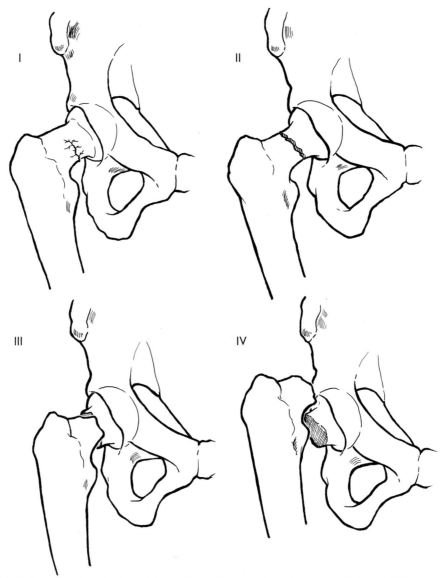

**Fig. 17-6.** Garden's classification of femoral neck fractures, including stages I through IV.

and prosthetic replacement. Various considerations are involved in deciding which option is best. Many surgeons routinely use prosthetic replacement, such as an Austin-Moore prosthesis (Fig. 17-8), hemiarthroplasty with a bipolar prosthesis, or total hip replacement. These options eliminate the problems of nonunion and avascular necrosis, which occur in up to 10% and 20% of cases, respectively, following internal fixation with late segmental collapse.[8] Prosthetic replacement is most commonly used in patients older than 70 years, while internal fixation is often attempted in patients younger than 50. Younger patients with a longer life expectancy who are treated with a fixed prosthesis can expect degeneration of the acetabulum due to cartilage trauma from a fixed prosthetic head, acetabular protrusio (protrusion of the head into the acetabulum), or component loosening eventually requiring total hip replace-

ment. Total hip replacement is often reserved following failure or complications of internal fixation or prosthesis in these younger patients.

Disadvantages of prosthetic replacement include prolonged operating time, postoperative dislocation, and difficulty in reoperation for mechanical failure or infection. The best results of internal fixation, which heals the fracture while avoiding avascular necrosis, are equal to or better than those of prosthetic replacement.

Patients undergoing internal fixation may have a sliding nail or compression screw and slide-plate device placed. After being driven into the femoral head, the screw can be tightened, bringing the fracture fragments together and providing compression, rigidity, and better healing rates. Pins may be added to prevent rotation. Another method is multiple parallel screw placement.

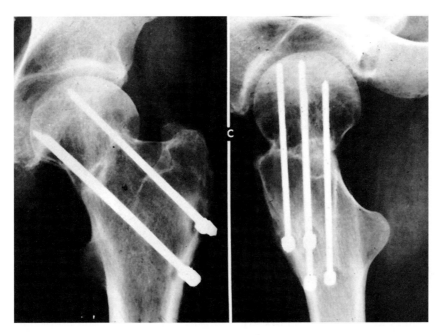

**Fig. 17-7.** Unstable femoral neck fracture fixed with Knowles pins, showing union after 1 year. (From Crenshaw AH, ed: Campbells Operative Orthopaedics, St. Louis, 1992, Mosby Year Book, p 939.)

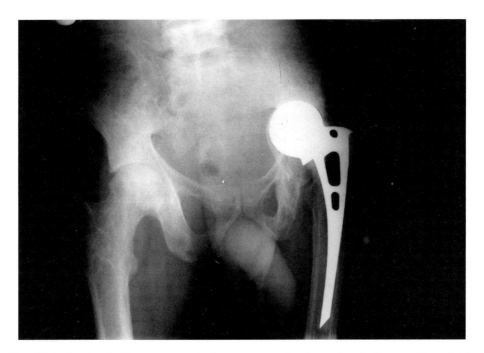

**Fig. 17-8.** An Austin-Moore prosthesis for treatment of a femoral neck fracture. Use of this prosthesis resulted in acetabular protrusio. (From Crenshaw AH, ed: Campbells Operative Orthopaedics, St. Louis, 1992, Mosby Year Book, p 934)

Patients undergoing hemiarthroplasty prosthetic replacement have a bipolar-type device placed that uses a stem designed to be compatible with polymethylmethacrylate cement. There is an acetabular component that fits into the acetabulum (Fig. 17-9). Total hip replacement is the proce-

dure of choice when there is preexisting rheumatoid arthritis or severe degenerative arthritis, or when converting from a failed hemiarthroplasty device. In these cases, the acetabular surface is replaced with a prosthetic device.

Femoral neck fractures resulting from high-energy

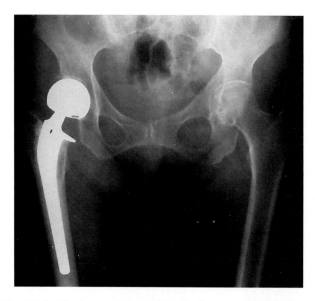

**Fig. 17-9.** Hemiarthroplasty with a bipolar prosthesis for treatment of a displaced femoral neck fracture. (From Crenshaw AH, ed: Campbells Operative Orthopaedics, St. Louis, 1992, Mosby Year Book, p 934.)

trauma in younger patients have a higher incidence of avascular necrosis and nonunion.[9] Studies have shown that multiple screw fixation obtains the lowest rates of nonunion and avascular necrosis. Bone grafting may also be used in these cases.

Complications of prosthetic replacement include infection rates of 5%, 12.5% mortality during the first month following surgery, and up to 20% mortality at 6 months.[10]

Pathologic fractures in the pelvic region occur as a result of malignancy or irradiation for malignancy. Impending fracture may be seen on radiography as an irregular line of increased density or sometimes as scattered areas of translucency in the femoral neck. Coxa vara deformity, in which the femoral neck becomes more horizontal to the femoral shaft, is often present. Metastatic pathologic fracture is an indication for hemiarthroplasty, while fractures from irradiation have better outcomes with more conservative approaches, as compared with fractures resulting from acute trauma. The decision is directed toward the functional status of the patient and life expectancy.

Initial emergency management, in addition to the diagnosis of the femoral neck fracture, includes examination to rule out additional trauma and a search for underlying medical conditions or predisposing factors leading to the fall or trauma. Additionally, medication for pain control and urinary catheter placement are often necessary. Orthopedic consultation is obtained. Traction is not useful in femoral neck fractures and may actually decrease the blood supply to the femoral head.

## INTERTROCHANTERIC FRACTURES

Intertrochanteric fractures of the femur differ from femoral neck fractures in several ways. The vascular supply to the

femoral neck and head is not affected and avascular necrosis is not a complication of intertrochanteric fractures. Periosteum is present and nonunion rates are much lower. However, more trauma is required to produce this type of fracture, leading to more complications. There is more blood loss in surrounding tissue, and the operative treatment is more extensive than for femoral neck fractures, with more difficulty in obtaining good reduction and stability. Generally, these fractures occur more often in osteoporotic bone and are usually comminuted, since they tend to occur in slightly older patients. Mortality in the first 3 months (16.7%) is more than twice that of femoral neck fractures. Most of these fractures occur in patients 66 to 76 years of age and are far more frequent in women than men.[9]

### Clinical presentation

The intertrochanteric fracture patient presents with a history of trauma, usually a fall. Pain is located at the groin, at or medial to the greater trochanter, and may radiate down to the midfemur area. Deformity may be present, and shortening and external rotation are present with displaced fractures. The patient cannot tolerate any passive or active movement of the hip. Neurovascular status is almost always intact; other injuries or preexisting conditions should be sought if deficits are present. Again, acute or chronic medical conditions may be present that predispose the patient to the trauma.

### Classification

There are several classification systems for intertrochanteric fractures, none of which is the most commonly accepted. Boyd and Griffin[11] classified these fractures into four groups (Fig. 17-10):

Type I:   Nondisplaced fractures along the intertrochanteric line

Type II:   Intertrochanteric line fractures but with comminution and displacement of additional fracture fragments

Type III:   Fractures extending from the lesser trochanter across the femoral shaft

Type IV:   Comminuted fractures of the trochanteric region and femoral shaft in two or more planes, often with spiral, oblique, or butterfly components

Kyle et al.[12] have also described four types (Fig. 17-11):

Type I:   Stable, undisplaced intertrochanteric fractures

Type II:   Stable, displaced intertrochanteric fractures with fracture of the lesser trochanter

Type III:   Greater trochanteric fractures with a posteromedial comminuted component and varus deformity

Type IV:   Type III fractures with an additional subtrochanteric fracture

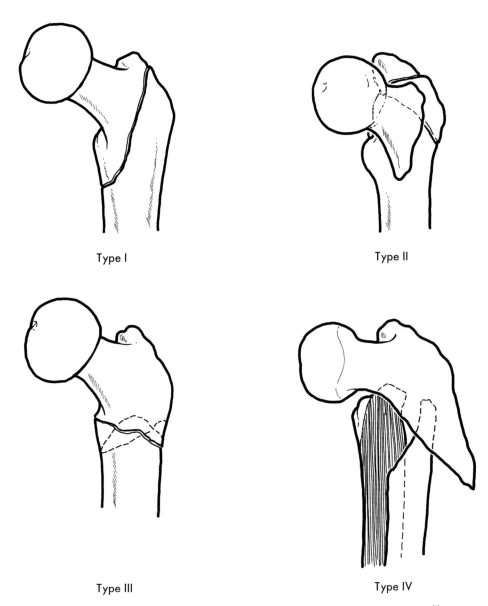

Type I

Type II

Type III

Type IV

**Fig. 17-10.** Boyd and Griffin's classification system of intertrochanteric fractures.[11]

Classification is important when discussing stability as well as surgical approaches for various fractures. Fractures with instability have shortening, varus of the neck-to-shaft angle, and fracture or collapse of the posterior component. A true lateral radiograph is required to evaluate this area.

## Surgical considerations

Intertrochanteric fractures are treated by internal fixation. Reduction of the fracture is carried out by either open or closed methods. Effective reduction to obtain stability is the most important factor in surgical management. To obtain this, the medial and especially the lesser trochanter and posterior components should have good contact. A number of fixation devices are then secured, such as a sliding nail or a compression screw inserted into the posterior aspect of

the femoral head (Fig. 17-12). Because there is medial collapse of the fracture fragments with healing, the "telescoping" nature of the screw into the side plate is important. This prevents the nail or screw from penetrating through the femoral head. If stable reduction is not obtainable, as may be the case in fractures with posterior and medial comminution, some surgeons may opt for osteotomy at the base of the greater trochanter and medial displacement of the femur, followed by insertion of a fixation device. This type of surgery, however, results in a poorer functional outcome. In pathologic fractures of this area, a femoral head prothesis is occasionally necessary if tumor also involves part of the femoral neck. Patients with intertrochanteric fractures usually have delayed weight-bearing, higher mortality, and poorer functional outcomes than patients with femoral neck fractures.

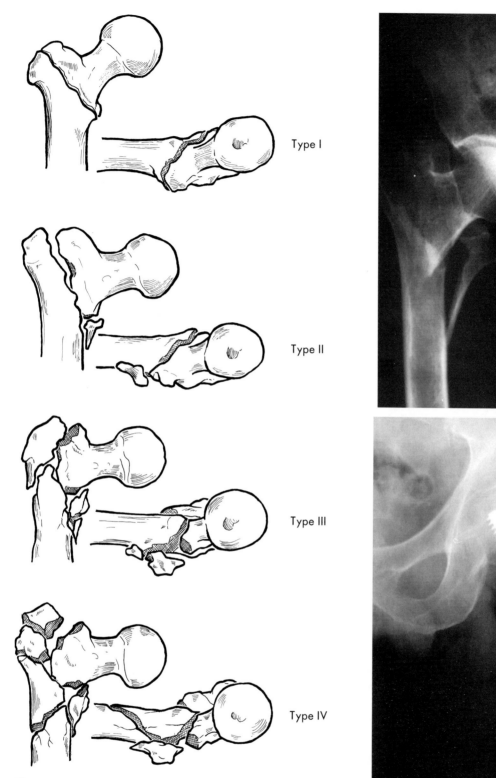

**Fig. 17-11.** Kyle et al.'s classification system of intertrochanteric fractures.[12]

Type I

Type II

Type III

Type IV

A

B

**Fig. 17-12. A,** Unstable intertrochanteric fracture, Boyd and Griffin type IV. **B,** Fixation of intertrochanteric fracture with a compression hip screw. (From Crenshaw AH, ed: Campbells Operative Orthopaedics, St. Louis, 1992, Mosby Year Book, p 901)

### Emergency management

In addition to diagnosis of the fracture, examination is necessary to rule out additional trauma and to look for underlying medical conditions. Preoperative evaluation may be started. Pain is managed and orthopedic consultation is obtained. Traction devices, such as Buck's traction device using 5 lbs of weight, may help to reduce pain (Fig. 17-13).

### HIP FRACTURES IN CHILDREN

Fractures of the hip area in children differ from those in adults in several respects. Bone and periosteum is stronger in children, and more severe trauma is required to produce fractures, which are then more likely to be associated with other, life-threatening injuries. In children, hip fractures occur without the degree of comminution or crushing seen in adult fractures, and often the periosteum remains intact, limiting displacement. The presence of the epiphyseal plate predisposes children to fracture and also to late complications of premature closure and angular deformity. The epiphysis of the lesser and greater trochanters and the femoral head fuse after puberty. The incidence of avascular necrosis of the femoral head is higher. Children, however, have a higher tolerance to bedrest and immobilization, making these treatment options more feasible.

### Femoral neck and intertrochanteric fractures

Colonna[13] proposed the following system for classifying femoral neck and intertrochanteric fractures in children (Fig. 17-14).

**Type I: transepiphyseal separations.** This condition occurs with or without dislocation of the femoral head from the acetabulum, but is most commonly seen with dislocation. Avascular necrosis and premature epiphyseal closure are sequelae seen in 80% to 100% of patients.[14] These require internal fixation surgically. Although closed reduction is attempted, open reduction is usually necessary. Fixation is obtained by the use of two to four smooth (nonthreaded) pins. Threaded pins increase the rate of premature epiphyseal closure and are avoided in children.[15] Threaded pins may be used in adolescents, since the capital femoral epiphysis contributes to only 15% of leg growth and premature epiphyseal closure occurring after age 9 years has minimal consequences.[16] Shortening is limited to less than 2 cm, depending on the patient's age at the time of closure.

**Type II: transcervical fractures.** Transcervical fractures, which are almost always displaced and thus unstable, are the most common type of hip fracture in children. Avascular necrosis is seen in 50% of these patients and is related to the degree of displacement.[17] The cause of the interruption of the blood supply is the same as in adult femoral neck fractures. Immediate reduction and fixation do not prevent its development, since the main factor is disruption of the blood supply at the time of the trauma. All type II fractures are treated surgically. Even nondisplaced fractures drift into coxa vara deformity if treated with spica cast immobilization, and nonunion rates are higher. Closed reduction is carried out with traction, abduction, and internal rotation, followed by open fixation with two to four

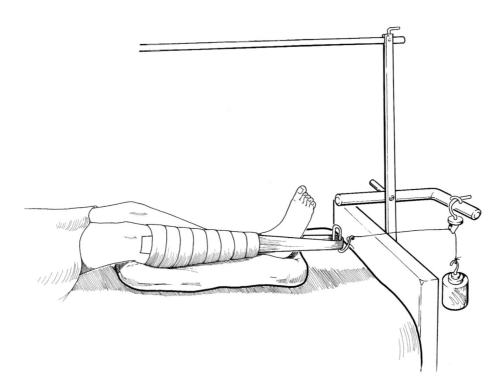

**Fig. 17-13.** Buck's traction device.

Type I                                           Type II

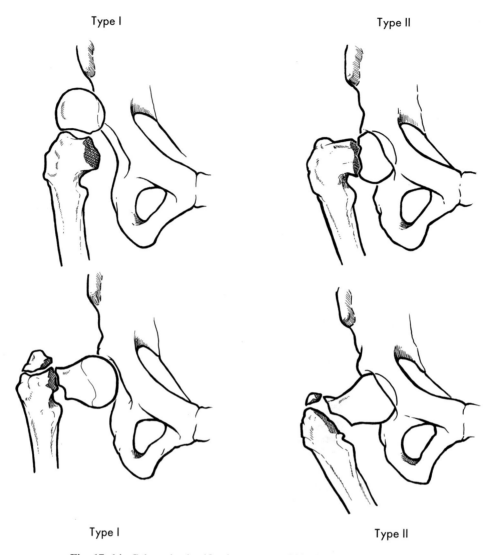

Type I                                           Type II

**Fig. 17-14.** Colonna's classification system of hip fractures in children.

Knowles pins or screws without crossing the epiphyseal line.

**Type III: cervicotrochanteric fractures.** These fractures are comparable to the fractures across the base of the femoral neck in adults, except that the rate of avascular necrosis is higher in children (20%). Treatment depends on the degree of displacement.[18] Nondisplaced fractures are treated with traction followed by abduction spica casting. Displaced fractures are treated with closed reduction and internal fixation with Knowles pins or cannulated hip screws without crossing the epiphyseal line.

**Type IV: intertrochanteric fractures.** These fractures differ from those in adults with regard to the degree of comminution and stability, and heal with higher union rates. They also heal with fewer complications than other fracture types in children. The fractures are reduced with traction for up to 3 weeks, and are then placed in an abduction spica cast for 6 to 12 weeks. In the adolescent, internal fixation is more likely to be used, with the nail or

screw not crossing the epiphyseal line. These fractures are complicated by an avascular necrosis rate of 0% to 14%.[17,18]

Pathologic fractures do occur in children and include involvement of tumors, such as unicameral bone cysts and fibrous dysplasia, and metabolic diseases, such as osteogenesis imperfecta. Stress fractures also occur and may be of two types: transverse fractures in the superior portion of the femoral neck (which may displace) and compression fracture in the inferior portion (which rarely displace). Transverse fractures are internally fixed with Knowles pins, and compression fractures are treated with non–weight-bearing management.[17]

The treatment of complications resulting from children's hip fractures is more difficult. The prognosis of avascular necrosis depends on the severity of the fracture type incurred. Treatment options include removal of internal fixation devices, bedrest, and surgery such as osteotomy and arthroplasty.

Coxa vara deformity causes shortening of the extremity. Significant varus or valgus deformity resulting from partial epiphyseal closure may be treated with subtrochanteric osteotomy.

Emergency management of hip fractures in children is largely limited to the evaluation and identification of other life-threatening injuries, pain control, and orthopedic consultation.

### Fractures of the lesser trochanter

Fractures of the lesser trochanter are avulsion injuries involving the iliopsoas tendon and are usually seen in adolescents (Fig. 17-15). They are caused by a forceful contraction of the muscle when the leg is in a fixed or extended position. Symptomatic treatment is adequate with crutch-walking and limited physical activity. Within 3 months, normal activity can be resumed. When the fracture involves a large degree of displacement (ie, greater than 2 cm), open reduction and screw fixation may be considered.

### Fractures of the greater trochanter

Fracture of the greater trochanter is also an avulsion injury that is usually seen in adolescence, but such fractures may occur at any age. The greater trochanter serves as the insertion point for most of the abductors and external rotators, including the gluteus medius and minimus, the piriformis, and the obturator internus and externus. Management is also conservative, with bedrest followed by gradual ambulation with crutches. With larger degrees of displacement (usually greater than 1 cm), operative reduction and internal fixation with compression screws may be considered. There are usually no long-term problems with isolated fractures of either trochanter.

## HIP DISLOCATIONS

Hip dislocations and fracture dislocations are orthopedic emergencies. High-energy trauma causes these injuries, with the most frequent cause being motor-vehicle accidents. The patient is often multiply traumatized and may have other, more life-threatening injuries.

In order to reduce late complications, reduction of this injury should take priority over other skeletal injuries. Most can be reduced in a closed fashion.

The hip can dislocate in one of three ways: anteriorly, posteriorly, or centrally. True central dislocation is rare but may occur through the floor of the acetabulum in patients with significant osteoporotic disease (Fig. 17-16). More commonly, a central dislocation occurs with a transverse fracture of the acetabulum, or with fracture of the anterior and posterior columns of the acetabulum. These fractures occur from lateral forces driving the head into the acetabulum.

### Posterior dislocations

Ninety percent of hip dislocations are posterior. They result from a high-energy force transmitted axially through the femoral shaft with the hip flexed at 90° or less and in neutral position. A common scenario is that of the knee striking the dashboard of an unrestrained occupant in a motor-vehicle accident. If the hip is adducted, dislocation without fracture may result, but if there is mild abduction or flexion less than 90°, the posterior wall of the acetabulum is at risk of fracture with a dislocating femoral head.

Femoral head fractures occur with posterior dislocations when force is transmitted axially when the hip is flexed less than 60°, driving the head against the firm posterosuperior acetabular rim.

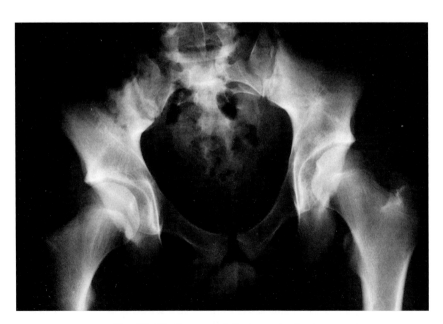

**Fig. 17-15.** Fracture of the lesser trochanter.

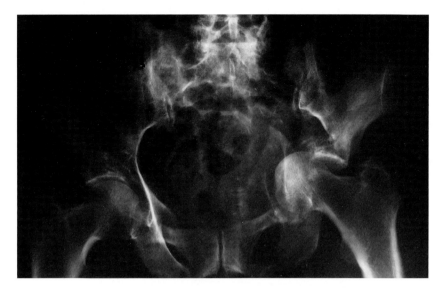

**Fig. 17-16.** Central dislocation with fracture of the acetabulum.

### Classification

The most widely used classification system is that of Thompson and Epstein.[19] Type 1 injury involves dislocation with or without minor acetabular fracture. These are stable after reduction; type 2 involves dislocation with a large single posterior acetabulum fragment. These are unstable after reduction; type 3 involves dislocation with severe comminution of the posterior acetabular rim; type 4 involves dislocation with fracture of the acetabular floor; and type 5 involves dislocation with fracture of the femoral head.

### Clinical presentation

In the awake patient with hip dislocation there is severe pain. The leg is in a position of adduction, flexion, and internal rotation (Fig. 17-17). If a large portion of the posterior acetabulum is fractured, the leg may be in a neutral position and the dislocation may not be clinically evident. In a multiply traumatized patient, an AP view of the pelvis is necessary to rule out this injury. The sciatic nerve runs directly posterior to the joint, and is commonly injured by fracture fragments or from contusion in a physiologic manner. Careful assessment of sciatic nerve function is necessary. Associated pelvic injuries may be present, as well as other orthopedic injuries in the same extremity, such as an anterior cruciate injury in the knee.

### Treatment

Reduction of the dislocated hip should be performed as soon as possible because a delay of greater than 12 hours increases the risk of avascular necrosis of the femoral head. Prior to reduction, the patient must be fully evaluated, and fractures of the femoral head and other fractures in the same extremity and sciatic nerve injury ruled out. These injuries may change the approach to reduction of the dislocation.

Most type 1 dislocations can be treated with closed reduction followed by Buck's traction. About 9% require open reduction due to nonreducibility or nonconcentric reduction, which is any joint widening or nonconcentric joint space that indicates the presence of osteochondral fragments in the joint space.[20] In irreducible dislocations, the femoral head has usually "button-holed" through the joint capsule. After closed reduction, CT scanning of the joint is performed to rule out intra-articular fragments and to identify any associated fractures in the joint. The patient is immobilized for 2 weeks using Buck's traction or a Thomas splint. Weight-bearing begins thereafter.

Type 2 through 5 fracture dislocations are usually treated surgically. Reduction is accomplished as soon as possible, often in a closed manner, which then allows preoperative evaluation, often including CT scanning, to assess for intra-articular loose bodies and associated pelvic fractures. The femoral head is kept in the acetabulum by Buck's traction during this time. Some type 2 dislocations are stable and do not require surgery, but weight-bearing may not be allowed for 6 weeks.

Postoperatively, weight-bearing in fracture types 2 through 5 is delayed for 3 to 6 months. Treatment varies for type 4 fractures that involve femoral head fracture. If good reduction is obtained, treatment may be nonsurgical. More commonly, internal fixation must be performed with screws or, in older patients, femoral head replacement.

Closed reduction may be attempted in type 1 dislocations or minor fracture dislocations using the Stimson technique (Fig. 17-18), and may be successful without the use of general anesthesia. The patient is placed face down on a table, with the affected extremity hanging in its flexed

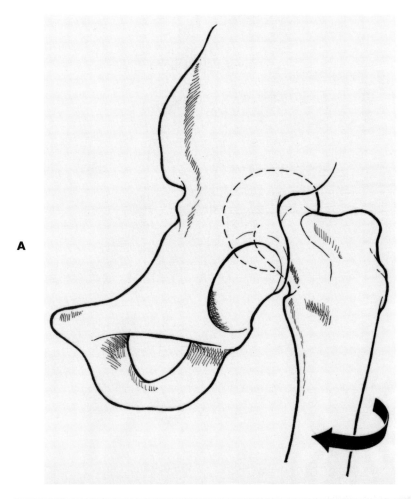

A

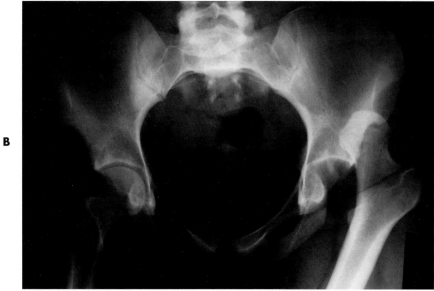

B

Fig. 17-17. A and B, Position of the femur in a posterior dislocation showing adduction and internal rotation.

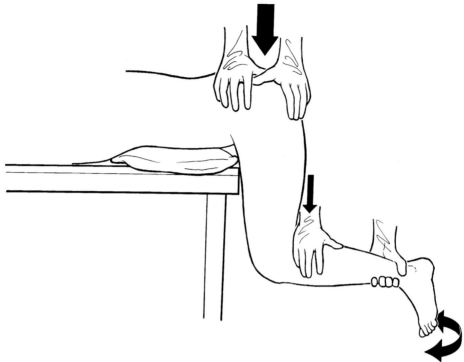

**Fig. 17-18.** The Stimson technique for reducing posterior dislocations.

position with flexion of the knee at 90°. The pelvis is supported while steady downward traction at the knee is maintained. The extremity is then gently rotated while an assistant pushes the greater trochanter forward toward the acetabulum. All maneuvers are gentle and repetitive maneuvers are avoided. Intravenous sedation is usually required.

The Allis maneuver may be attempted when the patient cannot be moved into a prone position (Fig. 17-19). While an assistant stabilizes the pelvis, the physician must usually stand on the stretcher to gain a mechanically advantageous position and apply traction in the axis of the deformity.[21]

### Anterior dislocations

Anterior dislocations of the hip comprise 10% of all hip dislocations. These are classified according to the position of the femoral head (Fig. 17-20). In anterosuperior dislocations, the femoral head is in the iliac or pubic position. Clinically, these dislocations present with the lower extremity in extension and external rotation. In anteroinferior dislocations (also called obturator dislocations), the extremity is flexed, externally rotated, and abducted. Each of these types may be associated with femoral head or acetabular fractures. Due to their close proximity to the anterior hip joint, the femoral nerve and vessels may be injured.

These injuries occur from accidents that involve forces that abduct, externally rotate, and extend the hip. An example is falling from a height and landing with the extremity in this position. The femoral head then rides over

or through the transverse acetabular ligament to lodge over the obturator foramen or the pubis.

### Treatment

Anterior hip dislocations can usually be reduced in a closed fashion (Fig. 17-21). Traction is supplied longitudinally to the femur with lateral force on the proximal thigh while the femoral head is pushed toward the acetabulum. Alternatively, reduction may be obtained by flexing both the knee and hip to 90°, then abducting the hip to 90° and moving the extremity in extension, adduction, and internal rotation in one slow and continuous movement. Intravenous sedation is usually required. Nonreducible dislocations may be caused by interpositioning of adjacent muscles and buttonholing of the head through the joint capsule, requiring open reduction. CT scanning is performed after reduction to search for intra-articular fragments and associated fractures. These dislocations are often seen with associated femoral head fractures.

### Emergency management

Early recognition and reduction of hip dislocations is necessary to reduce long-term complications, especially avascular necrosis (Fig. 17-22). Treatment of this injury takes priority over other skeletal injuries, but adequate assessment prior to reduction and definitive care is necessary, especially when other, life-threatening injuries may exist, as in the multiply traumatized patient. Other injuries

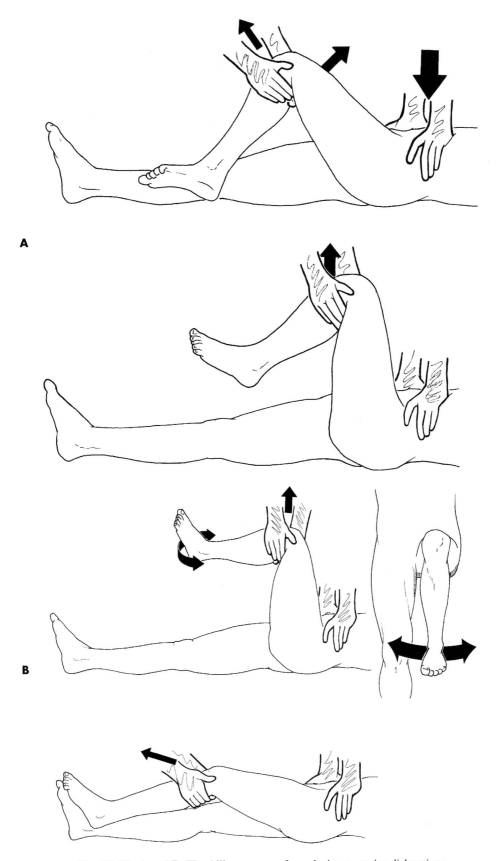

**Fig. 17-19. A** and **B,** The Allis maneuver for reducing posterior dislocations.

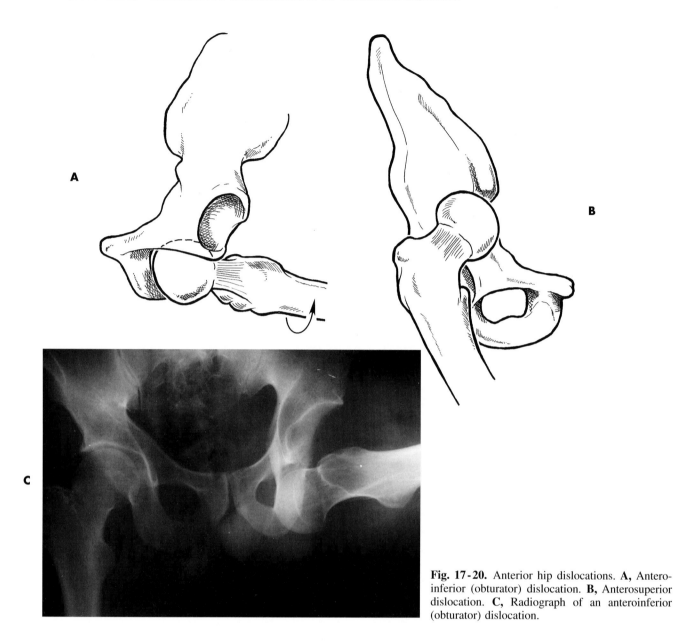

**Fig. 17-20.** Anterior hip dislocations. **A,** Antero-inferior (obturator) dislocation. **B,** Anterosuperior dislocation. **C,** Radiograph of an anteroinferior (obturator) dislocation.

of the extremity and pelvis must be recognized and their neurovascular status documented. Reduction is usually performed by the orthopedic surgeon or by a qualified emergency physician. Often only one attempt is made in the Emergency Department; if it is unsuccessful, many surgeons prefer that the next attempt be made in the operating room or in an open manner. If reduction in the Emergency Department is successful, Buck's traction may be applied. If there is obvious or suspected injury to the sciatic or femoral nerve, reduction attempts should not be made in this setting. Communication with the orthopedic consultant is necessary to optimize outcome.

**Complications**

Dislocations of the hip have high rates of associated complications. Overall avascular necrosis rates average 20%. Rates above 50% occur if reduction does not take place within 12 hours of injury.[9] Type 1 dislocations have the lowest avascular necrosis rate, while those requiring open reduction have higher rates. This complication is also influenced by the age of the patient and the severity of the injury. Clinical onset of avascular necrosis is on average 17 months; if no symptoms manifest in 2 years, it is unlikely to occur.[22]

Sciatic nerve injury has been reported to occur in 8% to 19% of acute dislocations. This injury occurs at the time of the dislocation due to the nerve being stretched over the femoral head or a portion of the fractured posterior acetabular wall. Severity is variable, as are recovery rates.

Traumatic arthritis occurs with an overall incidence of about 25%.[23] Clinical evidence may not develop for as long as 4 or 5 years after injury.

**HIP DISLOCATION IN CHILDREN**

Traumatic hip dislocations in children are rare. However, they occur more frequently than hip fractures. Falls have

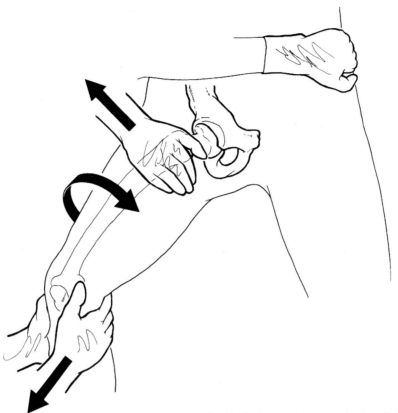

**Fig. 17-21.** Reduction of an anterior hip dislocation.

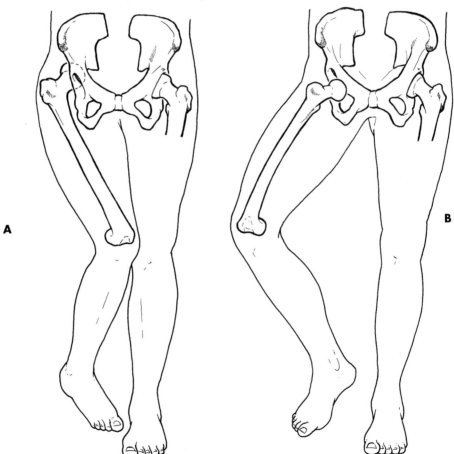

**Fig. 17-22.** Comparison of leg positions in hip dislocations. **A,** Posterior dislocation. **B,** Anterior dislocation.

caused dislocations with an incidence frequency of 50% in one series, with motor-vehicle accidents accounting for about 30%.[18] This is probably due to the pliability of the immature cartilage and the laxity of ligaments, especially in young children, in whom relatively minor trauma can cause dislocation. Recurrent dislocations may be a problem.

Treatment is similar to that of adult hip dislocations, and urgent, concentric reduction is necessary. The incidence of avascular necrosis is much less than that in adults, averaging 10%.[24] Long-term results reflect the severity of the injury and the timeliness of its reduction.

## HIP PAIN IN CHILDREN

Children and adolescents who present to the Emergency Department with a limp and pain in the hip, medial thigh, or knee may have a serious hip disorder. If there is no history of trauma, the differential diagnosis is expanded and may require more extensive testing in the acute setting.

### Slipped capital femoral epiphysis

When an adolescent presents with hip, thigh, or knee pain, slipped capital femoral epiphysis must be included in the differential diagnosis. This is a posterior slippage or separation of the epiphysis and may present with or without a history of trauma. Epidemiologically, this is a disease of prepubescence and occurs between the ages of 10 and 13 years in girls and 12 and 16 years in boys, the difference being due to the later growth spurt in boys. Seventy percent occur in boys, and obesity is a primary risk factor (greater than the 95th percentile for weight, which is present in 50% of the patients).[25] Other risk factors are being black and having an endocrine disorder. Slippage occurs bilaterally in one third of the patients. The etiology is unknown, but is probably multifactorial.[26]

Clinically, the patient presents with either knee or hip pain, and frequently has a history of minor trauma. A limp may be present or limited to physical activity. Often, an external rotation deformity is present, with loss of flexion and abduction, and the leg may be externally rotated when flexed. The patient may present with an "acute slip," with symptoms persisting for less than 3 weeks, or in a "chronic" condition, with symptoms for longer than 3 weeks, or "acute-on-chronic," a recent exacerbation from a minor trauma with symptoms for longer than 3 weeks.

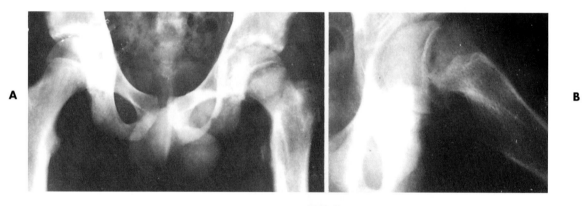

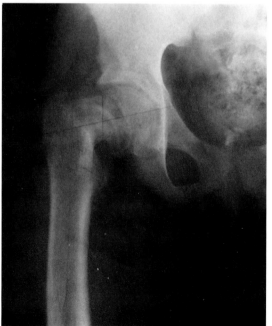

**Fig. 17-23. A** and **B,** Acute slipped capital femoral epiphysis with moderate slippage. **C,** Chronic slipped capital femoral epiphysis with varus deformity. (From Crenshaw AH, ed: Campbells Operative Orthopaedics, St. Louis, 1992, Mosby Year Book, p 1153, 1171.)

The diagnosis is made radiographically (Fig. 17-23). In the AP view, mild slipping occurs when the neck is displaced one third or less than the diameter of the femoral head. In moderate slipping, the displacement is between one third and one half the diameter of the head, and in severe slip, greater than one half the diameter. Angulation also occurs, with the head shaft angle deviating from the normal 145° to less than 30° in mild slip and greater than 60° in severe slip. "Pre-slip" is a radiographic abnormality of widening and irregularity of the epiphysis.

Once the diagnosis is made, the patient is kept non–weight-bearing, an orthopedic consultation is made, and the patient is admitted to the hospital. Surgical correction is achieved using fixation with Knowles pins, including patients with pre-slip. Reduction or manipulation with traction is generally not performed because it has been shown to increase the incidence of avascular necrosis. In patients with severe slip, pinning is performed to close the epiphysis (if it is still open), and an osteotomy (usually subtrochanteric) may or may not be performed to correct the deformity in the extremity.

Complications include chondrolysis, which is early loss of the width of the joint space. This is associated with deterioration of the joint over time, and is seen more often with depending on severity of the slip.

Avascular necrosis is seen in up to 15% of patients, and is also related to the initial severity of the slip.[27] There is a higher incidence with acute slippage compared with chronic slippage.

Additional operations are necessary in a high percentage of patients (up to 28% by age 50) due to degenerative changes.[28] These include primary hip replacement, but hemiarthroplasty and osteotomy may also be performed. Early recognition of this disease and proper surgical care have been shown to improve the long-term outcome and functional status of the patient.

## Legg-Calvé-Perthes disease

Legg-Calvé-Perthes disease is a disorder of the hip seen in children. It is caused by avascular necrosis of the femoral epiphysis with subsequent deformity of the femoral head. The term "coxa plana" is also used to describe this condition. The age of onset is typically between 4 and 9 years, but ranges from age 2 to 13 years.[29] Bilateral disease occurs in 10% to 20% of patients, and 80% of patients are boys.[30] The etiology of the necrosis is unknown but is believed to result from an interruption of the blood supply to the femoral neck, probably with multiple episodes of infarction. Children at risk have delayed skeletal maturation and are shorter than normal for their age.

The patient usually presents clinically with pain and a limp. The limp is antalgic and at first may only be seen with strenuous exercising. The pelvis may dip to the affected side. Pain is usually in the groin area and may radiate to the distal medial thigh. Occasionally only the knee is painful. Abduction of the hip and internal rotation are limited. The patient may stand with the affected leg in adduction, flexion, and external rotation. A history of trauma is usually absent but is not thought to be a precipitating factor in the disease.

Many other conditions must be considered in the differential diagnosis of this type of presentation, including transient synovitis, slipped capital femoral epiphysis, tumors, and infections that present with unilateral involvement. Epiphyseal dysplasia, hypothyroidism, and sickle cell disease may present with bilateral symptoms.[31] If radiographs are normal, the transient synovitis and septic arthritis are differential diagnostic possibilities; further tests are necessary, and aspiration of the joint is considered.

The diagnosis of Legg-Calvé-Perthes disease is made on the basis of the clinical history, physical examination, and radiographic findings (Fig. 17-24). The patient may present at any of the various stages, but those in the earliest stage of necrosis are rarely seen. Radiographs may show a bulging of the hip capsule due to synovitis, but they commonly show a small epiphysis and a more dense femoral head, with areas of radiolucency that represent areas of fracture of necrotic bone. This is called a *crescent sign,* and is often seen on a frog-leg lateral view.[27] As the disease process continues, the necrotic bone is crushed and fibrocartilage fills in the defect in an irregular manner. Lysis of bone and calcified cartilage lateral to the acetabulum may be present. The epiphysis deforms and the femoral neck widens, which in this stage is called fragmentation. Reossification of tissue follows fragmentation, and begins at the margin of the epiphysis until the entire epiphysis is reossified. This sometimes results in growth arrest of the femoral neck.

After reossification, the femoral head remodels continuously until the patient reaches skeletal maturity. One of four patterns of deformity is seen at maturity. In *coxa magna,* the femoral head is enlarged (usually spherically), and the femoral neck is widened. These patients are asymptomatic and usually do not progress to degenerative disease. In *coxa brevis,* the head and neck are shortened, and there is relative overgrowth of the greater trochanter as a result of premature closure of the epiphysis. This may occur in either central or lateral closure patterns. In the central pattern, the epiphysis is round; in the lateral pattern, the femoral head is tilted externally with an oval epiphysis and an acetabular deformity. In *coxa irregularis* the femoral head is collapsed and extruded laterally. A groove forms in the head from impingement by the acetabulum. These patients end up with decreased internal rotation and abduction. The least common deformity is *osteochondritis dissecans,* which is usually seen in late onset of the disease or in incomplete healing. These patients are usually asymptomatic.

The goal of treatment is to prevent deformity of the femoral head. The principles guiding this are maintenance of full range of motion and containment of the femoral head in the acetabulum. Patients presenting in the early stages require intervention with containment devices or via operative containment procedures. Patients who present in later

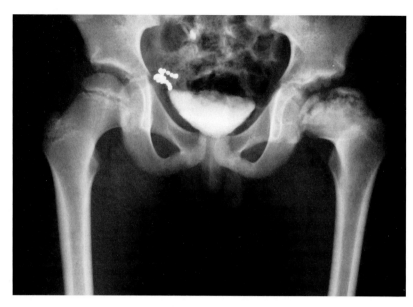

**Fig. 17-24.** Legg-Calvé-Perthes disease. This patient developed lateral subluxation of the femoral head and varus deformity.

stages generally require physical therapy with range-of-motion exercises unless significant pain is present, in which case other procedures may be necessary. Those who present near maturity may require procedures aimed at correction of the existing deformity. If diagnosis of the disease is made in an emergency setting, orthopedic consultation helps direct further evaluation, usually in an outpatient setting.

Prognosis is determined by age. Patients presenting at less than 6 years of age usually fare well. Prognosis is also related to the degree of necrosis, premature closure of the epiphysis, and deformity of the femoral head.[27] Osteoarthritis of the joint is a long-term complication, and 86% develop this condition by the age of 65.[32]

**Transient synovitis**

Transient synovitis is a self-limited, transient inflammatory condition found in younger children, usually 4 to 8 years of age, often with acute onset of hip pain and limp. There may or may not be a history of recent trauma. This sometimes occurs after a viral infection and may be immunologically mediated.[33] Painful limitation of range of motion is present, especially on internal rotation in abduction. Radiographs are normal, and the white blood cell count and the erythrocyte sedimentation rate may be normal or minimally elevated. This clinical presentation does not rule out septic arthritis, and further diagnostic tests, including joint aspiration, or close follow-up examinations may be necessary. Treatment consists of analgesic and limitation of physical activity. Pain is resolved and normal activity is resumed usually within 7 days. Rarely, the sequelae of avascular necrosis or Legg-Calvé Perthes disease may be evident within months of resolution, and these may be an indication for follow-up radiographic examination.

**Septic arthritis of the hip**

Septic arthritis may occur at any age in childhood and adolescence. It is found predominantly in children less than 3 years of age and in older, sexually active adolescents. In the neonate, there may be pseudoparalysis of the extremity and pain evident with diaper changes. In the ambulatory child, the common presentation is with pain and limp, usually always unilateral. Fever and lethargy or irritability are usually present except in the neonate, in whom fever may be absent and abdominal distention may suggest in intra-abdominal condition. The extremity may lie in flexion and external rotation. There may be multiple joints involved, most commonly the knee or ankle, but the hip is the most frequent sight in patients less than 5 years of age. Trauma is a preceding event in up to one third of patients.[34] Evaluation of this clinical picture includes radiography, a white blood cell count, an erythrocyte sedimentation rate, and joint aspiration. The radiograph is normal in up to 80% of children older than 1 year.[35] Both hips should be included for comparison on the radiographs, since a widening of the joint space is the earliest abnormality seen, and subluxation the most reliable finding, but these may be seen only in a late stage of the disease.

Leukocytosis may be seen in only one third of patients; a more reliable indicator is an elevated sedimentation rate. Joint aspiration for laboratory examination must be performed when this diagnosis is suspected. It is often performed under fluoroscopy, with contrast confirmation of entry into the joint space. Bacteriologic cultures are positive in over 80% of cases. Organisms may vary according to patient age, with those most commonly seen being *Staphylococcus aureus, Streptococcus,* and *Hemophilus influenza.*[36] Gonococcal arthritis may be present in adolescents.[37] Treatment consists of prompt and appropriate anti-biotic coverage and adequate pus drainage. The hip has the highest percentage of poor outcome of any infected joint; a high clinical suspicion of infection and prompt treatment may decrease the sequelae of avascular necrosis, loss or decrease of range of motion, limb length discrepancy, and residual deformity and arthritis.

### Osteomyelitis

Osteomyelitis of the femur may be clinically very similar to septic arthritis of the hip on presentation. It is most often seen in children 1 to 5 years of age with similar systemic symptoms and limb and localized bone pain. Leukocytosis may be present in up to 30% of patients, and an elevated sedimentation rate in 90%. Radiographs are abnormal in only 60% of patients, and the only finding present may be soft tissue swelling. Radionucleotide scanning is sensitive in 99% of patients and should be arranged or performed when this diagnosis is suspected.[38] Early orthopedic consultation is important for bone aspiration and culture prior to antibiotic treatment. *S. aureus* is the predominant organism found and may be associated with chronic sinusitis or mastoiditis. *Salmonella* species infection is associated with homogenous sickle cell disease. Infection tends to occur in the highly vascularized metaphysis with a proximity to growth centers, may predispose to interference in growth, and may, by direct extension, cause septic arthritis.

### Snapping iliopsoas tendon

Snapping iliopsoas tendon is a condition found in older adolescents and young adults. There is deep anterior groin or hip pain and often an audible snap associated with a variety of activities. Most patients experience this snapping when extending the hip from a flexed, abducted, and externally rotated position. Bursography has demonstrated a jerking movement of the iliopsoas tendon between the inferior iliac spine and the iliopectineal eminence, often with a bursitis of the iliopsoas bursa. Therapy consists of cessation of any activity that precipitates the pain and gradual stretching exercises that involve hip extension for 6 to 8 weeks. A minority of patients require a surgical procedure to correct the condition.[39]

## HIP PAIN IN ADULTS

Patients may present in the Emergency Department or Urgent Care setting complaining of hip pain without a history of acute injury. This should be distinguished from buttock pain because most often its origin is from the lumbosacral area and less often from vascular claudication with aortic-iliac occlusion. Pain related to the hip may be appreciated in the groin, medial thigh to the knee, and around the greater trochanter. Rarely, abdominal and retroperitoneal processes may refer pain to the hip with irritation of the psoas muscle.

### Greater trochanteric pain

Pain over the lateral aspect of the hip may also radiate down the lateral thigh. The two most common problems are tendinitis of the gluteus medius tendon as it inserts over the lateral aspect of the greater trochanter and bursitis of one or both of the bursae of the greater trochanter. Commonly, a history of overuse may be noted. The pain of tendinitis is felt with activity, and the pain of bursitis may be felt at night. Direct palpation localizes the tenderness usually at or just above the superior aspect of the greater trochanter. Effective management includes limitation of physical activity, exercises that strengthen the gluteal muscles, short-term use of nonsteroidal anti-inflammatory medications, and, occasionally, corticosteroid injection.

### Arthritis

Osteoarthritis is the most common form of hip disease and is involved in 19% of patients with symptomatic arthritis.[40] Hip involvement may occur alone, caused by primary osteoarthritis as a disorder of the articulating cartilage. Osteoarthritis may occur secondarily from previous trauma, congenital and developmental disorders, or previous inflammatory arthritis (Fig. 17-25). The onset is usually after 50 years of age and may start with unilateral involvement. Pain occurs with activity and is relieved by rest. With progression, pain occurs at rest and nocturnally, with joint stiffness followed by limp. The order of loss of range of motion is internal rotation, extension, abduction, adduction, flexion, and external rotation. Gluteal and quadricep muscle atrophy may be present. Characteristic radiographic changes are loss of the joint space, subchondral sclerosis, and osteophyte and cyst formation. Treatment consists of limitation of activity for acute flares, steroidal and nonsteroidal anti-inflammatory medication, and pain control. Surgery is an option for patients with severe pain or disability, and total hip replacement is the most commonly performed procedure.

## METASTATIC DISEASE OF THE HIP

The hip and femur are common sites of metastatic tumor involvement, being third in incidence following the spine and pelvis in bone metastasis. The incidence is increasing due to the longer survival of patients with cancers that commonly metastasize to bone, especially breast, prostate, lung, kidney, and thyroid cancers.[41] Myeloma and sarcoma may also involve this area. Pain is the presenting clinical feature, and the patient most often has a preceding cancer diagnosis. Bone lesions are most often seen on radioisotopic scanning but may be seen first on radiography as areas of bone destruction. The patient often presents with minor trauma and has evidence of pathologic fracture, which has been discussed previously. The rare patient may present with evidence of tumor involvement of the hip and may have an impending pathologic fracture. Coordination of care with the patient's oncologist and orthopedic surgeon is

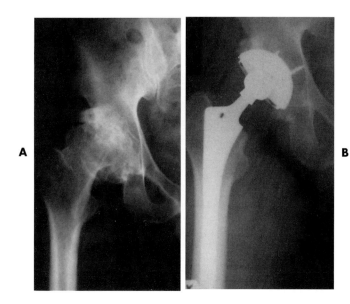

**Fig. 17-25. A,** Degenerative arthritis with deepening of the acetabulum and intra-articular osteophyte formation following Legg-Calvé-Perthes disease. **B,** The patient was treated with total hip prosthesis. (From Crenshaw AH, ed: Campbells Operative Orthopaedics, St. Louis, 1992, Mosby Year Book, p 507.)

necessary to determine subsequent treatment, which may include radiation therapy and/or prophylactic fixation. Pain control is indicated in acute management.

## AVASCULAR NECROSIS OF THE FEMORAL HEAD

Avascular necrosis of the femoral head in adults is a commonly recognized sequela to hip trauma, especially to fracture of the femoral neck and fracture-dislocation of the hip. Nontraumatic avascular necrosis has been recognized increasingly over the past 20 years. Several diseases and conditions have an association to its development, with steroid use being the most common. An idiopathic form is also recognized. This disorder is primarily seen in younger and middle-aged adults from age 20 to 50 years, and typically affects men more than women. Both hips are affected in 50% of patients.[42] This incidence reaches 80% in association with systemic steroid use. The risk of its development following steroid use seems to be highest in patients on long-term and high-dose treatment.

The etiology of the disease is unknown. Several theories have been postulated, including acute infarction or a compartment syndrome effect on the blood supply to the femoral head. Abnormal lipid metabolism and fat embolization to the femoral head and vascularity in steroid-associated avascular necrosis is also postulated. Pathologically, the earliest lesion seen is that of infarction in the subchondral region, followed by fracture of this bone, synovitis, and eventually collapse, which generates more areas of necrosis. Radiographically, the first lesions seen are areas of subchondral osteoporosis and/or sclerosis. A crescent sign may be seen, and there may be flattening of the femoral head. Finally, degenerative changes appear with narrowing of the joint space, osteophyte formation, and

cystic changes (Fig. 17-26). Its appearance at this stage often resembles chronic osteoarthritis. Clinically, the patient presents with groin pain, which often radiates to the medial thigh. The pain becomes worse with weight-bearing, and an antalgic limp may be present progressing to pain at rest. History of an associated illness or trauma in the past 2 years may be present. Range of motion may be normal, with limitation eventually occurring with increasing severity. The diagnosis is made with imaging techniques after initial radiographs are completed (Fig. 17-27). Radionucleotide scanning has a sensitivity of 80%. During the infarction stage, a cold spot can be seen in the femoral head, but is rarely seen in clinical practice because the evaluation is usually made on patients in a later stage of disease. The positive changes seen here are nonspecific, however, and are seen in other processes, such as arthritis, tumor, and infection. CT scanning is much more sensitive, and MRI has been shown to be the best imaging modality, with a sensitivity of 100%.[1]

The pathologic process is progressive, and nonoperative medical interventions do not halt its progression. Treatment is surgical, and total hip replacement is performed most commonly.

## TOTAL HIP REPLACEMENT

Total hip replacement is a procedure in which the native femoral head and neck are replaced with a metallic femoral prosthesis inserted into the femoral medullary canal and a polyethylene articulating surface is inserted into an enlarged articulating acetabular space. This procedure is used mostly in patients with severe osteoarthritis, but may also be used in patients with rheumatoid arthritis, avascular necrosis, and other degenerative diseases of the hip. Such patients may present with complications of the hip replacement.

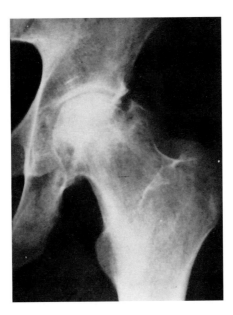

**Fig. 17-26.** Avascular necrosis of the femoral head 8 months following posterior dislocation of the hip, showing a narrow joint space with irregular surfaces and sclerosis of the head. (From Crenshaw AH, ed: Campbells Operative Orthopaedics, St. Louis, 1992, Mosby Year Book, p 950.)

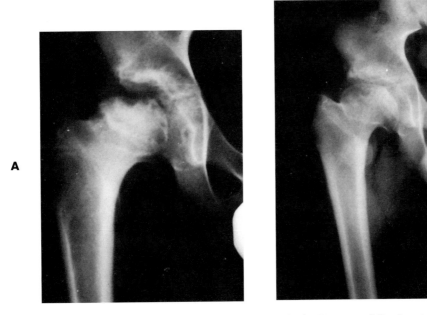

**Fig. 17-27.** Avascular necrosis of the femoral head. **A,** One year following transepiphyseal fracture. **B,** Four years after treatment showing shortened femoral neck from premature epiphyseal closure. (From Crenshaw AH, ed: Campbells Operative Orthopaedics, St. Louis, 1992, Mosby Year Book, p 1139.)

Dislocation is seen in less than 1% of patients with total hip replacement, and usually occurs within the first 6 months of surgery.[44] Inappropriate limb positioning may precipitate this dislocation, such as flexion beyond 90° and external rotation. Reduction can usually be done in the Emergency Department with mild sedation, but may require general anesthesia.

Loosening presents with pain in the hip area. This complication of the femoral or acetabular component may be evident radiologically, with bone absorption around the implants. Its incidence increases with time. Infection may occur, but is rare and has an incidence of less than 1%. Heterotopic ossification may occur in up to 70% of patients, but produces pain and limits function in less than 4%.[44]

## DISCUSSION

Knowledge and understanding of both the hip and the approach to the patient with hip trauma or pain is required for prompt diagnosis and treatment. Communication and coordination of care with the patient's orthopedic and primary care physicians will lead to the optimal functional outcome and will minimize complications.

## REFERENCES

1. Lang P, Genant HK, Jorgesen HE, Murray WR: Imaging the hip joint: computed tomography versus magnetic resonance imaging, *Clin Orthop* 274:135, 1992.
2. Ensign MF: Magnetic resonance imaging of hip disorders, *Semin Ultrasound CT MR* 2:288, 1990.
3. Alba E, Youngberg R: Occult fractures of the femoral neck, *Am J Emerg Med* 10:64, 1992.
4. Bentley G: The case for internal fixation of impacted femoral neck fractures, *Orthop Clin North Am* 5:729, 1974.
5. Ochs M: Surgical management of the hip in the elderly patient, *Clin Geriatr Med* 6:571, 1990.
6. Hirsch C, Frankel VH: Analysis of forces producing fractures in the proximal end of the femur, *J Bone Joint Surg* 42-B:633, 1960.
7. Garden RS: Stability and union in subcapital fractures of the femur, *J Bone Joint Surg* 46-B:630, 1964.
8. Ordway C, Levin PE, Dee R: Fractures of the pelvis and leg. In Dee R, Mango E, and Hurst C, ed: *Principles of orthopaedic practice,* New York, 1989, McGraw-Hill, pp. 1209-1242.
9. Russell TA: Fractures of the hip and pelvis. In Crenshaw AH, ed: *Campbells operative orthopaedics,* St. Louis, 1992, Mosby Year Book, pp. 895-987.
10. D'Arcy J, Devas M: Treatment of fractures of the femoral neck by the replacement with the Thompson prosthesis, *J Bone Joint Surg* 58-B:279, 1976.
11. Boyd HG, Griffin LL: Classification and treatment of trochanteric fractures, *Arch Surg* 58:853, 1949.
12. Kyle RF, Gustilo RB, and Premer RF: Analysis of 622 intertrochanteric hip fractures: a retrospective and prospective study, *J Bone Joint Surg* 61:216, 1979.
13. Colonna PC: Fractures of the neck of the femur in children, *Am J Surg* 6:793, 1929.
14. Canale ST: Fractures of the hip in children and adolescents, *Orthop Clin North Am* 21:341, 1990.
15. Griffen PP, Anderson M, and Green WT: Fractures of the shaft of the femur in children: treatment and results, *Orthop Clin North Am* 3:213, 1972.
16. Raju KK, Tepler M, Dharapak C, Perlman HS: Transepiphyseal fracture of the hips in children, *Orthop Rev* 13:33, 1984.
17. Canale ST: Fractures and dislocations in children. In Crenshaw AH, ed: *Campbells operative orthopaedics,* St. Louis, 1992, Mosby Year Book, pp. 1055-1248.
18. Mosely CF: Fractures and dislocations of the hip, *Acad Orthop Surg* 41:397, 1992.
19. Thompson VP, Epstein HC: Traumatic dislocation of the hip, *J Bone Joint Surg* 33:746, 1951.
20. Canale ST, Manugian AH: Irreducible traumatic dislocation of the hip, *J Bone Joint Surg* 61-A:1054, 1975.
21. Allis OH: *An inquiry into the difficulties encountered in the reduction of dislocations of the hip,* Philadelphia, 1896, Dornan Printer.
22. Stewart MJ, Milford LW: Fracture-dislocation of the hip: an end result study, *J Bone Joint Surg* 36-A:315, 1954.
23. Epstein HC: Posterior fracture-dislocation of the hip: long term follow-up, *J Bone Joint Surg* 5-A:1103, 1974.
24. Glass A, Powell HDW: Traumatic dislocation of the hip in children: an analysis of forty-seven patients, *J Bone Joint Surg* 43-B:29, 1961.
25. Kelsy J, Southwick WO: Etiology, mechanism and incidence of slipped capital femoral epiphysis. In *AAOS Instructional Course Lectures,* vol 21, St. Louis, 1972, Mosby, pp. 182-185.
26. Brenkel IJ, Wise DI: Slipped capital femoral epiphysis, *Br J Hosp Med* 45:140, 1991.
27. Lehman WB: Slipped capital femoral epiphysis. In Dee R, Mango E, and Hurst C, ed: *Principles of orthopaedic practice,* New York, 1989, McGraw-Hill, pp. 1101-1109.
28. Carney BT, Weinstein SL, and Noble J: Long-term follow-up of slipped capital femoral epiphysis, *J Bone Joint Surg* 73-A:667, 1991.
29. Tachdjran MO: *Pediatric orthopedics,* Philadelphia, 1990, WB Saunders, p. 934.
30. Wenger DR, Ward WT, Herring JA: Current concepts review: Legg-Calve Perthes disease, *J Bone Joint Surg* 73(5):778, 1991.
31. Bowen, JR: Legg-Calve-Perthes disease. In Dee R, Mango E, and Hurst LC, eds: *Principles of orthopaedic practice,* New York, 1989, McGraw-Hill, pp 1110-1122.
32. Mose K, Hjorth L, Ulfeldt M, et al: Legg-Calve-Perthes disease: the late occurrence of coxarthrosis, *Acta Orthop Scand* Suppl 169, 1977.
33. Salzman, et al: Chronic hip pain and limp in a 3-year-old girl, *Rev Infect Dis* 2:341, 1989.
34. Morrey BF, Bianco AJ, and Rhodes KH: Septic arthritis in children, *Orthop Clin North Am* 6:923, 1975.
35. Volberg EM, Sumner TE, Abraham JS: Unreliability of radiographic diagnosis of septic hip in children, *Pediatrics* 4:118, 1984.
36. Barton LL, Dunkle LM, and Habid FH: Septic arthritis in childhood, *Am J Dis Child* 141:898, 1987.
37. Lee AH, Chin AE, Ramanujam T, et al: Gonococcal septic arthritis of the hip, *J Rheumatol* 18:1932, 1991.
38. Faden H, Grossi M: Acute osteomyelitis in children, *Am J Dis Child* 145:65, 1991.
39. Jacobson T, Allen WC: Surgical correction of the iliopsoas tendon, *Am J Sports Med* 18:470, 1990.
40. Abyad A, Boyer JT: Arthritis and aging, *Curr Opin Rheumatol* 4:153, 1992.
41. Wilkins RM, Sim FH, and Springfield DS: Metastatic disease of the femur, *Orthopedics* 15:621, 1992.
42. d'Aubigne RM, Postel M, Mazabraud A, et al: Idiopathic necrosis of the femoral head in adults, *J Bone Joint Surg* 47-B:612, 1965.
43. Ficat RP: Treatment of avascular necrosis of the femoral head. In Hungerford DS, ed: *The hip: proceedings - 11th open scientific meeting of the hip society,* St. Louis, 1983, Mosby Year Book, pp. 279-295.
44. Quinet RJ, Winters EG: Total joint replacement of the hip and knee, *Med Clin North Am* 76:1235, 1992.
45. Berger PE, Ofstein RA, and Jackson DW: MRI demonstration of radiographically occult fractures: what have we been missing? *Radiography* 9:407, 1989.
46. Clift BA, Rowley DI: Hip replacement surgery, *Br J Hosp Med* 47:273, 1992.
47. Devas MD: Stress fractures of the femoral neck, *J Bone Joint Surg* 47-B:728, 1965.
48. Lavelle DG: Acute dislocations. In Crenshaw AH, ed: *Campbells operative orthopaedics,* St. Louis, 1992, Mosby Year Book, pp. 1349-1372.
49. Pitt JF, Lund PJ, and Speer DP: Imaging of the pelvis and hip, *Orthop Clin North Am* 21:545, 1990.
50. Sauser DD, Billimoria PE, Rouse GA, Mudge K: CT evaluation of hip trauma, *AJR* 135:269, 1980.
51. Stimson LA: *A treatise on fractures,* Philadelphia, 1883, HC Leas and Sons.
52. Wernstein SL: Legg-Calve-Perthes disease. In Morrissy RT, ed: *Pediatric Orthopaedics,* ed 3, Philadelphia, 1990, JB Lippincott, pp. 851-883.

# *18*

# Shaft Fractures of the Femur

*Timothy J. Crimmins*
*Ernest Ruiz*

The femur is the longest and strongest bone in the human body. It is surrounded by and attached to the most powerful muscles of the body. Fracture of this bone occurs only with considerable force. It is associated with significant morbidity and mortality that can be alleviated with proper initial and definitive care.

## EPIDEMIOLOGY

Femur fractures are relatively uncommon. They occur at a frequency of about 3 per 10,000 person-years in small children, and decrease in incidence during preadolescence. In adolescence, the incidence increases again, reaching adult levels secondary to motor vehicle injuries. This incidence is also about 3 per 10,000 person-years.[1] In all age groups, men suffer this injury about twice as frequently as women.[1,2]

The prototypical childhood fracture is that of a spiral midshaft fracture in the toddler as a result of a fall from a significant height. This is often the result of child neglect or abuse.[1,3] Dalton and associates[4] found that all common femur fracture types occur in abuse. In older children, the femur is most commonly fractured as a result of being struck by a motor vehicle, resulting in a transverse midshaft fracture of the femur. In adolescence and young adulthood, the most frequent mechanism of injury is a bending force applied to the femur in motor vehicle accidents. This high-energy trauma is commonly associated with fractures of the pelvis, intrathoracic trauma, intra-abdominal trauma, knee injuries, and head injuries. Motorcyclists may be struck from the side, resulting in extensive soft-tissue crush injury to the midthigh, with segmental or comminuted fractures of the femur. Gustilo[5] found in his series of open fractures of all bones that almost one third of Type III fractures occurred in motorcycle accidents.

Increasingly, gunshot wounds are another source of direct trauma to the femur, frequently resulting in spiral or transverse comminuted–type fractures of the femur.[6,7] Low-velocity, low-caliber weapons result in open, isolated femoral shaft fractures with considerable bone fragmentation. With close-range gunshot wounds or high-velocity weapons, there may be considerable soft-tissue damage often associated with vascular and nerve injury, although Bergman and associates[6,8] found that such wounds may heal well, as long as vascularity is preserved. Farm accidents, explosions, and tornadoes can inflict injuries to the femur, with segmental comminution and extensive soft-tissue damage. In the last decades of life, a slip and fall to the bent knee can result in a supracondylar or condylar femur fracture.

Pathologic fractures of the femur are relatively uncommon, but may result from metastases from breast, lung, or prostate carcinoma.[9] Primary bone tumors, such as osteogenic sarcomas, angiosarcomas, and chondrosarcomas, can result in pathologic fractures, but are rare causes of femur fracture.[9]

## ANATOMY

Figures 18-1 and 18-2 show the muscular attachments to the femur anteriorly and posteriorly. The pull of the muscles on the proximal and distal fragments of femur fractures results in patterns of displacement and angulation that are important factors in the definitive management of these cases.[10] Figure 18-3 summarizes these effects. Fractures

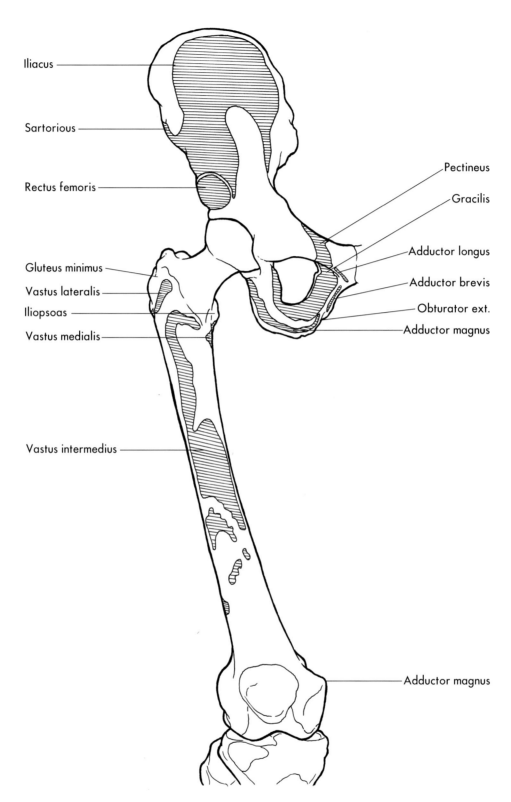

**Fig. 18-1.** Anterior view of the femur and hemipelvis, showing the sites of muscle origin and insertion. In addition, the tensor fascia lata, or ilio-tibial band, is inserted on the proximal tibia.

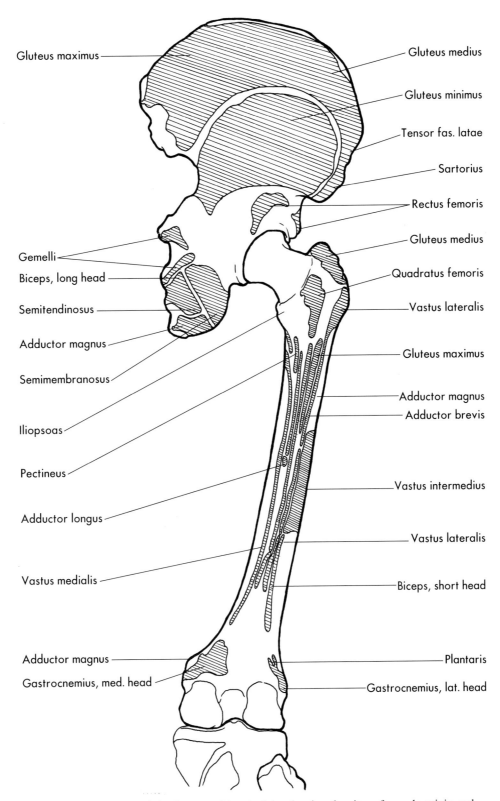

Gluteus maximus

Gluteus medius

Gluteus minimus

Tensor fas. latae

Sartorius

Rectus femoris

Gluteus medius

Gemelli

Biceps, long head

Semitendinosus

Quadratus femoris

Vastus lateralis

Adductor magnus

Gluteus maximus

Semimembranosus

Adductor magnus

Adductor brevis

Iliopsoas

Pectineus

Vastus intermedius

Adductor longus

Vastus lateralis

Vastus medialis

Biceps, short head

Adductor magnus

Plantaris

Gastrocnemius, med. head

Gastrocnemius, lat. head

**Fig. 18-2.** Posterior view of the femur and hemipelvis, showing the sites of muscle origin and insertion. The tensor fascia lata originates on the iliac crest and receives fibers of the gluteus maximus as it courses laterally to insert on the proximal tibia.

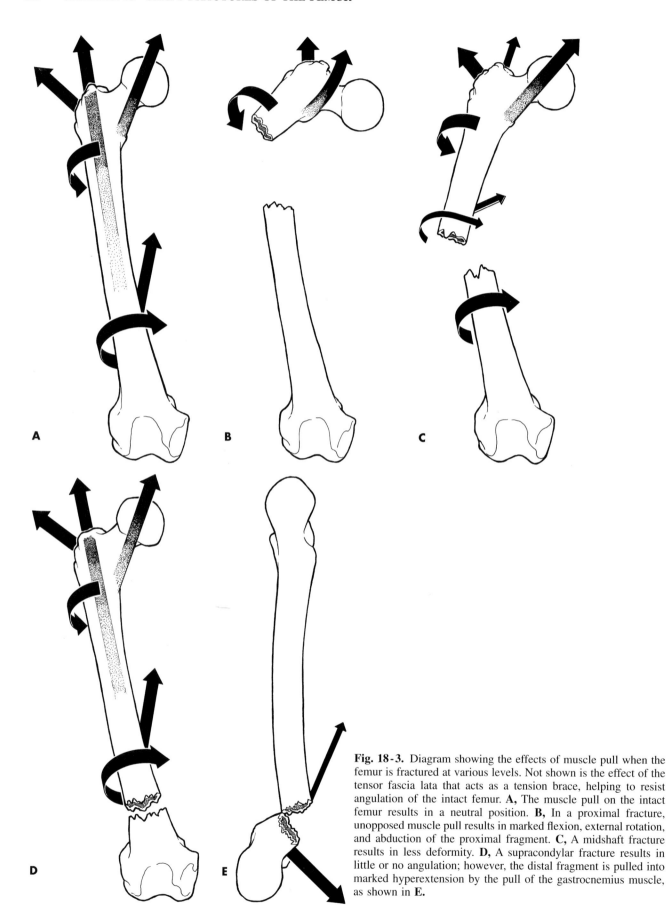

**Fig. 18-3.** Diagram showing the effects of muscle pull when the femur is fractured at various levels. Not shown is the effect of the tensor fascia lata that acts as a tension brace, helping to resist angulation of the intact femur. **A,** The muscle pull on the intact femur results in a neutral position. **B,** In a proximal fracture, unopposed muscle pull results in marked flexion, external rotation, and abduction of the proximal fragment. **C,** A midshaft fracture results in less deformity. **D,** A supracondylar fracture results in little or no angulation; however, the distal fragment is pulled into marked hyperextension by the pull of the gastrocnemius muscle, as shown in **E.**

of the proximal third of the femur put the proximal fragment in marked flexion, with abduction and external rotation secondary to the pull of the iliopsoas, abductors, and short external rotators. Muscle pull in midshaft (middle third) fractures pulls the proximal fragment in moderate flexion, lateral rotation, and abduction. In supracondylar fractures of the femur, the gastrocnemius muscle pulls the distal fragment in marked hyperextension.[10] When a patient with a proximal femur fracture is placed in traction, the distal fragment is brought into alignment by placing the thigh in 90° of flexion. With midshaft fractures, less flexion is needed. With supracondylar fractures, knee and thigh flexion is needed to align the proximal and distal fragments.

The femur itself has an anterior bow of approximately 10° in men and 15° in women. In small children, this bowing may be approximately 40°.[10] The shaft of the femur is thickened posteriorly along a line called the *linea aspera.* This thickening accommodates the attachment of thick fascial septa dividing the thigh into three compartments, as shown in Fig. 18-4. The three compartments—anterior, posterior, and medial—contain muscle groups and neurovascular structures, as listed in the box on page 429. The lateral aspect of the anterior compartment is covered by a strong and distinct thickening of fascia called the *tensor fascia lata,* or *iliotibial band,* of the thigh. This band provides a tension brace for the thigh, helping to prevent angulation. These three compartments are subject to the development of compartment syndromes secondary to hemorrhage, use of the pneumatic antishock garment (PASG), or to revascularization edema formation.[11-13]

The nutrient vessel of the femur usually originates from a single branch of the profundus femoris artery in the proximal third of the femur. This vessel penetrates the cortex of the femur posteriorly along the linea aspera.[10] Devascularization of the femur is not a common problem because of extensive collateralization of blood supply to the

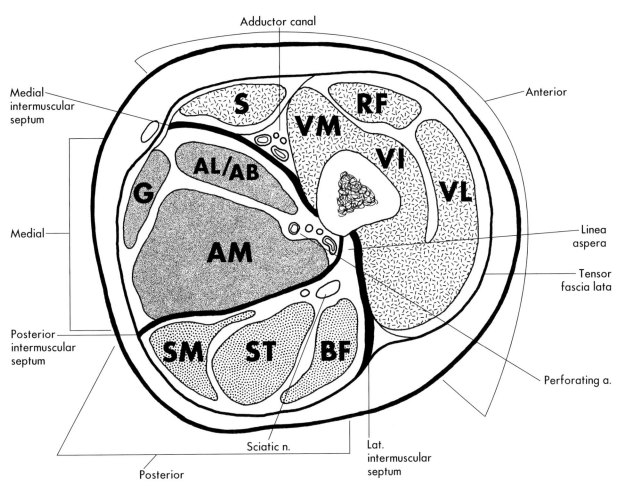

**Fig. 18-4.** Diagram of the thigh showing the three major compartments formed by fascial septa arising from the linea aspera of the femur. Note that the femoral artery lies in a space, called the adductor canal or Hunter's canal, formed by the sartorius and vastus medialis muscles and the medial septum. The quadriceps femoris, the great extensor muscle of the thigh, is composed of the rectus femoris, the vastus intermedius, the vastus medialis, and the vastus lateralis. Note that the vastus muscles almost encompass the femur from the trochanters to the condyles. *AL, AB, AM,* adductor longus, brevis, and magnus, respectively; *G,* gracilis; *SM, ST, BF,* semimembranosus, semitendinosus, and biceps femoris, respectively; *VM, VI, VL,* vastus medius, intermedius, and lateralis, respectively; *RF, S,* rectus femoris and sartorius, respectively.

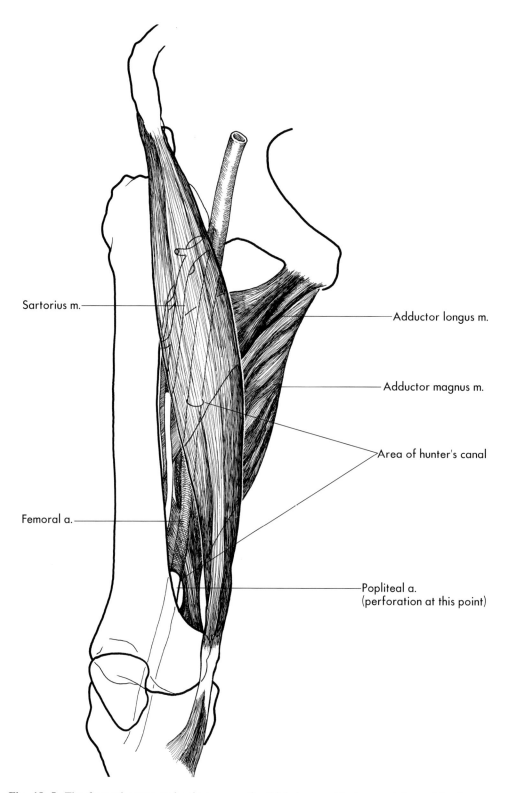

**Fig. 18-5.** The femoral artery and vein traverse the thigh in an adductor canal formed by the muscles of the anterior compartment and the medial intermuscular septum. This canal, also called Hunter's canal, ends with a perforation of the tendinous insertion of the adductor magnus muscle. The femoral artery then becomes the popliteal artery. At this point, it is especially vulnerable to shearing forces in blunt trauma.

**Contents of the three compartments of the thigh**

*Anterior compartment*

Muscles
    Quadraceps femoris
    Sartorius
    Iliacus
    Psoas
    Pectineus
Blood vessels and nerves
    Femoral artery and vein
    Femoral nerve
    Lateral femoral cutaneous nerve

*Medial compartment*

Muscles
    Gracilis
    Adductor longus, brevis and magnus
    Obturator externus
Blood vessels and nerves
    Obturator artery and vein
    Obturator nerve

*Posterior compartment*

Muscles
    Biceps femoris
    Semitendinosus
    Semimembranosus
    A portion of the adductor magnus
Blood vessels and nerves
    Branches of the profunda femoris artery and vein
    Sciatic nerve
    Posterior femoral cutaneous nerve

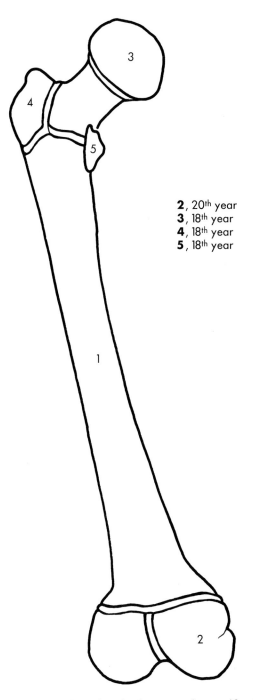

**2**, 20th year
**3**, 18th year
**4**, 18th year
**5**, 18th year

**Fig. 18-6.** Diagram illustrating the four secondary ossification centers of the femur and their approximate age of fusion.

periosteum, unless the periosteum is disturbed by trauma or ill-advised dissection at surgery.[14] Hemorrhage into the surrounding muscles after femur fracture is a well-known entity. However, recent reports cite low or no blood requirements in patients with isolated femur fractures.[15] This bleeding is commonly secondary to disruption of small perforating branches of the profundus femoris artery. The femoral artery in the thigh penetrates the tendinous insertion of the adductor magnus on the femur at the distal end of the adductor canal (Fig. 18-5), where it is subject to shearing forces in supracondylar femur fractures as well as in knee dislocation.[16]

The primary ossification center of the femur is the shaft. This center is ossified at birth, as is the secondary ossification center of the distal femur. Other secondary ossification centers are located in the greater trochanter, lesser trochanter, and head of the femur. These centers ossify at 2 to 5 years of age, 9 to 13 years of age, and 6 months of age, respectively.[10] The epiphyseal plates of the femur and their ages of fusion are shown in Fig. 18-6.[17]

## CLASSIFICATION

Several classification systems describe femoral shaft fractures, subtrochanteric femur fractures, and supracondylar femur fractures. The emergency physician should be prepared to describe the findings in detail. This is probably more important than trying to divine the correct classification of a particular femur fracture. Nevertheless, it is satisfying to be able to classify these fractures correctly;

Tables 18-1, 18-2, 18-3, and 18-4 are provided to give the emergency physician this opportunity.

Table 18-1 gives the Seinsheimer classification system for subtrochanteric fractures of the femur; Figure 18-7 provides examples.[18] Table 18-2 gives the Winquist classification system for comminuted femoral shaft fractures; Figure 18-8 provides examples.[19] Table 18-3 gives the AO (Arbeitsgemeinshaft für Osteosynthesefragen) classification system for supracondylar femoral fractures; Figure 18-9 provides examples.[20]

**Table 18-1.** The Seinsheimer classification system for subtrochanteric fractures of the femur

Nondisplaced fracture with less than 2 mm of displacement
Two-part fractures
   Two-part transverse femoral fracture
   Two-part spiral fracture with the lesser trochanter attached to the proximal fragment
   Two-part spiral fracture with the lesser trochanter attached to the distal fragment
Three-part fractures
   Three-part spiral fracture in which the third fragment includes the lesser trochanter
   Three-part spiral fracture in which the third part is a butterfly fragment
Comminuted fracture with four or more fragments
Subtrochanteric—intertrochanteric fracture with extension through the greater trochanter

**Table 18-2.** The Winquist classification system for comminuted femoral shaft fractures

Fracture with a small butterfly fragment comprising 25% or less of the width of the shaft
Fracture with a butterfly fragment comprising 25% to 50% of the width of the shaft
Fracture with a butterfly fragment wider than 50% of the width of the shaft
Severe comminution of an entire segment of bone
Fracture with segmental bone loss

**Table 18-3.** Arbeitsgemeinshaft für Osteosynthesefragen classification of supracondylar femur fractures

Extra-articular
   Avulsion of the medial or lateral epicondyle
   Simple supracondylar
   Comminuted supracondylar
Unicondylar
   Medial or lateral condyle
   Condyle fracture with extension proximally into the femoral shaft
   Posterior tangential fracture of one or both condyles
Bicondylar
   Intercondylar
   Intercondylar with a comminuted supracondylar component
   Severely comminuted bicondylar fracture

**Table 18-4.** The Gustilo classification of open fractures

| | |
|---|---|
| Type I. | Puncture wound ≤1 cm in diameter and is relatively clean |
| Type II. | Laceration longer than 1 cm without extensive soft-tissue damage, flaps, or avulsion, with a minimal to moderate crushing component |
| Type III. | Extensive damage to the soft tissues, including muscle, skin, and neurovascular structures |
| Type IIIA. | Adequate soft-tissue coverage of a fractured bone despite extensive soft-tissue laceration or flaps, or high-energy trauma irrespective of the size of the wound |
| Type IIIB. | Extensive soft-tissue injury loss with periosteal stripping and bone exposure |
| Type IIIC. | Open fracture associated with arterial injury requiring repair |

In general, femur fractures are described as being proximal third, middle third (midshaft), or distal third. The quality of the fracture itself is described as being transverse, spiral, or longitudinal. If the fracture is segmented and the segment is small, it is called a *butterfly fragment.* The fracture can be comminuted, and fragments can actually be missing; this is called *segmentation with bone loss.* In proximal third fractures, the lesser or greater trochanters can be separated. In distal fractures, the supracondylar fracture can be T'ed with a intercondylar fracture line. A degree of overriding is seen in femur fractures; the estimated length of this overriding or shortening is particularly important to the orthopedist who will manage a femur fracture in a child. Of course, distal and proximal fragment flexion and extension, angulation, and rotation are also important characteristics of the individual case.

Whether or not the fracture is open is also extremely important information. The Gustilo classification system for open fractures (Table 18-4) is very applicable to femur fractures and is widely used.[21] In this system, a type I injury has a puncture wound with a diameter of ≤1 cm and appears clean. Commonly, this injury is produced by a spike of bone without significant soft-tissue injury or crush. A type II injury has a laceration of >1 cm long, without extensive soft-tissue damage. There may be some crushing. Type III injuries involve extensive soft-tissue damage, including neurovascular injuries. This type is subdivided into three subcategories: type IIIA injury is present when there is extensive soft-tissue damage but there is adequate soft-tissue coverage of the fractured bone; type IIIB injury is present when there is extensive soft-tissue damage and loss, with periosteal stripping and bone exposure, usually with massive contamination; type IIIC injury is present when the open fracture is associated with arterial injury requiring repair.

The age of the patient, the length of time following injury, the mechanism of injury, any associated injuries, findings of the neurovascular examination of the involved extremity, and information regarding last meal and drug allergies will all be required by the orthopedic consultant.

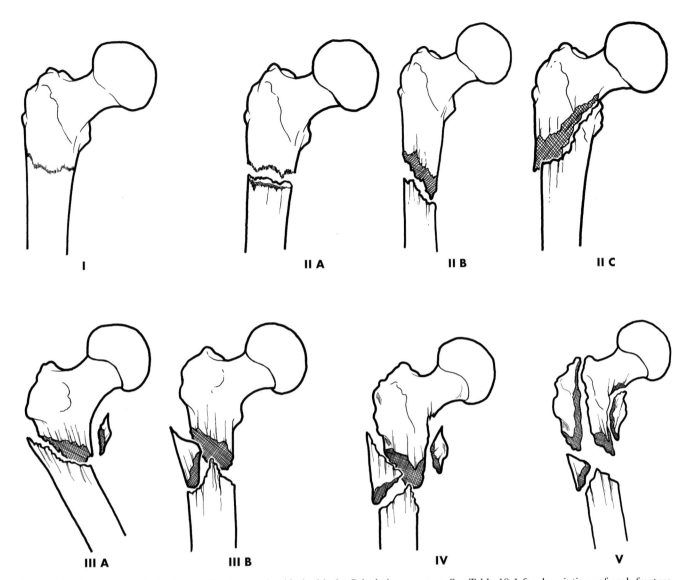

**Fig. 18-7.** Subtrochanteric fractures of the femur classified with the Seinsheimer system. See Table 18-1 for descriptions of each fracture type.

## INITIAL EVALUATION AND MANAGEMENT
### Prehospital care

Generally, femoral fractures are not overlooked in the field by prehospital personnel. The force required to fracture the femur is such that the possibility plainly exists at the scene. In extricating or moving patients (even comatose patients), the laxity and shortening of the femur is usually quite evident. If it is a relatively isolated injury, application of a traction splint is indicated. However, the pneumatic anti-shock garment (PASG) is also an adequate splint and may facilitate transfer and movement. It can be applied with more speed and ease than a traction splint. Traction should not be used when there is extensive tissue loss because additional injury may be incurred by vessels and nerves. Given the propensity for femoral shaft fractures to bleed, an intravenous line should be established en route to the hospital.

### Emergency department care

In the context of the ABCs of trauma management, femur fractures are readily detected during the primary and secondary surveys. A femur fracture can easily result in the loss of three units of blood, and this may be a factor in traumatic shock, although it is rarely the only one. If the fracture is open, broad-spectrum intravenous antibiotic coverage should be instituted.[22] Cefoxitin, a second-generation cephalosporin, is an acceptable choice; however, several other cephalosporins and β-lactamase–resistant antibiotics provide effective coverage as well. In penicillin-allergic patients, a combination of gentamycin and clindamycin provides good coverage.

Pulses should be assessed proximal and distal to the fracture and capillary refill checked and documented. Reduction of the fracture with traction may restore a pulse.

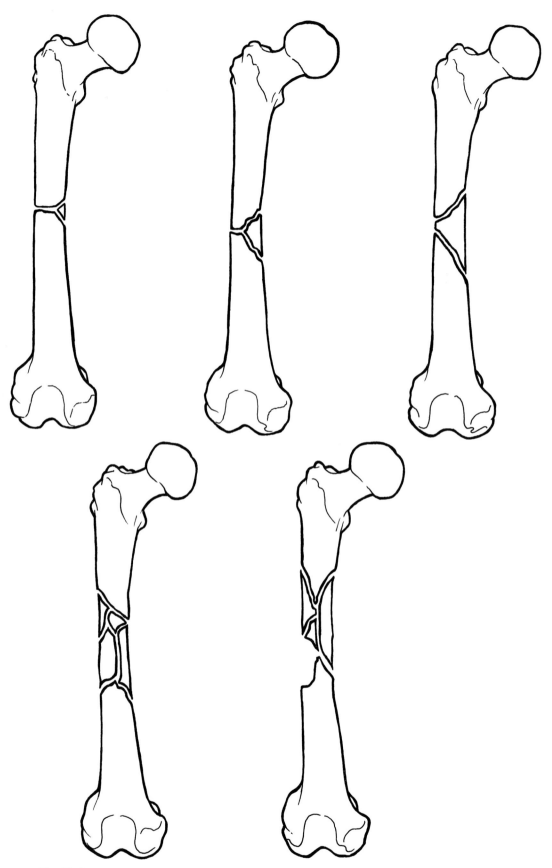

**Fig. 18-8.** Comminuted femoral shaft fractures classified with the Winquist system. See Table 18-2 for descriptions of each fracture type.

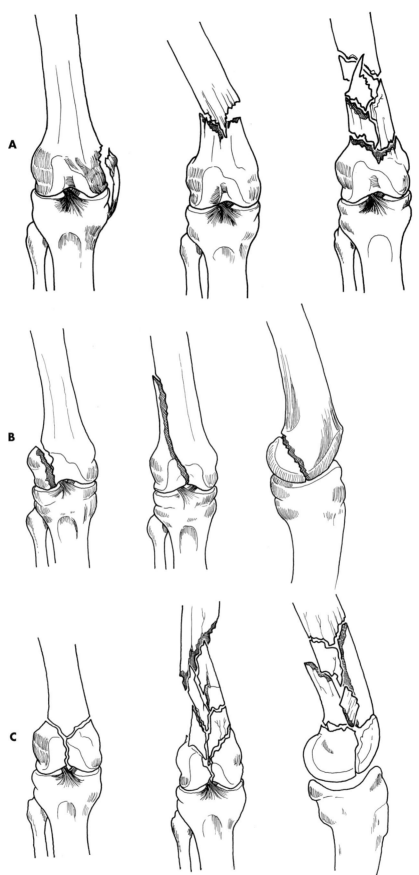

**Fig. 18-9.** Supracondylar femoral fractures classified according to the Arbeitsgemeinshaft für Osteosynthesefragen group (AO) system. See Table 18-3 for descriptions of each fracture type.

The patient's ability to move and feel the toes is important information. The extremity should be carefully palpated to detect possible elevated compartment pressures. Remember that loss of pulses and function distally is a very late effect of a compartment syndrome. The trauma team should be informed of any suspicion that a compartment syndrome may exist.

A Sager (Minto Research & Development, Redding, CA) or Hare (Dyna-Med, Carlsbad, CA) traction splint should be applied to restore length. See Chapter 2 for a description of these splints. Simply splinting a femur fracture reduces hemorrhage into the soft tissues of the thigh and greatly reduces patient pain and apprehension. A Sager-type splint is more compact and shorter that a Hare-type splint, and is more effective in a helicopter or a CT scanner. When traction is contraindicated, a plaster- or board-reinforced bulky dressing can be used. Toddlers and small children can be effectively splinted using this method.

Radiographs of the femur fracture are low priority in the acute resuscitation period. If the patient is unstable, they may have to be transferred to the operating room or a trauma center without obtaining radiograph results of a fractured femur. These films can be obtained later. Examples of femur fracture on radiograph are shown in Figs. 18-10, 18-11, and 18-12. When a patient with an open fracture is to be moved about the hospital or transferred to

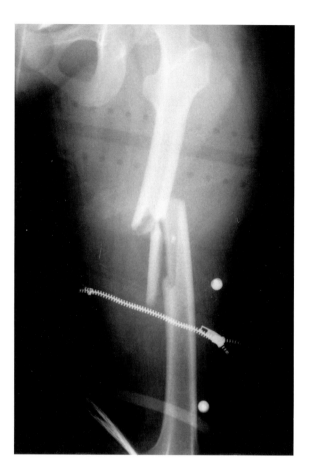

**Fig. 18-11.** Radiograph of a midshaft femur fracture.

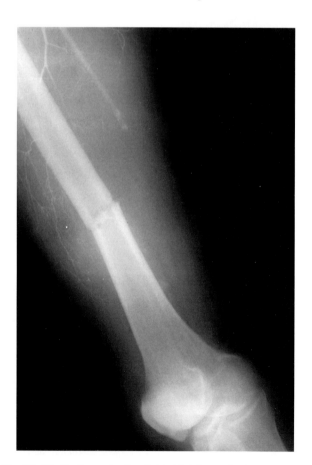

**Fig. 18-10.** Radiograph of a distal third femur fracture.

a trauma center, gauze sponges soaked with povidone solution should be applied to the wound and held in place with rolls of gauze or cotton. Of course, splinting should also be provided.

Consultation with an orthopedist should be obtained early. Frequently, fracture stabilization must precede the repair of vascular injury, to avoid disruption of a repaired vessel during reduction. Angiography should be considered when there may be major vascular injury. Careful documentation of pulses, bruits, thrills, and hematoma size are critical to good decision-making here.[23] The orthopedist must have the opportunity to help set priorities for each individual case.

**Assessment for child abuse**

Gross and Stranger[24] estimate that perhaps two-thirds of femur fractures occuring in a child's first year of life are a result of abuse. Dalton and associates[4] recommend that every child under 3 years of age with a femur fracture be admitted to the hospital unless the circumstances of the injury are extremely clear. Others point out that a 2-year-old can fracture a femur by running and tripping with a twisting motion.[25] Staheli[10] advises that suspicion of abuse should be aroused by the following: 1) the child is an infant; 2) the child is the firstborn; 3) there is pre-existing

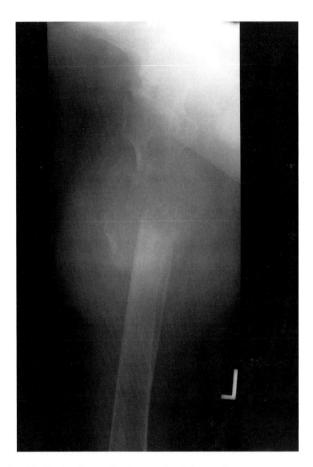

**Fig. 18-12.** Radiograph of a proximal femur fracture.

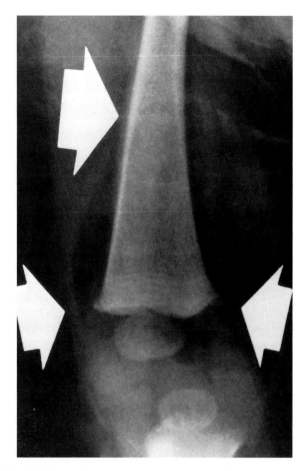

**Fig. 18-13.** Radiograph of an 11-month-old child showing chip fractures of the distal metaphyseal bone. There is also periosteal calcification along the shaft of the femur, indicating prior trauma. These injuries are very suspicious indications of child abuse. (From Campbell RM Jr: Problem injuries in unique conditions of the musculoskeletal system. In Rockwood CA Jr, Wilkins KE, and King RE, eds: *Fractures in children.* ed 3. Philadelphia, JB Lippincott, 1991. Used by permission).

brain damage; 4) the fractures are bilateral; 5) the fractures are subtrochanteric or there is a chip fracture of the distal metaphysis; 6) the family delays seeking medical care; and 7) additional trauma is present. An example of a distal metaphyseal chip fracture is shown in Fig. 18-13.[26]

## DEFINITIVE MANAGEMENT GUIDELINES

In general, the definitive management of femoral shaft fractures is guided by three observations: 1) traction methods of treatment yield acceptable but inferior results as compared with those achieved with internal fixation; 2) the use of plates in internal fixation may result in wound-healing problems because of the need for dissection of periosteum and muscle; and 3) closed intramedullary nailing affords good realignment of bone, rapid healing, and early mobilization.[27]

Femoral shaft fractures are usually fixed internally, immediately after resuscitation. When delays are unavoidable because of other injuries, traction is generally used to maintain alignment until the patient's condition permits surgery. External fixation may be an alternative, but this form of fixation is not always stable and may lead to contracture formation.[27]

Midshaft fractures are ideal for intramedullary nailing using a rod introduced just medial to the greater trochanter and directed down the shaft of the femur. The prototype is the Küntsher rod introduced in 1939.[28] Many styles of rods are available. Some have cutting edges and others require reaming of the marrow canal with a long drill bit prior to insertion. The rod can be inserted without exposing the fracture site, although this may be necessary when fragmentation is present. Figure 18-14 shows a radiograph of a femur nailed without an incision at the fracture site.

Proximal femur fractures (subtrochanteric) and supracondylar fractures generally require a combination of nails, lag screws, and plates to provide adequate fixation. Interlocking rods are those that have apertures that accommodate lag screws. Obviously, intraoperative fluoroscopy is usually necessary to ensure accurate reduction. When there is bone loss, bone grafts may be required to facilitate healing and afford adequate strength. Figure 18-15 shows a radiograph of a supracondylar femur fracture internally fixed with a nail and plate.

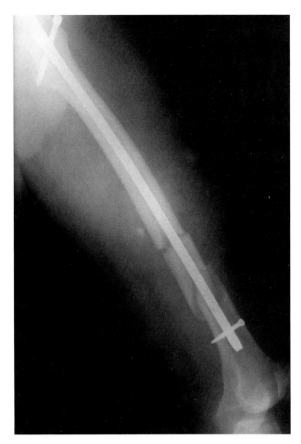

**Fig. 18-14.** Example of a midshaft femur fracture successfully nailed with closed technique.

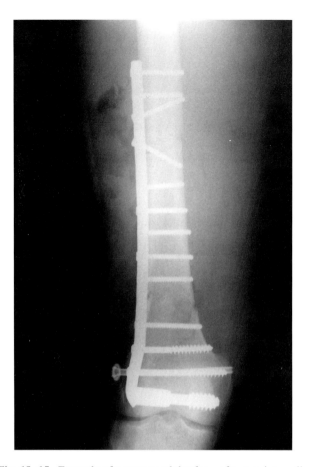

**Fig. 18-15.** Example of a supracondylar femur fracture internally fixed with a nail, screws, and a plate.

Children may be managed with traction or casting only. The rapid healing of these fractures combined with the ability of the growing bone to mold and gain length makes this form of treatment effective. In fact, an accurate reduction of a femur fracture in a small child results in overgrowth of the injured limb.[10] A degree of overriding of the bone fragments is desirable. A body, or Spica, cast is used in small children. In older children, carefully monitored skeletal traction may be used.

Open femur fractures are copiously irrigated during debridement and exploration. It is important that this occur as soon as feasible after injury. Type I and type II open fractures can be nailed immediately. Even type III fractures can sometimes be nailed immediately, in the judgment of some orthopedists.[27,29]

In general, the prognosis for full recovery is good in uncomplicated fractures of the shaft of the femur. Patients can usually ambulate within 2 weeks of injury, and return to normal activity within a few months.

## DISCUSSION

The emergency management of femoral shaft fractures is usually a satisfying experience for emergency physicians. The application of splints offers the patient a great reduction in pain and apprehension. Good and timely emergency department patient evaluation and management improves the immediate and ultimate outcome. The trauma surgeon and orthopedist are better able to make informed decisions when the emergency physician has competently assessed and stabilized the patient. As in all successful trauma resuscitation, teamwork and communication are key elements.

## REFERENCES

1. Hedlund R, Lindgren U: The incidence of femoral shaft fractures in children and adolescents, *J Pediatr Orthop* 6: pp. 47-50, 1986.
2. Nafei A et al: Femoral shaft fractures in children: An epidemiological study in a Danish urban population, 1977-86, *J Pediatr Orthop* 12: pp. 499-502, 1992.
3. Herndon WA: Child abuse in military population, *J Pediatr Orthop* 3: pp. 73-76, 1983.
4. Dalton HJ et al: Undiagnosed abuse in children younger than 3 years with femoral fracture, *Am J Dis Child* 144: pp. 875-878, 1990.
5. Gustilo RB, Mendoza RM, and Williams DN: Problems in the management of type III (severe) open fractures: A new classification of type III open fractures, *J Trauma* 24: pp. 742-746, 1984.
6. Bergman M et al: Femur fractures caused by gunshots: Treatment by immediate reamed intramedullary nailing, *J Trauma* 34: 783-785, 1993.
7. Hollman MW, Horowitz M: Femoral fractures secondary to low velocity missiles: Treatment with delayed intramedullary fixation, *J Orthop Trauma* 4: pp. 64-69, 1990.
8. Hollerman JJ, Fackler ML: Wound ballistics. In Tintinalli JE, Krome

RL, and Ruiz E, eds: *Emergency medicine: A comprehensive study guide.* ed 3. New York, McGraw-Hill, 1992.

9. Broos PLO, Rommens PM, and Vanlangenaker MJU: Pathological fracture of the femur: Improvement of quality of life after surgical treatment, *Arch Orthop Trauma Surg* 111: pp. 73-77, 1992.

10. Staheli LT: Fractures of the shaft of the femur. In Rockwood CA Jr, Wilkins KE, and King RE, eds: *Fractures in children.* ed 3. Philadelphia, JB Lippincott, 1991.

11. Flint L et al: Definitive control of mortality from severe pelvic fracture, *Ann Surg* 211: pp. 703-706, 1990.

12. Mubarak SJ, Hargens AR: *Compartment syndromes and Volkman's contracture.* Philadelphia, WB Saunders, 1981.

13. Schwartz JT Jr et al: Acute compartment syndrome of the thigh. A spectrum of injury, *J Bone Joint Surg* 71A: pp. 392-400, 1989.

14. Bucholz RW, Brumback RJ: Fractures of the femur. In Rockwood CA Jr, Green DP, and Bucholz RW, eds: *Fractures in adults.* ed 3. Philadelphia, JB Lippincott, 1991.

15. Cope AR, McGlove R, Sloan JP: Do we need cross-match blood in closed fractures of the shaft of the femur? *Injury* 20: pp. 27-28, 1989.

16. Wiss DA: Supracondylar and intercondylar fractures of the femur. In Rockwood CA Jr, Green DP, and Bucholz RW, eds: *Fractures in adults.* ed 3. Philadelphia, JB Lippincott, 1991.

17. Gray H, Goss CM: *Anatomy of the human body.* ed 29. Philadelphia, Lea & Febiger, 1973.

18. Seinsheimer F: Subtrochanteric fractures of the femur, *J Bone Joint Surg* 60A: pp. 300-306, 1978.

19. Winquist RA, Hansen ST Jr, and Clawson DK: Closed intramedullary nailing of femoral fractures: A report of five hundred and twenty cases, *J Bone Joint Surg* 66A: pp. 529-539, 1984.

20. Müller ME et al: *Manual of internal fixation techniques recommended by the AO group.* Schatzder J translator, New York, Springer-Verlag, 1979.

21. Gustilo RB: Principles of the management of open fractures. In Gustilo RB ed: *Management of open fractures and their complications.* Philadelphia, WB Saunders, 1982.

22. Kind AC, Williams DN: Antibiotics in open fractures. In Gustilo RM ed: *Management of open fractures and their complications.* Philadelphia, WB Saunders, 1982.

23. Cargile JS III, Hunt JL, and Purdue GF: Acute trauma of the femoral artery and vein, *J Trauma* 32: pp. 364-370, 1992.

24. Gross RH, Stranger M: Causative factors responsible for femoral fractures in infants and young children, *J Pediatr Orthop* 3: pp. 341-343, 1983.

25. Thomas SA et al: Long-bone fractures in young children: Distinguishing accidental injuries from child abuse, *Pediatrics* 88: pp. 471-476, 1991.

26. Campbell RM Jr: Problem injuries in unique conditions of the musculoskeletal system. In Rockwood CA Jr, Wilkins KE, and King RE, eds: *Fractures in children.* ed 3. Philadelphia, JB Lippincott, 1991.

27. Bucholz RW, Jones A: Current concepts review: Fractures of the shaft of the femur, *J Bone Joint Surg* 73A: pp. 1561-1566, 1991.

28. Kűntsher G: The intramedullary nailing of fractures, *Clin Orthop* 60: pp. 5-12, 1968.

29. Brumback RJ et al: Intramedullary nailing of open fractures of the femoral shaft, *J Bone Joint Surg* 71A: pp. 1324-1331, 1989.

# The Knee

*Kevin P. Kilgore*

The knee is the second most commonly injured major joint presenting to the emergency department for evaluation and treatment. Due to an increase in the number of deceleration injuries (from vehicular accidents and falls) as well as injuries from professional and recreational sporting activities, the number of knee injuries presenting to the emergency department for evaluation and therapy is increasing.

Consequently, the emergency department physician, family physician, and orthopedic surgeon can expect to be confronted with knee injuries frequently. Injury to the knee is a significant insult, and misdiagnosis potentially can lead to a life-long disability. Based on clinical investigations as well as the development of magnetic resonance imaging (MRI) techniques and arthroscopy over the past two decades, a more aggressive treatment philosophy has evolved for a number of knee injuries. The challenges in treating knee injuries lies in understanding the anatomic and functional intricacies of the knee, understanding the injuries that are possible, and differentiating benign injuries from those that are more ominous.

The essential canons applicable to the care of every patient are embodied in "the five A's."[1] These simple tenets create a rapport between physician and patient and allow the best recovery for the patient in the shortest time. First, *accept* the patient; make patients feel they are important and their maladies significant. Second, *avoid* expediency. Do not minimize an injury or affliction; and evaluate completely. Third, *adopt* the best methods by using techniques that allow for the most complete and expeditious recovery with the least morbidity. Fourth, *act* promptly. Once a diagnosis is made, a definite plan should be designed, discussed with the patient, and then enacted. Fifth, *achieve* perfection. To accomplish this goal, the physician must know what the objective is and then pursue that objective, persevering despite setbacks.

Descriptors used in depicting the knee are steeped in anatomic and orthopedic nomenclature, which is felt by many nonorthopedists to be a foreign language. Conversely, orthopedists feel unsure of the caregiver who cannot "speak the language" and are thus reticent to permit family physicians or emergency physicians the opportunity to treat knee injuries. These difficulties are compounded by the fact that there is a paucity of literature on orthopedic injury or disease in even the most prestigious emergency medicine journals.

## ANATOMIC CONSIDERATIONS

The knee is the largest and structurally the most complex synovial joint of the body. Due to its architectural and functional intricacies, the knee is subject to a large number of possible maladies. Considered a modified hinge joint with varying instant centers of motion, the knee is composed of three basic structural elements: 1) an osseous foundation, 2) ligamentous and meniscal stabilizers, and 3) surrounding muscle groups. Alone, these components are

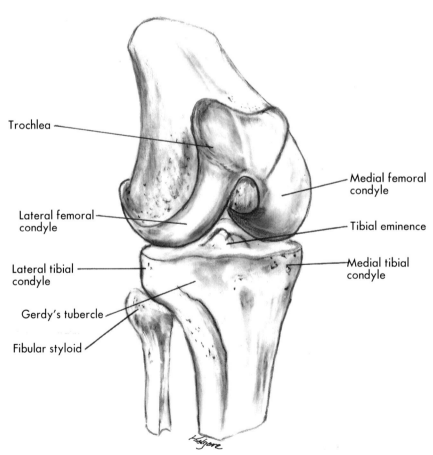

**Fig. 19-1.** Osseous foundation of the knee.

not capable of providing the necessary support or mobility to permit ambulation. Collectively, however, they provide a magnificent concert of stability and motion.

## Osseous foundation

The bony substructure of the knee is composed of the distal femur, tibial plateau, and patella (Fig. 19-1). At its distal extent, the femur broadens to form the lateral and medial femoral condyles. Both condylar surfaces are capped by hyaline cartilage and divided centrally by the intercondylar notch. The medial condyle is longer and more spherical in contour. At the anterior and central confluence of the condyles, a shallow groove called the trochlea, which facilitates engagement of the patella, is formed. The femoral condyles flatten along their posterior aspects, offering maximal flexion.

The proximal tibia flares in a similar fashion, forming the medial and lateral tibial condyles. Each condyle possesses a superior articular surface with a centrally located tibial eminence. Both tibial condyles possess a shallow central concavity (Fig. 19-2). Viewed sagitally, the tibial plateau slopes 10° downward as it continues posteriorly. Gerdy's tubercle is located along the anterolateral aspect immediately beneath the lateral tibial condyle. This excrescence acts as the attachment site of the iliotibial tract. The tibial tuberosity, which serves as the attachment site of the patellar tendon, is situated along the central anterior body of the tibia inferior to the tibial plateau.

The ovoid patella is the largest sesamoid bone of the body. Its posterior aspect consists of a medial and lateral facet separated by a median ridge and a smaller, odd facet present at its medial extreme (Fig. 19-3). The articular surface of the patella, like those of the femoral and tibial condyles, is covered by hyaline cartilage.

## The lateral compartment

The knee is supported laterally by a number of muscular elements. Superficially, the iliotibial band, iliotibial tract, and a portion of the lateral biceps femoris cross the knee joint to insert on Gerdy's tubercle (Fig. 19-4). The remaining elements of the lateral biceps femoris insert on the fibular head. The lateral head of the gastrocnemius origi-

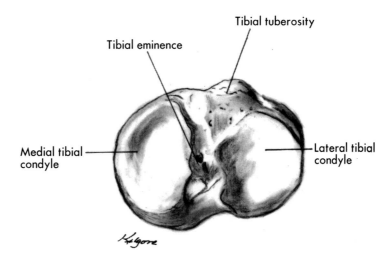

**Fig. 19-2.** Superior view of tibial plateau.

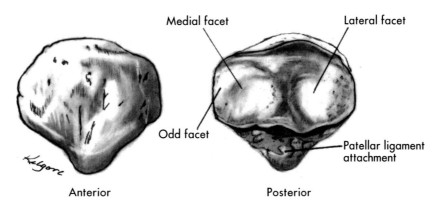

**Fig. 19-3.** Anatomy of the right patella.

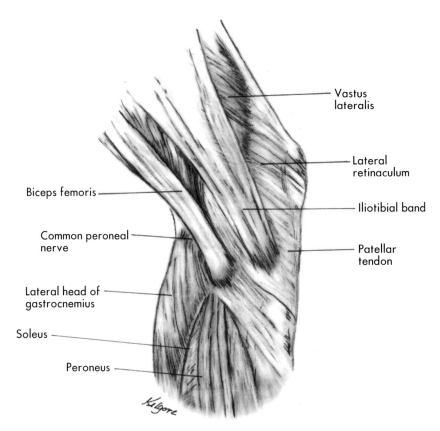

**Fig. 19-4.** Superficial anatomy of the lateral knee.

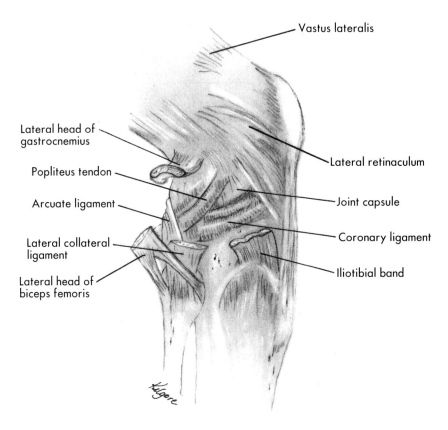

**Fig. 19-5.** Deep structures of the lateral knee.

nates along the posterolateral aspect of the lateral femoral epicondyle and spans the posterior aspect of the knee joint. Also arising from the lateral femoral epicondyle, the lateral collateral ligament courses distally 5 to 7 cm, deep to the iliotibial band and iliotibial tract, to attach on the anterosuperior aspect of the fibular head. As the lateral collateral ligament passes distally, it acts to divide the tendon of the lateral biceps femoris. This ligament is extracapsular and free of attachment to the joint capsule and meniscus (Fig. 19-5).

The lateral capsular ligament is divided into the anterior, middle, and posterior thirds. The thin, loose anterior one-third of the lateral capsular ligament lends little to the support of the knee joint. The middle third of this ligament arises inferior and deep to the popliteus origin at the lateral femoral epicondyle and courses to the lateral tibial epicondyle. This segment of the capsule provides a check reign against excessive anteromedial rotation.

Serving to buttress the posterior third of the lateral capsule, the popliteus muscle (Fig. 19-6) originates from the lateral femoral condyle, just below the attachment of the fibular collateral ligament. The intracapsular tendon wraps obliquely over the posterolateral joint line to insert on the posteromedial tibia. As the intracapsular popliteus tendon crosses the joint line, it passes through the polpiteal hiatus and then beneath the arcuate ligament, where it offers attachment to the lateral meniscus. The posterolateral third of the knee is also supported by the arcuate complex, which is a composite of the lateral collateral ligament, the posterior third of the capsular ligament, the arcuate ligament, and the popliteus tendon and its aponeurosis.

The lateral joint capsule also gives rise to the meniscofemoral and meniscotibial (coronary) attachments of the lateral meniscus. The sickle-shaped lateral meniscus is situated between the lateral femoral and the lateral tibial condyles (Fig. 19-7). The anterior and posterior horns of the meniscus are attached to the nonarticular tibial plateau. The lateral meniscus is thinner than that located medially and covers approximately two thirds of the lateral tibial condyle.

The intracapsular, extrasynovial anterior cruciate ligament (ACL) is a fan-shaped structure that is 11 mm wide and 31 to 38 mm long in the adult knee. This ligament takes its origin from the anteromedial tibial eminence and passes obliquely and cephalad to attach to the medial aspect of the lateral femoral condyle within the intercondylar notch. Some of the fibers of the anteromedial bundle of the ACL attach to the anterior horn of the lateral meniscus, while the posterior fibers blend into the posterior horn.

Two additional ligamentous structures are present in the

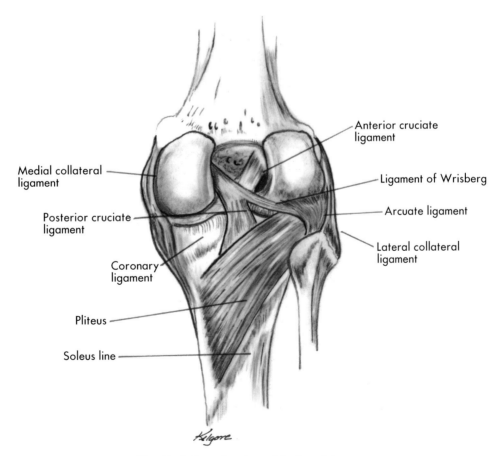

**Fig. 19-6.** Posterior view of the knee joint.

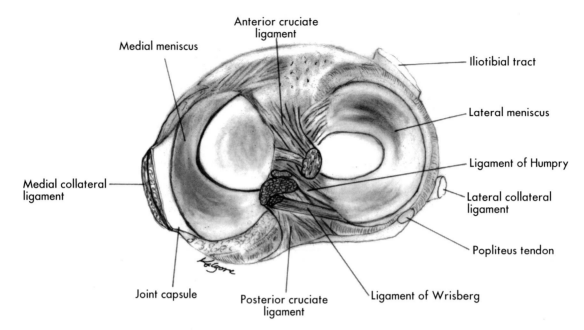

Medial meniscus

Anterior cruciate ligament

Iliotibial tract

Lateral meniscus

Ligament of Humpry

Medial collateral ligament

Lateral collateral ligament

Popliteus tendon

Joint capsule

Posterior cruciate ligament

Ligament of Wrisberg

**Fig. 19-7.** Ligaments and menisci of the knee joint.

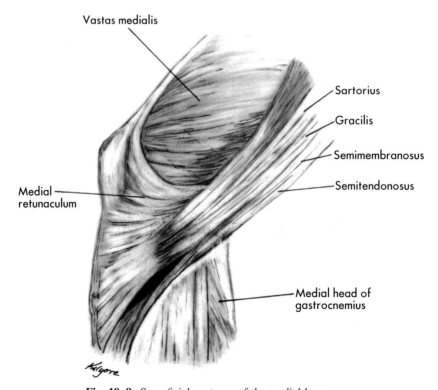

Vastas medialis

Sartorius

Gracilis

Semimembranosus

Semitendonosus

Medial retunaculum

Medial head of gastrocnemius

**Fig. 19-8.** Superficial anatomy of the medial knee.

lateral compartment (Fig. 19-7): the anterior meniscofemoral ligament (or Humphrey's ligament) and the posterior meniscofemoral ligament (or Wrisberg's ligament). Each of these ligamentous structures arises from the posterior horn of the lateral meniscus. Wrisberg's ligament runs behind the posterior cruciate ligament (PCL), while Humphrey's ligament runs along the anterior border of the PCL. These ligaments then attach within the intercondylar notch adjacent to the attachment of the PCL.

### The medial compartment

The most superficial supporting element of the medial compartment is the medial extensor retinaculum (Fig. 19-8). The pes anserinus group (the conjoining aponeurosis of the sartorius, gracilis, and semitendinosus muscles) crosses the medial aspect of the knee joint to attach at the antero-medial body of the tibia. The semimembranosus muscle divides into five arms that support the posteromedial segments of the joint capsule. One of these branches also contributes an attachment to the medial meniscus, which acts to draw the meniscus posteriorly with knee flexion. The tibial arm of the biceps femoris and the medial head of the gastrocnemius span the posterior aspect of the medial compartment, offering dynamic support to the posteromedial compartment.

The medial collateral and patellofemoral ligaments arise from the adductor tubercle of the femur immediately beneath the semimembranosus (Fig. 19-9). The patellofemoral ligament courses to the medial facet of the patella, offering restraint to lateral patellar subluxation. The medial collateral ligament is composed of a superficial and a deep layer.[2] The superficial leaf of the medial collateral ligament, which in the adult is 8 to 10 cm long, courses distally to insert into the proximal tibial metaphysis. The deep leaf of the medial collateral ligament is intimately attached to the medial capsular ligament (Fig. 19-7).

The anterior third of the medial capsular ligament, like its lateral counterpart, provides little in the way of joint stability. The middle third of this ligament lies immediately beneath the superficial medial collateral ligament and offers secondary restraint to abduction. The thicker posterior third of the capsular ligament, termed the posterior oblique ligament, is considered a secondary restraint to anteromedial rotatory motion.

The medial meniscus is two to three times thicker than the lateral meniscus and is more intimately attached to the joint capsule by the meniscofemoral and meniscotibial contributions from the medial capsular ligament.

The medial compartment is bound laterally by the PCL. The PCL is composed of two (posteromedial and anterolateral) bundles or fascicles. It arises from the lateral side of the medial femoral condyle, within the intercondylar notch, and runs posterior to the medial border of the ACL to insert on the tibial fovea.

### The anterior knee

Six muscles comprise the quadriceps femoris: the rectus femoris, the vastus medialis longus, the vastus medialis

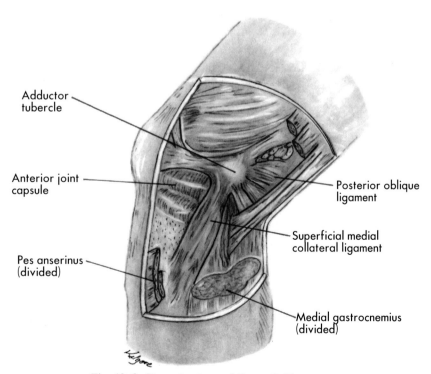

Adductor tubercle

Anterior joint capsule

Pes anserinus (divided)

Posterior oblique ligament

Superficial medial collateral ligament

Medial gastrocnemius (divided)

**Fig. 19-9.** Deep structures of the medial knee.

obliquus, the vastus lateralis, the vastus intermedius, and the articularis genu (Fig. 19-10). This collection of muscles converges to form the quadriceps tendon, which then inserts on the superior aspect of the patella.

The patellar tendon originates at the inferior pole of the patella and inserts distally on the tibial tuberosity. The patella is of critical importance to proper functioning of the extensor mechanism because it serves as a "pulley" for the quadriceps extension of the knee.

Sandwiched between the patella and the skin of the anterior knee is the prepatellar bursa. The infrapatellar bursa lies immediately posterior to the patellar tendon. The infrapatellar fat pad (of Hoffa) lies between the anterior joint space and the infrapatellar bursa (Fig. 19-11). Three redundant folds of synovium—termed infrapatellar, supra-

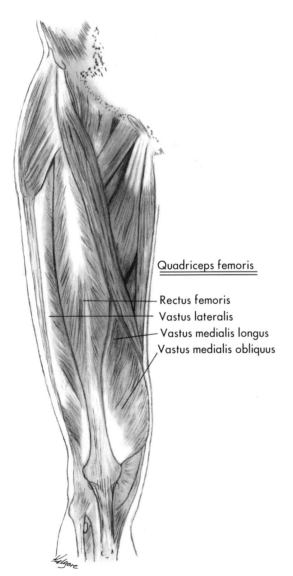

Quadriceps femoris

— Rectus femoris
— Vastus lateralis
— Vastus medialis longus
Vastus medialis obliquus

**Fig. 19-10.** Extensor mechanism of the knee. The quadriceps femoris is composed of the rectus femoris, the vastus medialis longus, the vastus medialis obliquus, the vastus lateralis, the vastus intermedius, and the articularis genu.

patellar, and medial plicae—are commonly found within the anterior knee joint (Fig. 19-12). These plicae are remnants of the knee's embryonic development.

## FUNCTIONAL ANATOMY

The knee joint is capable of six fundamental motions (three transitional and three rotational). Transitional motions include anterior-posterior drawer, medial-lateral translation, and distraction-compression of the joint surfaces. Rotational motions consist of flexion-extension, abduction-adduction, and internal-external rotation of the tibia. These motions are produced and modified through the complex interplay of the bony foundation, ligamentous stabilizers, meniscal stabilizers, and surrounding muscular assemblies.

The moderating mechanisms of the knee are considered either dynamic or static. The dynamic stabilizers, or restraints, of the knee are elastic and include muscular and ligamentous elements. The static, or inelastic, restraints of the knee are dependent on joint geometry, which generally increases as joint contact forces increase.

### Range of motion

Inasmuch as the knee is a hinge joint, motion is greatest in the sagittal plane, ranging from 0° when fully extended to 140° at full flexion. Little motion occurs in the transverse plane with full extension due to the interlocking mechanism of the longer medial femoral condyle with the medial meniscus. Rotational motion of the joint increases as the knee is flexed. Maximum rotation occurs at 90° of flexion, ranging from 0° to 45° of external rotation and 0° to 30° of internal rotation. When flexed beyond 90°, rotational mobility diminishes due to recruitment of muscular restraints. Varus and valgus mobility, in full extension, are essentially nil because of the stabilizing effect of the medial and lateral collateral ligamentous structures.

### Bony stability

If only the osseous structures are considered, the knee possesses little intrinsic stability. Because of the downward posterior slope of the tibial plateau, the knee is inherently unstable in the anteroposterior plane. Were it not for the ACL and the meniscotibial attachments of both the medial and lateral menisci, the femur would slide off posteriorly in full extension.

### Central stability

The centrally located cruciate ligaments are of prime importance to normal knee kinematics. The ACL is considered the primary restraint to anterior tibial displacement. This ligament is responsible for 85% of the total anterior constraint of the knee.[3] In addition, the ACL acts to blend the rotational and translational motion necessary for normal knee kinematics. Most authors recognize two nonparallel fascicles or bundles to the ACL.[4] The anteromedial bundle is taut while the knee is flexed, while the shorter postero-lateral bundle is relatively lax; in extension, both fascicles

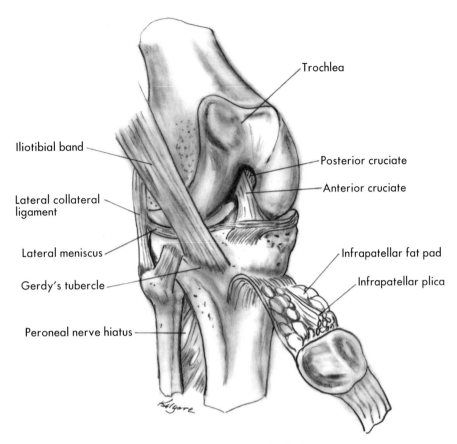

**Fig. 19-11.** Infrapatellar fat pad and plica.

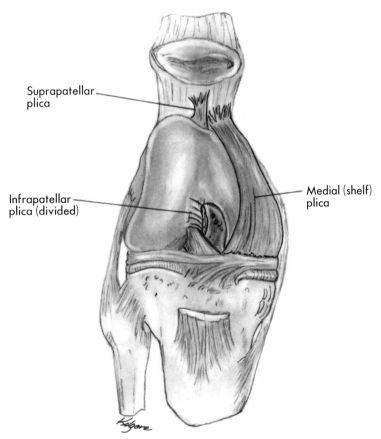

**Fig. 19-12.** Intrasynovial plica of the knee joint.

are equally burdened. The posterolateral bundle of the ACL is the first fascicle disrupted during hyperextension injury. The ACL is also credited as the primary restraint to internal tibial rotation as well as a secondary restraint to both valgus stress and external tibial rotation.[5]

The PCL is regarded as the central stabilizer of the knee joint. This structure accounts for 95% of the total posterior restraining force of the knee, and is thus considered the primary restraint to straight posterior drawer. It offers no restriction to anterior drawer motion.[6] Similar to its anterior counterpart, the PCL is composed of two bundles—anterolateral and posteromedial—which tighten in flexion and extension, respectively. Compared with the ACL the PCL possesses a greater cross-sectional area and twice the tensile strength.

Two other central ligamentous structures, Wrisberg's ligament and Humphry's ligament, have been identified in 80% of cadaveric studies. The ligament of Humphry runs along the anterior border of the PCL and is taut in knee flexion. The ligament of Wrisberg, by virtue of its more posterior location (coursing along the posterior border of the PCL), tightens in extension. With internal rotation of the tibia, both of these ligaments tighten, resisting posterior drawer translation.

### Medial ligamentous stability

The medial collateral ligament is considered the primary restraint to abduction stress (Fig. 19-13), contributing 78% of the total valgus restraint.[6] Should medial collateral ligament disruption occur, the cruciate ligaments become the primary restraints to an abduction stress. The medial collateral ligament (particularly the superficial leaf) also

offers the primary restraint to external tibial rotation in both flexion and extension of the joint.

### Lateral ligamentous stability

The lateral collateral ligament is considered the primary restraint to varus (abduction) stress (Fig. 19-14), contributing 69% of the total restraint.[6] The lateral collateral ligament becomes lax by 4% with flexion of the knee but relinquishes none of its stabilizing potential. This ligament is also considered a secondary restraint for internal and external tibial rotation. Other laterally positioned stabilizers of the knee include the popliteus and iliotibial band, which provide secondary restraint to internal and external tibial rotation as well as varus rotation in flexion.

### Menisci

Under normal circumstances, the menisci serve to 1) provide stability, 2) aid in lubrication, 3) act as shock absorbers, 4) prevent synovial impingement, 5) limit flexion and extension, and 6) provide an increase in joint congruity, which reduces contact stress. The wedge-shaped fibrocartilaginous medial and lateral menisci compensate for the incongruity between the femoral and tibial articular surfaces, effectively converting the tibial plateau into a "socket" joint. At the microscopic level, the collagen matrix of the meniscus is arranged at the periphery in a circumferential fashion, increasing its tensile strength in compression, while the midzone of the meniscus possesses a radial orientation, which acts to resist longitudinal splitting. The proteoglycan held within this collagen matrix serves to lubricate the joint surfaces.

The menisci have been shown to carry 60% of the total

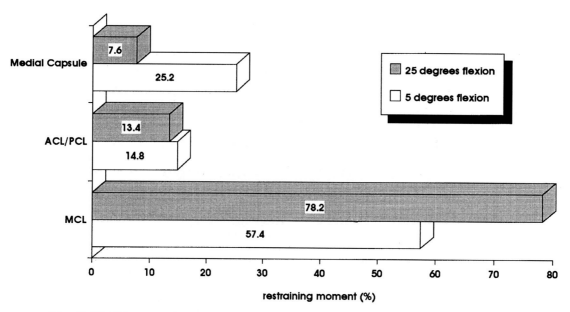

**Fig. 19-13.** Valgus restraining structures of the knee joint. This graph represents the structures responsible for valgus stability of the knee while at 25° and 5° of flexion. Each structure's relative contribution to this stability is represented in terms of percentage of total restraining moment.

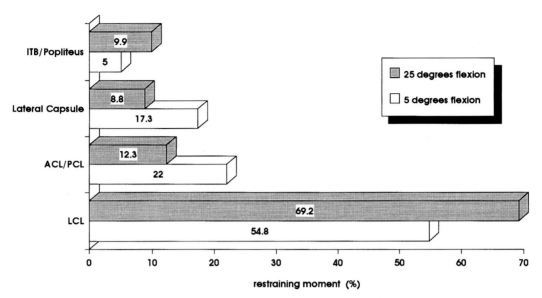

**Fig. 19-14.** Varus restraining structures of the knee joint. This graph represents the structures responsible for varus stability of the knee while at 25° and 5° of flexion. Each structure's relative contribution to this stability is represented in terms of percentage of total restraining moment.

load placed across the femorotibial joint in weight-bearing.[7] The menisci also serve to distribute weight over a broader area of the tibial plateau.

The thicker medial meniscus, coupled with the longer length of the medial femoral condyle, results in the so-called "screw-home" mechanism of the knee. This interlocking mechanism produces external rotation of the tibia when the knee is fully extended. Disruption of either meniscus invalidates the normal screw-home mechanism (explaining a lack of joint stability perceived by the patient having sustained meniscal injury during stance). This mechanism is "unlocked" by the action of the popliteus muscle, which also retracts the lateral meniscus as the knee is flexed beyond 90°. The popliteus is the only muscle capable of producing external tibial rotation of an extended knee.

### Anterior stability

The primary unit maintaining the femur on the tibia anteriorly is the patella and quadriceps femoris mechanism. Should some delay in contraction of the quadriceps occur, the PCL can provide the necessary check-reign. However, should the load be excessive or applied too rapidly, the PCL will fail. Compressive forces across the patellofemoral joint space are inordinately high.[8] Joint reaction forces across the patellofemoral joint during stair-climbing may be as high as 3.3 times body weight. This may increase to a value of 7.8 times body weight with deep knee bends.

### MECHANISM OF INJURY

The mechanisms of knee injury can be subdivided into two major types: microtrauma and macrotrauma.

### Microtrauma

Microtrauma is an overuse syndrome resulting from multiple submaximal insults, which ultimately produce an inflammatory response. Clinical presentations of microtraumatic injuries usually become apparent over time, and thus the patient does not recall a definite precipitating event. Specific forms of microtrauma include low load/high repetition, high load/low repetition, and excessive load/abnormal biomechanics. Microtraumatic injury occurs if there is a lack of conditioning (eg, strength or flexibility), improper technique, excessive fatigue, or if an exceptional degree of performance is required. Anatomic considerations such as alignment of the joint at the time of the injury or limb length inequality are also important determinates. Rehabilitative programs attempt to address these variables in order to avoid repeated injury.

**Manifestations of microtrauma.** Microtraumatic injury can present as sprain, strain, tendinitis, capsulitis, or pressure injury. Sprains occur secondary to stretching or tearing of a noncontractile unit such as a ligament or joint capsule. A strain results from the stretching or tearing of a contractile element or tendoperiosteal insertion of the muscle (Sharpey's fibers). Tendinitis is the result of tendon inflammation. Capsulitis occurs following capsular injury and inflammation. Pressure injuries, such as chondromalacia, result from repetitive loading of the articular surfaces followed by an inflammatory response and degradation of the articular cartilage surface.

### Macrotrauma

Macrotrauma occurs when the stresses applied to the joint are of sufficient amplitude to produce immediate symp-

**Table 19-1.** American Medical Association grading of muscular injury

| | |
|---|---|
| Mild | Local tenderness with minimal swelling, mild spasm, and little disability (1st degree or grade I) |
| Moderate | Local tenderness, swelling, ecchymosis, moderate muscle spasm, and moderate loss of strength (2nd degree or grade II) |
| Severe | Complete separation of muscle from muscle or muscle from tendon, marked pain, swelling, ecchymosis, and severe disability (3rd degree or grade III) |

From Committee on the Medical Aspects of Sports: *Standard nomenclature of athletic injuries,* Chicago, 1966, American Medical Association.

**Table 19-2.** American Medical Association grading of ligamentous injury

| | |
|---|---|
| Mild | Local tenderness with minimal swelling, no instability, and little disability (1st degree or grade I) |
| Moderate | Local tenderness, swelling, slight to moderate instability, and moderate disability (2nd degree or grade II) |
| Severe | Complete ligamentous disruption, marked instability, severe disability, tenderness, swelling, and hemarthrosis (3rd degree or grade III) |

From Committee on the Medical Aspects of Sports: *Standard nomenclature of athletic injuries,* Chicago, 1966, American Medical Association.

toms. Variables that appear important in macrotraumatic knee injuries include poor contact surface, improper footgear, suboptimal muscle strength, joint instability, and previous injury to that knee. Macrotraumatic injuries are either direct (contusion, producing a compressive injury) or indirect (resulting from rotation or distraction forces). The American Medical Association has attempted to provide a standardized grading system for strain injury to the contractile structures (Table 19-1) as well as for sprain injury to the noncontractile unit (Table 19-2).

## THE KNEE EXAMINATION

History-taking in patients with knee injuries is goal-specific, intended to determine the mechanism resulting in injury and the degree of disability. Physical examination of the knee is meant to appraise the presence or absence of pain, swelling, and instability. Ordering laboratory or radiographic evaluation before obtaining a history and performing a physical examination is inappropriate. A thorough interview and examination will yield more information at less cost than any of the ancillary studies.

It is also important for the treating physician to record specifically and concisely the information gathered in visitation with the patient. Some examiners use a worksheet to achieve consistency in the information obtained (Fig. 19-15). This allows the physician continuing with the patient's care to receive a clear picture what happened to the patient and why.

### The interview

As a rule, the history obtained in evaluating knee injuries is the most enlightening portion of the encounter because pain, muscular spasm, and the possibility of associated injuries usually limit the physical examination. The intent of the interview is to identify the mechanism of injury; determine the extent of injury and the resultant degree of disability; and delineate any previous injury to the knee. Reconstructing the events at the time of the injury allows the examiner to determine that one type of injury is more likely than another, and to tailor the examination accordingly.

Patients present as a result of either a memorable macrotraumatic event or a nonspecific microtraumatic event superimposed on an existing chronic problem. Patients are generally quite specific in describing the location of their discomfort at the outset. The history should include a description of the event. Was the knee flexed or extended at the time of injury? Was the knee weight-bearing? Was the foot internally or externally rotated? Was the force applied in a varus, valgus, rotatory, or hyperextending fashion?

Seventy percent of patients stating that they noted an audible pop or snap at the time of injury will disclose on arthroscopy a disruption of the ACL.[9] However, it has also been noted that approximately two thirds of patients sustaining an ACL tear hear no such sound.[5] Other possible causes of this sensation include patellar dislocation, meniscal tear, or osteochondral fracture.

The sensation of instability of the joint—described by the patient as a "giving way," "collapsing," or "buckling"—is common in those with chronic knee problems. This sensation is the result of quadriceps relaxation during weight-bearing or frank quadriceps weakness. It is actually a neurophysiologic reflex protecting the disrupted knee joint. In the acutely injured knee this historical element should prompt careful investigation.

The degree and timing of maximal swelling also offer clues to the type of injury sustained. Meniscal injury typically will produce maximal swelling during the initial 12 to 24 hours following injury. Conversely, ACL injuries, osteochondral fractures, peripheral meniscal tears, and patellar fractures generally swell appreciably within the first 12 hours postinjury. Excessive swelling occurs with significant ligamentous injury in only 25% of cases[2] because of the associated synovial and capsular disruption resulting in an extravasation of blood into the soft tissue surrounding the knee joint. Recurrent swelling with twisting or pivotal motion generally indicates meniscal or femorotibial pathology, while swelling reappearing after ascending or descending slopes generally denotes patellofemoral disorders.

It is also important to ascertain the extent and rapidity of disability. Could the individual continue the activity in

**LEFT    RIGHT**

Athlete:
Sport
Position
Non Athlete:     Job Description

Swelling: Immediate  Late  Degree     Aspirated     **WHAT**
Unable to walk: Immediate  Late     **HOW**
Exercises  Crutches  Taped  Cast     **WHEN**
Sitting  In/Out of Auto  Stopping     **WHERE**
Stairs:  Up  Down  Unable
Loss of Motion:  Related to
Giving  Catching  Popping  Locking  Twisting  Pivoting  Cutting
Swelling:  Degree  Recurrent  Related To
Pain  Location  Activity Related  Rest     Height  Weight

Initial Treatment: Dr.     Referred By:

HISTORY:

---

Date ___
Name ___     Chart No ___     Age ___  Sex ___

**Left**

Observation on entering:  Walking ☐  Limp ☐  Cane ☐  Crutches ☐
Observation on standing:

Normal  Varus  Valgus  Tiabia Vara P-3rd     **Alignment AP**
Tibial Torsion: Internal or External

Normal  Flexed  Hyperextended     **Alignment Lateral**

Patellae:
Patella Posture Sitting Flexed 90 degrees
Lateral  High     Patella Tendon Alignment
Bayonet  Q
Enlarged  Tender     Tibial Tuberosity
Dysplastic D-3rd     VMO - Leg Extended 45 degrees
Patella Mobility Passive - 45 degrees flexion
Hypermobile  Dislocates
Apprehensive  Tender     Patella Excursion on Extension Flexion
Lateral Slide Termninal or
Initial Crepitation/Plica
Painful Longitudinal - Transverse     Passive Patella Crepitation Knee Extended 0 Degrees
Painful  Medial-Lateral     Palpation Facets Patella
Medial Retinaculum  Quadriceps Tendon     Palpation About Patella
Patellar Tendon  Abnormal Contour
Swelling(synovitis) and Patella Ballottement
Mild  Moderate  Severe     Grade:  +Mild  ++Moderate  +++Severe

Ligamentous Instability:

| | | | | |
|---|---|---|---|---|
| Abduction Stress | Adduction Stress | | Abduction Stress | Adduction Stress |
| | | Hyperextended | | |
| | | 0 Degrees Ext | | |
| | | 30 Degrees Flexion | | |
| Anterior | Posterior | Drawer Test | Anterior | Posterior |
| | | Tibia Internally Rotated | | |
| | | Tibia Neutral | | |
| | | Tibia Externally Rotated | | |
| | | Lachman Test | | |
| | | External Rotation Recurvatum Test | | |
| | | Jerk Test | | |
| | | Palpation Painful | | |

Impression:

Degree of Recurvatum
Range of Motion     Painful on Forcing
Hip Motion, Normal - limited     Quadriceps tone
Hip Flexor Strength     Tight Heel Cords - degree
Tight Hamstrings - degree     Popping,catching, slipping
Tumor: lat, medial,popliteal     Pes Anserinus bursitis
Semimembranosus tentonitis     Fabella syndrome
Twisting - circle jog unilateral     Squating - duck walk

**Right**

Observation on entering:
Normal  Varus  Valgus  Tibia Vara P-3rd     **Alignment AP**
Tibial Torsion: Internal or External

Normal  Flexed  Hyperextended     **Alignment Lateral**

Patella Posture Sitting Flexed 90 degrees
Lateral  High     Patella Tendon Alignment
Bayonet  Q
Enlarged  Tender     Tibial Tuberosity
Dysplastic D-3rd     VMO - Leg Extended 45 degrees
Patella Mobility Passive - 45 degrees flexion
Hypermobile  Dislocates
Apprehensive  Tender     Patella Excursion on Extension Flexion
Lateral Slide Terminal or
Initial Crepitation/Plica
Painful Longitudinal - Transverse
Painful  Medial-Lateral     Palpation Facets Patella
Medial Retinaculum  Quadriceps Tendon     Palpation About Patella
Patellar Tendon  Abnormal Contour
Mild  Moderate  Severe     ++Moderate  +++Severe

**Fig. 19-15.** Knee interview and examination worksheet. (Modification of Hughston Clinic worksheet from Hughston, J.C.: *Knee ligaments: injury and repair.* St. Louis: Mosby-Year Book, Inc., 1993.)

which he or she was engaged, or was disability immediate? (Some individuals seemingly "shake off" or "walk off" the injury and continue play, later to discover a complete capsular tear that permits joint decompression.) Individuals sustaining a total diastasis of a ligamentous structure (grade III injury) also sustain disruption of pain-receptor fibers and thus experience surprisingly little joint discomfort.

Locking of the knee occurs in three forms: 1) pseudolocking, 2) recurrent locking, and 3) true locking. *Pseudolocking* is the sensation of locking in the absence of a mechanical cause. This is usually the result of effusion, pain, and muscle spasm. This restriction of joint mobility is generally seen in grade I and grade II ligamentous injuries. In *recurrent locking* the patient (who has sustained a displaced bucket-handle tear of the meniscus) will report a history of locking episodes in which the knee locks and unlocks, depending on the position of the joint. Less commonly, recurrent locking occurs due to an intra-articular loose body or a torn cruciate ligament that has become wedged between the condyle and meniscus. Individuals with this type of locking are able through some maneuver to "unlock" the joint and resume their activity. Joint locking immediately following injury indicates a "true" persistent locking event. *True locking* is the result of a mechanical block interpositioned between the meniscus and femoral condyle.

Individuals sustaining a significant injury report a lack of confidence in the knee joint. Joint instability is most commonly reported during activities of daily living such as going up or down stairs and getting into or out of a car, chair, or bed. Answers to these questions can queue the examiner to a significant injury when associated with a subsequent injury. Any antecedent therapies received should be included in the history.

### The examination

Physical examination of the knee is performed with specific attention to those portions of the examination that the history suggests as the possible site of pathology. It is *imperative* to establish a "measure of normal," which is easily obtained by performing the anticipated examination maneuvers on the unaffected, knee prior to examination of the affected joint. This technique serves to allay the fear that most patients have about examination of the injured knee by actually displaying the examination to the patient. Gentle examination is essential; overzealous or hurried testing will prompt protective muscular spasm and will result in an inaccurate examination. The patient should be observed on entry to the emergency department, and the use of any assistive devices (eg, crutches, cane, brace, wrap) should be noted.

The presence of a limp should always be considered abnormal. An antalgic (painful) limp, with its characteristic short-stance phase while weight-bearing on the injured side, is typically seen with knee injury. If hip joint motion is limited because of pain from injury or an inflammatory process, the normal neutral attitude of the pelvis and trunk during the swing-through phase of gait is disrupted. The patient appears to thrust the hip and trunk forward to continue forward progression. A short-limb limp will display a depression of the trunk and pelvis on the involved side during the stance phase. Weakness of the quadriceps femoris will also result in a characteristic limp. These individuals, who display a near-normal gait on level ground, will hyperextend the knee on stair-climbing, locking it into position during the stance phase. This is followed by an elevation of the pelvis of the uninvolved side as if to vault over the involved extremity.

Alignment of the joint is assessed in the standing, sitting, and supine positions. Patellar alignment should be noted. With the patient seated and the knees flexed 90°, the patellae normally point directly anteriorly and slightly upward. Observance of laterally facing patellae, patellar elevation, or patellar depression should be recorded. The quadriceps (Q) angle is the angle formed between two imaginary lines, the first line extending from the anterosuperior iliac spine to the midpoint of the patella and the second from the midpoint of the patella to the tibial tuberosity (Fig. 19-16). Normally the Q angle is less than 15° in women and less than 10° in men. Excessive Q angle measurements indicate possible patellofemoral problems. Atrophic changes of the quadriceps or gastrocnemius muscle groups signal a chronic disorder.

Joint swelling is an important finding indicating significant cruciate disruption in 90% of cases[10,18] when compared with operative findings. Generalized swelling normally signals an intra-articular site of injury. Localized swelling or ecchymosis indicates a local injury. The anterolateral and anteromedial extensor retinaculum, immediately adjacent to the patellar tendon, possesses the least-supporting tissue and is the best site to appreciate mild swelling. With the patient standing, the presence of a popliteal mass may be appreciated when viewing the posterior knee and suggests the existence of a Baker's cyst.

Range of motion of the knee, through both active and passive flexion and extension, is the next element of the examination, and any limitation should be recorded. Attempts to range the joint beyond what is comfortable to the patient are discouraged. If the knee is maintained in a locked position, this section of the examination should be omitted. The degree of hamstring tightness is tested if the injury is not too acute. This is accomplished (while the patient is in a supine position) by flexing both the hip and the knee to 90°, followed by maximal extension of the knee. Hamstring tightness is noted as an angle created by the anterior tibial surface and the horizontal plane, at the point where resistance to further extension of the knee is met (Fig. 19-17). Anterior knee pain is often the result of hamstring tightness in the absence of other pathology.[2]

The knee is then palpated for specific areas of abnormal temperature, effusion, induration, and tenderness. Palpation is generally the most helpful portion of the examination. It

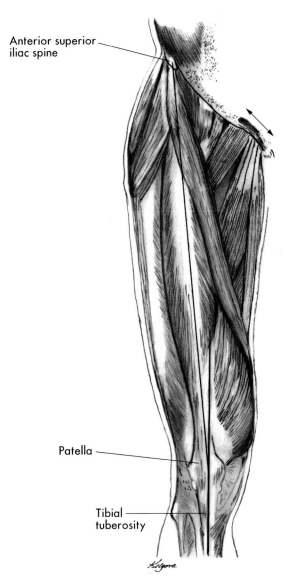

Fig. 19-16. Q-angle (quadriceps) determination technique. The Q angle is the angle formed between two imaginary lines, the first line extending from the anterior superior iliac spine to the midpoint of the patella and the second from the midpoint of the patella to the tibial tuberosity. Normally the Q angle is less than 15° in females and less than 10° in males.

is best to avoid the area cited by the patient as maximally tender until the end of this segment of the examination. Should the use of arthrocentesis with instillation of local anesthetic be anticipated, palpation must be done first because the anesthetic will obscure any tender areas. Specific areas of attention laterally include the lateral femoral epicondyles, the posterolateral corner of the joint line, and the fibular head. Medially, the joint line from anterior to posterior, and the medial femoral and tibial epicondyles should be palpated. Palpation of the quadriceps tendon, patellar tendon, patellar facets (Fig. 19-18), popliteus tendon, hamstring tendons, and popliteal fossa completes this portion of the examination.

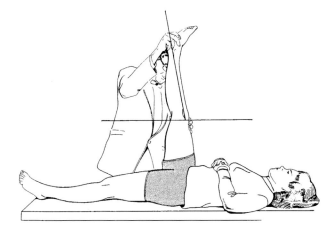

Fig. 19-17. Hamstring tightness testing. With the patient in the supine position on the examination table, both the hip and knee are flexed to 90°. The knee is then maximally extended until resistance is met. Should full extension not be attained, the angle formed by the horizontal plane and the anterior surface of the tibia is recorded. (From Hughston, J.C.: *Knee ligaments: injury and repair.* St. Louis: Mosby-Year Book, Inc., 1993.)

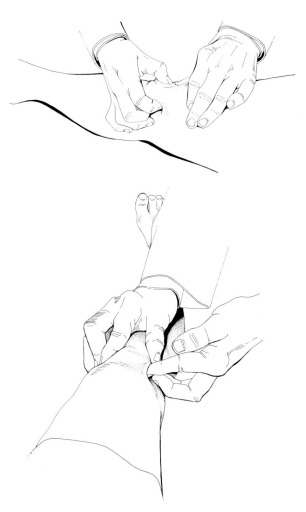

Fig. 19-18. Patellar facet palpation. The medial and lateral patellae are palpated for any evidence of tenderness, crepitance, or bony defect. (From Hughston, J.C.: *Knee ligaments: injury and repair.* St. Louis: Mosby-Year Book, Inc., 1993.)

To evaluate the knee for effusion or hemarthrosis, it is positioned in full extension, and the suprapatellar pouch is compressed by one hand. Concurrent palpation (using the other hand) of the medial and lateral parapatellar areas will evaluate fluid motion. An effusion is mobile, appearing and disappearing with suprapatellar pouch compression, while synovial thickening tends to be static and to possess a spongy quality when palpated.

The patellar compression test is performed with the patient in the supine position and the knee in 20° of flexion. The palm of the examiner's hand is used to depress the patella. Using a medial to lateral and proximal to distal motion (Fig. 19-19), the examiner seeks any evidence of crepitance or a "grinding" quality. Although classically used, this test is inconclusive in determining disruption of the posterior patellar surface or trochlea, or a patellar fracture. The knee must be in at least 20° of flexion to ensure patellar engagement with the trochlea and not the femoral metaphysis.

Passive lateral hypermobility of the patella is assessed with patient in a supine position. The examiner sits at the edge of the cart and the patient's hip is abducted and suspended over the examiner's thigh with the knee flexed 15° to 30°. With the quadriceps mechanism relaxed, the examiner then attempts to displace the patella laterally by applying laterally directed pressure to the medial patellar facet using his or her thumbs (Fig. 19-20). The test is positive if the quadriceps reflexly contract, a facial grimace appears, or abnormal laxity (compared with the opposite side) is noted. Should a positive response be received, it is

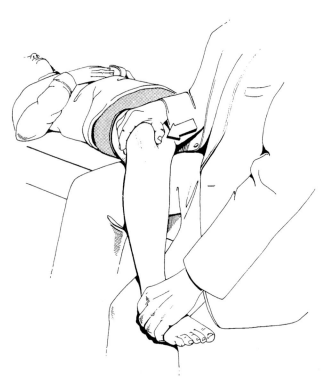

**Fig. 19-20.** Passive lateral hypermobility test of the patella. With the patient in the supine position on the examination table, the patient's hip is abducted and the leg is allowed to rest, suspended on the examiner's thigh. Once quadriceps relaxation is obtained the examiner applies a laterally directed force to the medial border of the patella, attempting to reproduce subluxation. (From Hughston, J.C.: *Knee ligaments: injury and repair.* St. Louis: Mosby-Year Book, Inc., 1993.)

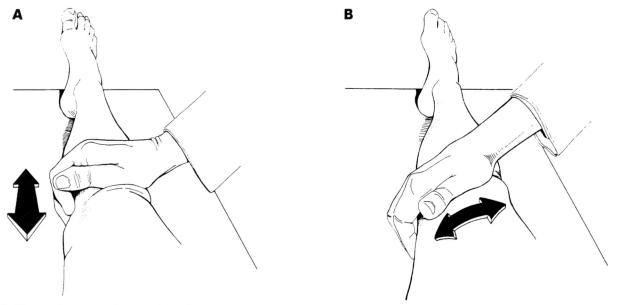

**Fig. 19-19.** Patellar compression test. **A** and **B,** With the patient in the supine position and the knee in 20° of flexion, the palm of the hand is used to depress the patella. Using a medial-to-lateral and proximal-to-distal motion, the examiner should seek any evidence of crepitance or grinding.

important to ask the patient if this sensation reproduces that experienced at the time of injury.

**Ligamentous stability testing.** A multitude of eponymonic ligament tests have been designed to assess the integrity of specific restraints of the knee. Knee stability tests can be divided into two broad types: those designed to test two-dimensional (anterior-posterior and medial-lateral) stability and those designed to examine rotatory (three-dimensional) stability. Pragmatically, all of the information necessary to arrive at the correct diagnosis can be derived from the anterior-posterior and medial-lateral stability tests. The joint's instability may then be stated as medially unstable (to valgus stress), laterally unstable (to varus stress), anteriorly unstable (to anterior drawer), or posteriorly unstable (to posterior drawer). Combined rotatory stability tests are designed to test multiple structures concurrently and rotational restrain soundness. While performing ligamentous testing of the knee joint some basic concepts must be kept in mind.[6]

- *Concept 1.* For each joint motion the knee possesses, there exist primary and secondary restraints (Table 19-3), which act in concert to restrict specific joint motion. The primary restraint also functions to protect the secondary restraints: it is "the first to go," and, once it is missing or deficient, the secondary restraints

are at risk of injury. A significant clinical laxity is index of significant primary restraint failure. A negative laxity test, however, means nothing.

- *Concept 2.* Clinical examination stresses are small compared with functional stresses. Stresses applied to the joint during clinical examination measure 10 to 20 pounds, while stresses applied to the knee during ambulation measure two to three times body weight. Therefore, stresses applied to the knee during strenuous activity are quite capable of unmasking clinically undetectable deficiencies of the primary and secondary restraints of the knee.

- *Concept 3.* Functional stability exists when the neuromuscular, ligamentous, and joint contact forces are capable of balancing the forces externally applied to the joint in question. This allows an explanation of the seemingly significant, clinically unstable injury that does not affect performance. It also lends credence to rehabilitation programs that facilitate a voluntary increase in the controllable element in the joint system, the neuromuscular unit.

- *Concept 4.* Physical examination of the joint is a subjective assessment that varies from one examiner to another and from day to day for a given examiner. It is also important to recognize that the "starting

**Table 19-3.** Primary and secondary restraints of the knee

| Applied stress | Knee position | Primary restraint | Secondary restraint |
|---|---|---|---|
| Valgus (abduction) | Extension | Superficial medial collateral ligament | Anterior cruciate ligament<br>Posterior capsule<br>Deep medial collateral ligament<br>Posterior cruciate ligament |
| | Flexion | Superficial medial collateral ligament | Anterior cruciate ligament<br>Posterior cruciate ligament |
| Varus (adduction) | Extension | Lateral collateral ligament | Anterior cruciate ligament<br>Posterior cruciate ligament |
| | Flexion | Lateral collateral ligament | Anterior cruciate ligament<br>Posterior cruciate ligament<br>Popliteus, iliotibial band<br>Lateral capsule |
| Hyperextension | | Anterior cruciate ligament | Posterior capsule<br>Posterior cruciate ligament |
| Anterior drawer | | Anterior cruciate ligament | Superficial medial collateral ligament |
| Posterior drawer | | Posterior cruciate ligament | Posterior capsule |
| External tibial rotation | Flexion | Superficial medial collateral ligament | Anterior cruciate ligament<br>Lateral collateral ligament<br>Popliteus<br>Posteromedial capsule |
| | Extension | Anterior cruciate ligament | Superficial medial collateral ligament |
| Internal tibial rotation | Flexion | Anterior cruciate ligament | Posterior cruciate ligament<br>Lateral collateral ligament<br>Popliteus<br>Iliotibial band |
| | Extension | Anterior cruciate ligament | Lateral collateral ligament<br>Popliteus<br>Iliotibial band<br>Posterior cruciate ligament |

point" or neutral position of an injured knee may be quite different from that of an uninjured joint (eg, additional restraints of the knee with ACL rupture may be due to muscle spasm, hemarthrosis of the knee joint, or meniscal tear with displacement).

In performing any of the following tests, the existence of a "firm" endpoint, even in the face of some instability, may be considered representative of a grade II injury, while a "soft" or "mushy" endpoint heralds the existence of a grade III injury. All of the tests, with the exception of Apley's compression and distraction tests, are performed on a supine patient with the patient's arms at his or her side. If these tests are performed with the patient in a seated position, the quadriceps mechanism obscures possible abnormalities.

***Two-dimensional tests.*** Abduction (valgus) stress testing is designed to assess the integrity of the medial collateral ligament. For this test, the patient is in the supine position and the examiner stands at the patient's side. The proximal hand (left, if examining the right knee and vice versa) is used initially to cradle the knee while the other hand grasps the forefoot. The hip is abducted slightly to allow the knee to dangle over the edge of the cart or table and the thigh is allowed to rest on the cart (Fig. 19-21). The knee is then flexed 60°, maintaining some support of the forefoot. The proximal hand is now used to stabilize the lateral knee joint. The hand grasping the foot is then drawn toward the examiner, abducting the lower leg in a gentle swinging motion. The arc of abduction should be small

initially and increase progressively until a firm endpoint is appreciated. Next, the knee is extended slowly while valgus force is applied at the foot in a pendulum motion. Particular attention is paid to the laxity that the knee displays in 30° of flexion and in full extension. The test is considered diagnostic of collateral ligament injury if medial joint space opening is noted (Fig. 19-22). Quadriceps relaxation must be present to perform a valid examination.

The adduction (varus) stress test is similar to the abduction study and is designed to assess the integrity of the lateral collateral ligament. For this test, the patient is in the supine position and the examiner at the patient's feet. The proximal hand (right, if examining the right knee and vice versa) is used initially to cradle the knee while the other hand grasps the forefoot. The hip is abducted to allow the knee to dangle over the edge of the cart or table while the thigh rests on the cart (Fig. 19-23). The knee is then flexed 60° while maintaining some support of the forefoot. The proximal hand is then used to stabilize the medial knee joint. The hand grasping the foot is then drawn toward the examiner in a gentle swinging motion, adducting the lower leg. The arc of adduction should be small initially and progressively increase until a firm endpoint is appreciated. Next, the knee is extended slowly while varus force is applied at the forefoot in a swinging motion. Particular attention is paid to the laxity that the knee displays in 30° of flexion and in full extension. This test is considered diagnostic of collateral ligament injury if lateral joint space

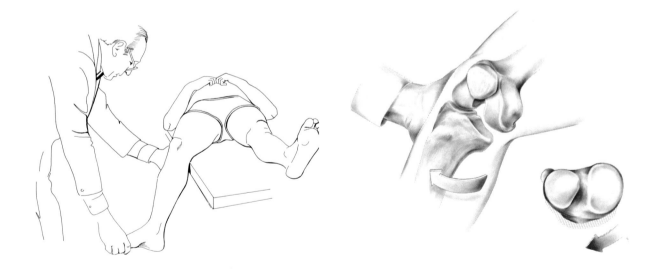

**A**    **B**

**Fig. 19-21.** Valgus (abduction) stress test. **A,** The patient is in the supine position, and the hip is abducted slightly. The forefoot is grasped and the knee is flexed to 30° with the lower leg suspended over the edge of the bed or cart. One hand offers resistance over the lateral joint line while the hand grasping the forefoot gently rocks the lower leg back and forth. This test is designed to elicit medial joint space opening, signifying medial collateral ligament disruption. Recorded information should include medial joint space widening at 30° and 0° of flexion. **B,** Anteromedial subluxation of the tibia when varus stress is applied. (From Hughston, J.C.: *Knee ligaments: injury and repair.* St. Louis: Mosby-Year Book, Inc., 1993.)

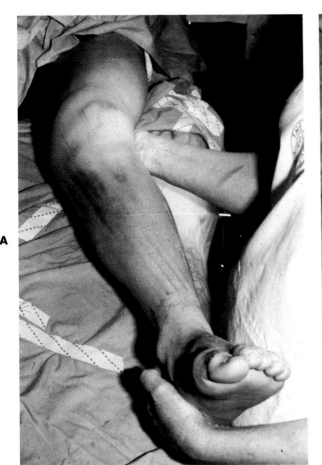
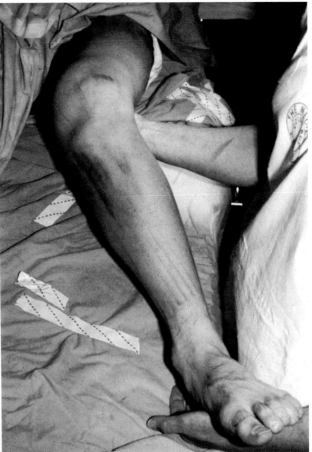

**Fig. 19-22.** Positive valgus stress test. **A,** This examination, performed with the patient under anesthesia, disclosed medial joint space opening on valgus stress testing at 0° of flexion. **B,** An even more significant test at 20° of flexion. This patient was found to have torn posterior cruciate and medial collateral ligaments. (From Hughston, J.C.: *Knee ligaments: injury and repair.* St. Louis: Mosby-Year Book, Inc., 1993.)

opening is noted. Quadriceps relaxation during the examination is imperative for a valid examination.

The Lachman test is felt by some to be the most sensitive test of ACL integrity, with a sensitivity of 87%[11] to 98%.[12] The patient is placed in a supine position with the arms across the abdomen. The knee is flexed 15° to 20° to allow relaxation of the hamstring group. The distal thigh is supported with one hand while the other grasps the proximal lower leg. The tibia is drawn forward (Fig. 19-24) in an attempt to displace it anteriorly. The test is felt to be positive if both tibial condyles demonstrate forward translation and the endpoint of forward glide of the tibia is not firm but is of an elastic nature. A false-negative test may occur if a bucket-handle tear of the meniscus blocks anterior translation of the tibia. Inasmuch as a false-positive test occurs as a result of PCL insufficiency, it is mandatory to exclude posterior instability before the Lachman test can be deemed positive.

Posterior cruciate ligament integrity is assessed using the posterior drawer and the gravity (or sag) tests. The posterior drawer test is performed with the patient supine, the hip flexed 45° to 60° and the knee flexed to 90°. The tibia is maintained in the neutral position and the foot rests flat on the cart, in neutral rotation, stabilized by the examiner's thigh. A posteriorly directed force is then applied to the proximal lower leg (Fig. 19-25). Should posterior translation of both tibial condyles be appreciated, PCL injury is probable.

The gravity, or sag, test is performed with the patient in a supine position. The hips are flexed to 45°, the knees to 90°, and the feet resting flat on the cart. Prominence of the tibial tuberosity of the injured extremity is compared with that of the uninjured side. The test is considered positive if the tibial tuberosity "sags" posteriorly (Fig. 19-26).

***Combined maneuvers.*** The external rotation recurvatum test is performed while the patient is in the supine

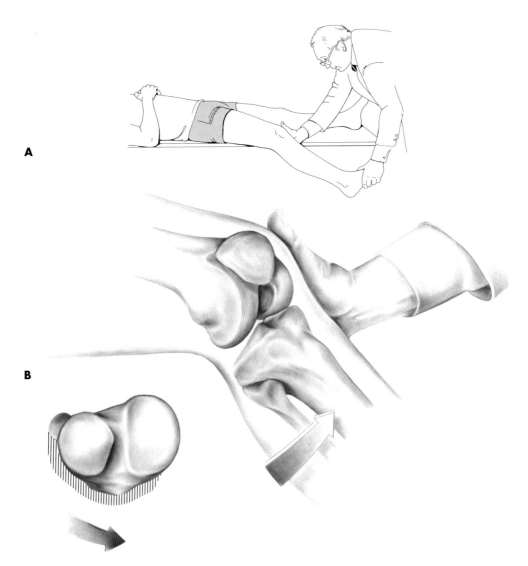

**A**

**B**

**Fig. 19-23.** Varus (adduction) stress test. **A,** The patient is in the supine position, and the hip is abducted slightly. The forefoot is grasped and the knee is flexed to 30° with the lower leg suspended over the edge of the bed or cart. One hand offers resistance over the medial joint line while the hand grasping the forefoot gently rocks the lower leg back and forth. This test is designed to elicit lateral joint space opening, signifying lateral collateral ligament disruption. Recorded information should include lateral joint space widening at 30° and 0° of flexion. **B,** Anterolateral subluxation of the tibia when varus stress is applied. (From Hughston, J.C.: *Knee ligaments: injury and repair.* St. Louis: Mosby-Year Book, Inc., 1993.)

position. The examiner grasps both great toes and lifts the entire lower extremity from the cart (Fig. 19-27), observing the knee for any degree of hyperextension or recurve. More importantly, external rotation of the tibial tubercle as the tibia rotates externally produces an apparent varus deformation of the knee that is indicative of posterolateral joint instability (Fig. 19-28).

The anterior drawer test, although not as sensitive to ACL injury as the Lachman or Noyes flexion-rotation drawer tests, is useful in demonstrating rotatory instability. This test is executed with the patient in the supine position with the hip flexed to 45° and the knee flexed to 90° to ensure hamstring relaxation (Fig. 19-29). The foot is in a

neutral position initially and is stabilized by the examiner's thigh. The examiner grasps the proximal tibial area, with the thumbs palpating the medial and lateral parapatellar joint line and the index fingers posteriorly palpating the hamstring for any lack of relaxation. If the hamstring group is taut, the patient is encouraged to relax. Once relaxation is attained, gentle anterior traction is applied. A jerking motion tends to encourage muscle spasm and pain, resulting in a false-negative test. This test is considered positive if the anterior translation of the tibial condyles is asymmetric with that of the opposite, uninjured knee. Should anterior translation be noted it is also important to note the quality of the endpoint. This test is repeated with the foot posi-

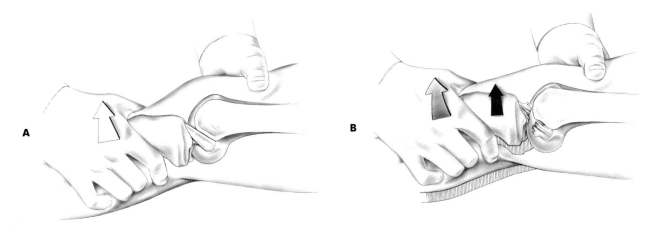

**Fig. 19-24.** Lachman test. **A**, With the patient in the supine position the knee is flexed 15° to 20°. The distal thigh is stabilized with one hand while the other hand grasps the proximal tibia and attempts to displace the tibia anteriorly. **B**, The appearance of Lachman test should the anterior cruciate ligament be disrupted. (From Hughston, J.C.: *Knee ligaments: injury and repair.* St. Louis: Mosby-Year Book, Inc., 1993.)

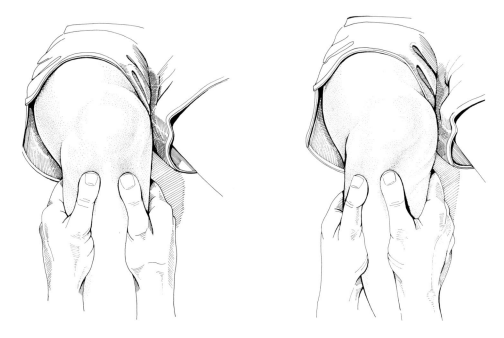

**Fig. 19-25.** Posterior drawer test. With the patient in the supine position, the hip is flexed 45° to 60° and the knee is flexed to 90°. The tibia is held in the neutral position and the foot rests flat on the cart. Using both hands, a push is applied to the tibia, attempting to produce a posterior translation. (From Hughston, J.C.: *Knee ligaments: injury and repair.* St. Louis: Mosby-Year Book, Inc., 1993.)

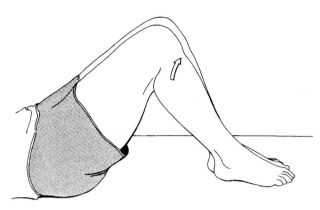

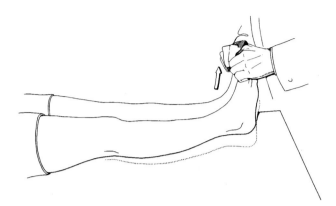

**Fig. 19-26.** Gravity (or sag) test. In the supine position the hips are flexed to 45° with the feet resting flat on the bed and the knees flexed to 90°. The knee is then viewed from the side for any evidence of loss of the tibial tuberosity prominence or anterior depression. (From Hughston, J.C.: *Knee ligaments: injury and repair.* St. Louis: Mosby-Year Book, Inc., 1993.)

**Fig. 19-27.** External rotation recurvatum test. In the supine position the great toe of each foot is grasped and entire leg is elevated from the cart, observing for any evidence of recurve of the lower extremity. (From Hughston, J.C.: *Knee ligaments: injury and repair.* St. Louis: Mosby-Year Book, Inc., 1993.)

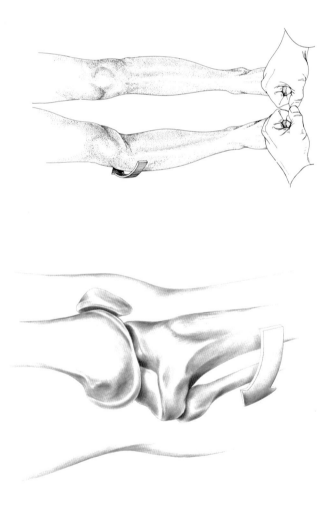

**Fig. 19-28.** External rotation recurvatum test. In addition to recurvatum external tibial rotation, this test is indicative of posterolateral knee injury. (From Hughston, J.C.: *Knee ligaments: injury and repair.* St. Louis: Mosby-Year Book, Inc., 1993.)

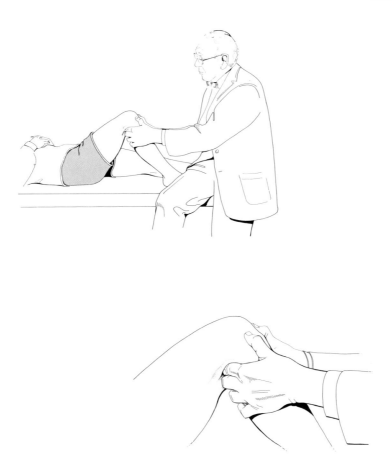

**Fig. 19-29.** Anterior drawer test. This test is performed with the patient in the supine position with the hip flexed to 45° and the knee flexed to 90°. The foot is placed in neutral and stabilized by the examiner's thigh. The proximal tibial area is grasped, with the thumbs palpating the medial and lateral parapatellar joint line and the index fingers palpating posteriorly. Gentle anterior traction is applied. The test is considered positive if there is anterior translation of the tibial condyles. (From Hughston, J.C.: *Knee ligaments: injury and repair.* St. Louis: Mosby-Year Book, Inc., 1993.)

tioned in 15° to 30° of internal and then external rotation. With translation occurring in neutral rotation, damage to the ACL is suspected. If instability is appreciated with the foot in external rotation, injury to the ACL and medial collateral ligament is suspected. In flexion and internal rotation, the posteromedial capsule is relaxed and thus is not subject to clinical stresses. Instability elicited while the foot is internally rotated generally indicates injury to ACL as well as to the lateral collateral ligament and arcuate complex. A false-negative anterior drawer test can occur when hemarthrosis, hamstring spasm, or displacement of a meniscus blocks anterior translation.

The Noyes flexion-rotation drawer test (Fig. 19-30) possesses elements of both the Lachman test and the pivot-shift test and is therefore useful in detecting both ACL and anterolateral rotatory instability. With the patient supine, the lower leg is elevated and suspended by the examiner's hand. The knee is flexed to about 20°, and the tibia is maintained in neutral rotation. ACL insufficiency allows the weight of the thigh to force the femur

posteriorly and, more importantly, to rotate externally, posteriorly subluxing the lateral femoral condyle. The patella appears to slide laterally within the trochlea, and the normal infrapatellar concavity appears flattened. Flexing the knee gently over a 10° range while applying downward pressure on the tibia reduces (internally rotates) the subluxed femur.

A variation of the posterior drawer test—the posterior drawer in external rotation—may also be useful to determine posterolateral instability of the knee joint. This examination is executed using the same patient position and maneuvers used in the posterior drawer test but the foot is externally rotated. A positive examination is evident when posterolateral translation of the tibia occurs (Fig. 19-31).

The Hughston jerk test is useful in assessing anterolateral rotatory instability and ACL insufficiency. With the patient in the supine position, the examiner grasps the foot, internally rotating the tibia, while the knee rests in 60° to 80° of flexion. The examiner's other hand is used to apply mild valgus stress immediately over the posterolateral

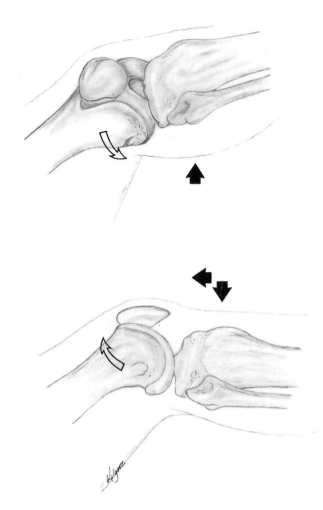

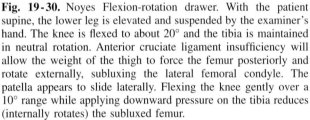

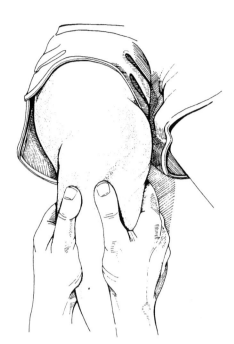

**Fig. 19-31.** Posterior drawer in external rotation. The posterior drawer position is utilized with the foot in slight external rotation. This test is considered positive if posterolateral tibial rotation is appreciated with a posterior push applied to the tibia. (From Hughston, J.C.: *Knee ligaments: injury and repair.* St. Louis: Mosby-Year Book, Inc., 1993.)

**Fig. 19-30.** Noyes Flexion-rotation drawer. With the patient supine, the lower leg is elevated and suspended by the examiner's hand. The knee is flexed to about 20° and the tibia is maintained in neutral rotation. Anterior cruciate ligament insufficiency will allow the weight of the thigh to force the femur posteriorly and rotate externally, subluxing the lateral femoral condyle. The patella appears to slide laterally. Flexing the knee gently over a 10° range while applying downward pressure on the tibia reduces (internally rotates) the subluxed femur.

aspect of the knee. The knee is then gently extended (Fig. 19-32). The test is positive if a sudden "jerk" occurs at the anterolateral corner of the tibial condyle and if there is pain along the anteromedial joint line.

Like the jerk test, the MacIntosh's pivot-shift test is useful in assessing anterolateral rotatory instability and ACL insufficiency. The examiner grasps the patient's foot, internally rotating the tibia, while the knee rests in an extended position. The other hand is used to apply mild anteromedially directed stress along the posterolateral joint line. The knee is then gently flexed to 30° (Fig. 19-33). A positive test is appreciated should a sudden jerk occur at the anterolateral corner of the tibial condyle. Relaxation of the hamstrings during this examination is imperative. The use of this test exclusively to determine anterolateral rotational instability is discouraged because ACL injury alone produces a positive pivot-shift test.

The Jakob reverse pivot-shift test is useful in delineating posterolateral instability in combination with PCL deficiency. With the patient supine, the hip and knee are flexed to 90°. The tibia is then rotated externally, and the knee is extended gradually while mild valgus stress is applied distal to the fibular head. A resolute "clunk" occurs as the femur subluxes forward on the moving tibia.

Evaluation of the meniscus is aided by the fact that the outer third of these structures possesses pain receptors, and pain elicited on palpation of the area in question offers a great deal of information. Meniscal testing classically includes range of motion through flexion and extension, McMurry's test, and Apley's compression test. In the acute knee injury, these tests are difficult to execute and may be omitted and held for later evaluation. The premise for performing these maneuvers is to drag the menisci over the femoral condyle.

Flexion and extension testing with the tibia in neutral rotation are the most elementary examinations of meniscal integrity. Any limitation in the range of motion, particularly with terminal extension or flexion, should raise the suspicion of meniscal injury.

McMurry's test is executed by maximally flexing the knee while applying external tibial rotation to test the medial meniscus, and internal rotation to test the lateral meniscus. The knee is then brought into full extension

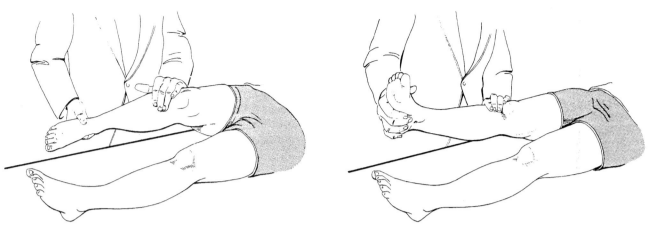

**Fig. 19-32.** Hughston jerk test. With the patient in the supine position, the examiner grasps the foot, internally rotating the tibia while the knee rests in 60° to 80° of flexion. A mild valgus stress is then applied immediately over the posterolateral joint. The knee is then gently extended. A positive test is present should a sudden "jerk" at the anterolateral corner of the tibial condyle and pain occur along the anteromedial joint line. (From Hughston, J.C.: *Knee ligaments: injury and repair.* St. Louis: Mosby-Year Book, Inc., 1993.)

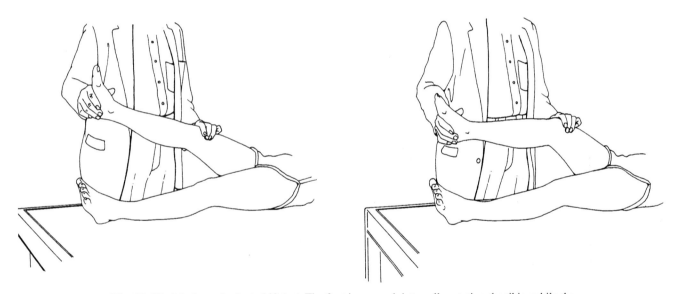

**Fig. 19-33.** MacIntosch pivot-shift test. The foot is grasped, internally rotating the tibia, while the knee rests in an extended position. An anteromedially directed stress is applied along the posterolateral joint line. The knee is then gently flexed to 30°. A positive test is appreciated should a sudden "jerk" occur at the anterolateral corner of the tibial condyle. (From Hughston, J.C.: *Knee ligaments: injury and repair.* St. Louis: Mosby-Year Book, Inc., 1993.)

while internal or external rotation is applied with one hand and the joint line is palpated with the other. A positive test elicits a painful pop or snap occurring over the medial or lateral joint line, depending on the meniscus being tested. A false-positive test can occur if a loose body or an ACL tear with a free-floating fragment is present in the joint. This test also frequently appears positive in adolescents and hyperextensile individuals who have no meniscal pathology.

Apley's compression test is primarily useful in demonstrating a tear of the posterior horn of the medial meniscus by entrapping the meniscus between the femoral condyle and tibial plateau. The patient is placed in the prone position, and the injured knee is flexed to 90°. One hand is placed in the popliteal fossa and the other grasps the sole of the foot. The foot is then rotated clockwise and counterclockwise while downward pressure is applied on the sole of the foot, much like a pestle in a mortar (Fig. 19-34). Pain is elicited if injury to the posterior horn of the meniscus exist and should be relieved when the sole of the foot is elevated (Apley's distraction test), while continuing to

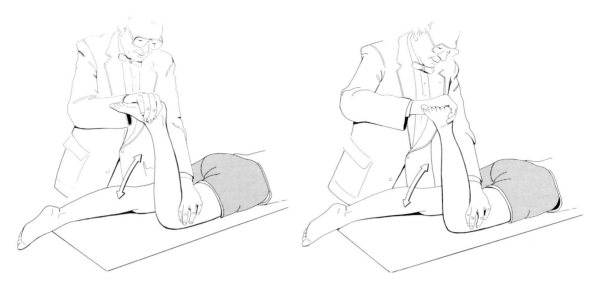

**Fig. 19-34.** Apley's compression test. The patient is placed in the prone position, and the knee is flexed to 90°. One hand is placed in the popliteal fossa and the other grasps the sole of the foot. The foot is then rotated clockwise and counterclockwise while downward pressure is applied on the sole of the foot, much like a pestle in a mortar. (From Hughston, J.C.: *Knee ligaments: injury and repair.* St. Louis: Mosby-Year Book, Inc., 1993.)

**Table 19-4.** Motor strength testing

| Movement | Muscle | Principal nerve supply |
|---|---|---|
| Flexion | Biceps femoris | Sciatic (L-5, S-1, S-2) |
| | Semitendinosus | Tibial portion of sciatic (L-5, S-1, S-2) |
| | Semimembranosus | Tibial portion of sciatic (L-5, S-1, S-2) |
| | Gastrocnemius | Tibial (S-1, S-2) |
| | Sartorius | Femoral (L-2, L-3) |
| | Gracilis | Obturator (L-2, L-3) |
| | Popliteus | Tibial (L-5) |
| Extension | Quadriceps femoris | Femoral (L-2, L-3, L-4) |
| Medial tibial rotation | Popliteus | Tibial (L-5) |
| | Semitendinosus | Tibial portion of sciatic (L-5, S-1, S-2) |
| | Semimembranosus | Tibial portion of sciatic (L-5, S-1, S-2) |
| | Sartorius | Femoral (L-2, L-3) |
| | Gracilis | Obturator (L-2, L-3) |
| Lateral tibial rotation | Biceps femoris | Sciatic (L-5, S-1, S-2) |

rotate the foot. If the patient experiences pain during the distraction test, injury to the medial collateral ligament or medial joint capsule, or both, should be suspected.

With such great attention paid to the ligamentous, meniscal, and osseous examinations, sensory-motor and vascular examinations are overlooked frequently in most texts and publications. Active hip, knee, and ankle joint range of motion must also be performed. Sensitivity of cutaneous dermatomes to light touch and pinprick offers clues to possible coexisting neurologic injury (eg, peroneal nerve palsy). The motor strength examination (Table 19-4) is performed by asking the patient to actively flex the knee, extend the knee, and internally and externally rotate the tibia, at which point his or her ability to resist the opposing motion can be ascertained. Popliteal, dorsalis pedis, and posterior tibialis arterial pulses should be felt for and compared with those of the uninjured limb.

**Radiographic evaluation.** Plain and stress radiographs in the assessment of knee injuries have been overused, and all too often a negative study is misleading. The history and physical examination should be trusted and should take precedence in the assessment of knee injury. Reasonable indications for requesting radiographs include an obvious deformity, crepitance noted on examination, the presence of a hemarthrosis, ACL instability, suspected open or penetration injury to the knee, lateral joint line tenderness, a

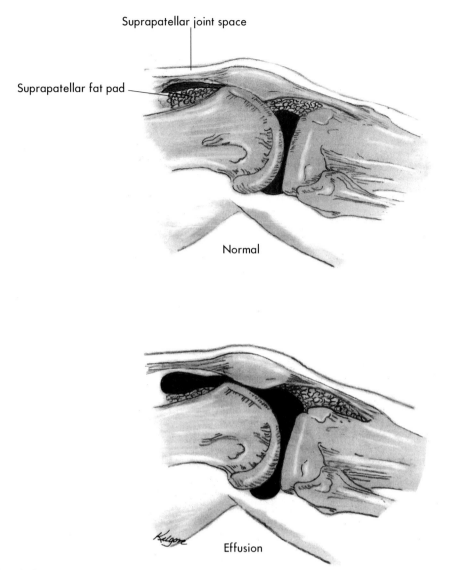

**Fig. 19-35.** Normal and distended joint space. The prefemoral fat pads appear prominent and the suprapatellar pouch is thin under normal circumstances. Joint effusion is evident with the loss of the fat pad and distention of the suprapatellar pouch.

possible loose body, and a young patient sustaining a knee injury.

A few subtle features of the knee radiograph aid the examiner in diagnosis. A joint effusion is identified by a widening of the space between the prefemoral and anterior suprapatellar fat pads (Fig. 19-35). This suprapatellar space is normally 3 to 5 mm wide on the lateral radiograph of the knee; with an effusion or hemarthrosis, this space distends to a centimeter or more. If no obvious fracture is evident, this finding suggests a significant ligament injury, and should also prompt the examiner to review the radiographs for a possible osteochondral fracture of the femoral condyle, patellar fracture, or tibial eminence fracture (Fig. 19-36). Free air within the knee joint (Fig. 19-37) appears as a radiolucency that rises to the highest point of the joint and, unlike the vacuum phenomenon, is not confined to the intra-articular areas of the joint. The presence of air within the confines of the knee joint (pneumoarthrosis) indicates an open-joint injury and mandates immediate orthopedic consultation and prompt treatment.

The presence of a prominent layering effect within the suprapatellar area on the cross-table lateral of the knee may be seen (Fig. 19-38). This is the result of fat layering out atop a collection of blood within the joint space (lipohemarthrosis). This finding is synonymous with the presence of an intra-articular fracture, most commonly involving the tibial condyle. A rarely seen finding termed *pneumolipohemarthrosis* occurs with an open-joint injury accompanying an intra-articular fracture. Radiographically, this appears as three distinct bands with a layer of free air and free fat anterior to a hemarthrosis.

Stress views in the adult population are of little benefit,

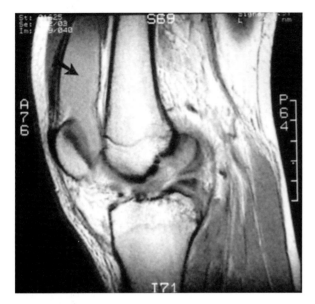

**Fig. 19-36.** Hemarthrosis of the right knee. Magnetic resonance imaging representation of a large generalized collection of blood within the joint space. Note the bulging of the suprapatellar pouch and posterior joint capsule. Note also the presence of a tibial eminence fracture.

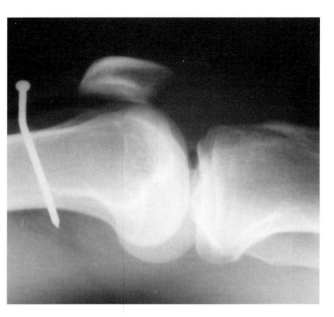

**Fig. 19-37.** Joint space free air due to penetrating injury. Note the presence of a penetrating foreign body and the suprapatellar radiolucency resulting from free air within the joint space.

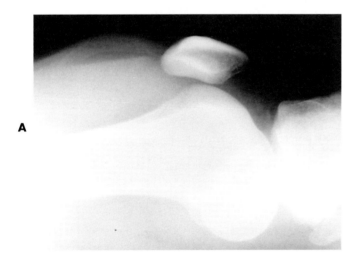

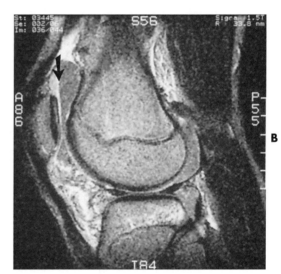

**Fig. 19-38.** Lipohemarthrosis of the knee joint. **A,** Radiograph demonstrating a superior radiolucent collection of fat in the suprapatellar pouch. **B,** Magnetic resonance imaging examination, demonstrating a layering effect of fat lying superior to an accompanying hemarthrosis. This finding is synonymous with an intra-articular fracture, usually of the tibial condyle.

yielding no more information than that already obtained during the physical examination of the knee. Stress views in the pediatric population have been appropriately suggested for delineation of physeal injury,[5] where the joint is clinically unstable and the site of instability and pain is at the physeal lines, not the joint line. In the immature skeleton, radiographic evaluation is more difficult to interpret. Anyone who evaluates pediatric trauma should be familiar with the growth plate appearance and closure charts.

**Special procedures.** Over the years, joint aspiration has

been underused. Some authorities believe that knee injuries with effusion or hemarthrosis should be aspirated using a sterile technique.[13-17] This procedure serves three purposes: 1) to remove a large intra-articular hematoma; 2) to detect the presence or absence of intra-articular fat; and 3) to allow a portal for instilling lidocaine and/or bupivacaine, providing analgesia and thus allowing a valid examination.

It is best to avoid selecting an entry portal that passes through infected or damaged skin (eg, eczema or psoriasis, burns). Arthrocentesis is contraindicated in an uncorrected bleeding diathesis (eg, anticoagulation, thrombocytopenia, hemophilia). If joint aspiration is deemed necessary, the underlying defect should be corrected first.

An arthrocentesis is performed adhering to the general principles of aseptic technique. The suprapatellar, lateral, or medial portal (Fig. 19-39) is selected, avoiding the area of maximum tenderness as stated by the patient. Practically speaking, the suprapatellar approach is the safest. The superior lateral pole of the patella is identified, and two fingerbreadths above the patella a skin wheal of 1% lidocaine is introduced subdermally. An 18-gauge needle is then introduced into the suprapatellar pouch and is directed along the posterior patella. Every attempt to remove all of the hemarthrosis should be made. After aspiration has been completed, 10 to 15 mm of 0.25% bupivocaine is instilled into the knee joint to afford pain relief and facilitate examination.

A hemarthrosis occurs in 90% of ACL disruptions.[10,18] Other, less common causes of hemarthrosis include patellar dislocation, osteochondral fracture, and peripheral meniscal tear. Aspiration of straw-colored synovial fluid casts doubt on the existence of an ACL injury, but is frequently present with longitudinal and radial meniscal injuries. Fat globules indicate the probability of intra-articular fractures and should prompt further radiographic investigation. Arthrocentesis can introduce air into the joint; if radiographs are desired, they should be obtained prior to arthrocentesis.

Magnetic resonance imaging has found its way into the armamentarium of noninvasive diagnostic modalities of knee afflictions. MRI portrays bone integrity well, including infiltrative processes of the bone marrow, osteochondritis dissecans, osteonecrosis, osteochondral fractures, stress fractures, bone bruises, and also nonosseous structures (menisci, collateral ligaments, and cruciate ligaments).[19] MRI appears sensitive to meniscal injury in 88% of cases (medial meniscus, 84%; lateral meniscus, 78%). In a study of 203 subjects, 198 patients met the indications for arthroscopy based on history and physical examination. These patients subsequently underwent MRI; and the findings indicated that arthroscopy had been indicated for only 52% of these patients.[20] MRI has essentially outmoded the use of arthrography.

## BASIC INITIAL TREATMENT

Priorities in assessment and treatment must be established. The patient sustaining multiple trauma, which includes a knee injury, requires a much more global assessment and resuscitative approach than the individual presenting with an isolated knee malady. Care of the patient presenting with a knee affliction or injury has three basic objectives: relief of pain and swelling, protection from additional injury or disease progression, and restoration of knee function.

### Relief of pain and swelling

Classical modalities used for the relief of pain and swelling are embodied in the mnemonic "RICE." Placing the knee at complete, non–weight-bearing *rest* allows contraction and coagulation of injured vascular structures. Rest also decreases the possibility of further injury and should be continued until the swelling has abated. The application of *ice* fosters vasoconstriction, retarding hematoma formation. The caveat in this treatment modality is that the application of ice for more than 15 minutes tends to precipitate pain and tissue damage (iatrogenic frostbite). Ice should be applied over the dressing for 15 minutes every 2 to 4 waking hours for the first 72 hours after injury. Heat also offers pain relief; however, its application is best delayed until after the first 72 hours; heat appears to be of greatest utility as a complement to a rehabilitation program designed for the patient.

The use of a *compressive* dressing is, in the author's view, the modality of greatest benefit in the early postinjury period. Ideally, this dressing affords mechanical compression, averting further bleeding without neurovascular compromise. This dressing should offer some degree of joint support and should prevent further injury. To this end, a number of commercially available knee immobilizers have been introduced. In the author's experience, however, "the splint that is made to fit everyone, fits no one."

A preferred alternative is a modified Robert Jones dressing incorporating coaptation splinting. Stockinet material, twice the length of the leg, is applied from groin to toe. Half of the excess stockinet is drawn into the groin area,

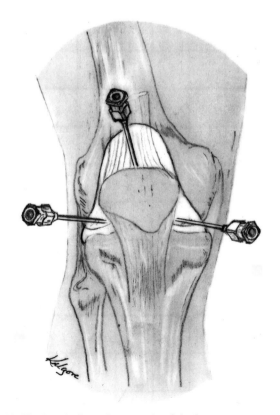

**Fig. 19-39.** Portals for arthrocentesis of the knee.

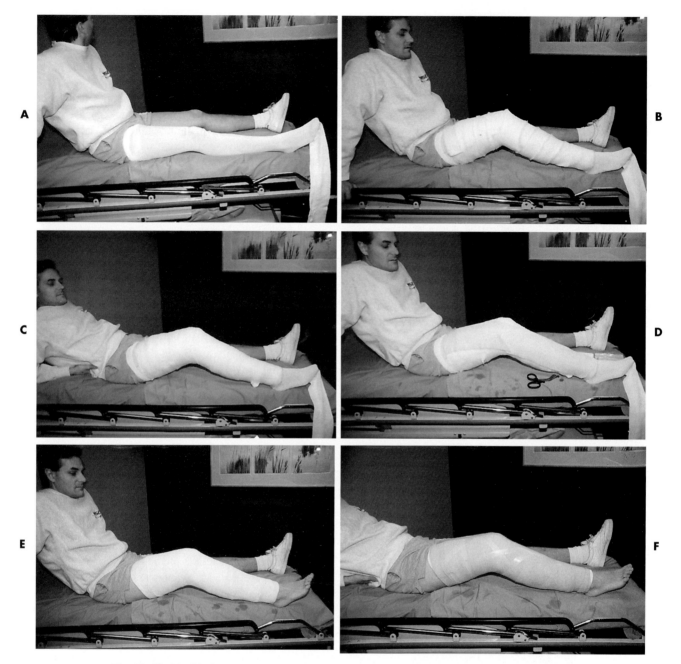

**Fig. 19-40.** Modified Robert Jones dressing. **A,** Stockingette application, in which twice the length of stockingette is applied. **B,** Cotton batting application. Four to six layers of uncompressed cotton batting are applied from ankle to groin. **C,** Webril application. Standard orthopedic softroll or webril is then applied to compress the previously applied cotton batting. **D,** Splinting material application. The splinting material of choice is applied to the medial and lateral surfaces of the compressive dressing and is maintained in place utilizing another layer of webril material. **E,** Stockingette inversion. The initially applied stockingette is then inverted over the compressive dressing and splints. An elastic wrap is applied over the entire affair and is taped into position. **F,** Completed modified Robert Jones dressing.

and the remainder over the end of the toes (Fig. 19-40A). Four to six layers of uncompressed cotton batting material are then applied (Fig. 19-40B). It has been the author's practice to use 4- to 6-inch widths of the batting material in single layers. Once applied, the batting is held in place by standard orthopedic soft-roll or webril (Fig. 19-40C). At this point, medial and lateral plaster or fiberglass coaptation splints are applied while the knee is maintained in 15° to 20° of flexion (Fig. 19-40D). An appropriate width of the splint material is selected according to the width of the patient's leg. The splinting material is then maintained in place by another layer of webril. The ends of the stockinet are then brought back over the padding and splint material, as one would turn a shirt sleeve inside out (Fig. 19-40E). An elastic compressive wrap is applied the length of the dressing (Fig. 19-40F). This dressing is allowed to remain in place until the patient is seen by his or her private physician (within the next 5 days if possible).

Patients should be instructed to *elevate* the extremity at or above heart level. This affords rest to the injured knee and also optimizes drainage of blood and edema from the injury site. Elevation should be continued until resolution of the swelling is achieved.

Pharmacologic agents at the disposal of the clinician for relief of pain fall into two general categories: nonnarcotic and narcotic. Nonsteroidal anti-inflammatory drugs (NSAIDs) are nonnarcotic agents useful in the treatment of mild to moderate pain associated with musculoskeletal injuries. Additionally, a decrease in synovial inflammatory response has been shown with the use of nonsteroidal agents both clinically and in vitro, and is thus indicated for the treatment of arthropathies. A 7- to 14-day course of NSAIDs generally is adequate in controlling postinjury inflammatory response. NSAIDs do have potential systemic side effects, however, including gastrointestinal, renal, respiratory, and hepatic toxicities. Contraindications to the use of NSAIDs include ongoing anticoagulant therapies, thrombocytopenia, peptic ulcer disease, asthma, and renal or hepatic failure. In the presence of diabetes mellitus, NSAIDs, which have been shown to decrease the peripheral cells' sensitivity to insulin, are contraindicated. In the asthmatic patient, nonsteroidal agents, including aspirin, may provoke an acute exacerbation of his or her reactive airway disease. Acetaminophen is most often useful for treating pain in the elderly or in those in whom NSAIDs are not recommended. If the patient's pain is significant and is corroborated by physical examination findings, narcotic analgesics are indicated and beneficial. Should a narcotic analgesic be used, the patient is cautioned about the fact that some sedation can be expected with the use of such agents. As a rule, analgesic therapy is used over the first 3 to 5 days following injury or as long as the patient has pain. The use of intra-articular corticosteroids is occasionally beneficial in treating osteoarthritis but should not be used in the acutely injured knee.[21]

### Protection of the injured joint

The second basic care objective is to guard the injured knee from further insult. This facet of care uses rest, abstinence from weight-bearing while using crutches, and immobilization of the involved knee. The use of casting in the acute setting can provoke neurovascular compromise as well as cause atrophic changes, which may then delay rehabilitation. The preferred initial immobilization is the use of the modified Robert Jones dressing. Once the acute phase of the injury has abated and rehabilitation has begun, the patient is fitted with one of the commercially available knee immobilizers and support is continued until the patient is able to achieve painless flexion of the knee to 90°.

### Rehabilitation

The third objective critical to the care of the injured knee is rehabilitation. This is generally a long process and one not easily monitored by an emergency department physician. Nevertheless, the physician initially caring for the patient needs to have some knowledge of knee rehabilitation principles in order to provide the patient with a few simple exercises and acquaint him or her with what might be included as part of follow-up therapies.

A knee rehabilitation program has two objectives: to restore normal range of motion and to strengthen the muscle groups serving the knee. All exercise programs are performed as the patient tolerates, and a physician or physical therapist is mandatory to allow monitoring of progress and fine-tuning of the program.

**Range-of-motion exercise.** Early restoration of physiologic range of motion is one key to any knee rehabilitation program. If range of motion is not regained early, normal function may never be achieved. In the isolated injury, range-of-motion exercises should be initiated when swelling has resolved. Passive flexion and extension are performed while the patient is prone with a small pillow beneath the involved knee (Fig. 19-41A). From a flexed position, the knee is allowed to extend against gravity. Assistance in extension is accomplished by placing the other leg over the heel of the involved leg. Downward pressure is applied by the uninvolved leg until full extension is attained. Flexion range of motion is performed in the same position. The knee is flexed, and the heel of the unaffected leg is placed under the anterior ankle of the involve leg to assist in flexion of the injured knee (Fig. 19-41B). It is suggested that alternating sets of 20 minutes be performed up to three times per day.

**Muscle strengthening.** Immobilization and disuse yield atrophic changes in the muscle groups responsible for knee motion. With as little as 4 days of immobilization, significant joint stiffness may be experienced. Should this element of rehabilitation be avoided, reinjury is inevitable. The critical factor in the success of an early mobilization program is the avoidance of repeated bouts of swelling, which will retard progress in a muscle-strengthening pro-

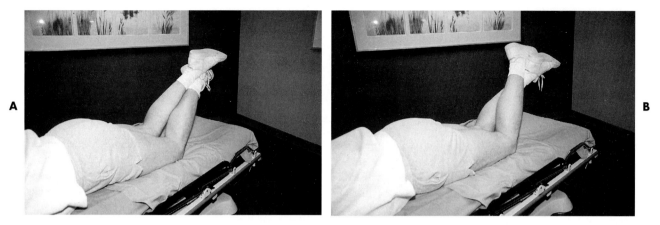

**Fig. 19-41.** Range-of-motion exercises. **A,** Knee extension exercise. To avoid the potential of knee stiffness, range-of-motion exercises are initiated as early as possible. In this photograph the injured right knee is extended. The uninjured leg offers resistance to tolerance during the extension exercise. **B,** Knee flexion exercise. Flexion exercise of the injured right knee is performed using the uninjured leg to apply resistance to flexion as tolerated by the patient.

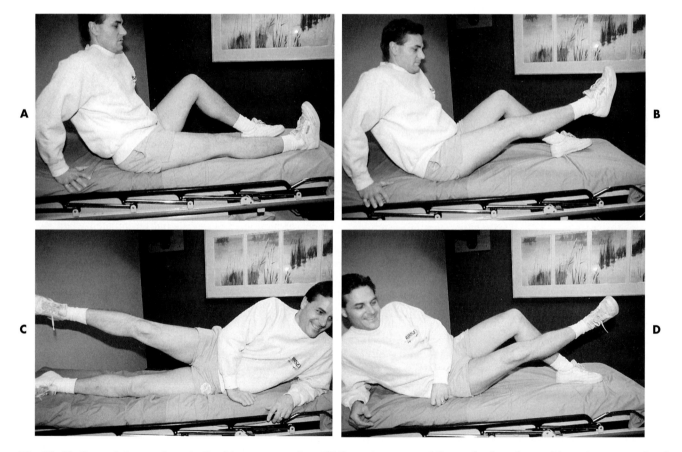

**Fig. 19-42.** Open-chain exercises. **A,** Quadriceps set exercises. While supine or seated flat on the floor the quadriceps is contracted and maintained for a count of 5 seconds. A "set" consists of 10 repetitions of this exercise. The patient is instructed to perform three sets daily. **B,** Straight leg-raising exercises. This is the most basic isometric, non–weight-bearing exercise and the most important in terms of avoiding atrophic changes. The patient raises the extended leg off the floor 10 to 12 inches and the leg is maintained elevated for a count of 5 seconds. This is repeated 10 times to equal a "set." Three sets should be performed daily. **C,** Abductor sets. To perform this exercise the patient is asked to lie on his or her side with the affected limb raised. The hip is then abducted against gravity 12 to 24 inches and is maintained abducted for a count of 5 seconds. Ten repetitions of this exercise is considered a "set" and three sets daily are suggested. **D,** Adductor sets. The patient is positioned on his or her side with the affected leg down. The unaffected leg is extended back out of the way. The patient lifts (adducts) the affected leg off the table, holding it adducted for a count of 5 seconds. This is repeated 10 times and constitutes a "set." Three sets should be performed daily.

gram. Exercise programs are, in fact, capable of accelerating the resolution of an effusion or hemarthrosis.

Muscle strengthening programs are separated into two major categories: *open chain* (non–weight-bearing) and *closed chain* (weight-bearing) exercises. Open-chain exercises are designed to combat the occurrence of disuse atrophy of the quadriceps group without excessively stressing the injured knee joint. This type of exercise is appropriately suggested during the patient's initial visit; however, any use of weight resistance (isotonic exercise) should be discouraged.

Open-chain exercises are begun as soon as possible. Regardless of the type of injury, a quadriceps setting exercise is generally the first exercise selected. This isometric exercise can be performed while the knee is supported in an immobilizer, cast, or elastic bulky dressing. In the sitting or supine position, the patient flexes the unaffected hip and knee (Fig. 19-42A). The affected quadriceps is then contracted and held for a 5-second count. Each set is composed of this maneuver performed 10 times; and three sets should be completed daily.

Straight-leg raises (Fig. 19-42B) are the most important exercise in the open-chain category. If it can be tolerated, this exercise is best done without the use of external supports or wraps. In a supine or seated position, the patient raises the affected leg 12 inches off the floor or table and holds this position for a count of 5 seconds. This maneuver is performed 10 times per set and three sets daily are suggested. If tolerable, leg raising in 30° of flexion is also performed. Synchronous with leg raising, a terminal quadriceps contraction, or "squeeze," is also encouraged in cases of meniscal, cruciate, and collateral ligament injury. In cases of patellar subluxation, symptomatic plica, Osgood-Schlatter disease, or any type of degenerative joint disease, terminal extension exercises are best avoided.

Hip abductor and adductor muscle groups should also be addressed in an early knee rehabilitation program. Abductor sets (Fig. 19-42C) are performed with the patient lying on his or her side, with the involved leg up. The leg is raised (abducted) 12 inches, is maintained in this position for 5 seconds, and then slowly lowered. Three sets of 10 repetitions should be performed daily. Adductor sets (Fig. 19-42D) are performed with the patient lying with the affected side on the floor or table. The unaffected leg is flexed behind the affected leg. The patient then lifts (adducts) the leg, holds for 5 seconds, and then slowly lowers the leg. Three sets of 10 repetitions should be performed daily.

A recent trend in knee rehabilitation has been to initiate closed-chain exercise, with tolerance of weight-bearing. These are isotonic maneuvers using the body's weight as resistance. The initial exercise in the closed-chain portion program is the partial squat (Fig. 19-43A). Standing with

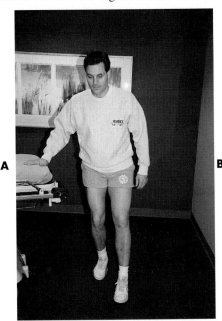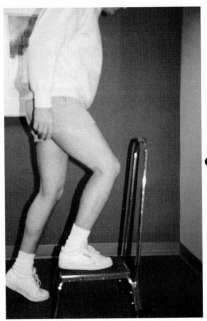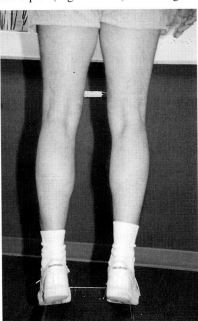

**Fig. 19-43.** Closed-chain exercises. **A,** Partial squat sets. While standing, the uninjured leg is extended forward. The patient then flexes the knee in a squatting fashion (to not more than 30°). Note that the patient needs to position him- or herself with side of injury next to the table. The hand on the affected side rests in the table offering support during this exercise. Ten repetitions of this exercise are performed to constitute a set. Three sets are performed daily. **B,** Step-up sets. The patient "steps up" on a 3- to 5-inch elevation, bearing weight on the affected knee. This is repeated 10 times per set and three sets daily are performed. **C,** Heel raises. Heel raises are designed to strengthen the gastrocnemius-soleus muscle groups. Using a table for balance the patient places his or her weight on the balls of the feet, the heels are then raised 3 to 4 inches off the floor and held for a count of 5 seconds. Ten repetitions of this exercise constitute a "set" and three sets should be performed daily.

the injured side next to a table, the patient places a hand on the table for balance. He or she then extends the unaffected leg. A shallow (30°) knee bend of the affected knee is performed. Ten repetitions three times per day should be performed. The program progresses to include step-up exercise (Fig. 19-43B), in which the patient steps up onto a low platform (6 to 8 inches), not allowing greater than 40° of knee flexion. The final element in the closed-chain category of exercises is the heel raise (Fig. 19-43C). This exercise is designed to strengthen the gastrocnemius-soleus group. Using a step or while on the floor, the patient supports him- or herself with an outstretched hand resting on a nearby table for balance. Then, placing the body weight on the balls of the feet, the patient raises his or her heels off the floor and holds this position for a count of 5 seconds. Three sets of 10 repetitions should be performed daily.

**Bracing.** Bracing is another facet of a rehabilitation program. It should never be the sole treatment of a knee injury; rather, it is only a small part of the rehabilitation program. Dispensing knee braces from an emergency department is not sound practice.

Brace selection is based on the type of injury being treated and the level of function required by the patient. Three basic types of brace exist: rehabilitative, prophylactic, and functional. For lateral knee injuries, studies have been unable to demonstrate a significant change in outcome by implementing bracing. Bracing ACL insufficiency is believed to have a definitive role in joint protection because of the appliance's ability to restrict full extension and protect the knee from external forces.[22] Protective bracing has an established role in the treatment of medial collateral sprains.[22] This facet of a rehabilitative program is best prescribed by an orthopedic surgeon.

## NONTRAUMATIC CONDITIONS
### Developmental and congenital conditions

Developmental deformities of the knee are quite common in children and are usually brought to the attention of the primary care physician by a concerned parent. There are multiple etiologies of congenital and developmental knee deformities (Table 19-5). It must be emphasized that all knee deformities in children should be evaluated relative to that child's age. Because they may appear concurrently, a distinction between frontal plane and rotational deformities needs to be made during evaluation. Most of these deformities are physiologic and spontaneously resolve with further growth and development. The interview should address family history, growth and development patterns, and nutritional problems. Screening procedures should include record of height, weight, and developmental percentile calculations. Examination includes a record of joint laxity, the femorotibial angle, and intercondylar or intermalleolar distances. Radiographic evaluation of angular deformities of the knee is indicated if 1) severe deformity

exists; 2) the deformity is asymmetric; 3) stature is below the fifth percentile; 4) other musculoskeletal abnormalities are noted; 5) the deformity is excessive; 6) a prior traumatic history exists; or 7) the family history is significant. Careful assessment with documentation, explanation and reassurance for the parents, and follow-up is sufficient for most patients.

**Physiologic genu varum.** Some degree of genu varum (bowlegs) is present in most children before 2 years of age.[23,24] Normal growth of the lateral femoral condyle is greater than that of the medial condyle during this time and is felt to give rise to this deformity. External hip and tibial rotation, also common during this time, is felt to accentuate the clinical appearance of the deformity. Early weight-bearing, certain childhood sitting positions, and obesity tend to accentuate this deformity, particularly when associated with external tibial rotation.

On examination, the knees appear widely spaced while the ankles are together. Pathologic genu varum should be considered when gait examination demonstrates ligamentous laxity of the lateral joint and a lateral thrust or lurch in the step-off and swing-through phases of gait. The unilateral appearance of this deformity in the child over 2 years of age with greater than 25° of unrelenting or progressive varum deserves special attention and radiographic evaluation because growth suppression or injury may be present.

**Genu valgum.** Genu valgum (knock-knee) is commonly viewed in children between the ages of 2 and 6 years. This is an angular deformity of the knee marked by wide separation of the ankles when the knees are together. The foot of the affected individual tends to evert, and a

**Table 19-5.** Etiologies of knee deformities

| |
|---|
| Physiologic |
|   Resolving |
|     Early infancy: lateral tibial bowing |
|     Late infancy: common tibial bowing |
|     Early childhood: common knock-knee |
| Pathologic |
|   Varus |
|     Tibia vara (Blount's disease) |
|     Physiologic genu varum (unresolved) |
|   Valgus |
|     Metaphyseal fractures of the tibia |
|     Hypoplasia of the lateral condyle |
|     Unresolved physiologic valgum |
|   Varus or valgus |
|     Trauma |
|       Malunion |
|       Partial physeal arrest |
|     Metabolic |
|       Rickets |
|       Renal disease |
|     Osteopenia |
|       Osteogenesis imperfecta |
|       Rheumatoid arthritis |

greater than normal laxity of the medial collateral ligament is present on examination. This deformity is usually bilateral. A strong familial tendency exists in the physiologic form. Genu valgum tends to be accentuated by early ambulation, particularly in obese children. Patellar dislocations occur commonly in these individuals due to an increase in function of the lateral extensor mechanism in association with the accentuated Q angle. Injury resulting from infection or trauma involving the lateral epiphysis of the distal femur or proximal tibia may retard normal growth and alignment and is also responsible for pathologic genu valgum.

Orthopedic referral is necessary in children who display a leg-length inequality, abnormal medial collateral ligament laxity, and an intermalleolar distance measurement of greater than 10 cm on radiographic evaluation. The use of medial heel wedges tends to increase the lateral ankle stresses if compensatory inversion of the foot is present and their use is discouraged.

**Genu recurvatum.** Genu recurvatum is a physical examination finding in which the knee appears to hyperextend. Due to their increased ligamentous laxity, genu recurvatum is more commonly seen in girls. This deformity may also be the result of avulsion of the tibial tubercle, fracture of the supracondylar femur, premature closure of the anterior tibial epiphysis,[22] surgery, or as a sequelae of poliomyelitis. This deformity in the pediatric age group is more commonly seen in arthrogryposis and myelodysplastic syndromes.

**Tibia vara.** This developmental disorder, commonly termed Blount disease, is the result of disorganized medial physeal and metaphyseal growth, causing a varus deformity of the knee. The disarray of the tibial metaphysis and physeal growth plate is felt to represent an osteochondrosis related to stress injury.[25] Medial tibial torsion and "intoeing" frequently accompany this deformity. Two distinct forms (infantile and juvenile) of tibia vara exist (Table 19-6). The incidence of tibia vara is higher in blacks and in the obese. A strong familial tendency exists.

Radiographs will demonstrate a collapse of the medial tibial metaphysis. A lateral translation of the tibia relative to the femur will also be present on the anteroposterior radiograph.

**Abnormal patellar position.** Patella alta is defined as an abnormally high-riding patella in relation to the femoral sulcus, while patella baja is an abnormally low-riding patella. Each of these entities represents a variety of extensor mechanism malalignment.

The positioning of the patella proximal to the femoral condyle in the resting extended knee suggests patella alta. Repeated episodes of patellar subluxation or habitual dislocation are associated with patella alta. Insall's radiographic technique[26] for the determination of patella alta appears to be the most practical for evaluation in the emergency department. Using standard lateral radiographs, the diagonal length of the patella is compared with that of the

patellar tendon (Fig. 19-44). A ratio of 0.8:1 or less indicates patella alta.

Patella baja is observed in quadriceps rupture, neuromuscular disease, such as poliomyelitis, and iatrogenically as the result of malpositioning of the tibial tubercle in a distal advancement procedure. Patients with patella baja generally present with a complaint of retropatellar pain resulting from patellofemoral chondrosis.

Primary care of these conditions includes relocation of the patella, should dislocation be present, as well as knee immobilization in extension, application of ice, and use of NSAIDs. Orthopedic referral should also be part of discharge planning for these patients because recurrence of subluxation or dislocation is common and is potentially correctable.

**Rachitic diseases.** Abnormalities in calcium or phosphorous metabolism result in defective mineralization of the bony osteoid. Rickets, due either to renal disease or to vitamin D–related metabolism, results in severe deformities of the weight-bearing bones. The hallmark of these diseases includes generalized growth suppression and osteopenia. Radiographic features include widening of the physis with cupping or flaring of the metaphyses, osteomalacia, and bowing of the diaphyseal segment of long bones. The varus deformity is seen more commonly in the vitamin D–related forms of rickets. Renal osteodystrophy, conversely, more commonly results in the development of a valgus deformity of the knee. In hypophosphatemic states, a fairly equal frequency of genu varus and genu valgus deformities occurs.[27] Both physical and radiographic findings are easily confused with those suggestive of child abuse. Abuse patterns, however, tend to be more isolated than those of rachitic diseases.

**Congenital meniscal disorders.** Discoid meniscus occurs more commonly in girls between the ages of 12 and 15 years.[28] This condition is a developmental malady in which the meniscus is discoid-shaped rather than semilunar. Discoid menisci tend to be bilateral and usually involve the lateral meniscus. This malformation presents with signs and symptoms characteristic of traumatic meniscal injury but without an associated effusion or history of a traumatic event.

Discoid menisci are particularly prone to the devel-

**Table 19-6.** Patterns of Blount's disease

| | Infantile | Juvenile |
|---|---|---|
| Age (years) | 1–3 | 6–18 |
| Bilateral | Yes | No |
| Symmetric | Yes | No |
| Physeal bridge | No | Sometimes |
| Anisomelia | Slight | Significant |
| Resolution | Sometimes | No |

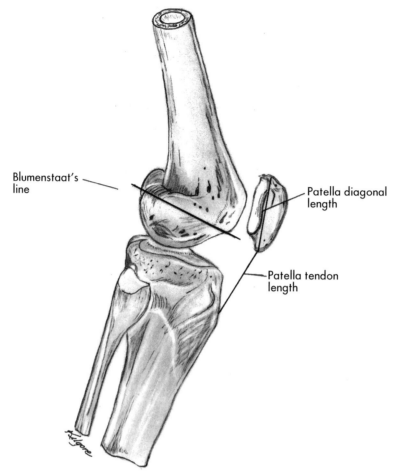

Blumenstaat's line

Patella diagonal length

Patella tendon length

**Fig. 19-44.** Patella alta (Insall-Salvetti technique). The ratio of patellar tendon length to the diagonal height of the patella is normally less than or equal to 0.8:1. If greater than this patella alta exists and extensor mechanism injury is common.

ment of radial meniscal tears. Presenting complaints include a popping noise with flexion and extension, muscle weakness, especially with pivotal motion, and a lateral aching sensation in the knee. Two distinct forms of discoid meniscus have been noted. In the complete form, which occurs more commonly, the meniscus covers the entire tibial plateau. This form of discoid meniscus retains the normal meniscofemoral and meniscotibial attachments and thus the patient tends to be asymptomatic. The Wrisberg type of discoid meniscus (Fig. 19-45) is deficient in its tibial attachments but retains its attachment to the ligament of Wrisberg. On extension of the knee, this ligament draws the posterior aspect of the meniscus into the intercondylar space, which limits extension and typically results in recurrent episodes of joint locking. An associated higher-than-usual fibular head may be noticed on physical examination and radiologic studies. Range of motion is generally limited and, during active range of motion, a loud click may be felt and heard. Because the discoid meniscus tends to be thicker than normal, radiographic examination may disclose a widened lateral joint space. Other radiographic features include a loss of the normal concavity of the lateral tibial condyle and hypoplastic changes of the anterolateral tibial

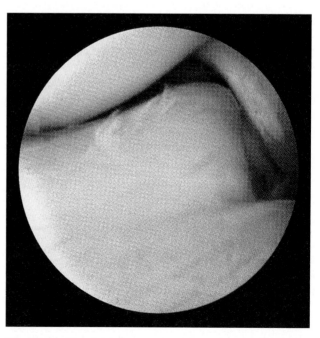

**Fig. 19-45.** Discoid meniscus. This arthroscopic presentation of a discoid lateral meniscus. Note that this dysplastic meniscus is displaced into the intercondylar notch (Wrisberg-type).

spine. If locking has occurred, orthopedic consultation is necessary. Treatment includes arthroscopic examination, and, if the peripheral rim is competent, an arthroscopic saucerization of the central discoid portion is performed, leaving a semilunar meniscus. If the Wrisberg variety is found, peripheral reattachment is performed in addition to saucerization.

# TRAUMATIC CONDITIONS
## Intra-articular fractures

**Chondral and osteochondral fractures.** Chondral and osteochondral injuries are present in 20% of hemarthrotic knees. Chondral injuries consist of a fracture of the articular surface involving the cartilaginous articular surface without subchondral bony involvement (Fig. 19-46). Osteochondral fracture involves both articular cartilage and subchondral bone.

The mechanism producing osteochondral fractures is either exogenous or endogenous. The exogenous mechanism involves a shearing blow applied directly to the knee. Those fractures produced endogenously (Fig. 19-47) are the result of combined compression and rotatory forces acting on a weight-bearing knee in flexion. The endogenous mechanism appears to be more common in adults. The injury typically occurs during a sporting event, with

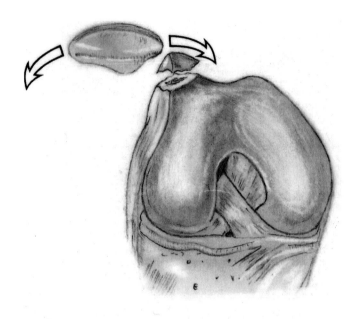

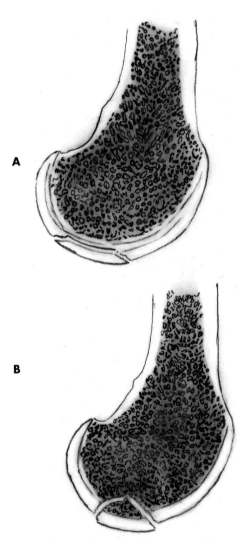

**Fig. 19-46. A,** Chondral fracture. This type of fracture results when compressive or rotatory forces are dispersed along the "tidemark" between calcified and uncalcified cartilage. Note subchondral bone is spared. This type of injury is generally seen in adults. **B,** Osteochondral fracture. In the child and adolescent the subchondral bone is violated in addition to the chondral surface.

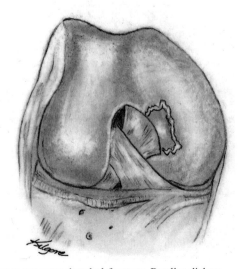

**Fig. 19-47.** Endogenous osteochondral fracture. Patellar dislocations produce a shearing force against the lateral femoral condyle, resulting in an osteochondral fracture. This event may occur either at the time of dislocation or with spontaneous reduction. The site of fracture is non–weight-bearing. The medial femoral condyle is particularly prone to osteochondral fractures. Shear forces are applied with combined running and cutting maneuvers.

patients commonly reporting an abrupt onset of severe pain and swelling and an immediate inability to bear weight. An accompanying "snap" is sometimes heard at onset. Approximately 20% of patients subsequently give a history of suffering locking episodes. On examination, the knee at rest is generally held in 15° to 20° of flexion. Tenderness over the medial or lateral femoral condyle or over the midpatella is present on palpation, and any attempt to flex or extend the knee produces discomfort.

Osteochondral fractures seldom involve the tibial plateaus. This is believed to be due in part to the protective function of the menisci. Over time, chondral and osteochondral fractures result in an intraarticular loose body that can be seen on radiography. Treatment of osteochondral and chondral fractures includes arthroscopic removal of the fragment if less than 1 cm; if the fragment is larger than this and a bed of bleeding subchondral bone is visualized during arthroscopy, replacement and fixation of the fragment with Kirschner wire or minifragment screws are indicated. Fixation is contraindicated if operative intervention is delayed for 10 days or longer, since fibrocartilage replacement of the defect has begun.

**Tibial eminence fractures.** Tibial eminence fractures are not uncommon and occur in up to 15% of all tibial plateau fractures.[29] This injury occurs uncommonly in children, with an incidence of three cases per 100,000 children annually. Vehicular accidents and sporting injuries are the most common causes of this fracture, which involves rotation, hyperextension, and varus-valgus stresses. The ratio of anterior tibial eminence fractures to posterior tibial eminence fractures is 10:1.[30]

The most commonly accepted classification scheme bases the severity of injury on the degree of tibial spine displacement viewed radiographically (Fig. 19-48).[30] In a small percentage of patients 2% to 4%), more commonly in children, tibial spine fractures are identifiable on routine radiographs (Fig. 19-49). These fractures are not synonymous with cruciate injury; however, cruciate insufficiency is a likely accompanying injury in the presence of a tibial eminence fracture. In children, fractures of the tibial spine occur more commonly than cruciate disruption. The same stress that produces an ACL injury in adults results in an avulsion injury of the tibial spine in children. This is due to failure of the subchondral bone at the apophyseal insertion of the cruciate in children.

Historically, patients report an immediate disability and swelling of the knee. If displacement of the fracture fragment occurs the patient will state a locking history. Examination discloses a painful hemarthrosis and limitation in terminal flexion and extension that exacerbates the patient's discomfort. Should the hemarthrosis be tense and limit examination, arthrocentesis for evacuation of hematoma and instillation of local anesthetic offers immediate relief of pain, permitting a valid examination and painless splint application. This technique is also useful should stress views be desired to assess the proximal tibial physis.

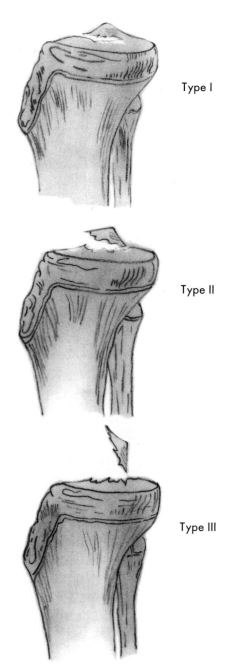

Type I

Type II

Type III

**Fig. 19-48.** Classification of tibial eminence fractures. Meyers-McKeever classification of tibial eminence fractures based on the anatomic location of the fracture fragment. Type I is avulsion with slight displacement; type II is avulsion with elevation of the anterior border with the posterior border of the fragment acting as a hinge; and type III is avulsion with complete dissociation from the fracture bed and possible rotation.

Type I and type II tibial eminence fractures are treated closed, splinting the knee in 10° of flexion. Type III fractures generally require open reduction and internal fixation using suture material or interfragmentary screw fixation. Casting of type III fractures is done with knee in 10° to 20° of flexion. Displacement of the fracture fragment will result in nonunion or malunion.

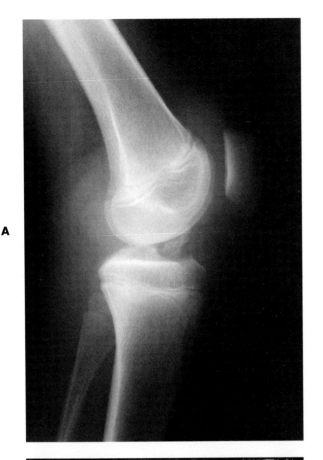

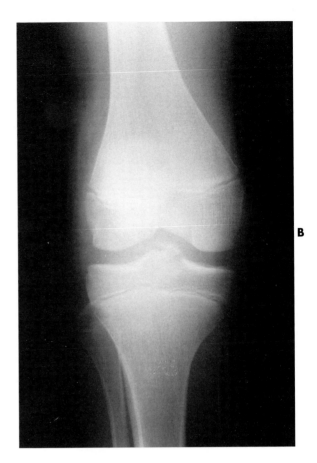

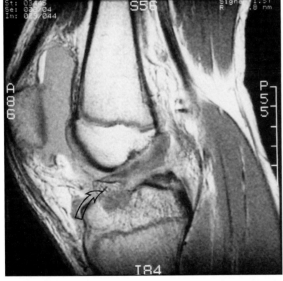

**Fig. 19-49.** Type III tibial eminence fracture. **A** and **B**, Antero-posterior and lateral radiographs of the right knee demonstrating a type III medial tibial eminence fracture. Note the degree of anterior displacement of the avulsed fracture fragment. **C**, Magnetic resonance imaging of type III tibial eminence fracture. Magnetic resonance imaging of the same patient demonstrating a significant lipohemarthrosis, avulsion of the medial tibial eminence with comminution of the avulsed fragment (see "x"), and an intact anterior cruciate ligament.

**Patellar fractures.** Fractures of the patella occur commonly, accounting for 1% of all skeletal injuries. However, only 1% of all patellar fractures occur in the pediatric population.[29] This is believed to be due to the cushioning effect of the cartilaginous surface of the patella in children. The diagnosis of patellar fracture in the immature skeleton is a difficult challenge because of developmental variations and the cartilaginous nature of the pediatric patella.

Fractures of the patella are classified as transverse, longitudinal, or stellate (Fig. 19-50), and result from either indirect or direct injury. An indirect injury occurs when the inherent strength of the patellar substance is exceeded by the tension applied by its musculotendinous attachments. Patients generally relate a history of a stumbling episode or fall in which they attempt to catch themselves. Massive quadriceps contraction occurs and once the patella is fractured, the dysfunctional quadriceps mechanism yields to the weight of the body and the fall is completed. With this mechanism, the fracture orientation is transverse with varying degrees of comminution. Most importantly, disruption

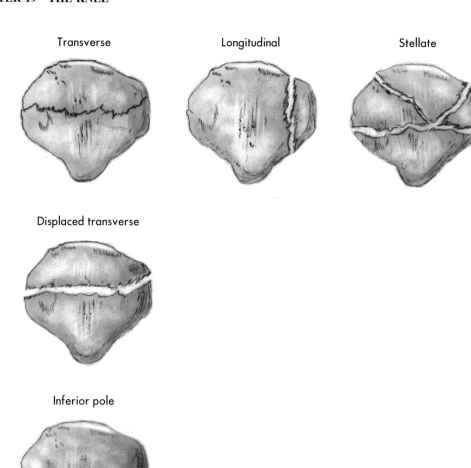

Transverse          Longitudinal          Stellate

Displaced transverse

Inferior pole

**Fig. 19-50.** Patellar fracture classification. Three broad types of patellar fractures occur: transverse, longitudinal, and stellate. Subcategories of each of these types are dependent on the location of the fracture line and the degree of distraction of the fracture fragments.

of the quadriceps expansion is present, allowing for separation of the fracture fragments.

The most common mechanism of patellar fracture is that of a direct blow to the anterior aspect of the knee, which results in a longitudinal or stellate type of fracture. These fracture patterns tend to spare the medial and lateral quadriceps expansion, and there is generally little distraction of the fracture fragments. The lack of quadriceps expansion involvement also explains why the patient is able to extend the knee without a great deal of discomfort.

Oblique and transverse types account for the majority of patellar fractures, followed by comminuted stellate fractures and longitudinal fractures. Despite its subcutaneous location, an undisplaced fracture line of the patella is often difficult to appreciate; point tenderness is the only remarkable examination finding. Soft tissue bleeding tends to extravasate into the subcutaneous tissue; large hemarthroses can also occur and may require aspiration for relief of pain. To determine the integrity of the quadriceps mechanism, active extension of the knee must be evaluated against gravity. Should the patient be unable to perform this

maneuver, some form of extensor mechanism injury exists and radiographic evaluation is indicated.

Radiographic assessment of patellar fractures should include anteroposterior, lateral, and skyline (or axial) projections. Transverse fractures are best seen on lateral views (Fig. 19-51). Marginal longitudinal fractures of the patella, which tend to be undisplaced with the knee in extension, are best visualized on the skyline view. In both adult and pediatric patients, a medial margin fracture cues the examiner to the possibility of an accompanying lateral patellar dislocation. Patellar tomography is indicated for the delineation of elusive fractures (those not well demonstrated on planar films) or in the event that bipartite patella is discovered.

A bipartite patella can easily be mistaken for a fracture of the patella in the face of historical patellar injury. This developmental abnormality occurs when the patellar ossification centers do not coalesce, resulting in an apparent separation of the patella. The accessory ossicle is located generally at the superolateral corner of the patella, at the insertion of the vastus lateralis. Inferiorly and laterally

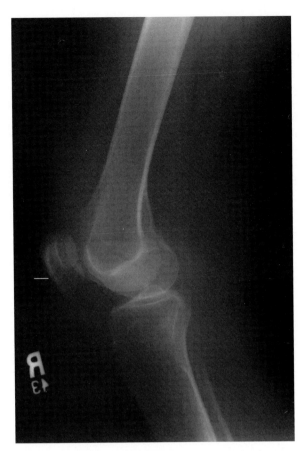

**Fig. 19-51.** Inferior pole patellar fracture. Attempting to catch herself while stumbling, this patient noted her knee buckling followed by completion of her fall. Note the presence of the minimally displaced transverse fracture of the lower pole of the patella. The fracture line is best demonstrated on the lateral projection.

located ossicles have also been described. When repetitive microtraumatic events result in microfractures of the synchondrosis that separates the ossicles, patients without recollection of a specific traumatic event report a pain pattern consistent with patellar fracture. Bipartite patella is best displayed on the anteroposterior view of the knee and is most often discovered coincidentally. Unlike an acute fracture, in which the fracture line is sharply demarcated, radiographs demonstrate an ill-defined sclerotic border. If tenderness is appreciated on examination over the area of synchondrosis, management initially consists of immobilization for 3 weeks. Persistent pain occasionally occurs, for which surgical intervention can be performed (excision of small fragments or osteosynthesis of larger fragments). Orthopedic referral for follow-up evaluation is necessary.

Preservation or restoration of the extensor mechanism is the primary goal in the treatment of patellar fractures. In general, nonoperative therapy yields good results. Cylindric casting (from the groin to the supramalleolar area) or a modified Robert Jones dressing is indicated if the quadriceps mechanism is intact and there is less than a 4-mm

separation of fracture fragments and/or less than 4 mm of articular surface step-off. Protective weight-bearing with crutch support is allowed after 3 days. Operative intervention is advocated 1) if an open fracture exists; 2) if fracture fragment separation exceeds 4 mm; 3) if more than 4 mm of articular surface step-off exists; 4) if an osteochondral fracture is present; or 5) if a longitudinal or marginal fracture is discovered. If operative therapy is indicated, orthopedic evaluation should be sought.

### Dislocation and subluxation

**Patellar subluxation.** Patellar tracking abnormalities are common. The pathomechanics of this entity are that of patellar hypermobility in either the medial or lateral direction. Medial patellar instability is considered rare; when seen, it is usually related to hyperextensile states, neuromuscular disease, or excessive patellar-medializing surgery. The patient has no recollection of knee deformity during these episodes but states a significant lack of confidence in the knee joint stability. Examination of the knee demonstrates a positive passive patellar hypermobility test and medial retinacular tenderness. If passive subluxation of the patella is greater than 50% of the patellar width, instability is probable. Findings following patellar subluxation are less pronounced than for those of patellar dislocation. Arthroscopic studies have demonstrated the presence of chondrosis of the medial patellar facet in 94% of the cases studied. This area correlates with the area where the patella contacted the lateral femoral condyle as it subluxed laterally.[31]

If recurrent, patellar subluxation is treated primarily with a quadriceps-strengthening program, with particular attention paid to the development of dysplastic oblique fibers of the vastus medialis. It is treated secondarily with lateral patellar support. Should patients suffer a recurrence despite a diligent rehabilitation program, operative intervention may be necessary. Surgical management of recurrent patellar subluxation includes lateral retinacular release, proximal extensor mechanism realignment (alone or in combination), or proximal and distal patellar realignment. The lateral retinacular release, at present, appears to be the initial procedure of choice.

**Patellar dislocation.** Acute patellar dislocation is by definition a complete lateral displacement of the patella. Dislocation assumes some degree of disruption of the medial patellar retinaculum. Individuals with any form of patellofemoral malalignment are at risk of patellar dislocation. Specific patellofemoral disorders include hypoplasia of the lateral femoral condyle, shallow femoral trochlea, increased quadriceps angle, patella alta, laterally faced patellar position, and vastus lateralis contracture.

The most common history is that of a direct blow to the medial aspect of the patella or a pivotal motion, away from the involved side, on a semiflexed knee. A rapid contraction of the quadriceps ensues, placing stress on the medial retinaculum, which yields, allowing the patella to slide laterally over the lateral border of the trochlea and lateral femoral condyle. On attempting to extend the knee, the patient will experience an increase in pain and thus tend to maintain the knee in a flexed position.

If the patella remains unreduced, the knee appears obviously deformed, with the patella situated lateral to the lateral femoral condyle. Should the patient present with reduction accomplished spontaneously, he or she generally says the knee "dislocated" and, with extension, "slipped back into place." During this description, the patient commonly reports a prominence of the medial aspect of the joint. This occurs because the anterior contour of the knee changes so dramatically due to the loss of the patellar shielding of the medial femoral condyle.

Tenderness is present on palpation at the lateral border of the patella as well as over the lateral and medial patellar retinaculum. The medial femoral condyle is easily palpated. Any attempt to extend the knee generally is met with adamant protest. Unlike medial collateral ligament injury, the joint capsule is disrupted in patellar dislocation, the resultant hemarthrosis extravasates into the surrounding soft tissue, and a generalized swelling appears rapidly over the entire knee.

It is important to remember that the primary injury involves a tearing of the medial patellar retinaculum. This injury usually occurs at its patellar insertion. An accompanying avulsion fracture of the superomedial pole of the patella may be evident on radiography. Osteochondral fractures of the lateral femoral condyle, the posterior patellar articular surface, or both, may occur with patellar dislocations.

Radiographic studies should include anteroposterior, lateral, and oblique views, with the addition of either a Hughston, sunrise, or silhouette view of the retropatellar surface.

Treatment is initially directed at relocation of the displaced patella. Ordinarily, reduction is accomplished easily by simple extension of the knee. Reduction is quite painful, and pain relief should be afforded the patient prior to the procedure. The combined use of benzodiazepine sedation and narcotic analgesia is a time-honored means of obtaining enough pain relief to perform relocation. Alternatively, arthrocentesis with instillation of 10 to 15 ml of lidocaine and bupivacaine (1:1) has found favor. This technique 1) affords excellent procedural anesthesia; 2) allows examination of joint fluid for fat droplets, alerting the examiner to a possible fracture; 3) provides postprocedural analgesia for 6 to 8 hours; and 4) avoids prolonged sedation (which may delay discharge). In the hypersensitive or hysterical adolescent, general anesthesia is occasionally required to perform reduction. Following reduction, the primary site of injury, the medial retinaculum, is palpated for any defect. A bulky compressive dressing and knee immobilizer or modified Robert Jones dressing is applied. Postreduction radiographs should be obtained, with particular attention paid to the position of reduction and the possibility of accompanying osteochondral fracture.

***Habitual patellar dislocation.*** Habitual dislocation implies repeated lateral patellar dislocation with each knee flexion cycle. This entity usually appears in childhood, unlike recurrent dislocation, which usually occurs in adolescence. Contracture of the quadriceps mechanism, in particular the vastus lateralis, is generally the underlying pathology of this type of dislocation. Examination of the habitual dislocating knee will demonstrate a significant passive lateral hypermobility test and a characteristic inability to manually maintain the patella in the midline with knee flexion. Basic initial care is directed to maintenance of extension, for which splinting in conjunction with non–weight-bearing crutch ambulation is appropriate. Orthopedic referral is sought for consideration of surgical mobilization of the quadriceps and patellar centralization.

***Recurrent patellar dislocation.*** By definition, recurrent patellar dislocation includes intermittent periods of patellar instability, with intervening asymptomatic periods of relative patellar stability. This malady generally occurs during adolescence but may occur in childhood. Girls are more frequently affected than boys. As a rule, the younger the child is at the time of initial dislocation, the more significant the underlying pathology and the greater the likelihood of recurrent dislocations. Of children suffering dislocation of the patella, only one third do not experience recurrence. One study demonstrated that children younger than 14 years who sustained dislocation had a 60% incidence of redislocation, while only a 30% recurrence rate occurred in those between 19 and 28 years of age.[32] A persistent dislocation is uncommonly seen on examination. Diffuse parapatellar tenderness and a positive passive lateral hypermobility test, which reproduces the patient's discomfort, is present. The presence of a significant hemarthrosis suggests the possibility of osteochondral fracture, which occurs in 10% of cases.

Significant radiographic features for recurrent patellar dislocation include dysplastic changes of the patella and lateral femoral condyle and the existence of an osteochondral fracture. Radiographs of the hip should be considered if the patellar radiographs are normal, since slipped capital femoral epiphysis and osteogenic sarcoma of the femur or tibia may present with knee pain, similar to patellar dislocation.

Initial treatment includes limitation of knee flexion with either a commercially available immobilizer or a modified Robert Jones dressing. Adolescent patients may be instructed in quadriceps exercise. Referral for orthopedic consultation is indicated because recurrence is frequent. In the young child, surgical intervention such as lateral retinacular release, medial plication, or patellar tendon transfer may be necessary. If an osteochondral fracture smaller than 1 cm is identified, arthroscopic removal is suggested.[29] If the fragment is larger than 1 cm, reduction and fixation are indicated.

**Femorotibial dislocations.** This rare but potentially devastating injury, which results from a violent force applied to the knee, is generated by vehicular accidents (two thirds of all cases), sporting accidents, falls, or a crushing injury to the extended knee. The relatively low incidence of knee dislocation is felt by some authors[32] to be due to the possibility that emergency medical technicians, during extrication and preparation of the patient for transport, may unknowingly facilitate a reduction of the dislocation. Thus complaints of knee pain in the multiple-trauma victim require ligamentous structure examination. Obesity has been proposed as a predisposing factor for knee dislocations. Total disruption of the posterior capsule, as well as disruption of the ACL and PCL, must occur before there is complete dislocation.

Of particular importance is the anatomy of the posterior popliteal space, where the popliteal artery is proximally

tethered to the femur at the adductor canal of Hunter and distally by the fibrous arch of the soleus muscle (Fig. 19-52). With dislocation of the knee, the popliteal artery is brought under tension and is subject to injuries ranging from thrombosis with transverse intimal tears (Fig. 19-53) to formal rupture. Intimal injury occurs more commonly with anterior dislocation while rupture of the vessel results more commonly from posterior dislocation. Hemarthrosis may be either significant or minimal, depending on the degree of capsular tearing.

Some general precautions need mention. First, the patient suspected of having sustained a dislocation of the knee must be assumed also to have sustained injury to the popliteal artery and/or the peroneal nerve. Second, absence of distal pulses should alert the examiner to the possibility of a knee dislocation and an accompanying popliteal artery injury. Third, the presence of distal pulses and normal capillary refill does not eliminate the possibility of popliteal arterial injury, and finally, if diminished distal pulses are present, arterial spasm must not be considered the etiology until proven so by arteriography.

Because this injury is the result of significant trauma, primary survey followed by resuscitation should be performed, with reduction of the dislocation included under this heading. Reduction should precede radiographic examination of the knee, even if fracture is suspected. If the popliteal artery is in fact lacerated, repair within 6 to 8 hours is mandatory in an attempt to avoid irreversible muscle necrosis and a resultant amputation. Studies have demonstrated that without surgical intervention to treat the popliteal artery injury, the amputation rate is 86%, while surgical intervention yields a limb salvage rate of 89%.[33] Peroneal nerve injury has been observed in 25% to 40% of

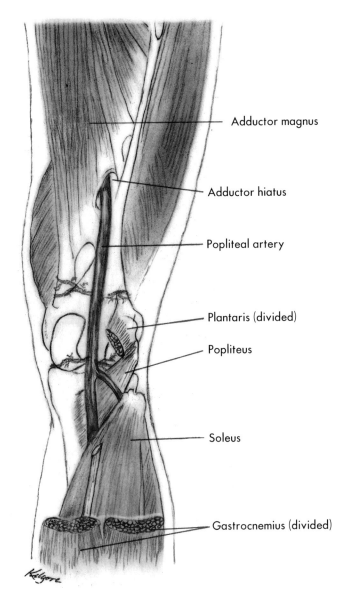

**Fig. 19-52.** Anatomy of the popliteal fossa. The popliteal fossa is bound inferiorly by the two muscle bellies of the gastrocnemius and plantaris—laterally by the lateral head of the biceps femoris and medially by the tendon of the semimembranosus. The profunda femoris artery enters the popliteal fossa via the adductor hiatus to become the popliteal artery.

Labels (Fig. 19-52): Adductor magnus; Adductor hiatus; Popliteal artery; Plantaris (divided); Popliteus; Soleus; Gastrocnemius (divided)

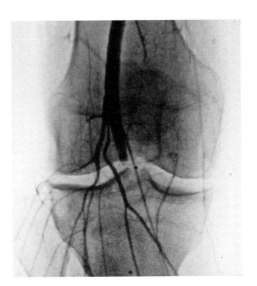

**Fig. 19-53.** Intimal tear of the popliteal artery. This arteriogram demonstrates normal filling of the superior geniculate and superior segment of the popliteal artery with an abrupt discontinuation of popliteal arterial filling and an absence of the inferior geniculate tributaries.

knee dislocations. Associated knee injuries include ligamentous disruption and fractures of the fibular head, tibial shaft, tibial plateau, patella, and supracondylar femur. Care must be taken to avoid overzealous or repetitive examination, since iatrogenic, secondary injury is possible.

Complications of knee dislocation include compartment syndrome, due to either tissue necrosis or massive crush injury, as well as acute tubular necrosis secondary to rhabdomyolysis and its accompanying myoglobinuria.

Anterior dislocations of the knee (Fig. 19-54) account for 30% to 50% of the knee dislocation cases reported in the literature.[33] The usual mechanism of injury is that of hyperextension of the knee, generally occurring when an opponent or the bumper of an automobile strikes the anterior aspect of the knee. This form of dislocation is accompanied by the highest incidence of vascular injury[33] and the greatest number of nerve injuries. Contact injury producing hyperextension of the knee initially disrupts the ACL,[34] then the posterior capsule, and finally the PCL. Kennedy[32] noted that posterior capsular rupture occurs at

30° of hyperextension. Should the hyperextension continue to 50° the popliteal artery will fail.

Reduction of an anterior knee dislocation is performed initially by application of longitudinal traction, either by an assistant or through the use of a Hare traction device. The posteriorly displaced femur is then drawn forward by the examiner over the more anteriorly situated tibial condyles. Hyperextension of the knee is absolutely contraindicated. Following reduction, a well-padded posterior splint is applied with the knee in 10° to 20° of flexion. Visual and tactile access points should be maintained to allow subsequent assessment of neurovascular status. In the grossly unstable knee, which frequently subluxes despite splinting, immediate casting or the application of an external fixation device will maintain the joint reduction. The latter appliance is particularly appropriate if surgical exploration of the popliteal artery is anticipated.

Posterior dislocation (Fig. 19-54) of the knee joint generally occurs as the result of a crushing injury, resulting in total disruption of the quadriceps mechanism. The most

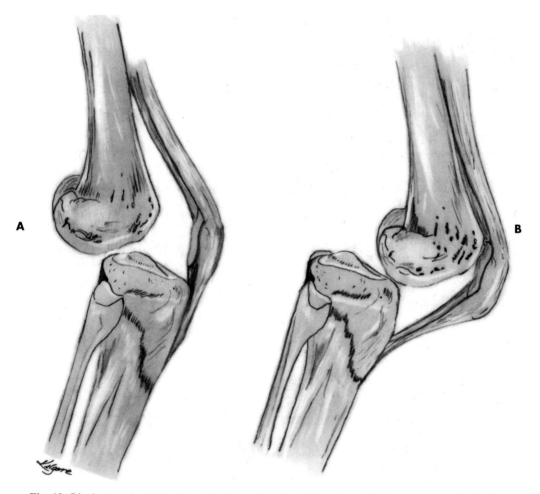

**Fig. 19-54. A**, Anterior dislocation of the knee. Anterior dislocations of the knee account for 30% to 50% of the reported cases. The usual mechanism of injury is that of hyperextension. This form of dislocation is attended by the highest incidence of vascular and nerve injuries. **B**, Posterior dislocation of the knee. Posterior knee dislocations occur as the result of a crushing injury, which causes total disruption of the quadriceps mechanism. Accompanying rupture of the patellar tendon may also occur.

common history is one in which the tibia strikes the dashboard of a decelerating vehicle, retropulsing the tibia. An accompanying rupture of the patellar tendon has been demonstrated experimentally.[32] If a crush injury is discovered and patellar tendon rupture appreciated on examination, the possibility of posterior knee dislocation must be considered. Reduction is accomplished by the application of longitudinal traction, either by an assistant or through the use of a Hare traction device. The posteriorly displaced tibia is then drawn forward by the examiner, beneath the anteriorly displaced femoral condyles. Hyperextension of the knee is absolutely contraindicated if posterior knee dislocation is suspected or proven.

Medial dislocation of the knee can occur when simultaneous valgus and rotational forces are applied to a semiflexed knee. This type of dislocation may be associated with supracondylar and tibial plateau fractures. Peroneal nerve injury commonly accompanies this type of injury.

Lateral and posterolateral knee dislocations occur as a result of concurrent varus and rotatory stresses. Peroneal nerve injury is a common concurrent injury. The posteriorly displaced tibia, occurring with this form of dislocation, will tear the peroneal nerve. Irreducibility of this type of dislocation is commonly encountered.[35]

Rotational dislocation of the knee generally does not involve rupture of the PCL. Instead, this ligament becomes the axis about which the tibia rotates. Once disrupted, the medial capsule may allow a "button-hole" protrusion of the medial femoral condyle, necessitating open reduction.

Indications for arteriography (see box on this page) following suspected knee dislocation include the following:

---

**Indications for popliteal arteriography**

*Popliteal arteriography*

Unknown status of the popliteal artery with a history suggesting dislocation with or without distal pulse abnormality

Presence of an expanding popliteal mass

Gross generalized ligamentous instability with a history suggestive of knee dislocation

Penetrating wound of the popliteal fossa or high-velocity weapon insult to the knee

---

1) an unknown status of the popliteal artery, with a significant history, with or without normal distal pulses; 2) the presence of an expanding popliteal mass; 3) the presence of a significant mechanism of injury with demonstrable ligamentous instability of the knee; and 4) penetrating injury to the popliteal fossa or high-velocity weapon injury to the knee. Contraindications to arteriography include the known presence of a popliteal laceration and an expected delay of more than 6 hours in obtaining a completed arteriogram. Should this be the case, an intraoperative "one-shot" femoral percutaneous arteriogram after reduction of the dislocation can be obtained to assess vascular patency and to direct further surgical exploration.

### Soft tissue injuries

**Bursal injuries.** A number of bursae are present about the knee (Fig. 19-55). These structures facilitate frictionless

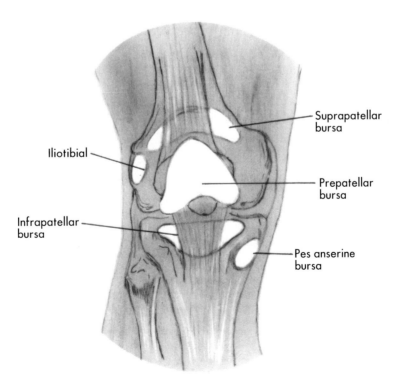

Iliotibial

Infrapatellar bursa

Suprapatellar bursa

Prepatellar bursa

Pes anserine bursa

**Fig. 19-55.** Bursa of the knee. Five major bursae are present about the knee joint, providing for muscular motion over the bony prominence about the joint.

motion of the musculotendinous structures over the joint. Once inflamed or irritated from repetitive motion, injury, or infection, these structures may become painful and restrict joint motion. The critical focus must be directed toward differentiation of septic from nonseptic etiologies.

Bursal infections tend to affect young and middle-aged individuals who are actively engaged in labor. Traumatic inoculation (puncture or abrasion) of the bursa is the most common mechanism, although hematogenous seeding does occur rarely. *Staphylococcus aureus* is the causative agent in 80% to 90% of septic bursitis cases. Penicillin resistance is common. Affected individuals are generally febrile with marked tenderness of the bursa. The skin overlying the bursa will generally appear erythematous and warm to the touch. An abrasion or puncture site over the bursa may or may not be evident. Range of motion of the knee is usually painless except in the extremes of flexion and extension. Diagnosis is based on clinical suspicion. Should clinical suspicion of infection be high a needle aspiration of the bursal fluid may be undertaken to obtain a specimen for culture and sensitivity studies. Treatment of bursal infections consists of antibiotic therapy and possible surgical drainage. Antibiotic therapies include oxacillin, either intravenously or orally, or, in the penicillin-allergic patient, intravenous vancomycin or oral erythromycin.

Nonseptic bursitis primarily affects those older than 40 years of age. Prolonged direct pressure irritation and arthropathy (eg, rheumatoid, gout, pseudogout) are the major causal factors that result in an inflammatory response of the bursa. Classically, rest has been prescribed; however, to avoid the perils of disuse and excessive stiffness, the early initiation of range-of-motion exercises is now favored.

***Prepatellar bursitis.*** Prepatellar bursitis, or "housemaid's knee," commonly occurs in persons who kneel for long periods of time (ie, housekeepers, wrestlers). These patients generally present with acute painful swelling of the anterior aspect of the patella, without an associated joint effusion. The function of the prepatellar bursa is to allow the skin to slide freely over the knee. With inflammatory prepatellar bursitis, the patient seldom reports pain. However, if pain is a prominent symptom in the presentation, septic bursitis should be considered.

Treatment consists of the use of NSAIDs (if not contraindicated), padding of the knee, and restriction of the precipitating activity. Occasionally, posterior splinting is employed. Aspiration of the bursa, followed by application of bulky compressive dressing, is employed to relieve pain in individuals who do not respond to more conservative therapy or for the purpose of ruling out an infectious etiology. Infection is not uncommon and the clinician must maintain a high index of suspicion in caring for the patient with prepatellar bursitis.

With repeated bouts of inflammation and irritation, the bursa becomes thickened and develops a chronic bursitis that is recalcitrant to conservative treatment. In such cases, orthopedic follow-up for possible bursectomy is indicated.

***Iliotibial band bursitis.*** A common affliction of long-distance runners, iliotibial band bursitis occurs as a result of repetitive rubbing of the iliotibial band over the lateral femoral condyle and its adjacent bursa. Clinically, tenderness is appreciated over the lateral femoral condyle, and may extend distally to Gerdy's tubercle. Swelling over the lateral aspect of the knee may also be evident.

Treatment generally begins with restriction of activity, avoidance of repetitive joint loading, and the use of NSAIDs, ice, and muscle-stretching exercises. Swimming may be employed as an alternative form of exercise for the avid runner who feels he or she must continue to exercise.

***Pes anserinus bursitis.*** Another problem confronting the clinician in caring for the runner is that of pes anserinus bursitis. Like iliotibial band bursitis, this condition is due to repetitive motion, with resultant irritation or direct trauma to the conjoin sartorius, gracilis, and semitendinosus tendons. On clinical examination, swelling and tenderness are present 4 to 5 cm below the medial tibial joint line.

Activity restriction, avoidance of repetitive joint loading, and the use of NSAIDs, ice, and muscle-stretching exercises are the initial treatment plan. Swimming may be employed as an alternative form of exercise. Orthopedic follow-up for possible excision is indicated in cases in which the patient experiences recurrence that has not responded favorably to more conservative modalities.

***Infrapatellar bursitis.*** Repeated dropping to the knees (eg, in wrestlers or laborers) or people engaged in repetitive jumping activities (eg, competitive divers and basketball players) may result in painful swelling of the infrapatellar bursa. Localized swelling and erythema distinctly separate from the prepatellar area and joint space are seen in the infrapatellar region. Pain is elicited with direct pressure, with passive knee flexion, and on complete active extension of the knee. This entity is easily confused with patellar tendinitis; however, the tenderness in infrapatellar bursitis occurs over a broader area than does that in patellar tendinitis.

Treatment includes rest, the application of ice, padding or splinting, and the use of NSAIDs. Recurrence is common; for repetitive episodes, orthopedic consultation for possible bursal excision should be sought.

***Popliteal cysts.*** The classic "Baker's cyst" is a bursitis of the semimembranosus (medial gastrocnemius) bursa, lying between the semimembranosus and medial head of the gastrocnemius tendon. Initially, the patient may appreciate a small soft tissue mass of the popliteal space, which may or may not be followed by varying periods of heaviness or aching of the posterior knee. The mass frequently disappears with flexion of the knee, only to reappear with extension. Since this bursa frequently communicates with the joint space, symptoms may be transitory. Conversely, should the mass be persistent, it generally heralds some form of internal joint derangement, and orthopedic referral should be sought. Classically, popliteal cysts are associated with tears of the posterior horn of the medial meniscus.

Other atypical locations of popliteal cysts involve the bursa lying between the lateral head of the gastrocnemius and the lateral biceps femoris. This cystic structure is capable of dissection and rupture, and usually results in hemorrhage. Cysts may become massive, mimicking the lower extremity swelling of deep vein thrombosis.

**Extensor mechanism injury**

***Sinding-Larsen-Johannson disease.*** This syndrome was initially presented in 1921 by Sinding-Larsen.[36] It occurs most commonly in adolescent males aged 10 to 13 years. Initially, it was believed to represent an inflammatory process and a resultant osteonecrosis, and consequently was termed an epiphysitis, apophysitis, and osteochondritis. It is currently believed to be an overuse syndrome caused by repetitive stresses resulting from a traction phenomenon along the proximal attachment of the patellar tendon. This traction apophysitis is felt to be the pediatric equivalent of jumper's knee in the adult.

Sinding-Larsen-Johansson disease is frequently seen in patients with cerebral palsy, who, by walking in a crouched position, sustain excessive loading of the patellar tendon. These patients present with tenderness and swelling over the inferior pole of the patella that is exacerbated by deceleration and jumping activities. Radiographic changes include radiopaque infrapatellar ossification, which, if followed over a period of time, appears to coalesce with the patella.[37] The approximate duration of the disease ranges from 3 to 12 months; no disability should be anticipated.

The initial treatment consists primarily of rest. Rigid immobilization yields no benefit over rest alone. Ice application, isometric quadriceps exercise, and anti-inflammatory agents are also used in early conservative management. In the refractory case, orthopedic referral is indicated. The use of local steroid injections is not recommended because tendon degeneration may be precipitated and little long-term benefit is gained.

***Jumper's knee: patellar tendon rupture and patellar tendinitis.*** Rapid acceleration and deceleration activities occurring during competitive sports concentrate considerable stress on the patellar tendon. Jumper's knee, or patellar tendinitis, represents an overuse syndrome, analogous to tennis elbow and Achilles tendinitis. It is characterized by microtears of the patellar tendon at its site of attachment along the inferior pole of the patella. This syndrome is most commonly seen in basketball players and competitive divers, and results from an unexpected extensor load accompanied by forceful contraction of the quadriceps, basically "overloading" the extensor mechanism.

Universally, the presenting complaint is that of pain, which generally recurs with practice or competition. Because the onset is insidious, few patients are able to recall a specific traumatic incident responsible for their pain. Interestingly, right-handed individuals usually present with left knee discomfort, and vice versa. The history commonly discloses that the pain is reproduced with deceleration or (less commonly) acceleration. Other exacerbating activities

include bicycling, squatting, and ascending or descending stairs. Patellar tendinitis is most often confused with chondromalacia patella and plica syndrome; a distinction is necessary because treatments do differ.

Tenderness that is well circumscribed to the patellar tendon is present on examination. With the knee in full extension, palpation immediately below the inferior pole of the patella almost always elicits a pain response. Occasionally, a small amount of swelling is also encountered in this area.

No radiographic changes have been documented consistently in those who have experienced symptoms for less than 6 months. However, in individuals with symptoms for longer than 6 months, the lateral knee radiographic examination is helpful, demonstrating a decreased bone density along the inferior pole of the patella, suggesting hyperemia or disuse. In those having symptoms for 1 to 2 years, there is an area of increased density in the patellar tendon, which is due to fibrocartilage production. Ossification may be seen inferior to the patella in patients experiencing symptoms for over 2 years.

The initial treatment is rest, because symptoms are produced when the patient is engaged in activity. No benefit over rest alone is gained by rigid immobilization with knee immobilizers or cylinder casting. Ice application, isometric quadriceps exercise, and anti-inflammatory agents are also used in early conservative management. In refractory cases orthopedic referral for possible surgical debridement of the tendon is indicated. The use of local steroid injections is not recommended because further tendon degeneration may be precipitated and little long-term benefit is gained.

Total patellar tendon rupture is a catastrophic event and will be remembered vividly by the patient. Patients experience a sudden, sharp pain and an inability to extend the knee. There is usually a palpable defect or gap of the patellar tendon, which may be masked by hematoma and swelling. A high-riding patella with palpable increased mobility is the pathognomonic sign of patellar tendon rupture. Lateral radiographic evaluation will display an obvious elevation of the patella (Fig. 19-56). This injury deserves orthopedic consultation, since early repair offers excellent results.[38]

***Quadriceps tendon injury.*** Disruption of the trilayered quadriceps tendon occurs as the result of an abrupt reflex contraction of the quadriceps against the body's weight. Case scenarios include the weekend softball player who slides into second base with the knee held in a semiflexed position and comes into contact with the fixed base, or the 60- or 70-year-old individual who stumbles or slips and reflexively attempts to avoid the fall. Injury may be partial or complete, starting in the anterior-central segments and progressing to involve the more medial and lateral fibers. Partial tears generally involve only the superficial layer of the tendon whereas complete tears involve all three layers. A tear of the suprapatellar synovial membrane occurs concurrently with a complete rupture. Factors predisposing

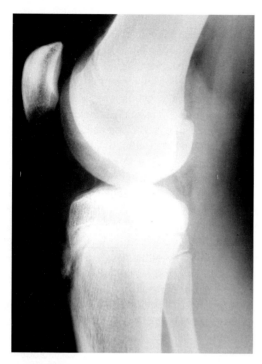

**Fig. 19-56.** Patellar tendon rupture. Lateral radiographic projection demonstrating patella alta. Note the elevation of the patella (Insall-Salvetti ratio of 0.55:1).

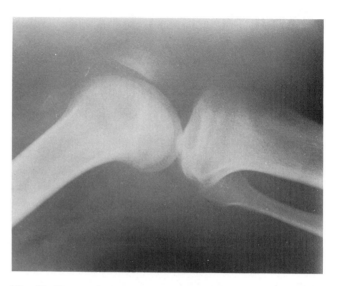

**Fig. 19-57.** Quadriceps tendon rupture. Lateral x-ray projection demonstrating a lower than normal position of the patella (patella baja). (From Hughston JC. Knee Ligaments: Injury and Repair. St. Louis: Mosby-Year Book, Inc., 1993: 92.)

an individual to injury of the quadriceps tendon include obesity, increasing age, prior injury to the tendon substance, degenerative arthritis, atherosclerosis, diabetes mellitus, nephritis, hyperparathyroidism, and gouty arthropathy. The patient suffering quadriceps tendon rupture vividly recalls a sharp, stabbing pain. If there is a complete tear, the pain tends to be short-lived. Incomplete tears that are treated result in persistent pain that is exacerbated by ascending stairs or inclined planes and a sensation of buckling of the knee with simple ambulation.

A large hemarthrosis and/or ecchymosis over the suprapatellar area may be seen. The results of ligament stress tests are normal. The most important finding present on physical examination is the patient's inability to extend the knee against gravity while in a sitting position. In the case of complete rupture, the patient is able to stand but cannot walk. The injured patella may be "low riding" (patella baja) and more freely movable than the uninjured patella. A palpable cleft, produced with quadriceps retraction, is usually 2 to 5 cm in breadth; however, this may be masked by hematoma in the acute period. A visible cleft of the skin over the anterior suprapatellar thigh is present after an 8- to 12-week healing period. A paucity of swelling and normal radiographic evaluation may lead to a misdiagnosis of sprain. Radiographic examination is generally normal, with the exception of a lower positioning of the patella on lateral projection (Fig. 19-57). On occasion radiography will demonstrate a small bony avulsion from the superior pole of the patella.

Treatment of complete rupture of the quadriceps tendon is operative[36] and involves reapproximation of the severed tendon, necessitating orthopedic consultation. Cylinder casting in full extension for a period of 5 to 6 weeks is indicated in selected patients with partial disruption who lack 10° to 15° of extension.

**Ligamentous injury of the knee.** In general, ligamentous injuries in both adults and children are managed the same. Pure ligamentous injuries of the knee do occur occasionally in the immature skeleton.[39] Because the ligamentous structures about the knee possess a greater tensile strength than the physeal plates, children are more likely to sustain growth plate injuries, especially with translational mechanisms. The incidence of pediatric ligamentous injury, to which the primary care community has become more vigilant, has increased.[39] The presence of a fracture about the knee by no means precludes the possibility of associated ligamentous injury in both of these populations.

*ACL injury.* The ACL is held as the primary restraint to both anterior drawer and hyperextension.[6] It also determines the blend of translational motion between the femur and tibia required for normal knee kinematics. Most authors recognize two fascicles or bundles to the ACL.[4] The anteromedial bundle is taut while the knee is in flexion. The posterolateral bundle is relatively lax while the knee is in flexion; and in extension both fascicles are equally burdened. Because most ACL injuries occur while the knee is in some degree of flexion, it would follow that the anteromedial bundle of this ligament appears to be at the greatest risk of injury. Conversely, the posterolateral bundle is more likely to be injured if hyperextension of the knee occurs. The ACL also functions as a secondary restraint to both valgus and varus stresses.

**Table 19-7.** Initial symptoms of anterior cruciate
ligament insufficiency

| Symptom | Incidence (%) |
| --- | --- |
| Knee motion decrease by 24 hours | 96 |
| Knee swelling within 6 hours | 90 |
| Knee "gave way" | 90 |
| Unable to continue play | 88 |
| Immediate knee pain | 85 |
| Heard a pop or snap at outset | 65 |

From Paulos L, Noyes FR, Malek M: A practical guide to the initial
evaluation to the initial evaluation and treatment of knee ligament injuries,
*J Trauma* 20:498, 1980.

A number of significant clues to ACL injury (Table 19-7)
can be elicited from the patient during the interview and
examination process. Acute disruption precipitates a
guarded or painful range of motion (94%), instantaneous
disability (85%),[40] acute hemarthrosis (90%),[16] and an
audible pop or snap (65%).[41] Patients report varied histories
resulting in ACL disruption. The most commonly reported
mechanism of injury is a vertical deceleration event, such
as during a fall or after retrieving a rebound, which result in
the hyperextension of an already extended knee. This injury
also occurs when an individual unknowingly steps into a
hole with the knee in full extension or suddenly decelerates
while attempting to perform a lateral "cutting" movement.
ACL disruption offers a memorable instability of the knee
and an inability to continue any activity. Significant swelling ensues within the next 12 hours.

The Lachman test has proven to be the most reliable and
clinically the least painful test for determination of ACL
insufficiency. Noyes et al.[6] have advocated the use of the
flexion-rotation drawer test for evaluation of both ACL
insufficiency and anterolateral rotatory instability in the
acute care setting. In the presence of ACL insufficiency, the
anterior drawer test is the least sensitive at demonstrating
anterior tibial translation. Performance of the pivot-shift or
jerk tests in the presence of hemarthrosis is generally next
to impossible.

Hemarthrosis occurs in 90% of ACL disruptions.[31]
Other, less common causes of hemarthrosis include patellar
dislocation, osteochondral fracture, and peripheral meniscal
tear. Aspiration of straw-colored synovial fluid casts doubt
on the existence of an ACL injury, but is seen with
longitudinal and radial meniscal injuries.

Twenty-four percent to 39% of all ACL injuries involve
partial disruption of the ligament. Progression of an ACL
injury has also been well documented. Fruensgaard and
Johannsen[42] demonstrated that 51% of arthroscopically
proven partial ACL tears progressed to a complete injury
over a 17-month follow-up period. Studies have delineated
the "critical mass" necessary to avoid progression of the
ACL to total failure. Noyes et al.[43] demonstrated that if
three fourths of the ligament is intact, no progression

occurs, but if only one fourth of the ligament remains
undisrupted, there will be an eventual failure rate of 86%.

Associated meniscal disruption originating at the time of
ACL injury has been widely acknowledged. Clinical investigations have reported a 41%[44] to 68%[45] incidence of
concurrent ACL disruption and meniscal injury. Chronic
repetitive subluxation of an ACL-deficient knee results in a
de novo meniscal injury or extension of an existing meniscal injury.

The incidence of collateral ligament injury associated
with ACL disruption ranges from 21%[18] to 40%.[23] In the
chronically ACL-deficient knee the incidence of meniscal
pathology ranges from 85% to 91%.[46] Associated injuries
to the articular cartilage have been reported in 23% of acute
ACL injuries and in 54% of chronic ACL injuries.[45]

Planar radiographs offer no information regarding the
integrity of the radiolucent ACL. A number of indirect
findings, which, when present, suggest disruption of the
ACL have been described. Avulsion fracture of the origin of
the ACL, the anteromedial tibial eminence, signals possible
disruption. The lateral capsule sign (Segond's fracture)
represents an avulsion of the anterolateral tibial tubercle
(Gerdy's tubercle) by the iliotibial band (Fig. 19-58). This

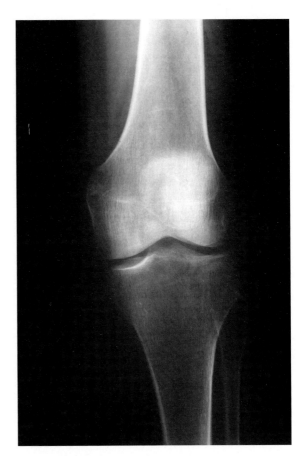

**Fig. 19-58.** Segond's fracture ("lateral capsular sign"). This
represents an avulsion of the anterolateral (Gerdy's) tibial tubercle
by the iliotibial band. This fracture has a significant association
with accompanying anterior cruciate ligament injury.

radiographic finding indicates an injury to the middle third of the lateral capsule and a significant possibility of ACL disruption.[47] A depth of 1.5 mm of the lateral condylopatellar sulcus (Fig. 19-59), termed the *deep lateral femoral notch,* is also useful as an indirect radiographic sign of ACL disruption.[48]

Magnetic resonance imaging is ideally suited for the delineation of knee ligamentous injury and reveals fractures previously undetected by routine radiographic study. In one series of patients undergoing MRI for evaluation of ACL disruption,[19] a 56% incidence of occult bone bruise injury involving the posterolateral tibial plateau was found. Formal ACL disruption on MRI demonstrates a loss of the normal parallel margins of the ligament within the intercondylar notch area (Fig. 19-60).

Isolated ACL injury (Fig. 19-61) need not uniformly undergo surgical stabilization. Many individuals can be treated conservatively with rehabilitative programs, bracing, and a redirection in recreational activities, with the patient conceding his or her instability.

Indications for operative intervention include a grossly unstable knee (ie, gross unstable jerk and pivot-shift tests), combined ACL and medial collateral ligament rupture, avulsion of the anterior tibial eminence, and the professional athlete with an isolated ACL injury. Instability of the

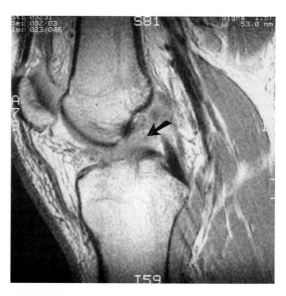

**Fig. 19-60.** Magnetic resonance imaging demonstrating anterior cruciate ligament disruption. Note the disarray of the normal parallel cruciate fibers. Synovitis and hemorrhage are implied by the irregularities of Hoffa's fat pad.

joint is the major determinate, and age is not a limiting factor in determining operability.

*PCL injury.* The PCL is viewed as the primary stabilizer of the entire knee and the primary restraint to posterior drawer translation. Most PCL injuries result from either automobile accidents or sporting activities. PCL injury has been estimated to occur in 20% of all knee injuries.[49]

Cadaver studies have demonstrated two predominant mechanisms of PCL injury: 1) a concentrated posterior displacement of the tibia on the femur while the knee is held in a flexed position and 2) an abrupt hyperextension of the knee. The site of injury appears to be the midsubstance of the PCL in 76% of cases (femoral avulsion in 36% to 55% of cases, and tibial avulsion in 22% to 42%).[19] Injuries to other structures that concurrently accompany PCL injuries include medial collateral ligament (50%), posteromedial joint capsule, ACL (65%), and meniscal injuries (30%).

Diagnosis of PCL injury is difficult and is fraught with a number of caveats. The patient cites little in the way of immediate instability, but rather describes a sensation of the femur "slipping off" the tibia, and medial joint line discomfort. The presence of a tense hemarthrosis assumes an intact joint capsule and is generally mistaken for an ACL tear. The anterior drawer sign frequently is appreciated as positive if the PCL is deficient; this is due to an erroneous starting position of the examination (with the tibia initially subluxed posteriorly). Care must also be taken in positioning the tibia in neutral position while performing the posterior drawer sign, since internal rotation tightens the intact ligaments of Wrisberg or Humphry, producing a false-negative test. The sag test appears to be the most reliable clinical test for determining PCL disruption (90% specificity).[49]

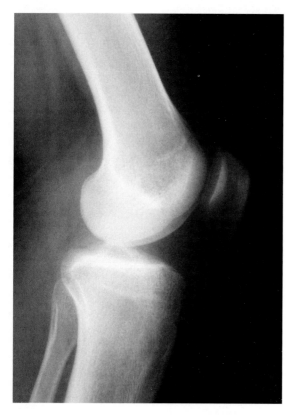

**Fig. 19-59.** Deep lateral femoral notch sign. This lateral radiograph demonstrates a 1.5-mm defect in the lateral femoral sulcus. This finding is useful as an indirect indicator of anterior cruciate ligament disruption.

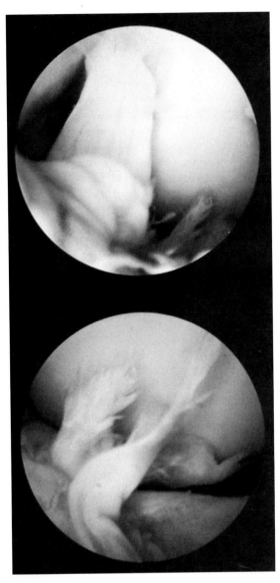

**Fig. 19-61.** Arthroscopic representation of an anterior cruciate ligament disruption.

Tibial avulsion of the PCL presents as tenderness and swelling of the popliteal fossa. Radiographic examination may disclose avulsion fracture of the ligament's proximal or distal attachment; however, with midsubstance disruption, radiographs add little information to that obtained through physical examination. Due to its relative importance to joint stability and the high incidence of associated joint structure injury, orthopedic consultation is required in cases of PCL injury. Early surgical repair has been advocated by some authors.[5] Others[2] feel that isolated injuries of the PCL can be managed conservatively with bracing and a rehabilitation program. If associated structures are disrupted, however, combined instabilities will result, and the patient should undergo surgical repair of the PCL and its associated structures.[50] Tibial plateau avulsion injuries in combination with PCL disruption require direct repair. Midsubstance PCL injury involves reconstruction with a free or vascularized musculotendinous graft.

*Medial collateral ligament injury.* The patient with a medial collateral ligament disruption reports a lateral blow to a slightly flexed knee at the time of injury. He or she may also state some element of twisting motion (such as when stepping into a hole or when in a skiing accident). The major component of this injury is a valgus stress. The most important physical finding favoring this diagnosis is that of medial joint space opening with valgus stress applied at 30° of flexion. Injury is graded using the American Medical Association guidelines of ligamentous injury (Table 19-1), with particular attention given to the presence or absence of a firm endpoint to valgus stress. Palpation of the medial joint reveals tenderness along the course of the medial collateral ligament. The anterior drawer test in external rotation demonstrates an anterior subluxation of the medial tibial condyle. Patellar instability occurs in approximately 20% of patients with medial collateral ligament disruption, resulting from concurrent vastus medialis rupture.

Routine radiographs including valgus stress views add little information to that obtained by physical examination. Should accompanying injury (eg, ACL, PCL, or meniscal injury) be suspected after examination, MRI or arthroscopic examination with the patient under anesthesia is indicated.

Philosophies of treatment for isolated medial collateral ligament injuries have changed dramatically over the past decade, with a move away from traditional surgical repair to one of functional bracing.[51,52] Currently, a functional range-of-motion brace has been suggested as the best treatment modality for grade II and grade III injuries of the medial collateral ligament.[52] This bracing limits extension to 30° and flexion to 90°, and the patient initially is maintained non–weight-bearing.

The possibility of multiple structural injury underscores the importance of the initial examination and diagnosis. Should the examination unveil excessive valgus instability (which suggests posterior oblique ligament disruption) in combination with medial collateral ligament injury, or ACL disruption combined with medial collateral ligament injury, surgical intervention is indicated. Peripheral medial meniscal tears occur more commonly in association with isolated medial collateral ligament injury, while midsubstance injuries of the medial meniscus accompany combined ACL and medial collateral ligament disruption.[53]

*Lateral collateral ligament injury.* The lateral collateral ligament is the primary restraint to varus deformity of the knee. Secondary restraints include the lateral capsular ligaments, the arcuate complex, and the popliteus muscle. Injuries to these structures tend to occur in combination and are seldom isolated. It is common for disruption of the ACL or PCL to occur with varus injury once the lateral collateral ligament has failed. Typically, the mechanism of injury is a blow to the anteromedial aspect of the knee, with resultant varus and hyperextension deformation of the knee joint. The entire posterolateral complex is disrupted, including the lateral collateral ligament, lateral capsular ligaments, arcuate complex, popliteus muscle, and ACL.

Diagnosis of this type of injury is difficult. Specific tests that should be performed include the adduction (varus) stress test at 30° of flexion, the external rotation recurvatum test, and the anterior drawer test with the foot internally rotated. Six percent of routine radiographs may demonstrate a fracture of the proximal fibula, suggesting lateral collateral avulsion injury, and possibly a fracture of the anterolateral tibial condyle or lateral capsular sign. The latter finding should also prompt the examiner to suspect an injury to the ACL.[47] The next step in evaluating such an injury is MRI. Examination with the patient under anesthesia and/or arthroscopic examination may be needed if MRI is not available.

Grade I and grade II isolated lateral collateral ligament injuries are treated primarily using either a modified Robert Jones dressing or a well-padded knee immobilizer. Treatment ordinarily includes early functional bracing in conjunction with a rehabilitation program. If the injury is believed to be an isolated grade III injury of the lateral collateral ligament, or if associated structural instability is appreciated, surgical intervention is indicated[12] and orthopedic consultation is requested.

**Meniscal injuries.** The menisci are imperative for normal knee kinematics and are no longer felt to be expendable. The incidence of meniscal injury in the general population has been estimated at 60 per 100,000, with sporting activities producing two thirds of these injuries. In men, the incidence of meniscal injury appears to peak from ages 21 to 40, while in women peak incidence occurs between the ages of 11 and 20.[54] The adolescent with a meniscal injury is typically more likely to have sustained synchronous ligamentous injury when compared with the adult. As a result of the magnitude of force necessary to produce meniscal injury, attendant ligamentous injuries are common.

The lateral, middle, and medial geniculate arteries supply the perimeniscal plexus, which is limited to the peripheral 10% to 30% of the medial meniscus and 25% of the lateral meniscus. The central marginal two thirds of the menisci derive nutritional support by simple diffusion from the synovial fluid. In order for meniscal injury to heal, vascular communication between the site of injury and this peripheral plexus must exist. Since 52% of acute meniscal injuries are reported as peripheral in location, attempts at repair are reasonable and in fact have met with a 75% to 80% healing rate.[55]

The lateral meniscus is more mobile than its medial counterpart. This is explained by its lack of attachment to the lateral collateral ligament and an interruption in the capsular attachment that occurs at the popliteal hiatus. Laterally, the capsular attachments do not fasten the lateral meniscus as rigidly as do those found medially. This greater mobility in the anteroposterior direction is believed in part to protect the lateral meniscus from injury. Statistically, the

medial meniscus sustains injury twice as often as is its lateral counterpart.

The history associated with meniscal injuries usually involves a cutting, squatting, or twisting maneuver. Displacement of a meniscal fragment may result in a complaint of locking, usually in 30° of flexion and at the time of injury. Joint line tenderness and an incomplete range of motion (limited terminal flexion and extension) are noted by both the patient and the examiner. An associated hemarthrosis is present in virtually all medial meniscal injuries and in half of all lateral meniscal injuries. The sensation of giving way is due to a displacement of the meniscal tissue

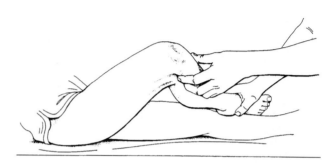

**Fig. 19-62.** Palpation of the posterolateral joint line. To detect a possible tear of the lateral meniscus the patient's affected knee is flexed and the hip is externally rotated, allowing the leg to rest atop the lower leg of the unaffected side. This produces opening of the lateral joint space. The examiner then palpates the joint line for any tenderness. (From Hughston, J.C.: *Knee Ligaments: injury and repair.* St. Louis: Mosby-Year Book, Inc., 1993.)

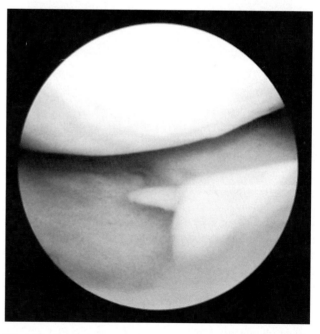

**Fig. 19-63.** Radial meniscus tear. Arthroscopic presentation showing a small radial tear of the anterior one third of the medial meniscus. (From O'Connor RL: *Arthroscopy.* Kalamazoo, MI: The Upjohn Co, 1977.)

with compression and rotation of the joint. Patients suffering a lateral meniscal injury report a morning stiffness and instability with reproduction of pain on pivoting and turning. Should a chronic meniscal injury be present, noticeable quadriceps atrophy will be present on examination.

Joint line tenderness is an important finding in cases of meniscal injury. Because 81% of meniscal injuries involve the peripheral posterior meniscus,[23] palpation of the posterior joint line cannot be neglected (Fig. 19-62). McMurry's test is positive in 70% of patients with demonstrable meniscal injury. Apley's compression test can also claim only a 70% accuracy.

There are five basic patterns of meniscal injury. Radial tears or "parrot beak" injuries account for 20% of meniscal

injuries (Fig. 19-63). This form of tear originates from the central edge of the meniscus and radiates peripherally. A 5-mm tear is necessary to produce symptoms. This pattern generally involves the middle third of the lateral meniscus. Although less common, radial tears can also occur in the medial meniscus but they tend to involve the posterior third of this structure. The term *root tear* implies a radial tear of the posterior horn of the lateral meniscus and is associated with a concurrent disruption of the ACL.

The bucket-handle tear (Fig. 19-64) occurs more commonly in younger patients. A significant incidence of coexisting ACL disruption occurs with this type of meniscal lesion, and the medial meniscus is involved three times more often. Large tears of this type are capable of central displacement into the intercondylar notch (Fig. 19-65), resulting in clinical locking of the knee. Smaller tears, particularly those of the posterior third of the meniscus, are unstable and result in symptoms of meniscal injury but lack a history of locking.

Flap tears (Figs. 19-66 and 19-67) are vertical tears of the meniscus and occur as the result of extension of a radial tear or detachment of the anterior (or posterior) attachment of a remnant of the central meniscal edge of a bucket-handle injury.

Horizontal cleavage tears (Figs. 19-68 and 19-69) arise at the peripheral margin of the meniscus, separating the meniscus into superior and inferior pieces. Parameniscal cysts are most often associated with horizontal cleavage tears (Fig. 19-70).

Complex tears are the most common pattern of meniscal injury, and are responsible for 30% of all meniscal injuries.[55] Individuals shown to have this type of injury are generally between 40 and 50 years of age, and concurrent

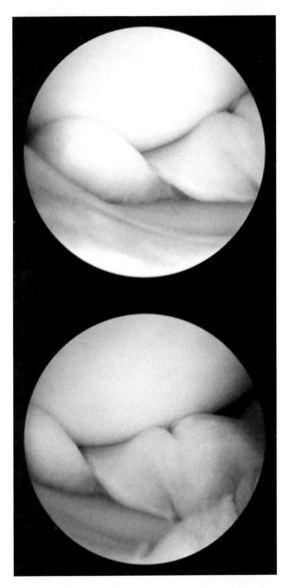

**Fig. 19-64.** Bucket handle tear. Arthroscopic presentation of a bucket-handle tear of the medial meniscus showing displacement of the anterior rim (*top*) and main body near the posterior meniscotibial attachment (*bottom*). (From O'Connor RL: *Arthroscopy.* Kalamazoo, MI: The Upjohn Co, 1977.)

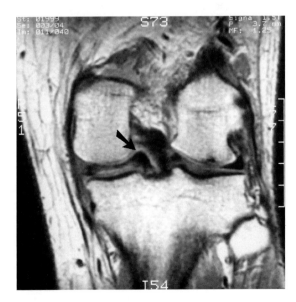

**Fig. 19-65.** Bucket-handle tear. Magnetic resonance imaging representation of a bucket-handle tear of the medial meniscus. Note the displacement of the fragment into the intercondylar notch.

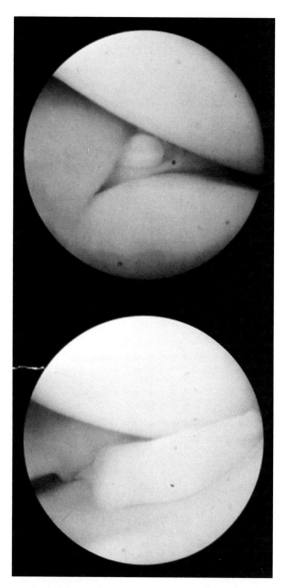

**Fig. 19-66.** Flap tear of the meniscus. Arthroscopic presentation of a flap tear of the medial meniscus. With internal rotation of the tibia (*top*) the torn segment is trapped between the remaining intact meniscus. External rotation (*bottom*) of the tibia dislocates the flap. (From O'Connor RL: *Arthroscopy.* Kalamazoo, MI: The Upjohn Co, 1977.)

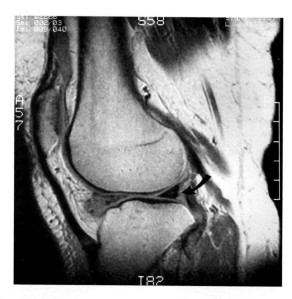

**Fig. 19-67.** Flap tear of the meniscus. Magnetic resonance imaging presentation of a flap tear of the posterior horn of the lateral meniscus.

ligamentous injury generally is not present. This pattern of meniscal injury represents a degenerative process in which there is also degeneration of the articular cartilage of the knee joint.

Injury to the peripheral 3 mm of the meniscus results in tearing of the perimeniscal capillary plexus and the development of a hemarthrosis. Approximately 26% of meniscal injuries demonstrate some degree of peripheral involvement. This type of injury is most amenable to surgical repair. Diagnostic arthrocentesis in knees sustaining the more centrally located radial or longitudinal meniscal tears yields a straw-colored synovial aspirate. Conditions often confused with meniscal injury include plica syndrome,

popliteal tendinitis, intra-articular loose bodies, osteochondral fractures, fat pad impingement, meniscotibial ligament strain, discoid meniscus, inflammatory arthritis, synovitis, and synovial tumors.

Meniscal pathology has been identified in 85% of knees studied for chronic ACL deficiency.[46] Anteromedial rotatory instability of the knee can be expected if the patient has sustained disruption of the medial meniscal attachment to the posterior oblique ligament with concurrent ACL insufficiency.

Since the menisci are radiolucent, planar radiographs offer little in terms of diagnostic assistance. With the advent of arthroscopy and MRI, the role of arthrography has become a topic of debate. Since operative intervention is indicated when multiple structures of the knee are disrupted and a significant incidence of associated injuries occur concurrently with meniscal injuries, MRI and arthroscopy appear to offer the most assistance in determining the extent of knee injury.

Treatment directives in the care of meniscal injuries are relatively limited. The patient with a locked knee should be splinted in a position of comfort, and no attempt to reduce the lock should be attempted until orthopedic consultation is received. Over the last decade, philosophies of treating meniscal injuries have changed dramatically, and a more aggressive approach has been undertaken to facilitate an expedient repair. To accomplish this, early orthopedic consultation and direction in further evaluation and operative intervention are needed.

**Miscellaneous conditions**

***Chondromalacia patellae.*** Chondromalacia patellae is a common degenerative malady resulting from overuse, trauma, or disturbances of the patellar function. The under-

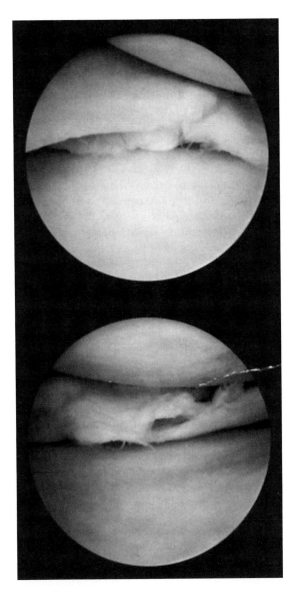

**Fig. 19-68.** Horizontal cleavage tear of the meniscus. Arthroscopic presentation of a horizontal cleavage tear of the left medial meniscus. (From O'Connor RL: *Arthroscopy*. Kalamazoo, MI: The Upjohn Co, 1977.)

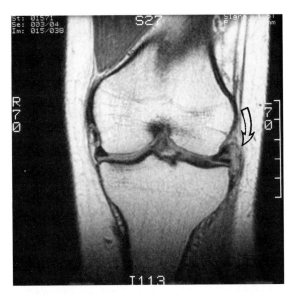

**Fig. 19-69.** Horizontal cleavage tear of the lateral meniscus. Note the bulging of the lateral joint capsule and the diamond-shaped defect of the peripheral midsubstance of the lateral meniscus.

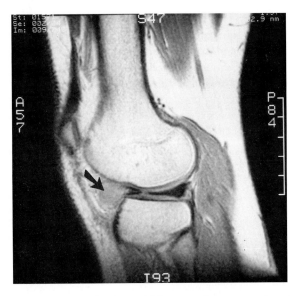

**Fig. 19-70.** Parameniscal cyst. This magnetic resonance imaging presentation demonstrates an anteriorly located parameniscal cyst dissecting through Hoffa's infrapatellar fat pad. A peripheral horizontal cleavage tear of the anterior aspect of the lateral meniscus.

lying pathomechanics of chondromalacia involves an abnormal patellar tracking mechanism. Causes of abnormal tracking include recurrent subluxations (51%), idiopathic dislocations (30%), posttraumatic dislocations (10%), recurrent dislocations (4%), and postoperative dislocations (5%).[56] A deterioration or "wearing" of the patellar articular cartilage occurs[57] and presents in four degrees of severity: grade I involves softening of the articular surface with fibrillation of the cartilage; grade II, fissuring; grade III, erosion of the articular cartilage; and grade IV, a cartilaginous deficit extending to the subchondral bone.[58]

With chondromalacia patellae, pain is usually appreciated at the extremes of flexion and extension as well as during extension against resistance. It is most frequently reported to occur after sitting for long periods of time, during stairway ascent, and transiently after exercise (swelling and pain). Pain is produced as the quadriceps tendon causes the tender patella to engage the trochlear surface of the femur. Findings on physical examination include crepitance with passive motion of the patella and a positive "apprehension" test. Of particular concern to the clinician is the extent of quadriceps wasting (the oblique fibers of the vastus medialis in particular), which commonly occurs.

Chondromalacia patellae has become a "wastebasket" diagnosis and is indiscriminately used for any anterior parapatellar pain syndromes. Other clinical entities that may be confused with chondromalacia patellae include prepatellar bursitis, pes anserinus bursitis, fat pad syndrome, generalized synovitis (rheumatoid, villonodular, and infectious), meniscal lesions, ligamentous instability, and osteochondritis dissecans.

Treatment consists of a 6-week program of open-chain exercises, ice application, and anti-inflammatory agents, which may control symptoms in the early stages. Some investigators[31] prefer to use aspirin initially in the treatment; their studies have demonstrated a relative lack of chondromalacia after 6 weeks of preoperative salicylate therapy at the time of arthroscopy, compared with an untreated control group, which had a 91% incidence of chondromalacia. If progression is encountered, intervention requires arthroscopic debridement and occasionally a patellar realignment procedure for which early orthopedic referral is indicated.

*Plica syndromes.* Synovial plicae represent the remnants of the septae, which act to divide the three divisions of the embryonic knee. Within the knee there are three such plicae: the infrapatellar plica or ligamentum mucosum, the suprapatellar plica, and the medial (shelf) plica (see Fig. 19-12). The infrapatellar plica is the most common plica identified on anatomic dissection and during arthroscopy. The infrapatellar plica proceeds from the intercondylar notch to the infrapatellar fat pad. When inflamed, it may be a source of irritation, and on arthrography it may be confused with the ACL. Otherwise, it is of little clinical significance.

The suprapatellar plica is a crescentric fold of synovium located between the suprapatellar bursa and the joint space proper. Arising from the posterior surface of the quadriceps tendon, it attaches to the lateral and superomedial wall of the joint. Should the suprapatellar plica be large, it is capable of harboring an intra-articular loose body within its folds (Fig. 19-71). Pressure injury, with erosion or fibrillation of the medial femoral condyle or patellar articular surface, is another sequelae of the suprapatellar plica.

The medial (shelf) plica passes inferiorly and obliquely over the anteromedial joint space to insert into the synovium, which sheathes the medial infrapatellar fat pad. Arthroscopic studies have demonstrated the presence of a medial patellar plica in 18.5% to 55% of subjects.[59] With a direct blow to the anterior knee, the subsequent effusion, hemorrhage, and synovitis result in thickening and fibrosis of the plica (Fig. 19-72) and loss of its inherent extensibility. Because the medial patellar plica spans the joint, this loss of extensibility may produce a "bowstring" effect with knee flexion. Impingement of the medial femoral condyle and the medial facet of the patella may then result in groove formation of the femoral condyle or chondromalacia (commonly noted with a thickened medial patellar plica). On flexion and extension of the knee the fibrous plica will sublux, resulting in a clicking or snapping noise that is appreciated by the patient. Symptoms of pain and pseudolocking are also disclosed during the interview. The plica is easily palpable at the medial aspect of the patella.

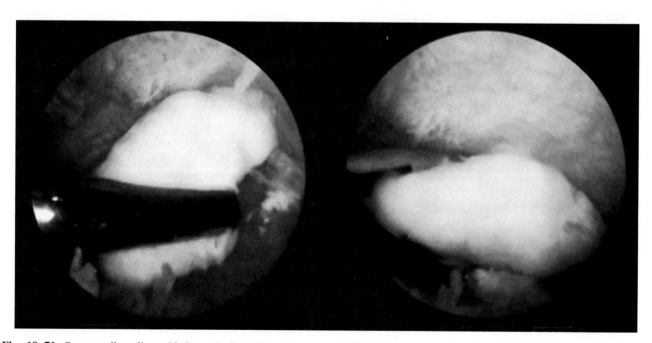

**Fig. 19-71.** Suprapatellar plica with loose bodies. Arthroscopic presentation of an osteocartilaginous loose body discovered in the suprapatellar pouch during arthroscopic removal. (From O'Connor RL: *Arthroscopy.* Kalamazoo, MI: The Upjohn Co, 1977.)

With the knee in flexion, the index and long finger palpate along the medial border of the patella. The knee is then gently extended, and the examiner hears a snapping sensation as the plica rolls over the anteromedial femoral condyle (Fig. 19-73). A positive apprehension test may also be present as the plica snaps beneath the examiner's fingers. If the patient perceives this sensation, it is important to ask whether the sensation reproduces his or her pain. This entity is frequently misdiagnosed as chondromalacia patellae or patellar subluxation.

***Infrapatellar fat pad impingement.*** This uncommon condition is due to impingement of the large pad of fat (Hoffa's fat pad) that lies posterior to the patellar tendon (see Fig. 19-11). This entity typically affects females in

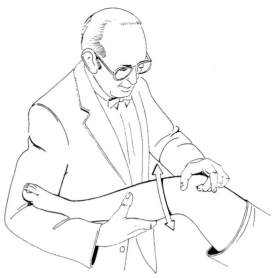

**Fig. 19-73.** Maneuver for detection of medial plica. The affected knee is flexed and cradled by the examiner's arm and hand. The knee is then flexed while the other hand is used to displace the patella medially. A snapping or popping sensation is appreciated as the plica is caught between the opposing articular surfaces. (From Hughston, J.C.: *Knee ligaments: injury and repair.* St. Louis: Mosby-Year Book, Inc., 1993.)

their teens and early twenties. Symptoms are generally noticed when the knee is moved into extension during activity; patients also note that symptoms are relieved with flexion and rest. The patient may also appreciate some swelling and repeated effusions during these acute episodes. Enlargement of this fat pad can be the result of posttraumatic swelling, premenstrual syndrome, anterior displacement by a concurrent bucket-handle tear of the medial meniscus, or anterior spur formation caused by osteoarthritis.

The major thrust of treatment is quadriceps-strengthening exercises (particularly if atrophy of the quadriceps is present), heel-lift exercises, and NSAIDs. Should chronic repeated episodes be encountered despite these conservative modalities either splinting in 15° to 20° of flexion or surgical excision may be necessary.

## DISCUSSION

An understanding of the anatomy and functional intricacies of the knee is central to the diagnosis and care of knee injuries. By using this information the physician is able to understand what structures may be injured, why certain mechanisms produce specific injuries, and what physical examination maneuvers will best display the suspected malady.

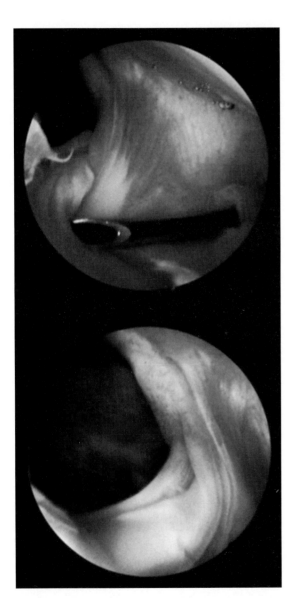

**Fig. 19-72.** Thickened hemorrhagic medial shelf plica. Arthroscopic presentation of a thickened medial (shelf) plica. Note the vascular engorgement of the supporting synovium. (From O'Connor RL: *Arthroscopy.* Kalamazoo, MI: The Upjohn Co, 1977.)

## REFERENCES

1. O'Donoghue DH: Treatment of acute ligamentous injuries of the knee, *Orthop Clin North Am* 4(3):617, 1973.
2. Hughston JC: *Knee ligaments: injury & repair.* St. Louis, 1993, Mosby-Year Book, Inc.

3. Butler DL: Ligamentous restraints in the human knee: anterior-posterior stability, *Orthop Trans* 2:161, 1978.

4. Bessette GC, Hunter RE: The anterior cruciate ligament, *Orthopedics* 13:551, 1990.

5. Marshall JL, Rubin RM: Knee ligament injuries: a diagnostic and therapeutic approach, *Orthop Clin North Am* 8:641, 1977.

6. Noyes FR, Grood ES, Butler DL et al: Clinical laxity tests and functional stability of the knee: biomechanical concepts, *Clin Orthop* 146:84, 1980.

7. Metcalf RW: The torn medial meniscus, In Parisien JS, ed: *Arthroscopic Surgery* 1988, pp. 93.

8. Hungerford DS, Barry M: Biomechanics of the patellofemoral joint, *Clin Orthop* 144:9-15, 1979.

9. Feagin JA: The office diagnosis and documentation of common knee problems, *Clin Sports Med* 8:435, 1989.

10. De Haven KE: Diagnosis of acute knee injuries with hemarthrosis, *Am J Sports Med* 8:9, 1980.

11. Jonsson T, Althoff B, Peterson L et al: Clinical diagnosis of rupture of the anterior cruciate ligament: a comparative study of the Lachman test and anterior drawer sign, *Am J Sports Med* 10:100, 1982.

12. Noyes FR, Mooar PA, Mathews DS et al: The symptomatic anterior cruciate deficient knee. Part I: The long-term functional disability in athletically active individuals, *J Bone Joint Surg* 65-A:154, 1983.

13. Ivey FM Jr: Evaluating acute knee injuries, *Am Fam Physician* 22:122, 1982.

14. Jain AS, Swanson AJG, and Murdoch G: Haemarthrosis of the knee joint, *Injury* 15:178, 1983.

15. Mariani PP, Puddu G, and Ferretti A: Hemarthrosis treated by aspiration and casting: how to condemn the knee, *Am J Sports Med* 10:343, 1982.

16. Paulos L, Noyes FR, and Malek M: A practical guide to the initial evaluation to the initial evaluation and treatment of knee ligament injuries, *J Trauma* 20:498, 1980.

17. Rand JA: The role of arthroscopy in the management of knee injuries in the athlete, *Mayo Clin Proc* 59:77, 1984.

18. Noyes FR, Bassett RW, Grood ES, et al: Arthroscopy in acute traumatic hemarthrosis of the knee, *J Bone Joint Surg* 62-A:687, 1980.

19. Kaplan PA, Walker CW, Kilcoyne RF et al: Occult fracture patterns of the knee associated with anterior cruciate ligament tears: assessment with MR imaging, *Radiology* 183:835, 1992.

20. Boeree NR, Ackroyd CE: Assessment of the menisci and cruciate ligaments: an audit of clinical practice, *Injury* 22(4):291, 1991.

21. Turek SL: *Orthopaedics: principles and their applications,* ed 4, Philadelphia, 1984, JB Lippincott Co.

22. Morton KS, Starr DE: Closure of the anterior portion of the upper tibial epiphysis as a complication of tibial shaft fracture, *J Bone Joint Surg* 46-A:570, 1964.

23. Hardaker WT, Garrett WE Jr, Bassett FH: Evaluation of acute traumatic hemarthrosis of the knee joint, *South Med J* 83(6):640, 1990.

24. Salenius P, Vankka E: The development of the tibiofemoral angle in children, *J Bone Joint Surg* 57-A:259, 1975.

25. Cook SD, Lavernia CJ, Burke SW et al: A biomechanical analysis of the etiology of tibia vara, *J Pediatr Orthop* 3:449, 1983.

26. Insall J, Salvati E: Patella position in the normal knee joint, *Radiology* 101:101-104, 1971.

27. Mankin HJ: Rickets, osteomalacia and renal osteodystrophy: Part II, *J Bone Joint Surg* 56-A:352, 1974.

28. Helfet AJ: *Disorders of the knee,* Philadelphia, 1963, JB Lippincott.

29. Rockwood CA Jr, Kaye EW, and King RE: *Fractures in Children,* ed 3, 1991, JB Lippincott, p. 1222.

30. Meyers MH, McKeever FM: Fracture of the intracondylar eminence of the tibia, *J Bone Joint Surg* 41-A:209, 1959.

31. Oglivie-Harris DJ, Jackson RW: The arthroscopic treatment of chondromalasia patellae, *J Bone Joint Surg* 66-B:660, 1984.

32. Kennedy JC: Complete dislocations of the knee joint, *J Bone Joint Surg* 45-A:889, 1963.

33. Green NE, Allen BL: Vascular injuries associated with a dislocation of the knee, *J Bone Joint Surg* 59-A:236, 1977.

34. Grigis FG, Marshall JL, and Almonajem ARS: The cruciate ligaments of the knee joint: anatomical, functional and experimental analysis, *Clin Orthop* 106:216, 1975.

35. Meyers MH, Moore TM, and Harvey JP Jr: Traumatic dislocations of the knee: followup notes, *J Bone Joint Surg* 57-A:430, 1975.

36. Sinding-Larsen CA: A hereto unknown affliction of the patella in children, *Acta Radiol* 1:171, 1921.

37. Medlar RC: Sinding-Larsen-Johansson disease, *J Bone Joint Surg* 60-A:1113, 1978.

38. Siwek CA: Rupture of the extensor mechanism of the knee joint, *J Bone Joint Surg* 63-A:932, 1981.

39. Clanton TO, DeLee JC, Sanders B et al: Knee ligament injuries in children, *J Bone Joint Surg* 61-A:1195, 1979.

40. Torg JS, Conrad W, and Kalen V: Clinical diagnosis of anterior cruciate instability in the athlete, *Sports Med* 4:84, 1976.

41. Fetto JF, Marshall JL: The natural history and diagnosis of anterior cruciate ligament insufficiency, *Clin Orthop* 147:29, 1980.

42. Fruensgaard S, Johannsen HV: Incomplete ruptures of the anterior cruciate ligament, *J Bone Joint Surg* 71-B:526, 1989.

43. Noyes FR, Mooar LA, Moorman CT III: Partial tears of the anterior cruciate ligament progression to complete ligament deficiency, *J Bone Joint Surg* 71-B:825, 1989.

44. Cerabona F, Sherman MF, Bonamo JR, and Sklar J: Patterns of meniscal injury with anterior cruciate tears, *Am J Sports Med* 16:603, 1988.

45. Indelicato PA, Bitters ES: A perspective of lesions associated with ACL insufficiency of the knee: a review of 100 cases, *Clin Orthop* 198:77, 1985.

46. McDaniel WJ, Dameron TB: Untreated ruptures of the anterior cruciate ligament, *J Bone Joint Surg* 62-A:696, 1980.

47. Woods GW, Stanley RF, and Tullos HS: Lateral capsular sign: x-ray clue to a significant knee instability, *Am J Sports Med* 7:27, 1979.

48. Cobby MF, Schweitzer ME, and Resnick D: The deep lateral femoral notch: an indirect sign of a torn anterior cruciate ligament, *Radiology* 184:855, 1992.

49. Clendenin JB, DeLee JC, and Heckman JD: Interstitial tears of the posterior cruciate ligament of the knee, *Orthopedics* 3:764, 1980.

50. Parolie JM, Bergfeld JS: Long-term results of non-operative treatment of isolated posterior cruciate injuries in the athlete, *Am J Sports Med* 14:35, 1986.

51. Indelicato PA: Non-operative treatment of complete tears of the medical collateral ligament of the knee, *J Bone Joint Surg* 65-A:323, 1983.

52. Mok DW, Good C: Non-operative management of acute grade III medial collateral ligament injury of the knee, *Injury* 20:277, 1989.

53. Fetto JF et al: Medial collateral ligament injuries of the knee: a rationale for treatment, *Clin Orthop* 132:206, 1978.

54. DeHaven KE, Linter DM: Athletic injuries: comparison by age, sport and gender, *Am J Sports Med* 14:218, 1986.

55. Neumann RD: Traumatic knee injuries, *Primary Care* 19:351, 1992.

56. DeHaven KE, Dolan WA, and Mayer PJ: Chondromalacia patellae in athletes: clinical presentation and conservative management, *Am J Sports Med* 7:5, 1979.

57. Ficat R, Hungersford D: Disorders of the patello-femoral joint, Baltimore, 1977, Williams & Wilkins.

58. Cailliet R: *Knee pain and disability,* Philadelphia, 1973, FA Davis.

59. Patel D: Plica as a cause of anterior knee pain, *Orthop Clin North Am* 17:273, 1986.

60. Aichroth P: Osteochondritis dissecans of the knee: a clinical survey, *J Bone Joint Surg* 53-B:440, 1971.

61. Baker CL Jr, Norwood LA, Hughston JC: Acute combined posterior cruciate and posterolateral instability of the knee, *Am J Sports Med* 12:204, 1984.

62. Bomberg BC, McGinty JB: Acute hemarthrosis of the knee: indications for diagnostic arthroscopy, *Arthroscopy* 6:221, 1990.

63. Dee R, Mango E, and Hurst LC: *Principles of Orthopedic Practice,* New York, 1988, McGraw-Hill, pp. 1054-1058, 1267-1270, 1283-1330.

64. DeHaven KE: Diagnosis of acute knee injuries with hemarthrosis, *Am J Sports Med* 8:9, 1980.

65. Donaldson WF, Warren RF, and Wickiewicz T: A comparison of acute anterior cruciate ligament examinations, *Am J Sports Med* 13:5, 1985.

66. Finsterbush A, Frankl U, Matan Y et al: Secondary damage to the knee after isolated injury of the anterior cruciate, *Am J Sports Med* 18:475, 1990.

67. Flanagan JP, Holmes CF, and Schenck RC: Primary care of the acutely injured knee, *J Musculoskel Med* 9:29, 1992.

68. Gray DJ: Prenatal development of the human knee and superior tibiofibular joints, *Am J Anat* 86:235, 1950.

69. Hallen LG, Lindahl O: Lateral stability of the knee joint, *Acta Orthop* 36,2:12, 1965.

70. Halpern AA: Tendon ruptures associated with corticosteroid therapy, *West J Med* 127:378, 1977.

71. Hansson LI, Zayer M: Physiologic genu varum, *Acta Orthop Scand* 46:221, 1975.

72. Henry JH: Conservative treatment of patellofemoral subluxation, *Clin Sports Med* 8:261, 1989.

73. Hughston JC: Classification of knee ligament instabilities: 1. The medial compartment and cruciate ligaments, *J Bone Joint Surg* 58-A:159, 1976.

74. Hughston JC, Andrews JR, Cross MJ, et al: Classification of knee ligament instabilities: 2. The lateral compartment, *J Bone Joint Surg* 58-A:173, 1976.

75. Indelicato PA, Pascale MS, and Huegel MO: Early experience with the Gore-tex polytetrafluoroethylene anterior cruciate ligament prosthesis, *Am J Sports Med* 17:55, 1989.

76. Insall J, Goldberg V, and Salvati E: Recurrent dislocation and the high-riding patella, *Clin Orthop* 88:67, 1972.

77. Keene JS: Diagnosis of undetected knee injuries: interpreting subtle clinical and radiographic findings, *Postgrad Med* 85:153, 1989.

78. Lichman HM: Computerized blood flow analysis for decision making in treatment of osteochondritis dissecans, *J Pediatr Orthop* 8:208, 1988.

79. Marks PH, Goldenberg JA, Vezina WC et al: Subchondral bone infarction if acute ligamentous knee injuries demonstrated on bone scintigraphy and magnetic resonance, *J Nucl Med* 33:516, 1992.

80. Marshall JL, Baugher WH: Stability examination of the knee: a simplified anatomic approach, *Clin Orthop* 146:78, 1980.

81. McCabe CJ, Ferguson CM, and Ottinger LW: Improved limb salvage in popliteal artery injuries, *J Trauma* 23:982, 1983.

82. McKeag DB, Roy SP: The complexities of diagnosing acute soft tissue knee injuries, *Emerg Med Rep* 6:1, 1985.

83. Mink JH, Deutsch AL: Occult cartilage and bone injuries of the knee: detection, classification and assessment with MR imaging, *Radiology* 170:823, 1989.

84. O'Donoghue DH: Treatment of acute ligamentous injuries of the knee, *Orthop Clin North Am* 4:617, 1973.

85. O'Donoghue DH: An analysis of the end results of surgical treatment of major injuries to the ligaments of the knee, *J Bone Joint Surg* 37-A:1, 1955.

86. O'Donoghue, DH: Surgical treatment of fresh injuries of the major ligaments of the knee, *J Bone Joint Surg* 32-A:721, 1950.

87. Roberts JM, Lovell WW: Fractures of the intercondylar eminance of the tibia: Proceedings of AAOS, *J Bone Joint Surg* 52-A:827, 1970.

88. Rothenberg MH, Graf BK: Evaluation of acute knee injuries, *Post-grad Med* 93:75, 1993.

89. Schenck RC Jr, Rodriguez F: Office evaluation of the acutely injured knee, *J Musculoskel Med* 9:55, 1992.

90. Scott SG: Current concepts in the rehabilitation of the injured athlete, *Mayo Clin Proc* 59:83, 1984.

91. Scott WN: *Arthroscopy of the knee,* Philadelphia, 1990, WB Saunders, p. 176.

92. Simont WT, Sim FH: Current concepts in the treatment of ligamentous instability of the knee, *Mayo Clin Proc* 59:67, 1984.

93. Slocum DB, James SL, Larson RL et al: Clinical test for anterolateral rotatory instability of the knee, *Clin Orthop* 118:63, 1976.

94. Speer KP, Spritzer CE, Bassett FH III et al: Osseouys injury associated with acute tears of the anterior cruciate ligament, *Am J Sports Med* 20:382, 1992.

95. Sweetham R: Corticosteroid arthropathy and rupture, *J Bone Joint Surg* 51-B:397, 1969.

96. Szalay MJ, Hosking OR, and Annear P: Injury of knee ligament associated with ipsilateral femoral shaft fractures and with ipsilateral femoral and tibial shaft fracture, *Injury* 21:398, 1990.

97. Templeman DC, Marder RA: Injuries of the knee associated with fractures of the tibial shaft, *J Bone Joint Surg* 71-A:1392, 1989.

98. Unverferth LJ: The effects of local steroid injections on tendon, *J Sports Med* 1:31, 1973.

99. Vellet AD, Marks PH, Fowler PJ et al: Occult posttraumatic osteochondral lesions of the knee: prevalence, classification and sequellae evaluated with MR imaging, *Radiology* 178:271, 1991.

100. Warrren LF: The prime stabilizer of the medial side of the knee, *J Bone Joint Surg* 56-A:665, 1974.

101. Wilson-MacDonald J, Dodd C, and Cockin J: Arthroscopy in the acute knee injury: a prospective controlled trial, *Br J Accid Surg* 21:165, 1990.

# The Tibia and Fibula

*Paul R. Haller*
*Carson R. Harris*

## ANATOMY

Support for weight bearing in the lower leg is provided by the tibia, and to a lesser extent, the fibula. Because of their unique position, nerves and the vessels to the foot are susceptible to injury when violence to the tibia and fibula occurs. Also, because the bones and their tough connective tissues divide the lower leg into four compartments, increased tissue pressure in these compartments can damage nerves and vessels.

### Bones and ligaments

The tibia has a triangular cross-section in its path from the knee to the ankle. Its subcutaneous location anteriorly predisposes it to injury from anterior or medially directed forces, making it the most commonly fractured long bone in the body. It is the major weight-bearing bone, carrying 83% to 94% of the load.[1,2] Because of its thick cortex and large diameter, a significant amount of violence is required to injure the tibia. The shaft of the tibia is connected to the fibula by the interosseous membrane, a tough sheet of connective tissue running the length of the shaft of the tibia and fibula. The proximal tibia is splayed outward from the shaft as it nears the articular surface with the femur. The joint surface is made up of the medial and lateral plateaus that articulate with the medial and lateral femoral condyles. The lateral plateau is the smaller of the two; because of this, and because it is higher than the medial plateau, the lateral plateau is more commonly fractured than the medial plateau. Greater violence must occur for the medial plateau to fracture.

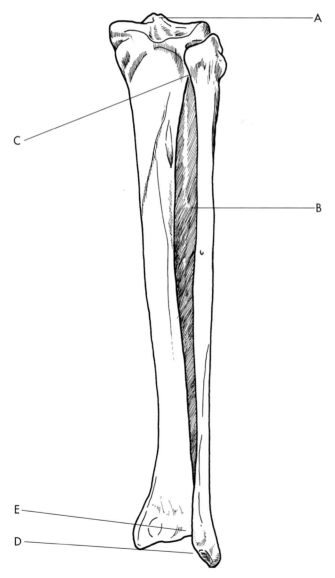

**Fig. 20-1.** Posterior view of the bones of the lower leg. **A,** Intercondylar eminence; **B,** Interosseous ligament; **C,** Proximal tibial-fibular joint; **D,** Fibulotalar joint; **E,** Distal tibial-fibular syndesmosis.

Menisci cover the periphery of the joint surface of the plateaus. The medial meniscus is smaller, covering less of the joint surface than the lateral. Between the medial and lateral plateau, the intercondylar eminence protrudes superiorly. This is not an articular surface; rather, it is the site of attachment for the anterior cruciate ligament. The joint surface of the tibia overhangs the interosseous membrane laterally. Inferior to this, the posterior lateral surface of the tibia articulates with the fibular head (Fig. 20-1). The distal tibia articulates with the talus inferiorly and the fibula laterally. The medial portion of the tibia extends past the talus to form the medial malleolus, and the middle section of the tibia forms the weight-bearing tibial-talar joint. The distal tibia and fibula are held together by the ankle syndesmosis, a series of ligaments that lie inferior to the interosseous membrane. Loss of the integrity of these ligaments may occur in a tibial shaft fracture, with resulting laxity and incompetence of the ankle joint.

The fibula courses lateral and posterior to the tibia in its path from the proximal tibia to the talus. It bears little weight, and function is minimally affected by its loss. Its inferior portion has a large facet—the lateral malleolus—for articulation with the talus, and a smaller facet for articulation with the tibia.

The knee joint is stabilized by the medial collateral ligament that attaches to the proximal tibia and the lateral collateral ligament, which in turn connects with the fibular head. The cruciate ligaments are named for their articulation to the tibia. The anterior cruciate ligament attaches to the intercondylar eminence; its function is to prevent forward movement of the tibia on the femur. The posterior cruciate ligament attaches on the posterior aspect of the tibia; this ligament prevents the tibia from sliding backward on the femur.

The interosseous ligament is a thick membrane in the form of a plane between the anterior-medial border of the fibula and the lateral border of the tibia. It starts just below the height of the proximal tibiofibular joint and extends the length of the tibia and fibula to the ankle.

### Nerves and vessels

The popliteal artery is a continuation of the femoral artery. After it exits the popliteal fossa, it splits in two: the anterior tibial artery crosses over the interosseous membrane and runs on the anterior surface of that structure. The other branch of the popliteal artery is the posterior tibial artery, whose path runs along the posterior aspect of the interosseous membrane to the medial part of the ankle where its patency can be evaluated in the foot as the posterior tibial artery. The integrity of the anterior tibial artery is assessed by the strength of the dorsalis pedis pulse in the foot.

The leg is innervated by the peroneal, sural, and tibial nerves. Each nerve provides motor funtion to a group of muscles responsible for a specific movement of the foot and is sensory to an area of the foot. The sural nerve courses through the superficial posterior compartment where it innervates the soleus, gastrocnemius, and plantaris muscles. This group's action is to plantar flex the ankle. The lateral heel is the sensory field of the sural nerve. The tibial nerve controls the muscles that plantar flex the toes (ie, flexor digitorum longus, flexor hallucis, and tibialis posterior). It provides sensation to the sole of the foot. The peroneal nerve courses just lateral to the upper pole of the fibula. After swinging anterior to that bone, it bifurcates into the superficial and deep peroneal nerves. The superficial peroneal nerve provides motor control to the peroneus brevis and longus muscles, which are everters of the foot. Sensory fibers of the superficial peroneal nerve extend from the lateral aspect of the foot. The deep peroneal nerve is sensory to the webspace between the first and second toes. Its motor action is to dorsiflex the ankle and toes.

## Compartments

The lower leg is divided into four compartments by bone and connective tissue. Because of the inelasticity of these dividers, pressure caused by edema or blood within one or more of these compartments may increase to the point of ischemic damage to the muscles and nerves within. This increased tissue pressure effect is called compartment syndrome. The resultant ischemic damage to muscles may result in permanent loss of function. Although compartment syndrome and its sequela (Volkmann's contracture) were initially described involving the upper extremity, they more

frequently occur in the leg. This ischemia can be prevented with timely diagnosis and treatment.

The four compartments in the lower leg run parallel to the tibia and fibula. Each is surrounded by bone or connective tissue, and each contains specific muscle groups, nerves, and vessels. A cross-section of the midshaft of the leg shows that the tibia is connected to the medial fibula by the interosseous membrane (Fig. 20-2). Attached to the fibula anteriorly is the anterior peroneal (crural) septum, which, with the posterior peroneal (crural) septum and the fibula itself, circumscribes the lateral compartment. The lateral compartment, which lies just superficial to the fibula, houses the superficial peroneal nerve (sensory to the lateral dorsum of the foot) and muscle responsible for eversion of the foot. No major vascular structure lies within this compartment.

The anterior compartment is surrounded by the interosseous membrane, the tibia medially, and the fibula and anterior crural septum laterally. It contains the muscles responsible for gross dorsiflexion of the ankles and toes. The anterior tibial artery and veins run within this compartment to the dorsal pedal artery, where they can be clinically assessed. The deep peroneal nerve supplies motor function to the anterior compartment (dorsiflexion of ankle and toes), and its sensory zone is the web space between the first and second toes.

The two posterior compartments are divided by the intermuscular septum. The superficial posterior compart-

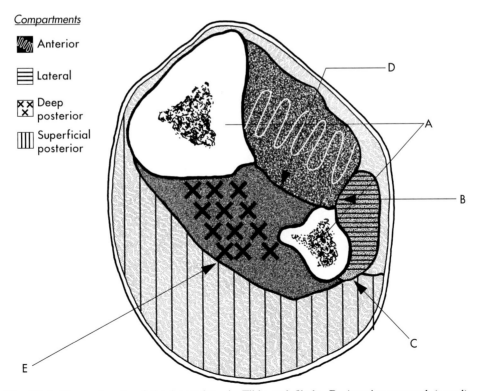

*Compartments*

▨ Anterior

▤ Lateral

⊠ Deep posterior

▥ Superficial posterior

**Fig. 20-2.** Compartments of the lower leg. **A,** Tibia and fibula; **B,** Anterior peroneal (crural) septum; **C,** Posterior peroneal (crural) septum; **D,** Interosseous ligament; **E,** Intermuscular septum.

ment contains the gastrocnemius, soleus, and plantaris muscles, which are responsible for plantar flexion of the ankle. The sural nerve extends through this compartment to the lateral heel, where it provides sensation. There are no major arteries in this compartment. Because the superficial posterior compartment is the most distensible, it is the least likely to develop a compartment syndrome.

The deep posterior compartment contains muscles responsible for plantar flexion of the toes (ie, flexor digitorum longus, flexor hallucis longus, and tibialis posterior). The tibial nerve provides motor control to these muscles and is responsible for sensation over the sole of the foot. The deep posterior compartment also contains the posterior tibial artery, the integrity of which can be assessed in the ankle (Table 20-1).

## COMPARTMENT SYNDROME

In 1881, Volkmann described what is now recognized as the sequela of untreated compartment syndrome: irreversible contracture of the hand caused by ischemic processes in the forearm. The *sine qua non* of compartment syndrome is increased tissue pressure within a closed space. If persistent and untreated, this increased pressure can cause permanent damage to the muscles within the compartment and the nerves that traverse it. The lower leg is divided into four compartments by bones and fascia. This connective tissue is relatively inelastic, providing the environment for compartment syndrome. As the skull allows a fixed amount of brain swelling before herniation through the foramen magnum occurs, the compartments of the leg also allow a limited increase in size before tissue pressure rises, resulting in hypoperfusion and cell damage. The relative inability of the compartment to expand can be accentuated by iatrogenic methods such as the application of antishock trousers, constrictive dressings, or tight casts.

Within the compartment, tissue pressure rises if there is an increase in the volume in the compartment. Two scenarios lend themselves to increased compartment volume: hemorrhage into the compartment and swelling of the muscles within. In the first instance, for example, fracture of the tibia with lacerations of the small vessels can lead to elevated intracompartmental pressures as a result of clotting within the compartment. In the second case, it is common for muscle edema to occur after ischemic muscle regains its blood supply. During the ischemic period, fluid leaks through damaged basement membranes and capillaries,

causing edema. When the blood flow resumes, the edema continues because of damaged capillaries. Hence, compartment syndrome secondary to vascular damage typically occurs several hours after restoration of blood flow to the area. Similarly, the incompetent capillaries accompanying burns cause increased tissue pressure that has the potential for ischemic muscle and nerve damage.

Increased tissue pressure within a compartment leads to hypoperfusion of the muscles and nerves on a microvascular level. Increased tissue pressure resulting in decreased venous return affects the pressure gradient at the capillaries, causing inadequate blood flow through nutrient capillaries. Pressures sufficient to cause capillary insufficiency do not approach the systolic or diastolic blood pressure; thus the major vessels traversing the compartment continue to maintain easily detectable pulses despite the tissue damage ongoing within that compartment.

### Mechanism of injury

For compartment syndrome to develop, all that is required is an injury sufficient to cause tissue swelling or hemorrhage. This can occur from blunt trauma to the lower leg; normal bony films should not lull the physician into a false sense of security. If the leg has been ischemic secondary to vascular injury, as seen in popliteal artery damage associated with posterior knee dislocation, the swelling usually occurs after the restoration of blood flow. Likewise, an unconscious patient whose supine positioning has led to temporary ischemia of an extremity may develop elevated tissue pressures after restoration of blood flow.

External devices that restrict compartment size, such as casts or antishock trousers, can increase the risk of compartment syndrome development.

### Signs and symptoms

The first sign of compartment syndrome in an alert patient is pain. Unfortunately, many of these patients already have a reason for pain, such as a fracture of the tibia or fibula. The pain that is secondary to a compartment syndrome may incorrectly be attributed to this injury. In compartment syndrome, the pain is usually greater than what would be expected, given the already documented injury. For example, the radiographs are normal but the pain is refractory to medication, or an increasing amount of analgesia is required for something that seems to be a minor injury. Such circumstances should lead the physician to consider the development of compartment syndrome. Pain occurring

**Table 20-1.** The four compartments

| Compartments | Nerve | Sensation | Muscle group | Artery |
|---|---|---|---|---|
| Lateral | Superficial peroneal | Lateral foot | Evertors of foot | |
| Anterior | Deep peroneal | Web space of 1st and 2nd toes | Dorsiflex ankle and toes | Anterior tibial |
| Superficial posterior | Sural | Lateral heel | Plantar-flex ankle | |
| Deep posterior | Tibia | Sole of foot | Plantar-flex toes | Posterior tibial |

at a site distant from the fracture may also indicate compartment syndrome.

The pain of compartment syndrome is typically exacerbated by the passive movement of the muscles within that compartment. When the muscle is spherically shaped, it takes up the smallest volume; as it passively stretches, it increases its volume within the compartment, exacerbating the pain. Similarly, the pain of compartment syndrome may be exacerbated by manually compressing the compartment.

Neurologic changes can be seen early in compartment syndrome. These may include numbness in the foot or toes. Sensation in the distribution of the nerve that courses through the affected compartment may be compromised, as may be the motor function of that nerve (Table 20-1).

Although we compulsively check the pulses when evaluating trauma to the extremity, in compartment syndrome this is a nearly useless task. Because tissue ischemia is a microvascular phenomenon, the blood flow through the major vessels in the compartment frequently remains normal, despite the occurrence of irreversible muscle and nerve damage. An absent pulse would more likely be a clue to possible major vascular damage, not compartment syndrome. Because the loss of distal pulses occurs late or not at all in compartment syndrome, once the patient has reached this point the physician has most likely missed the best opportunity for intervention.

### Diagnosis

The gold standard for the diagnosis of compartment syndrome is measurement of tissue pressure within the affected compartment. The basic apparatus is shown in Fig. 20-3A. By way of a three-way stopcock, a manometer is connected by tubing to a saline-filled syringe and to a needle. The needle is inserted into the muscle of the compartment (insertion into a tendon or fascia gives a falsely elevated reading). Air bubbles are flushed from the needle and tubing. A syringe plunger is then slowly depressed. As saline is injected into the compartment, the manometer records the amount of pressure required to inject into the compartment. Kits are commercially available that simplify the equipment set-up (Fig. 20-3B).

Accurate measurements from all four compartments can be quickly obtained with this apparatus. The anterior, lateral, and superficial posterior compartments are easily accessible for measurement. A reliable method of reaching the deep posterior compartment is to insert the needle medially just posterior to the tibia with the needle directed to the center of the leg at that level. When the needle tip is near the center of the leg it will be in the deep posterior compartment. The normal tissue pressure is 0 mm Hg. Normal tissue pressure, as measured alone or with commercial electronic manometers, is usually about 10 mm Hg. The pressure elevation and its duration (especially the latter) are the critical determinants of tissue ischemia and irreversible damage. Using an animal model, Rorabek and Clarke[3] found that elevated tissue pressures that were relieved within 4 hours of onset did not result in irreversible

nerve damage, whereas elevations of 12 hours caused permanent conduction abnormalities. In a retrospective study of patients with acute compartment syndrome, Sheridan and Masten[4] found that 31% of patients treated within 12 hours had residual functional deficits; by contrast, patients treated after 12 hours had greater than a 90% incidence of residual deficits, and 20% required amputation. Pressures high enough to cause compartment syndrome typically range from 40 to 60 mm Hg, or are 30 mm Hg less than the diastolic blood pressure. Tissue pressures higher than 30 to 40 mm Hg warrant fasciotomy to relieve the pressure, and those between 20 and 30 mm Hg may be closely observed clinically, with repeat measurements in 1 to 2 hours if indicated.

Tissue pressure readings should be obtained more liberally in patients whom the physician will not be able to follow clinically, such as those with head injuries, drug or alcohol intoxication, or those undergoing general anesthesia for treatment of associated injuries.

### Treatment

Once the diagnosis of compartment syndrome is made, action should be immediate. A conservative initial approach would include removal of restrictive dressings and elevation of the affected extremity to reduce swelling. Casts of the leg may be split or removed. If conservative treatment fails to restore tissue pressures to an appropriate range, the definitive treatment is fasciotomy, to release the constriction causing the elevated tissue pressures. Because permanent nerve and muscle damage can result from prolonged ischemia (more than 4 hours), fasciotomy must be prompt. The trauma surgeon's linear incision into the compartment fascia is left open, with secondary closure at a later date. Depending on degree of swelling, grafting may be necessary to close the fasciotomy defect.

## INJURIES IN ADULTS
### Tibial plateau fractures

Most car bumpers are approximately 20 inches from the ground, which is the same distance from the sole of an adult's foot to the proximal tibia. Tibial plateau fractures most frequently occur after a car-pedestrian accident, with a medially directed force. They constitute 1% of all fractures and are disproportionately higher in the elderly. Because the tibial plateau is the articular surface for a major weight-bearing joint, optimal treatment of these fractures is critical for ambulation without residual stiffness in the knee or degenerative joint disease.

**Mechanism of injury.** Sheer forces or axial loading are the two causes of fracture of the tibial plateau. The bumper fracture is a classic example of an injury caused by sheer forces. The car bumper strikes the outside of the knee, creating a valgus deformity and a depressed or split fracture of the lateral tibial plateau when the femoral condyle is driven into it. As the femoral condyle is compressing the plateau, the lateral meniscus (which covers a larger portion of the plateau than does the medial meniscus) may be

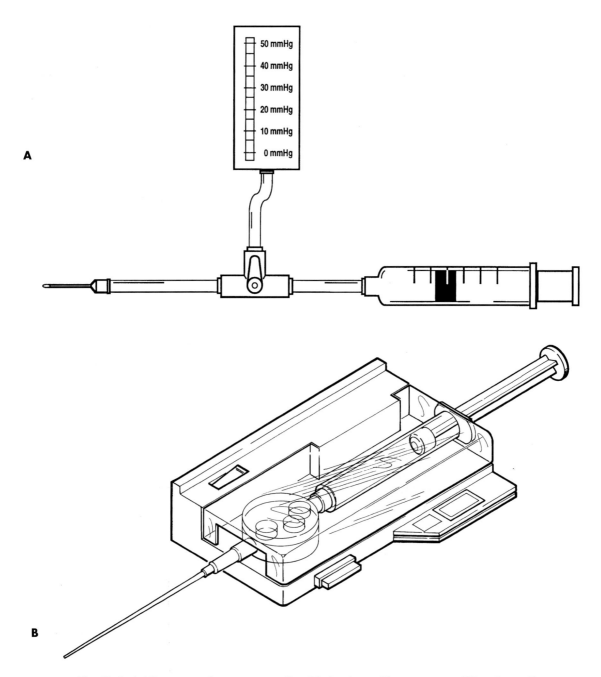

**Fig. 20-3. A,** Three-way valve connects a saline-filled syringe with a monometer. When the needle is inserted into the compartment, the amount of pressure necessary to inject saline into the compartment is determined. **B,** Compartment pressure monitor. The pressure required to inject 1 ml of saline into the compartment is easily measured with a commercial kit.

crushed. This same valgus force can also stress the medial collateral ligament and possibly the anterior cruciate ligament, resulting in a tear in one or both of these. Although some authors believe that, for tibial plateau fractures to occur, an intact medial collateral ligament is necessary to act as hinge, up to 20% of plateau fractures have been found to have associated ligament damage.[5] Hence, the bumper injury typically involves the fracture of the lateral plateau and possible involvement of the medial collateral ligament, anterior cruciate ligament, and lateral meniscus.

Lateral plateau injuries constitute approximately 50% of all tibial plateau fractures.

Similarly, a sheer force directed from the medial side of the knee toward the lateral produces a varus stress, with the medial femoral condyle compressing the medial plateau. Because the medial plateau is stronger than the lateral, this plateau fractures less frequently; the presence of a medial plateau fracture suggests that a much greater force caused the injury. The deformity caused by this stress tests the strength of the lateral collateral ligament; if this ligament ruptures, the posterior cruciate ligament becomes susceptible to tearing. As before, the femoral condyle may damage the meniscus as it is driven into the medial plateau. Fractures of the medial plateau (which comprise 10% to 23% of all plateau fractures) are frequently associated with damage to the lateral collateral ligament, posterior cruciate ligament, or medial meniscus.

Tibial plateaus can also be fractured by heavy axial loading, such as that caused by a fall from a significant height. Compression of the plateau again results from the femoral condyle being driven down into the plateau. With enough velocity, the result can be a shattering of one or both plateaus into numerous pieces. An axial load can also result in a fracture of both tibial plateaus in an inverted Y pattern.

Characteristics of the tibia play a role in the type of fracture that occurs. Younger patients have a stronger cortex, and the fracture that results is more often a splitting of a part of the plateau away from the tibia. With age and loss of calcium, depressed fractures with the crumbling of the bone and loss of height of the plateau become more common.

**Signs and symptoms.** The patient presents with pain and tenderness over the fracture site. Weight-bearing is usually not possible. A hemarthrosis may be present. If aspirated and fat particles are found in the fluid, it is pathogenic of a fracture. Varus or valgus stress can reproduce the mechanism injury, and, although painful, can reveal the presence of associated injuries to the collateral ligaments. The integrity of the anterior cruciate ligament and posterior cruciate ligament should also be assessed.

**Radiology.** Anteroposterior (AP) and lateral radiographs should be supplemented by oblique views, if plateau fracture is suspected. An oblique view in internal rotation demonstrates the lateral plateau, and the oblique with external rotation defines the medial. An additional view that may be useful has been described by Moore.[6] An AP view with the knee in 10° to 15° flexion shows the plateaus as a flat surface and allows for measurement of depression. Tomography in the anterior-posterior or lateral planes can also be used to define the degree of depression of the fracture fragments. CT scanning may be needed for preoperative evaluation of complicated fracture. The CT scan can be used to develop a three-dimensional picture of the tibia.

**Diagnosis.** There have been several attempts to classify fractures of the tibial plateau. These systems are primarily oriented toward optimal treatment methods. Because tibial plateau fractures entail considerable morbidity and chronicity, they should be managed by orthopedic surgeons. The focus here is on the identification of fracture patterns, to allow the emergency physician to communicate with the orthopedic surgeon.

Fractures of the plateau can be described by their location, the amount of displacement, the number of fracture fragments, and the type of fracture. Tibial plateau fractures can be either *split*, with a vertical fracture line separating a fragment of bone from the tibia (Fig. 20-4A), or *depressed*, with the articular surface being pressed into subcortical bone (Fig. 20-4B). Split fractures tend to occur in young patients with strong calcified subcortical bone, and elderly patients tend to suffer depression fractures associated with osteoporosis. Both split and depression

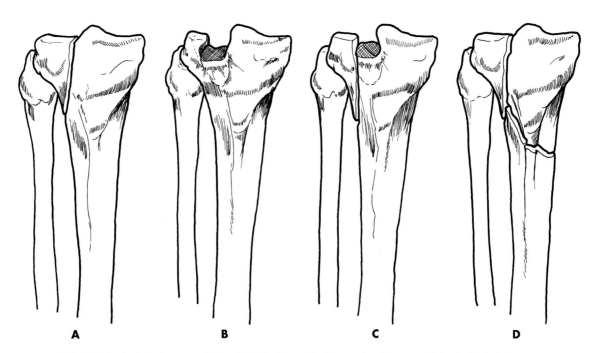

**Fig. 20-4. A,** Split fracture of lateral tibial plateau. **B,** Depression fracture of lateral tibial plateau. **C,** Split and depression fractures of lateral tibial plateau. **D,** Split fracture of the tibial plateau with separation from the diaphysis.

fractures can occur on the same plateau (Fig. 20-4C). The medial condyle is less frequently fractured than is the lateral. Fractures can occur in both plateaus simultaneously, producing an inverted Y pattern. The fracture plane may separate the metaphysis of the tibia from the diaphyses (Fig. 20-4D). Another fracture variation involves a break near the tibial intercondylar eminence, which is an extra-articular injury. When evaluating tibial plateau fractures, the physician must pay close attention to the possibility of associated soft-tissue injuries; collateral ligaments, cruci-ates, and menisci are frequently damaged with the force necessary to sustain a plateau fracture. Collateral ligament injury likely would be on the opposite side of the fractured plateau. A thorough evaluation of disability of the knee is vital to planning treatment.

**Treatment.** Historically, these fractures have been treated with casting. The major drawback with this method was the residual decreased range of motion in the knee (legs that had been casted for more than 1 month typically had as little as 70° range of motion). Open reduction and internal fixation of these injuries has become more com-mon. With the early immobilization allowed by open reduction and internal fixation, residual stiffness is less of a problem. Thus, the goal of treatment now is anatomic reduction and early motion. Achieving these goals requires excellent alignment of the joint, joint stability (ie, intact ligaments), and a maximal amount of articular surface available for weight-bearing.

Management of these fractures is directed by the ortho-pedic surgeon. After other injuries are attended to, the orthopedist should be consulted when the patient is still in the emergency department. Long leg splinting and nonweight-bearing provide temporary support to the leg and may reduce pain and swelling.

### Proximal tibial-fibular dislocation

The proximal tibia-fibular joint allows anterior-posterior movement of the fibula with flexion and extension of the knee and also allows for external rotation upon dorsiflexion of the ankle. This joint can sustain an isolated injury, typically in sports, or can be injured when the tibia is fractured.

**Anatomy.** The superior tibial-fibular joint is situated on the posterior-lateral aspect of the tibia, on the underside of the shelf of the lateral-tibial plateau. The capsule that envelopes this joint is thicker on its anterior aspect than its posterior. Several ligaments provide support to the joint. The anterior tibial-fibular ligament extends upward and obliquely from the anterior head of the fibula to the posterior aspect of the lateral tibial condyle. The biceps femoris tendon passes anterior to this ligament and inserts into the lateral side of the head of the fibula (Fig. 20-5). The lateral collateral ligament of the knee also provides support by attaching to the head of the fibula. The posterior tibial-fibular ligament is a single broad band passing ob-liquely upward from the fibular head to the lateral tibia

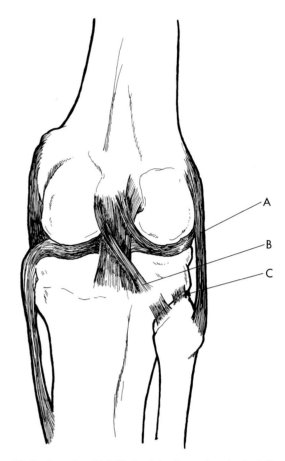

**Fig. 20-5.** Superior tibial-fibular joint (posterior view). **A,** Lateral collateral ligament; **B,** biceps femoris tendon; **C,** posterior tibial-fibular ligament.

condyle. It is reinforced by the popliteus tendon that also crosses the joint posteriorly.

There are two variations of the bony interface between the proximal fibula and tibia. The joint surface may be either horizontal or oblique[7] (Fig. 20-6A). Horizontal joints (less than 20° angle) are characterized by bony interfaces that are circular and planar, laying underneath and behind a projection on the lateral head of the tibia.[6] The position of the tibia provides some joint stability by preventing forward displacement of the fibula. Oblique joints (20° to 70° angulation) (Fig. 20-6B) are more variable in their inclina-tion and the configuration of the joint surface. Their joint surfaces are less able to accomodate rotational stresses and these joints are more likely to dislocate. The normal position of the proximal tibial-fibular joint on radiograph shows the medial aspect of the fibula overlying the lateral aspect of the tibia. The lateral view best defines the angle of the joint surface (horizontal or oblique), with the entire head of the fibula overlying the lateral tibia. The common peroneal nerve lies adjacent to this joint. Its path extends from the superior-posterior fibula, around the neck of that bone just distal to the fibular head and continues in an anterior-lateral position. The common peroneal nerve di-vides into the superficial peroneal nerve which is sensory to

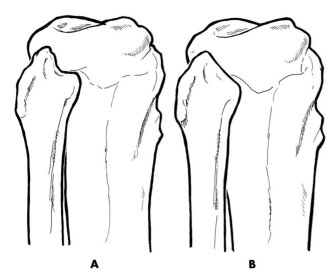

**Fig. 20-6. A,** Horizontal proximal tibial-fibular joint. **B,** Oblique proximal tibial-fibular joint.

the lateral aspect of the foot and provides motor control of eversion. The deep peroneal nerve, which is the other division of the common peroneal nerve, tracks in the anterior compartment of the shin and provides sensation to the web space between the first and second toes. Motor fibers of the deep peroneal nerve controls dorsal flexion of the ankle and toes. Thus, damage to the common peroneal nerve as it arches around the fibular head would result in sensory losses in the first web space and the lateral aspect of the foot, and motor findings would include foot drop and inability to evert the foot.

**Mechanism of injury.** Injuries to the proximal tibial-fibular ligament may follow one of four patterns: 1) anterior-lateral dislocation; 2) posterior-medial dislocation; 3) superior dislocation; or 4) chronic instability.

**Anterior-lateral dislocation.** Anterior-lateral dislocation of the proximal fibula with relation to the tibia is the most common type of injury to this joint. It is caused by the contraction of the peroneal and anterior muscles of the leg

when the leg is flexed (flexion allows the lateral collateral knee ligaments and biceps femoris to relax, thus making this joint susceptible to lateral movement). The fibula swings lateral and then anterior to the fibula (Fig. 20-7A), where it comes to rest. This injury is most frequently sustained when playing sports, such as a fall with the knee flexed under the player. Alternately, the athlete may be externally rotating the body with the planted foot inverted and plantar flexed. Typically, there are associated injuries, such as a fracture or a dislocation of the ankle or hip, or a disruption of the distal femoral epiphysis. Fractures or crush injuries of the tibial shaft may also be seen.

**Signs and symptoms.** On presentation the patient complains of pain on the outer aspect of the knee that is worsened with movement of the knee or dorsiflexion or inversion of the ankle. The pain may also localize to the lateral popliteal fossa due to stretch of the biceps tendon. Dysesthesia in the distribution of the peroneal nerve (eg, lateral foot, web space of the first and second toes) may occur secondary to stretching.

On physical examination, the fibular head is in a prominent position anterior to the tibia. The biceps tendon may stand out as a tense cord. Sensation and motor should be tested particularly with reference to the peroneal nerve (eg, dorsiflexors and evertors of the foot, sensory as previously mentioned). This injury is not always as obvious as shown in the series presented by Ogden[8]; one-third of the time, this diagnosis was not made at the initial presentation.

**Radiology.** The radiographic picture will show the fibular head laying anterior to the tibia on the lateral view and the AP view would demonstrate a lateral shift to the fibula.

**Treatment.** Reduction of the dislocation can usually be accomplished closed with local or general anesthesia. With the knee flexed and the foot dorsiflexed and inverted, direct pressure is applied to the fibular head in an attempt to reduce the subluxation. An alternative position is external rotation of the foot with the knee flexed; again direct pressure is applied to the fibular head. After successful

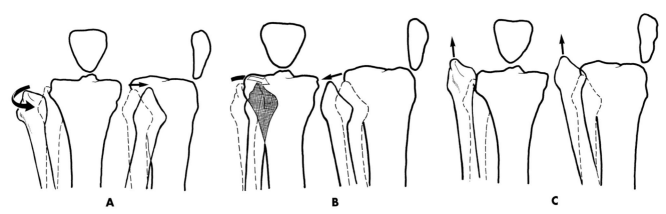

**Fig. 20-7. A,** Fibular head is dislocated anteriorly (best appreciated on the lateral view) and laterally (seen on AP film). **B,** Posterior and medial displacement of the proximal fibula with respect to the tibia. **C,** Superior dislocation of the proximal fibula.

reduction, the injury is treated with immobilization of the knee for a 3-week period. Some patients may go on to develop chronic arthritis or subluxation; thus, referral to an orthopedist is appropriate.

**Posterior-medial dislocation.** Posterior-medial dislocation of the fibular head may be secondary to direct trauma (ie, being hit by the bumper of a car) or due to a twisting injury. There is usually significant damage to the anterior aspect of the tibial-fibular joint capsule, the mobility caused by this allows the biceps femoris tendon to pull the fibular head posteriorly and medially. The lateral collateral ligament of the knee is frequently damaged at the same time (Fig. 20-7B).

Posterior medial dislocation is often best treated operatively with surgical repair of the ligamentous damage at the same time as the reduction of the joint. Persistent symptoms after conservative treatment is common.

**Superior dislocation.** The fibular head can be displaced superiorly if there is injury to the ankle or in the setting of a fractured tibial shaft (Fig. 20-7C). The treatment for this dislocation is aimed at correction of the tibial shaft or ankle injury.

**Chronic instability.** Chronic instability of the proximal tibial-fibular joint is defined as excessive symptomatic anterior-posterior movement without frank dislocation. It is commonly seen in children and teens, particularly those with joint hypermobility (eg, generalized joint laxity or associated with muscular dystrophy). Patients complain of pain along the lateral aspects of the knee and lower limb which can be reproduced by direct pressure on the fibular head (ie, pushing it forward or medially). Typically this is a self-limited condition that resolves with skeletal maturity. In adults it can be treated with 3 weeks of knee immobilization.

## Fractures of the tibial shaft

Although the tibial shaft appears to be a rather simple structure, the evaluation and management of its fractures is quite complex. The reason for this is not so much the tibia itself, but rather the injury causing the damage. A wide range of trauma can occur in tibial shaft fractures, from low-velocity falls causing greenstick fractures in children to high-velocity (eg, motor vehicle accident) crush injuries with comminution of the tibial shaft and degloving injury to the soft tissues in adults. This variety of injuries, given the high frequency of fractures of the tibial shaft, taxes the emergency physician's skills.

**Mechanism of injury.** Injuries causing tibial shaft fractures typically do so by either indirect (torsional) mechanisms or by a direct blow to the tibia. The small amount of muscle and soft tissue protecting the anterior and medial aspects of the tibia predispose to a fracture from direct trauma.

In children, falls from low heights and other low-velocity injuries such as sports are the most frequent causes of tibial fractures. Motor vehicle accident is the next most common cause of injury, such injuries being associated with a higher level of trauma. Children are also susceptible to specific injury patterns, such as bike spoke injuries or child abuse.

A greater amount of trauma is involved when the fibula is fractured in addition to the tibia. Isolated tibial shaft fractures in children are more commonly caused by a torsional trauma (eg, twisting on a planted foot), and the tibia-fibula fractures result from higher-velocity mechanisms.

In adults, crush injuries may be the result of industrial accidents or motor vehicle accidents, as when the tibia is caught between two car bumpers. Direct violence tends to cause a transverse or comminuted fracture line, and indirect violence causes oblique or spiral fractures. Low-velocity gunshot wounds can cause tibial fractures with a minimum of soft-tissue injury, unlike wounding from high-powered weapons, which cause significant damage to the surrounding tissue as the bullet passes through the leg.

**Signs and symptoms.** The finding of tibial shaft fracture is determined primarily by mechanism of injury. If the patient has fallen from a significant height, a closed-head injury or a hypotension may dominate the clinical picture. In contrast, the skier who tried to turn on a planted ski and sustained a boot-top fracture may accurately localize the fracture site. The patient complains of pain and, because the tibia is the weight-bearing bone in the lower leg, is unable to ambulate. In contrast, an isolated fibula fracture may not prevent ambulation.

In tibial shaft fractures, the extent of soft-tissue injury plays a critical role in determining treatment and predicting outcome. Because of this, the examination must be thorough. Dorsal pedal and posterior tibial pulses are evaluated, as is sensation. Lacerations or degloving injuries of the skin are searched for circumferentially. Persistent blood and drainage from a small laceration suggests this cut was caused by bone. Boggy areas under the skin suggest hematoma.

**Radiology.** The AP and lateral films should include the views of the ankle and knee when the tibial shaft has been fractured. Although the greenstick fracture in children may show a minimal displacement, a fracture of the tibial shaft in adults is rarely subtle radiologically. A fracture may be simple (ie, transverse), spiral or oblique, butterfly, or comminuted.

**Diagnosis.** When tibial shaft fractures are suspected, treatment should begin before radiographic evaluation. After circulation, motion, and sensation (CMS) evaluation, the leg should be immobilized with a radiolucent splint. Injuries to the soft tissue, such as degloving, abrasions, or lacerations, are noted. With adequate analgesia, the patient undergoes radiographic evaluation with the splint still in place. Adequate splinting prevents movement of the sharp edges of the bone and further injury to the soft tissue. Resting the leg on a pillow does not constitute immobilization, as the radiologist will likely remove all pillows.

In 1958, Ellis[9] devised a classification scheme that effectively determines optimal treatment methods and predicts outcome. Ellis defined three groups of tibial shaft injuries: mild, moderate, and severe. A mild injury is not angulated or displaced with a small degree of comminution or a minor wound opening. Moderate injuries involve total displacement of the tibial fragments or angulation, with a small degree of comminution or an open wound. Severe injuries are those including a complete displacement of the fracture fragments with major contamination or a major open wound. Ellis found a healing time of 10 weeks for minor wounds, 15 weeks for moderate wounds, and 23 weeks for major wounds. Delayed union occurred in 60% of the major injuries, 23% of the moderate injuries, and 2% of the minor injuries. Subsequent studies have corroborated the importance of grading soft-tissue damage when evaluating tibial fractures.

There have been many classification schemes developed for tibial shaft fractures. As no one scheme has demonstrated superiority over the others, it is perhaps best to just describe the injury. Important factors to be noted in the description include: 1) if the injury is open or closed, 2) the amount of soft-tissue damage to the leg; 3) the presence of associated injuries; 4) the amount of energy involved in the accident; 5) if the fibula has remained intact; and 6) the pattern of the fracture line itself (eg, oblique, spiral, transverse), its location in the tibia, and the number and position of fracture fragments. With this information, appropriate treatment can begin.

**Treatment.** Just as the severity of tibial shaft fractures covers a wide spectrum, so do the treatment options. In low-velocity injuries, such as in children who have fallen and sustained an isolated greenstick fracture, conservative treatment with reduction and casting may be sufficient. If the fibula is intact and there is no interruption in the continuity proximal or distal tibial-fibular joint, then shortening of the leg is unlikely to occur. Rotation of the fracture fragments can be prevented by a long leg cast.

Open fractures require tetanus prophylaxis and prompt irrigation and debridement of the wounds. Parenteral antistaphylococcal antibiotics are administered to prevent wound infection. Definitive care of tibial shaft fractures falls under the realm of the orthopedic surgeon working in consultation with the trauma specialist. Because the amount of trauma necessary to fracture tibias is high, the potential for compartment syndrome or vascular injury exists. It is good practice to admit all proximal tibia shaft fracture patients for close observation. If the soft-tissue loss or destruction is excessive, serial debridements may be necessary, with subsequent grafts required for closure. If conservative measures are unable to obtain or hold adequate alignment of the tibial shaft fracture fragments, operative techniques such as internal rodding or external fixation are necessary.

## Fibular fractures

Isolated fibular fractures are relatively uncommon. When the fibula is fractured, it is usually in association with the tibia. The more severe the trauma, the greater the likelihood of an associated fibular fracture. The intact fibula with the interosseous membrane will tend to act as a stabilizer or internal splint for tibial fractures. Also, whenever the fibula is not involved in fractures of the tibia, the prognosis is better. In general, the clinician may intuit by the presence of a fibular fracture that a significant amount of force has been imparted to the leg.

**Mechanism of injury.** The usual mechanism for an isolated fracture of the fibula is direct trauma to the lateral aspect of the leg. Because the fibula only bears approximately 15% of the standing weight,[1,2] in many instances, the patient is able to walk if no associated tibial fracture exists. When significant external rotational forces are involved in the injury, a proximal spiral fracture of the fibula is usually seen. With significant internal rotation injuries to the lower leg or ankle, fractures involving the distal fibula may be noted. For further discussion of distal fibula fractures, see Chapter 21, *Ankle Injuries.*

**Stress fractures.** The fibula is the second most common site for stress fractures. The typical runner's fracture involves the distal fibula a short distance above the ankle. Stress fractures involving the proximal fibula may occur but are rare.[10] Runners with anatomic discrepancies that produce an abnormal gait are usually at greater risk of developing a stress fracture. Conditions leading to stress fractures in the athlete include hyperpronation, variation in leg length, and varus or valgus deformities of the knee. Another common profession other than athletics that may produce stress fibular fractures is ballet.[11]

**Signs and symptoms.** The patient will generally give a history of trauma with immediate pain in the area of the fracture. Ambulating may be possible if there is no concomitant tibial fracture. Occasionally, the patient will state that the pain radiates the entire length of the fibula either spontaneously or whenever palpated. On examination, there may be swelling and ecchymosis in addition to marked tenderness over the fracture site. The physician must not omit the neurovascular examination when evaluating the patient in the emergency department suspected fibular fracture.

**Diagnosis and radiology.** Examination and radiographs must include the entire fibula when a fracture is suspected. Following inspection, the length of the fibula should be palpated. The emergency physician must keep in mind the possibility of compartment syndrome when the patient presents with a crush injury to the leg and consider appropriate compartment pressure determination. Many stress fractures may be identified by plain radiographs; however, when these are nondiagnostic, bone scan, CT scan, or MRI may yield the diagnosis.

**Treatment.** Treatment is usually directed toward reducing activity and avoiding strenuous lower extremity workouts in stress fractures. Of course, more severe fractures of the fibula should be seen in the emergency department by an orthopedist and definitive treatment can be initiated. Splinting of the fractured extremity with a stirrup splint, nonweight-bearing, and referral to the orthopedist are often prescribed for nondisplaced or minimally displaced fibular fractures. Diagnosis can be ascertained by bone scan. This particular diagnostic procedure can determine the presence of a stress fracture as early as several days after the insult when plain radiographs may be unremarkable.

**Complications.** Complications involving the neurovascular complex are rare in isolated fibular fractures. Probably the most common nerve injury involves the peroneal nerve, which may be contused or stretched from significant direct trauma proximally.[12]

### Achilles' tendon rupture

As the linkage responsible for the plantar flexion of the foot that occurs when the soleus and gastrocnemius muscles contract, the Achilles' tendon plays a crucial role in ambulation. Rupture of this tendon occurs less frequently than other large tendons, such as the shoulder cuff and the quadriceps, but it nonetheless accounts for about one-fifth of all major tendon ruptures.

The injury typically occurs in a 20- to 40-year-old man who participates in sports on a sporadic basis (ie, the "weekend warrior"). Rupture can occur either after a sudden forceful plantar flexion of the foot by the gastrocnemius as in sports, or unexpected dorsal flexion of the ankle such as misjudging a step on a staircase. The patients at increased risk for Achilles' tendon rupture include those with rheumatoid arthritis, systemic lupus erythematous, or prior systemic steroid use. Patients who have received prior injection of local steroids in the Achilles' tendon are also more prone to rupture.

**Signs and symptoms.** The patient often presents after hearing a pop or a snap when running or jumping. Patients complain of a sudden inability or weakness with plantar flexion of the foot.

The Achilles' tendon commonly ruptures 2 to 6 cm proximal to its attachment on the calcaneus. It is this site that is the poorest vascular supply. On physical exam, the patient may have a gap in the tendon at this site, detectable visually or by palpation. If considerable soft-tissue swelling exists or there is a large hematoma in this area, the gap may be obscured. There are several maneuvers that can be done to support the diagnosis of Achilles' tendon rupture. The Thompson-Dougherty test,[13] described in 1962, involves having the patient kneel down or lie supine on the gurney when the examiner squeezes the midportion of the calf on the affected side. With an intact Achilles' tendon, the foot will plantar flex in response to this squeeze. No movement of the foot is strongly suggestive of acute rupture. If there is an observable gap between the ends of the Achilles' tendon, this maneuver would widen that gap. A second test in evaluation of the achilles tendon is the heel rise test which assesses the ability of the patient to walk on tip-toes. With complete rupture of the Achilles' tendon, patients are unable to perform this maneuver. Although the posterior tibial tendon and peroneal muscles can provide some plantar flexion in the setting of Achilles' tendon rupture, the patient cannot support his weight without an intact Achilles' tendon. In the knee flexion test, the patient is placed prone on the examining table with his or her foot extending over the table at the ankle joint. The patient is then instructed to flex the knee to 90°. If the gastrocnemius is still tethered to the calcaneus, the foot will plantar-flex during this arc due to the insertion of the head of the gastrocnemius proximal to the knee joint. Disruption of the Achilles' tendon allows the foot to assume a dorsiflexed position during this arc. A final method of evaluation of this tendon is the needle test. With the patient again prone, a 25-gauge needle is inserted through the skin of the calf just medial to the midline. The insertion site is 10 cm proximal to the calcaneus and the needle is inserted perpendicular to the skin. The needle is advanced through the skin until resistance is met—entrance into the Achilles' tendon without transfixing it. The examiner then plantar-flexes and dorsiflexes the foot. If the Achilles' tendon is intact, the needle will move with the examiner's plantar flexion and dorsiflexion of the foot. Disruption of the tendon would result in no movement of the needle.

**Radiology.** To the dismay of the emergency department physician, this lesion does not show on plain radiographs. The diagnosis can be accurately made clinically. Radiologic evaluation could include either ultrasonography (which is not terribly sensitive), CT scanning (which would be more useful if longitudinal reconstructions were done), or MRI scanning. The MRI examination generates quality pictures of the ligaments and surrounding tissue, but its cost is often prohibitive.

**Treatment.** The goal of treatment is to return the patient to the level of functioning comparable with that prior to injury. Surgical repair of the ligament has been compared with conservative treatment in which the lower leg is casted in plantar flexion and frequent cast changes are made to the point where the ankle is in a neutral position after 6 weeks of immobilization. Some have advocated surgical treatment as a method of reducing the incidence of recurrent rupture, and others claim conservative therapy produces similar results if the period immobilization is long enough (ie, 12 weeks). In the emergency department, the patient may be immobilized with a cast or a Robert Jones dressing with the foot plantar-flexed and the patient referred to an orthopedist.

### Stress fractures

Significant repetitive trauma can result in stress fractures. This is typically seen in the young patient such as the athlete, military recruit, or ballet dancer. The fracture may involve the tibia or the fibula. They also are commonly found in the metatarsals of the foot. In military recruits, the fracture most frequently involves the upper one-third of the tibia, most often on the posterior medial aspect. Ballet dancers more frequently develop fractures slightly lower on the tibia, typically in the middle one-third. Fractures in young athletes are prone to the distal one-third of the tibia.

Just above the ankle is the area of the fibula most often is affected; this is usually seen in runners.

The patient presents with pain. The pain initially would occur with running and increase during exercise. If left unheeded, the pain would progress to the point where it occurred throughout the day, unrelieved by rest. Although this pain is similar to shin splints, with stress fractures, the exam often localizes the pain to a focal site on the bone perhaps with overlying erythema and swelling. This is as opposed to shin splints where the tenderness is less dramatic and more diffuse over the anterior leg.

Radiographs taken to search for stress fractures typically are negative if taken within the first 2 weeks of injury. A radiologic diagnosis can only be made in the first few weeks with a bone scan. When radiograph results are positive, findings on radiographs would include a localized periosteal reaction or endosteal thickening. A faint radiolucent line may be seen involving one or both cortices.

There are a range of treatment options available. In all cases, exercise must be stopped. Crutches will make ambulation much less painful. In some cases, this is sufficient treatment; other patients may require casting. Follow-up with a sports medicine specialist or an orthopedist would also be appropriate.

### Shin splints

The term *shin splints* is a phrase that perhaps means more to the layman than the physician. It is a nonspecific term that encompasses a number of different disease processes. Because these different processes are often lumped together, the literature on diagnosis and treatment is rather muddled. One definition of shin splints would be recurrent pain in the lower legs that occurs during exercise and resolves with rest. It is typically seen in athletes, often early on in the training period. Frequently running on a hard surface is involved, such as an indoor track or frozen ground. The pain—a dull ache—is diffusely located over the anterior and lateral leg.

There are perhaps several different diseases that constitute this entity, such as inflammation of the interosseous membrane, chronic anterior compartment syndrome, inflammation of the attachment of the posterior tibial muscle along the posterior aspect of the tibia, or irritation of the anterior tibia muscles attachment at the anterior border of the tibia.

The emergency department evaluation of patients with such complaints could be quite straightforward; examination to rule out the presence of compartment syndrome and Achilles' tendonitis. Radiographs may be ordered to exclude the possibility of occult fracture. Stress fractures typically will not be detectable within 2 to 4 weeks after the onset of symptoms unless a bone scan is included in the radiologic evaluation.

The treatment for shin splints includes heat, nonsteroidal anti-inflammatory drugs (NSAIDS), and rest. The patient often will have a recurrence of symptoms if the precipitat-ing activity is begun too soon. Often shin splints will disable an athlete for an entire season. Thus, referral to a sports medicine specialist or orthopedist is appropriate, with instructions to the patient not to resume activity until cleared by the specialist.

## PEDIATRIC INJURIES
### Proximal epiphyseal fractures

**Mechanism.** Injuries to the proximal growth line of the tibia are uncommon, accounting for less than 1% of all epiphyseal injuries. This is likely a result of its anterior protection by the downward extension of the tibial tubercle and the position of the fibula, providing support from lateral forces. Although the epiphysis can be injured by direct forces (ie, a car bumper) children are more likely to sustain an injury here secondary to forced abduction or hyperextension of the tibial shaft against a fixed knee. This indirect mechanism is commonly seen in adolescents playing sports such as football.

**Signs and symptoms.** According to the Salter classification, fracture of the growth line itself (ie, in the same plane) is a Salter I. Here, the patient presents with pain, swelling, and tenderness over the epiphysis. Radiographs in a Salter I fracture may be normal (in up to one half of the patients) or may show some displacement. Typically, the proximal tibia is normal in its relation to the femur but the tibial diaphysis (shaft) has moved either posteriorly or medially. Anterior displacement of the shaft is prevented to a large extent by the tibial tuberosity and the fibula prevents lateral movement of the diaphysis. Significant shift of the tibial shaft away from the fibula would indicate associated damage to the interosseous ligament. If a Salter I fracture is suspected, stress radiographs may be obtained to show opening of the epiphyseal line. This is perhaps best done under the direction of an orthopedist. A more common injury to the proximal epiphysis is the Salter II fracture, where the fracture plane runs along the growth line and extends distally into the shaft of the tibia. Again, the vast majority of the displacement is determined by the anterior tibial tuberosity and the fibula, resulting in posterior or medial displacement of the tibial shaft with respect to the epiphysis. An additional finding could be valgus deformity. Salter III injuries are less common. Here, the fracture extends proximally from the growth line into the joint. Interarticular extension is more common on the lateral plateau than the medial and may be associated with a tear of the medial collateral ligament. Salter IV and V fractures are unusual.

There are several injuries that may occur with proximal tibial epiphyseal fracture. Although the proximal fibular growth line is usually intact, the fibular shaft itself is frequently broken. Fibular neck fractures may be accompanied by damage to the peroneal nerve as it travels around the fibular shaft. Ligamentous injury to the medial collateral ligament, and less often the lateral collateral ligament, can occur, particularly if the mechanism was a blow from the lateral side (ie, a football player being clipped). The most severe potential injury accompanying tibial epiphyseal fractures is vascular. Posterior displacement of the tibial shaft can damage the popliteal artery as it is held tightly against the proximal tibia. Thus, evaluation of this injury should include careful attention to the vascular status of the leg.

**Treatment.** Treatment of these fractures include the involvement of an orthopedist. Salter I fractures that are not displaced can be managed with immobilization of the limb and crutch walking. Fracture with displacement requires reduction, which can be performed closed. If the line extends into the weight-bearing joint, optimal alignment may require open reduction. Salter II and III fractures are often difficult to maintain a reduction with closed methods, and these also may eventually come to surgical therapy.

Unless these injuries are accompanied by the previously mentioned neurologic or vascular problems, outcome is generally good. Fractures that do not involve the articular surface tend to have better long-term results. The injury may lead to premature closure of the growth line, but most commonly this has occurred in a teenager and subsequent growth problems are minimal. In the younger child, premature growth line closure would lead to more pronounced sequela.

### Proximal tibial metaphyseal fractures

This injury frequently results from a direct force applied to the outside of the extended knee, resulting in a fracture of the medial aspect of the proximal tibia just distal to the growth line. Typically the child is 3 to 6 years of age. The radiographic findings include a greenstick fracture with an open cortex on the medial side along with lateral angulation of the distal aspect of the tibia. Occasionally, there will be an accompanying plastic deformity of the fibula; more likely the fibula will remain intact.

There are two serious problems with this injury—the first is vascular. The susceptible vessel is the anterior tibial artery as it passes through the interosseous membrane at the level of this fracture. Delay in recognition of the injury to this artery can result in Volkman's contracture necessitating a delayed amputation. The second sequela to proximal metaphyseal fractures is residual deformity. Follow-up radiographs during the treatment phase often show a progression from initial adequate alignment to valgus deformity. The subsequent valgus deformity may be secondary to initially unrecognized inadequate reduction. At times optimal reduction is not possible because of soft-tissue entrapment in the fracture line. An alternative etiology of the deformity is the fracture on the medial aspect of the tibia resulting in accelerated growth in the medial part of that bone with respect to the lateral aspect of the tibia, leading to valgus deformity.

Treatment of this fracture can often be accomplished in a closed fashion if there is adequate (ie, general) anesthesia. It is appropriate to warn the parents of the possibility of subsequent valgus deformity. If the orthopedist is unable to obtain satisfactory reduction with closed techniques, an open approach is indicated. After reduction, the patient is placed in a long leg cast for a minimum of 6 weeks.

### Osgood-Schlatter disease

This condition of the knee was first described in the literature by Osgood and Schlatter in 1903. The anatomic lesion is a partial separation of the tibial tuberosity at the patella tendon insertion (Fig. 20-8). It is a common occurrence in adolescents with a history of knee pain, especially those involved in junior sports. This condition is primarily seen in boys, but is becoming more prevalent in girls now that they are participating more in junior and little-league sports activity. The sports most commonly responsible are football, soccer, basketball, gymnastics, and ballet.[5] Osgood-Schlatter lesions are generally unilateral but can be bilateral in 25% to 30% of patients.[12,14]

Osgood-Schlatter disease is caused by repeated submaximal stress and contraction of the quadriceps during periods of rapid growth (8 to 13 years of age in girls; 10 to 15 years of age in boys) and involves a pulling away or

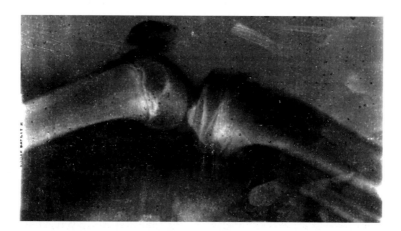

**Fig. 20-8.** Lateral radiograph demonstrating classic appearance of Osgood-Schlatter lesion in an adolescent boy.

traction of the tibial tuberosity. The lesion is often referred to as *traction apophysitis*. Although originally thought to be secondary to avascular necrosis at the tibial tuberosity ossification center, histologic studies support a traumatic cause. Repetitive quadriceps contraction transmits sufficient stress to cause a partial avulsion fracture through the ossification center, leading to the development of Osgood-Schlatter disease. The lump that is commonly seen on physical exam is caused by the hypertrophic bone formation in the patellar tendon.

**Diagnosis.** Clinically, Osgood-Schlatter disease is associated with swelling, pain, and tenderness just below the knee, with the patient typically in his or her early teen years. Symptoms are aggravated by kicking, running, jumping, kneeling, and climbing. The patient may give a history of increased pain at the knee when climbing or descending stairs. The symptoms are generally better when the patient is at rest and not involved in sports activity. On physical examination of the knee and leg, swelling and extreme tenderness are noted at the tibial tuberosity. On extension of the knee against resistance or stressing the quadriceps, the patient will have pain in the same area of complaint.

**Radiology.** Although the diagnosis can usually be made by history and physical examination, radiographs are helpful in the symptomatic patient. A lateral view of the involved knee flexed at approximately 30° will give the optimum figuration of the tibial tuberosity. Because of the limitations of plain radiographs to evaluate soft tissues and tendons, ultrasound has been used by some to further define abnormalities of these structures. Also, by using ultrasound, the child is less exposed to radiation. The sonographic characteristics of the Osgood-Schlatter lesion was described by Lanning[15] as soft-tissue swelling anterior to the tibial tubercle, elevation of the tubercle from the tibia, and thickening of the distal patellar tendon. Other modalities, such as three-phase bone scintigrams, CT scans and MRI may be utilized to evaluate the abnormalities of this disease.[14]

**Treatment.** Treatment has been controversial, in that some believe that no treatment is needed, and others advocate splinting and discontinuing the sports activity that leads to the symptoms. Frequent application of cold compresses, NSAIDs, and knee immobilization, in addition to improving the flexibility of the lower extremities, is the more standard approach to management.[16] To prevent atrophy of the quadriceps muscles, the patient should be instructed in straight-leg raises and quadriceps sets. Operative management that involves drilling the tibial tuberosity in patients with severe symptoms offers good pain relief, but the residual bony defect is not altered.[17] The author recommends the conservative and standard approach involving rest and physical therapy.

**Prognosis and complications.** The majority of patients will have spontaneous resolution of their symptoms, but the prognosis for Osgood-Schlatter disease is not always good, especially when untreated. Patients with the diagnosis may experience symptoms well into adulthood. This appears to be particularly true in patients with persistent abnormality of the tibial tubercle.[17] Rarely, recurvatum of the knee may develop as a complication of Osgood-Schlatter disease resulting from premature closure of the proximal tibial epiphyseal plate.[17,18]

### Fracture of the tibial tuberosity

Injuries to the tibial tuberosity may be acute or chronic in nature. Both occur predominantly in adolescent males. Chronic injury to the tibial tuberosity is previously discussed as the Osgood-Schlatter lesion. Symptoms often are gradual in onset (over weeks to months), the patient is able to ambulate without difficulty, and the physical exam is unremarkable. However, in acute tibial tuberosity fractures, there is a specific precipitating event, dramatic pain, and swelling along with tenderness over the tibial tuberosity, often with an inability for the patient to walk.

**Anatomy.** Ossification of the proximal tibia begins in two areas. The primary ossification center develops just proximal to the epiphyseal line, and one or more secondary ossification centers develop in the area that will subsequently become the tibial tuberosity (Fig. 20-9). With maturation, the secondary ossification centers coalesce with each other and then merge with the primary ossification center. Eventually, the epiphysis closes and the proximal tibia is completely calcified. Fractures of the tibial tuberosity can occur in any of three places: 1) between the secondary ossification centers; 2) between the primary and secondary ossification centers; or 3) through the epiphyseal line propagating proximally into the articular surface of the knee[19] (Fig. 20-10).

The quadriceps muscle is responsible for extension of the knee. The patellar ligament encases the patella and attaches at the upper anterior tibia at the site of the tibial tuberosity and just distal to this. With avulsion of a piece of the tibial tuberosity, there may be a tear of this ligament on the attachment to the more distal tibia, thus allowing displacement of the fragment of the tibial tuberosity. This tear of the patellar ligament would then allow proximal displacement of the knee cap (patella alta). The patellar ligament is also supported by fibers that extend medially and laterally from the patella to attach near the tibia condyles. If these ligaments remain intact, the knee can still be actively extended by the quadriceps despite fracture of the tibial tuberosity and rupture of the distal attachment of the patellar ligament.

**Mechanism.** The typical patient is a 14- to 16-year-old boy who is participating in sports. During forcible contraction of the quadriceps against resistance (ie, jumping) the tibial tuberosity is fractured or avulsed and the distal patella ligament is disrupted.

**Signs and symptoms.** The patient recalls the event quite vividly, with a sudden onset of pain. At times, the picture may be muddled by this event occurring in a patient with a prior history of Osgood-Schlatter–type symptoms.

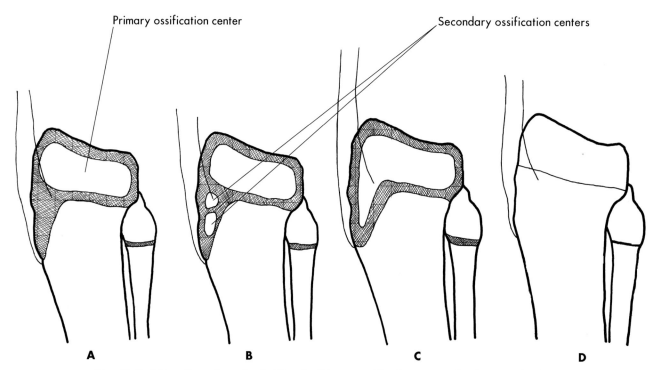

**Fig. 20-9.** Maturation of proximal tibia. **A,** Primary ossification center develops proximal to epiphyseal lines; **B,** one or two secondary ossification centers; **C,** secondary ossification centers coalesce with each other and with primary ossification center; **D,** closure of epiphyseal line.

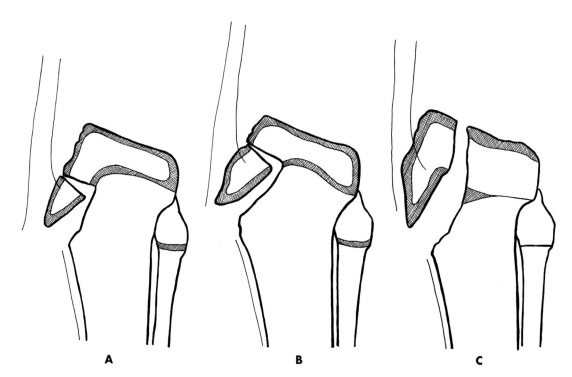

**Fig. 20-10.** Ogden's classification of tibial tuberosity fractures. **A,** Type I—fracture between secondary ossification centers; **B,** type II—fracture splitting secondary ossification centers from primary ossification center; **C,** type III—fracture into articular surface of the knee.

Swelling and tenderness over the site of the fracture and crepitance or movement of the fracture fragment itself may be felt. If the fracture extends into the knee joint (Salter III), hemarthrosis often is present. The patient may not be able to actively extend the knee. Other times, full extension of the knee is possible. Spasm of the hamstring muscles may be present, resulting in the knee being flexed at 20° to 40°.

**Radiology.** The lateral film of the proximal tibia best displays the injury. Ogden[19] describes three types of injuries based on the position of the fracture plane (Fig. 20-10). In a type I fracture, the plane extends anteriorly through the secondary ossification centers. There is minimal displacement of the bone fragments. Type II injuries are transverse fractures of the tibial tuberosity at the same height as the epiphysis, again propagating to the anterior surface of the tibia. Here, there is more damage to the patellar ligament and also more displacement of the tibial tuberosity. Type II fractures may in addition involve fractures through the secondary ossification centers (ie, type II may be accompanied by type I). A type III fracture extends from the tibial tuberosity proximally through the epiphysis and into the articular surface of the knee. These would alternatively be classified as Salter III fractures. Radiographically, the amount of displacement and size of fracture fragments can be underestimated if the secondary ossification centers are poorly calcified. On the other hand, if the skeleton has matured to the point of closure of all growth lines, then fractures of the tibial tuberosities are uncommon.

Type III fractures often extend into the joint space just anterior to the tibial spine, again best visualized on the lateral films. Films may show hemarthrosis, and with type II injury, the patella may be high riding.

**Treatment.** Type I fracture with minimal displacement of the fracture fragments can be treated conservatively. With the hip flexed and the knee extended, the fracture fragment is simply pushed back into place. The knee is then immobilized with a long leg cast with molding of the cast aimed at pushing the patella distally. Type II and III fractures frequently undergo open reduction and internal fixation. This allows optimal reduction of the fracture fragments. Often times, a flap of periosteum is found entrapped underneath the fracture fragment. Hardware is then used to maintain the reduction.

With good treatment, the outlook for these patients is excellent, with most of these youths able to return to preinjury status. As the injury occurs primarily in patients who are near skeletal maturity, there are minimal problems with premature closure of the growth plates causing subsequent deformity of the legs or leg-length discrepancy.

### Tibial-fibular shaft fractures

The most common fracture of the leg involves the shaft of the tibia or fibula. Typically, a rotational force is applied to the lower leg (ie, the child is turning on a planted foot, resulting in a spiral fracture). Less often, direct force such as that in a fall or a motor vehicle accident leads to fracture; here, the fracture line tends to be transverse or in a butterfly pattern. Child abuse is most likely to result in fracture of the humerus with fracture of the tibia as the second most common occurrence.

Fractures of the tibia may be either complete or incomplete (greenstick). Most frequently, they involve the middle to distal one-third of the tibia, as in the younger child, this section of bone is less mature. If the tibia alone is fractured, there will often be a varus deformity but the intact fibula will prevent shortening. Conversely, if the fibula also has a complete fracture, there may be shortening of the bony fragments. Greenstick fractures of the tibia itself are not prone to shortening. Although some greenstick fractures are readily apparent, more subtle injuries can also occur, perhaps with the fracture apparent only on one of the views. With complete fracture of the tibia, the fibula may undergo a plastic type of deformity, or bowing, without obvious fracture line. This may be easier appreciated with comparative views of the uninjured leg.

The patient presents in a variety of ways. In the younger child a known history of trauma may be lacking; exams can show tenderness, swelling, or erythema over the fracture site. With complete fracture of the tibia, the child will not be able to walk, although a patient with a greenstick fracture may still be ambulatory. The treatment approach depends on the fracture itself, extent of soft-tissue damage, and presence of associated injuries. These fractures tend to heal quite well with delayed union almost never seen (the exception to this is in the multiple trauma victim with a closed-head injury). Simple fractures with adequate alignment and no other injuries can be casted; after several days, weight bearing may commence depending on the patient's comfort. Oblique fractures of the tibia with an intact fibula tend to be pulled into valgus deformity by the flexors of the toes and ankles. These muscles can be neutralized to some extent by casting with the knee flexed and the foot, plantar-flexed. When both the tibia and fibula are fractured, shortening can occur. Although bayonette opposition of other long bones is a treatment goal, in the lower leg, reduction should be nearly anatomic in terms of the length of the bony fragments. Similarly, although the forearm and femur can remodel angular deformities in the tibia, this does not happen at the same extent.

Isolated fractures of the fibula have usually occurred after a direct blow to the lateral side of the leg. If there is no associated injury of the tibia (with particular attention to the epiphysis), fibula fractures heal quickly with immobilization and early ambulation.

### Toddler's fracture

Torsion force applied to the foot can result in this spiral fracture of the distal one-third of the tibia. Classically, this occurs in a child just learning how to walk, but the age limit may be up to 6 years of age. The child may have twisted (ie, to evade parents) on a planted foot. Other times, specific traumatic event cannot be recalled. The parents present with a fussy or irritable child or one who is limping.

Examination of the child may be difficult, depending on his or her age. In the cooperative child, tenderness can be appreciated over the fracture site. Radiographs performed in the emergency department can show a spiral fracture of the distal one-third of the tibia with an intact fibula. The oblique fracture may be subtle and detectable only on one of the film views. Indeed, initial films may be negative, and the correct diagnosis made 2 weeks after the injury as a result of callous formation around the fracture site and reabsorption of calcium along the fracture line.

Treatment for fracture involves a long leg cast for 2 to 4 weeks with weight bearing as tolerated. As initial films results often are negative, the decision to treat can be made on a clinical rather than a radiographic basis.

### Bicycle-spoke injuries

This accident occurs when a child is given a ride on a bicycle. The child's foot becomes wedged between the frame of the bike (ie, the front fork) and the rotating spokes of the wheel. This may be the result of a fall or the sudden braking of the wheel caused by the foot may result in a crash. Additional injury can result from an extrication of the entrapped foot if the attendant merely reverses the rotation of the wheel to free the foot. The primary problem with bicycle-spoke injuries is the extent of damage to the soft tissues of the foot that has sustained a crush injury after being wedged between the fork of the bike and the wheel. Additionally, the spoke may have caused a laceration, typically over the malleoli or Achilles' tendon.

On presentation, the foot may appear normal or there may be only mild abrasions or injuries to the soft tissue. Over the ensuing 24 to 48 hours, the true extent of soft-tissue damage becomes apparent and full-thickness loss of the soft tissue may occur. Lacerations that initially were sutured will usually dehisce around this time. Although the child may be able to walk on the leg, fractures are common and all children who have a bicycle-spoke injury should have radiographs taken.

Traditional treatment of these injuries includes elevation, immobilization with a loose bulky dressing, and admission to the hospital. Reevaluation 1 to 3 days after the injury may determine if grafting is indicated. Parents should be warned at the initial evaluation the potential for wound complications.

## DISCUSSION

Injuries to the tibia or fibula cover a diverse spectrum. The proximal tibia is an articular surface for a major weight-bearing joint; thus, injuries to this area are often complicated by a subsequent degenerative joint disease. The tibial shaft itself is unique in that its subcutaneous position

provides little protection from anterior or medially directed forces; thus, fractures of the shaft are frequent. The management of a shaft fracture is determined more by the extent of damage to the soft tissue and the amount of energy involved in the accident than the type of diaphyseal fracture. Isolated injuries to the fibula are uncommon, and treatment of fibular injuries are more directed by the nature of the damage to the tibia than the fibula.

There are a number of soft-tissue complications that can occur in the lower leg, even without a fracture. Compartment syndrome secondary to blunt trauma may threaten the leg, as can injury to the popliteal artery as it exits the popliteal fossa. The relatively subcutaneous position of the common peroneal nerve in its course near the proximal fibula predisposes to a traumatic neuropathy. Children are subject to a number of injuries that are not seen in adults. Young adults may sustain acute or chronic injury to the tibial tuberosity, and they may also fracture the tibia because of rotational forces applied when playing sports.

## REFERENCES

1. Lambert KL: Weight bearing function of the fibula, *J Bone Joint Surg* 54A:507-513, 1972.
2. Takebec K, Nakagawa A, Miwami H, Kanazawa H, Hirohata K: Role of the fibula in weight bearing, *Clin Orthop* 184:289-92, 1984.
3. Rorabeck CH, Clarke KM: The pathophysiology of the anterior tibial compartment syndrome: An experimental investigation, *J Trauma* 18:299, 1978.
4. Sheridan GW, Masten FA: Fasciotomy in the treatment of acute compartment syndrome, *J Bone Joint Surg* 58:112-115, 1976.
5. Delamarter R, Hohl M: Ligament injuries associated with tibial plateau fractures, *Clin Orthop* 250:226-233, 1990.
6. Moore T, Harvey P: Roentographic measurement of tibial plateau depression due to fracture, *J Bone Joint Surg* 56A:155-160, 1974.
7. Ogden JA: The anatomy and function of the proximal tibiofibular joint, *Clin Orthop* 101:186-91, 1974.
8. Ogden JA: Subluxation of the proximal tibiofibular joint, *Clin Orthop* 101:192-197, 1974.
9. Ellis H: Disabilities after tibial shaft fractures, *J Bone Joint Surg* 40B:190-197, 1952.
10. LaCroix H, Keeman JN: An unusual stress fracture of the fibula in a long distance runner, *Arch Orthop Trauma Surg* 111:289-90, 1992.
11. Kozlowski K, Azouz M, and Hoff D: Stress fracture of the fibula in the first decade of life, *Pediatr Radiol* 21:381-383, 1991.
12. Dunn JF Jr: Osgood-Schlatter disease, *Am Fam Pract* 41:173-176, 1990.
13. Thompson TC, Doherty TH: Spontaneous rupture of tendon of Achilles': A new clinical diagnostic test, *J Trauma* 1:126, 1962.
14. Rosenberg ZS et al: Osgood-Schlatter lesion: Fracture or tendonitis: Scintigraphis, CT, and MR imaging features, *Radiology* 185:853-858, 1992.
15. Lanning P, Heikkinen E: Ultrasonic features of the Osgood-Schlatter lesion, *J Pediatr Orthop* 11:538-540, 1991.
16. Haber EC: Osgood-Schlatter disease (letter), *Am Fam Pract* 43:400-405, 1991.
17. Krause BL, Williams JP, Catterall A: Natural history of Osgood-Schlatter disease, *J Pediatr Orthop* 10:65-68, 1990.
18. Lynch MC, Walsh HPJ: Tibia recurvatum as a complication of Osgood-Schlatter's disease: A report of two cases, *J Pediatr Orthop* 11:543-544, 1991.
19. Ogden JA, Tross RB, and Murphy MJ: Fractures of the tibial tuberosity in adolescents, *J Bone Joint Surg* 62A:205-215, 1980.

# Ankle Injuries

*Carson R. Harris*

Ankle injuries continue to challenge the emergency physician. Each day an estimated one in 10,000 persons sustains an injury to the ankle.[1] These injuries occur most commonly as a result of sports accidents (especially in volleyball, basketball, football, and racquetball), but can also occur as a result of simple activities of daily living, and present acutely and subacutely to the emergency department. Although most of the ankle injuries seen in the emergency department are soft tissue injuries rather than significant bony injuries chronic disability and instability may result.[2]

This chapter reviews ankle anatomy, specific injuries and their mechanisms, clinical findings seen in the emergency department, and various approaches to the management of ankle injuries

## ANKLE ANATOMY

There are three bones and three important collateral ligament groups in the ankle (Figs. 21-1 and 21-2). The bones that form the ankle joint are the tibia, fibula, and talus. The ligaments of the ankle include the lateral collateral, the medial collateral, and the interosseous ligaments. The medial (deltoid) ligament complex is relatively thick and strong, and extends from the medial malleolus to the talus, calcaneal, and navicular bones in a triangular fashion (Fig. 21-2A). This complex stabilizes the joint during eversion and prevents subluxation. It consists of the tibionavicular, tibiocalcaneal, and anterior and posterior tibiotalar ligaments.

The lateral collateral ligaments permit a significant amount of inversion and stress compared with the deltoid complex. This complex consists primarily of the anterior talofibular (ATFL), posterior talofibular (PTFL), and calcaneofibular ligaments (Fig. 21-2B), which function to prevent anterior and lateral subluxation of the talus. The PTFL is the strongest of this complex, and a significant amount of joint trauma is required to rupture it.

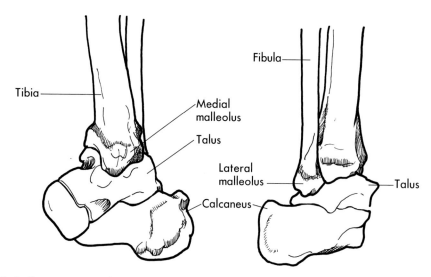

**Fig. 21-1.** Bony anatomy of the ankle in medial and lateral views.

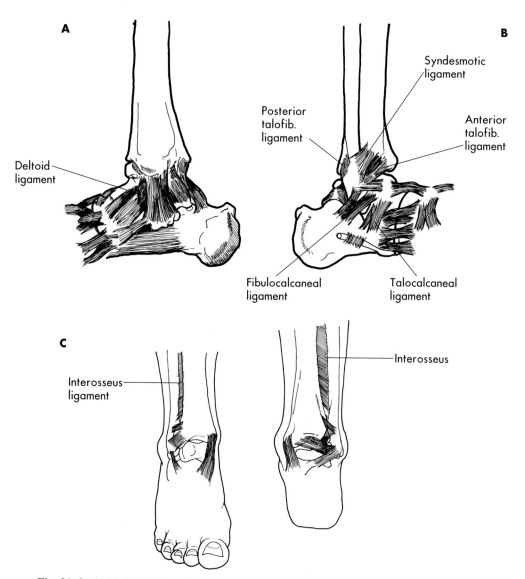

**Fig. 21-2. A,** Medial, **B,** lateral and, **C,** anteroposterior views of the ankle ligaments.

Other important structures associated with the ankle joint include the interosseous ligament, which connects the tibia and fibula proximally, and by the tibiofibular syndesmosis, which connects the bones distally (Fig. 21-2C). The fibers of these ligaments are only minimally extensible and help to maintain the connection between the fibula and tibia. The tendons of the peroneus muscles pass distally and inferiorly to the lateral malleolus with the peroneus brevis inserting at the base of the fifth metatarsal and the peroneus longus inserting along the plantar surface of the foot (Fig. 21-3). These muscles originating from the lateral aspect of the fibula assist the lateral collateral ligaments in stabilizing the ankle. The peroneus brevis and peroneus longus are instrumental in pronating and everting or abducting the foot.

The range of motion of the ankle joint allows for dorsiflexion and plantar flexion, internal and external rotation, and inversion and eversion (Fig. 21-4). Normal range of motion varies but is approximately 20° of dorsiflexion to 30° of plantar flexion. Adduction-abduction is approximately 10°, and internal and external rotation of the joint is about 17°.

The undersurface of the tibia is vaulted and smooth. The term *plafond* (or ceiling) refers to the inferior articular surface of the tibia. This surface is broader anteriorly than it is posteriorly and is longer on its lateral side than medially. It is continuous with the medial malleolus and ends laterally at the syndesmosis with the fibula.

## HISTORY AND PHYSICAL EXAMINATION

The patient's history is an extremely important part of the evaluation of the ankle injury. Questions should be directed toward defining the mechanism of injury and the immediate symptoms and signs following the injury. Typically, the patient will simply state that he or she "twisted" the ankle or foot. It is important to know the approximate position of the foot at the time of injury, ie, whether it was plantar-flexed or dorsiflexed. There are several points of the history that should be addressed, including the patient's activity, the position of the foot at the time of injury, the rotation of the ankle or the mechanism causing the injury, and the patient's symptoms immediately after the injury. Equally important is his or her symptoms at the time of presentation to the emergency department. It should be remembered that injury to adjacent areas may accompany the ankle injury, and the emergency physician should not neglect to ask about joints above and below the primary injury site.

The activity in which the patient was engaged when injury occurred may allow the emergency physician to anticipate the severity of the injury prior to the physical examination. This activity can give the physician an idea of the approximate amount of force that was imparted to the ankle structures. One may expect that the twisting of the ankle while walking or stepping from a curb would be less severe than if the injury had occurred while the patient was sky-diving or if he or she fell from a roof.

The foot's position when the injury occurred may suggest which structures of the ankle joint are injured. A plantar-flexed or dorsiflexed position is usually related in the history. In sporting events or running the position of the foot is generally plantar-flexed at the time of injury. A significant injury to the ankle may also occur with the foot in the neutral position. This may be especially true in those

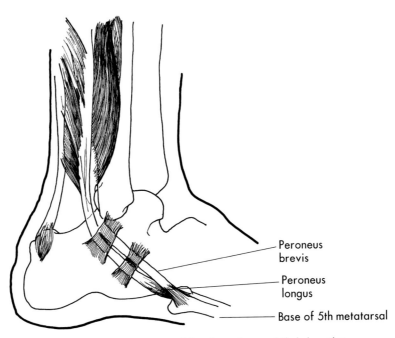

**Fig. 21-3.** Course of the peroneus longus and brevis tendons and their insertion.

Peroneus brevis

Peroneus longus

Base of 5th metatarsal

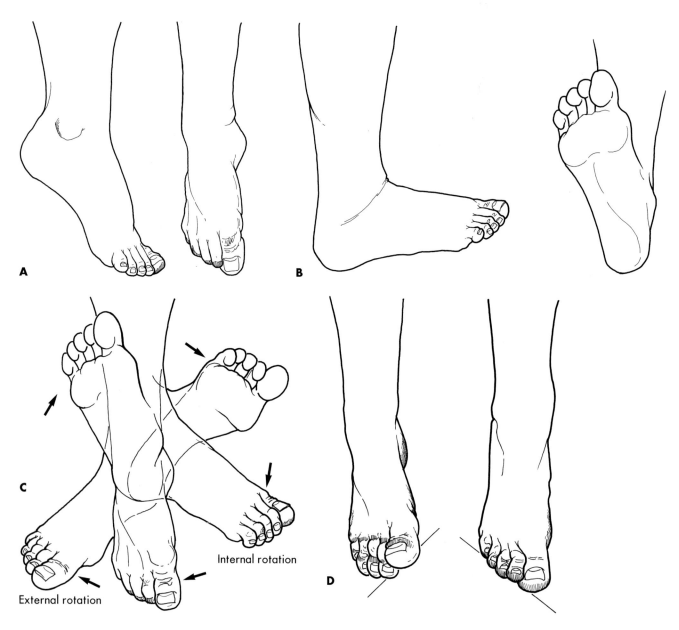

**Fig. 21-4.** Ankle range of motion. **A,** Plantar flexion. **B,** Dorsiflexion. **C,** Internal and external rotation. **D,** Eversion and inversion.

having a weakened joint subsequent to a previous significant ankle injury.

The mechanism causing the injury may be crucial in diagnosing ligamentous injuries in the emergency department. Knowing whether the ankle was overly inverted, everted, supinated, or impacted can also assist the emergency physician in defining the possible injured bony and ligamentous structures, as discussed above. In many instances the patient will state that a snap or popping was felt when the injury occurred. The significance of this has been inconsistent in my experience, in that a rupture of the ligament is not always associated with this finding in the history.

Symptoms immediately after the injury should be elic-ited, especially regarding the ability of the patient to bear weight after the injury. This information has been correlated with the presence of more significant ankle fractures when associated with ankle swelling, although the clinician should bear in mind that there are patients who may continue to walk on the injured ankle and still have a fracture. Chances are minimal that such patients will have a significant fracture or ligament rupture requiring more aggressive emergency department therapy and expeditious follow-up.

When examining the ankle, the physician should have a systematic approach, and this approach should be used consistently regardless of the initial presentation. The author's preferred approach is to expose the injured lower

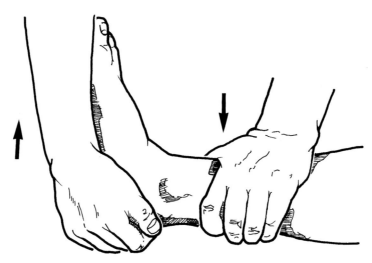

**Fig. 21-5.** Anterior drawer test.

extremity; inspect for gross abnormalities; palpate for tenderness and the presence of pulses; and stress specific ligamentous structures for laxity.

Many fractures have been missed because the clinician failed to examine the areas above and below the injury site. In addition, other structures neighboring the ankle should be considered for possible injury, ie, the Achilles, peroneal, and posterior tibial tendons. When presenting with an ankle injury, the patient's entire leg should be exposed from knee to toes. Examination should begin away from the injured ankle with the knee. The most common injury at the knee associated with an ankle injury is fracture of the proximal fibula. Exposing both the injured and uninjured lower extremities can assist the physician in recognizing subtle differences in size, discoloration, and ligamentous laxity.

During the inspection phase of the examination, which begins at the knee and progresses to the foot, any discoloration, swelling, skin breaks, or deformity should be documented. The injured extremity should then be palpated, noting the location of tenderness, crepitus, and the presence or absence of pulses (in some institutions, the use of a Doppler stethoscope is routine in evaluating the presence of a pulse in the injured extremity). The fibula should be palpated along its entire length. The lateral and medial malleoli are palpated for bony tenderness, as is the base of the fifth metatarsal. A fracture at the base of this bone (Jones or Dancer's fracture) must be suspected in patients with inversion injuries and tenderness at this location (see Chapter 22 for further discussion). Palpating for tenderness at the primary collateral ligaments (ATFL, deltoid, and fibulocalcaneal) is also very important. The emergency physician should attempt to determine which ligamentous structures have been injured.

Both the dorsalis pedis and posterior tibial pulses should be palpated. Palpation for neurovascular compromise is extremely important early in the examination in cases of gross ankle dislocation. If pulses are absent, it is considered an orthopedic emergency and the dislocation should be reduced as soon as possible by the emergency physician or orthopedist if one is immediately available.

Generally, after palpating the injured part of the ankle, radiographs are obtained. If no fracture is seen, most clinicians will elect to stress the ligaments on the initial visit to assist in defining the extent of injury. Complete rupture of certain ligaments will produce laxity. The primary stress tests that can be done in the emergency department are the talar tilt and the drawer tests. A third test that can be performed in the emergency department is the squeeze test (not to be confused with the Thompson squeeze test for Achilles tendon rupture discussed in Chapter 20).

The anterior drawer test is performed to examine the integrity of the ATFL (Fig. 21-5). The technique for this test involves grasping the heel in one hand and applying a posterior force to the lower tibia with the other hand while pulling forward on the heel. This maneuver should also be done on the uninjured ankle to compare the amount of laxity. The test is considered positive when significant displacement of the foot (more than 1 to 2 mm discrepancy between the affected and unaffected ankles) from the tibia is noted.

The ATFL may also be examined by the talar tilt test (Fig. 21-6). The patient's foot is plantar-flexed and inverted by the examiner. This test cannot be carried out without imparting discomfort to the patient with an inversion injury. A positive test is demonstrated when there is a difference in laxity when compared with the normal ankle. The significance of a positive test will depend on the presence of a significant previous injury to either ankle.

The squeeze test is not frequently given in the emergency department and is performed to determine the presence of a syndesmotic injury. As shown in Figure 21-7, the emergency physician places his or her hand approximately

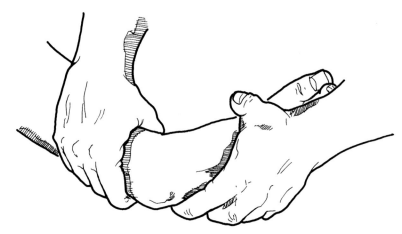

**Fig. 21-6.** Talar tilt test.

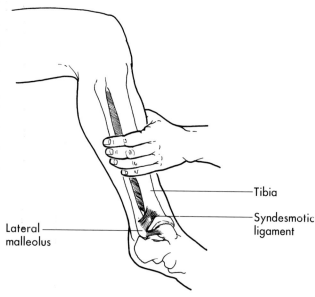

Lateral malleolus

Tibia

Syndesmotic ligament

**Fig. 21-7.** Squeeze test.

15 to 20 cm (6 to 8 inches) below the knee and squeezes the tibia and fibula together. If the patient has injured the syndesmotic ligament, he or she will complain of pain in the ankle when this test is applied.

## APPROPRIATE USE OF RADIOGRAPHY IN ANKLE INJURIES

Approximately 15% of all trauma radiographs are obtained for ankle injuries.[3] The incidence of an ankle fracture significant enough to change patient management is estimated to be less than 15%.[4] That is, 85% of patients receiving radiography could be treated as though they had sprains, while the remainder will have significant injuries that require more aggressive or immediate treatment.

Patients' expectations that they will receive radiographs in the emergency department after presenting with an ankle injury, coupled with the emergency physician's fear of litigation for missing a fracture, has led to an extraordinary number of radiographs being ordered. The cost of diagnosis and rehabilitation has been an issue in emergency medicine for some time, and approaches $900 million per year.[5] One of the important contributing factors to this cost is the use of radiography. It is difficult to say what percentage of patients requesting radiographs who do not receive them, eventually do have them taken at another institution. Radiographs tend to serve three purposes: documentation of the presence or absence of pathology, diagnosis, and assistance with disposition and treatment. The controversy lies in whether the emergency physician's treatment and the patient's outcome will be altered based on the radiographic findings.

Numerous studies[4,6-12] have attempted to reduce the overuse of ankle films by establishing objective clinical criteria for determining the presence of a significant injury. These studies generally show that ankle radiographs are unnecessary in patients with minimal pain or swelling after an acute, isolated injury.

It also appears that patients over the age of 50 years have a risk of sustaining malleolar fractures.[4] This correlation is thought to be associated with the presence of osteoporosis in this age group. In addition, Sujitkumar et al.[9] concluded that even when moderate or severe pain and swelling were present, they were not reliable indicators of significant ankle trauma, the primary reason being the difference in the examiner's perception of "moderate" and "severe" when such studies are performed. Using a more objective approach, the presence of ankle fractures has been correlated with bimalleolar diameter ratios.[12] Ankles with a significant fracture (ie, those requiring surgical intervention and/or cast immobilization) tend to have a bimalleolar ratio greater than 1.065. The diameter is measured with calipers from the lateral malleolus to the medial malleolus on both the injured and uninjured ankles. The busy emergency department physician may find this impractical and much more easy to simply order radiographs.

In many busy emergency departments, there are occasions when the patient may be triaged to the radiology department by the triage nurse based on history and little or no physical examination. This is usually done in an attempt to expedite the patient's progress through the emergency department, but does little to serve the patient and is an unnecessary contributor to the overuse of radiography. Specific guidelines for the triage personnel for the evaluation of extremity injuries necessitating radiography are beneficial to the optimal use of these films. British studies examining the use of radiography of acute ankle injuries tend to support the policy of "no ankle swelling, no x-ray."[7,9,10]

There are no recent clinical studies proving 100% specificity and sensitivity of a clinical presentation that directs the clinician to radiograph the ankle. Some clinical variables that appear to be consistent in determining clinically significant injuries necessitating radiography in patients with pain at the malleoli include the following: patient age over 50 to 55 years, an inability to bear weight for four steps either immediately after injury or in the emergency department, or bony tenderness at the posterior edge or inferior tip of the involved malleoli.[4] Use of these criteria could reduce the number of ankle radiographs obtained in the emergency department and could expedite patient care without altering management or outcome. Once it has been determined that the patient does not have clinically significant findings indicating a fracture, that patient can be treated and released with follow-up. If, however, the patient is referred inappropriately to radiology, awaits radiographs, returns with his normal films (usually interpreted by the radiology resident and emergency physician), the patient has not only had an extended stay in the emergency department, but has also incurred an additional charge for radiographs. Thus, a brief and directed physical examination as well as judicious use of clinical judgment acquired from training and experience is advocated.

Most studies attempting to limit the use of ankle radiographs have included primarily adult patients. The pediatric patient may deserve a lower index of suspicion for fracture. This group of patients tends to get radiographed more often for their injuries, in part due to the insistence of the parents and the comfort level of the emergency department physician of his or her examination. Children's ligaments have a tendency to be somewhat stronger than the bony attachment. Therefore, it may be prudent to document the presence of a chip fracture in children who appear to have a significant ankle injury (ie, swelling, bruising, tenderness, and refusing to walk on the injured extremity) or a history of significant trauma to the ankle.

## Standard views

Standard radiographic ankle views include the anteroposterior (AP), lateral, and mortise views. The mortise view is taken with the foot internally rotated approximately 10°, placing the medial and lateral malleoli in the same horizontal plane. This view allows optimal visualization of the joint and the relationship of the bony elements.[13] In some institutions, five views are obtained routinely (AP, lateral, mortise, internal oblique, and external oblique). The oblique projections are obtained with the leg internally and externally rotated at 45°, and are designed to clarify subtle or occult fractures that could easily be missed in the routine AP and lateral films.

The number of radiographic views necessary to diagnose ankle injury has been evaluated by surveying US and non-US radiologists. An average of 2.9 views were taken in the United States, compared with an average of 2.5 views taken in non-US countries.[6] In this study of 242 patients with ankle injuries, in which up to four views were taken, 29% were noted to have fractures, and all fractures could be diagnosed on either the AP and/or lateral films. The authors concluded that patients with point tenderness and ankle swelling could be diagnosed sufficiently by obtaining AP and lateral views only, thereby reducing the number of radiographs by nearly 60%. These findings were substantiated later by Wallis,[11] in a larger sample of patients (n = 954), who found that all "major fractures" could be diagnosed with AP and lateral views only.

After taking the history and conducting the physical examination, the emergency physician should decide whether radiographs will further aid in his or her management decisions. In ankle injuries with minimal symptoms and signs, therapy is rarely altered by radiographic findings.[14] The emergency physician must consider the costs to the patient, not only in terms of time and money, but also in terms of exposure to radiation.

In those patients who have injuries that are highly suspicious for a fracture, the standard views (AP, lateral, and mortise) should be obtained. If the history and physical examination suggest fractures at the proximal fibula (discussed later in this chapter) or base of the fifth metatarsal, appropriate radiographs must be taken of these areas as well.

Careful and systematic scrutiny of the films should allow the emergency physician to identify significant fractures. When viewing the ankle films, one should start from the soft tissue and then proceed inward to the bones. Significant soft tissue swelling over certain structures around the ankle, ie, Achilles or peroneal tendons, may portend an injury. Each bone constituting the ankle must be inspected carefully to avoid overlooking subtle cortical breaks, especially in areas of ligament attachments. The articulating surfaces of the various bones must be scrutinized for the presence of asymmetry and fractures.

## Computed tomography and magnetic resonance imaging

Computed tomography (CT) and magnetic resonance imaging (MRI) in the diagnosis of acute ankle injuries are not only impractical emergency medicine tools but they are also relatively costly for the patient. Proper evaluation of ligamentous integrity generally can be achieved by history and physical examination, plain films when indicated, and, if necessary, the use of stress radiographs. Although CT and MRI are noninvasive methods of better defining ligamentous injuries, these tests involve a considerable amount of time and expense to the patient. The MRI has received extensive use in evaluating injuries to the knee ligaments and tendons, but has had relatively limited use in ankle injuries.[15] Its popularity for defining ankle ligament injuries without invasive techniques is growing, however, and these images can assist the orthopedist in management of these injuries. The ordering of such examinations is best left to the specialty physician providing definitive follow-up care.

### Stress films

Stress views of the ankle are generally performed to document and diagnose acute ligament rupture and ankle joint stability. Because emergency physicians do not provide follow-up in most instances, very little is gained from these films toward management decisions by the emergency physician in the acute setting.

Stress films must be taken while the patient is relaxed and without fear of impending pain. Nerve blocks or local anesthetic injected into the joint prior to applying stress is

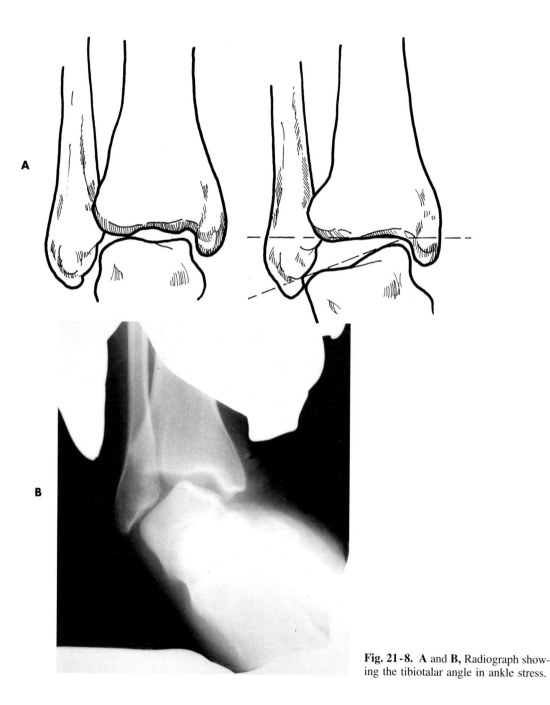

**Fig. 21-8. A** and **B,** Radiograph showing the tibiotalar angle in ankle stress.

helpful in many cases and can reduce the amount of muscle-guarding, which creates a false-negative test. In the inversion stress view, the heel is held fixed and pressure is applied medially to the lateral aspect of the ankle. This stress may be applied manually or by the use of an ankle stress device. The tibiotalar angle is measured, with lines drawn along the tibial plafond and the dome of the talus (Fig. 21-8). Stress is applied in the same manner to the contralateral side because of the variability in laxity. Angles greater than 10° to 15° of the uninjured ankle are highly suggestive of ligamentous injury. Any angulation greater than 25° is thought to be abnormal.[16] Unfortunately, approximately one third of patients have had previous sprains to the opposite ankle.[17] Attempts to compare angle discrepancies may be of little benefit in these patients and other diagnostic modalities should be used.

It should be remembered that normal alignment on lateral and AP views does not rule out significant injury because of stiffness caused by swelling, and pain (or fear of pain) leading to muscle guarding. Because of this, and the possibility of significant previous injury to either ankle, the reliability of stress films is questionable, and they are of little value to the emergency physician. These films should be reserved for the patient with a chronically unstable ankle and should be performed by the specialist considering repair of the ligament. They are relatively contraindicated in the presence of a fracture and should not be taken in children with acute ankle injuries because of the open epiphysis, where a Salter I fracture may exist.

## SPRAINS

Ankle sprains account for 30% to 50% of all reported injuries among sports teams.[2,18] Even the routine demands of daily living supply a great deal of force to the ankle and are occasionally sufficient to result in ligamentous injury.

Most sprains are considered to be minor injuries, but they can lead to chronic symptoms and disability in 25% to 40% of cases.[2] The ankle sprain should be diagnosed only after more serious injuries are excluded with thorough physical examination and radiography when appropriate. Some patients may be left with years of recurrent injury and limitation of recreational activity.

Ankle sprains are generally classified as mild (grade I), moderate (grade II), or severe (grade III). The grade I sprain is a stable injury that is associated with minimal signs and symptoms and, pathologically, with overstretching of the ligament or minimal tearing. Grade II injuries tend to show more obvious symptoms of swelling, pain, tenderness, and ecchymosis, and they involve more extensive injury to the ligament fibers. Joint instability can be seen with a grade II sprain but is more likely to be seen in grade III injuries. A grade III injury is typically a near-complete or complete rupture of the ligament accompanied by severe pain, swelling, and ecchymosis, with loss of function and abnormal joint motion (see the box on this page).[2] These patients, of course, have a more serious

---

### Ankle sprains

**Grade I**

*Clinical findings:* mild pain and swelling; no instability
*Probable pathologic injury:* ligament stretching or minimal tear (<25% of fibers)
*Emergency department treatment:* rest, ice, compression wrap, elevate, early mobilization
*Referral:* PMD in 1 to 2 weeks as needed (discharge instruction regarding home care)

**Grade II**

*Clinical findings:* moderate symptoms with obvious swelling, ecchymosis, and minimal laxity*
*Probable pathologic injury:* more extensive tear, usually 25% to 75% of fibers torn)
*Emergency department treatment:* rest, ice, elevate rigid splinting†
*Referral:* orthopedist, sports medicine clinic, or physical medicine clinic in 1 week

**Grade III**

*Clinical findings:* marked swelling, pain, tenderness, ecchymosis, and laxity*
*Probable pathologic injury:* more than 75% of fibers torn
*Emergency department treatment:* rest, ice, elevate, rigid splint (preferably plaster or fiberglass)
*Referral:* orthopedist in one half to 7 days‡

*Consider radiographs in suspected grade II and III injuries.
†Commercial splints are available to limit eversion and inversion motion.
‡Referral for severe sprains will vary according to the institution. The emergency department physician should discuss timing of referral with the consulting orthopedist because of the controversy regarding operative versus nonoperative management.
Adapted from Wilkerson LA: Primary Care: Clin Office Pract 19:377-390, 1992

---

injury with a high potential for chronic disability, and deserve more aggressive management and referral.

### Lateral ankle sprains

Approximately 85% of ankle sprains involve the lateral collateral ligaments, with the remaining 15% involving the deltoid or tibiofibular ligaments.[19] This disproportionate split is due chiefly to the bony design of the ankle, which tends to allow more inversion rather than eversion. The most common ligament involved is the ATFL, which is known as the weakest of the three lateral ligamentous support structures of the ankle. The second ligament to be injured in the lateral complex is the calcaneofibular ligament, and, finally, the PTFL. Biomechanical studies have shown the calcaneofibular ligament is approximately 2.5 times stronger than the ATFL when maximally stressed, while the PTFL can support twice the stress of the ATFL.[20] The progression of injured structures with inversion trauma is the tearing first of the anterior lateral capsule, then the ATFL, and finally the anterior tibiofibular ligament. With more severe stress, the calcaneofibular ligament is torn and finally, but uncommonly, the PTFL (Fig. 21-9). Approximately 20% of ATFL injuries will have associated calcaneofibular ligament tears.[18]

**Mechanism of injury.** The patient may be engaging in sports, dance, or routine walking. In the non–sports-related injury, the patient is usually stepping off a curb or down a stair. When the muscles fail to respond quickly enough to

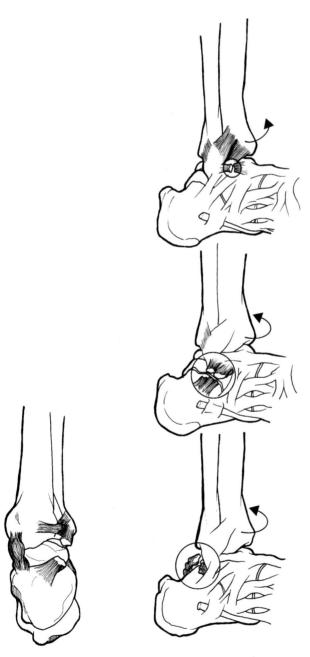

**Fig. 21-9.** Progression of lateral ligament complex ruptures during inversion injury: anterior talofibular ligament first, then calcaneofibular ligament, then posterior talofibular ligament.

support unexpected stress, the ligaments and/or their attachments may be partially or completely disrupted. Five times the body weight is transmitted across the ankle joint during heel strike.[2] Thus, the force imparted on these ligaments is extraordinary during the majority of sporting activities. The usual mechanism of injury leading to lateral ankle sprains is supination, which is essentially a combination of plantar flexion, inversion, and adduction. In addition, the lower leg is rotated laterally.

**Clinical presentation.** Patients with ankle sprains may present with a history of twisting the ankle or the ankle "giving way" while engaging in a sporting activity or a simple daily routine. Patients may also relate a popping or tearing sensation. With milder sprains the patient may be able to continue his or her usual activity with increasing pain that then prompts them to seek medical attention. In more severe sprains, the patient will usually seek medical care immediately because of severe pain, swelling, and instability on ambulating. Tenderness and swelling will appear near and around the lateral malleolus with subsequent ecchymosis showing at the anterolateral ankle depending on the degree of the sprain and time of presentation. Symptoms at the proximal leg may indicate a more severe injury as discussed previously. The patient should be questioned regarding pain or tenderness in this area.

**Diagnostic evaluation.** After an adequate history, a directed physical examination should be performed. The ankle should be inspected for swelling, discoloration, and deformity. It should then be palpated for point tenderness, especially over bony ankle prominences, the base of the fifth metatarsal, and ligamentous structures. The ankle should also be palpated for pulses (dorsalis pedis, posterior tibial arteries). In all degrees of acute sprains, ankle pain is aggravated by stressing the involved ligaments. If the patient can tolerate it, a talar tilt and anterior drawer test (anterior-posterior stress) can be done. The latter tests may require an ankle block with anesthesia around the peroneal nerve as it travels inferiorly to the lateral malleolus.

Minor acute sprains (grade I) or injuries with minimal symptoms and findings can be managed without any further evaluation beyond history and physical examination. Moderate sprains (grade II), which are generally more symptomatic, should be evaluated closely with decisions made regarding whether the ankle should be radiographed. Severe, grade III injuries should be radiographed to exclude a significant bony injury requiring more immediate orthopedic intervention. Because these injuries typically present with more dramatic findings, careful evaluation should be carried out (as with all injuries).

**Management.** Although lateral ankle sprains are relatively common, treatment still remains controversial for the more severe injuries. Minor grade I and some grade II sprains can achieve a more rapid recovery by early mobilization after a period of 48 to 72 hours of rest, ice, compression, and elevation (RICE). Grade III sprains should probably be treated with 3 to 6 weeks of casting and aggressive rehabilitation depending on age, occupation, and activity level.

In grade I injuries, the patient should be instructed to decrease activity or use a cane to allow the injured ligament to rest. For grade II and grade III sprains, the use of crutches is recommended and the patient is directed not to bear weight on the injured ankle for 48 to 72 hours. This allows the joint to rest and reduces the chance of reinjury.

The application of ice to the acutely injured ankle is a typical recommendation, with the patient instructed to place some type of barrier between skin and ice, usually a plastic bag. Adding a small amount of water to crushed ice will help the ice bag conform to the ankle. Use of towels as a barrier has been discouraged because of their tendency to insulate the skin and decrease the cooling effect. Because prolonged application of ice can lead to cold injury, ice should be applied for periods of 15 to 20 minutes every 2 or 3 hours. It has been postulated that ice may actually contribute to an increase in swelling of the injured area when used alone (without compression or elevation). This reasoning was suggested after animal studies demonstrated an increase in swelling once cooling was discontinued and perfusion increased.[21] After 48 hours, treatment with cryotherapy is thought to retard wound healing. Heat therapy should be started at that time. Physical therapists at our institution recommend cold therapy in the majority of sprains as long as swelling exists.

Wrapping and/or splinting of the lateral ankle sprain is the recommended approach. A medial-lateral or short-leg stirrup splinting must be applied to give support to the involved structures and to reduce pain. The application of posterior splints to the acutely sprained ankle does not provide adequate immobilization. The various splinting techniques are discussed in Chapter 4. Grade I sprains may be treated with simple elastic bandage wrapping or an elastic ankle brace. Occasionally it is prudent to prewrap the ankle with Webrill (Kendall, Mansfield, MA), Kling (Johnson & Johnson Medical Inc., Arlington, TX), or Kerlex (Kendall) gauze before applying the elastic bandage. The prewrap material can absorb any moisture or perspiration that may occur in addition to adding extra padding. Ready-made splints specifically designed for ankle sprains are available and are used primarily for mild to moderate sprains. These allow the patient to wear ordinary footwear while still receiving lateral and medial support to the ankle. Severe sprains require a more stable support, which can be achieved by placing the patient in a short-leg Robert Jones splint employing a thick cotton padding (see Chapter 4).

An important part of emergency medicine management is to begin the process of patient education at the initial visit. The four elements of treatment (RICE) must be emphasized in addition to the importance of follow-up and the need for additional physical therapy either at home or as prescribed by a physiatrist or family physician. The patient must be informed at the initial emergency department visit of the possibility of reinjury and future precautions during sporting activities (additional ankle support) to prevent reinjury.

**Follow-up and rehabilitation.** After determining whether an injury requires immediate or timely orthopedic intervention, consultation or follow-up should be arranged for the patient. To avoid chronic disability, the patient should be referred for physical therapy or instructed in methods of home therapy to rehabilitate the injured ankle. From the emergency physician's viewpoint, unless the emergency department is prepared to provide extended follow-up, the patient should be referred to an orthopedic surgeon, psychiatrist, family medicine physician, or sports medicine specialist. Occupational medicine clinics are also a referral alternative for patients whose job performance may be affected by the injury. Return-to-work assessment can be done at the initial follow-up, and a prescription for physical therapy may be given through this clinic.

Grade I sprains should be given at least one follow-up visit on an as-needed basis, either to a clinic designed to manage such injuries or to an emergency medicine follow-up clinic. Such injuries should be reevaluated in 1 to 2 weeks. At this time, the patient's healing status is reassessed. The patient is either referred for further evaluation by the specialty clinic or is taught range-of-motion exercises and gait training. If the pain has decreased by 50% or more after a period of rest, usually 24 to 48 hours on crutches with ice, compression, and elevation, the patient should be instructed in techniques to strengthen the muscles that contribute to ankle stabilization. Over half of the patients with recurrent ankle sprains tend not to have significant ankle laxity, but rather peroneal muscle weakness.[22] A common exercise used to strengthen these muscles, which involves no special equipment or weights, is for the patient to write the alphabet with his or her foot without moving the hip or knee joints. Patients with grade I sprains generally are able to return to normal activity in 1 to 2 weeks; however, complete healing may take 4 to 6 weeks.[2]

Early mobilization of the ankle (within 1 to 2 weeks) in these injuries results in maintaining full range of motion of the ankle and reducing stiffness and subsequent morbidity.[5,23,24] The patient should then be instructed to begin a more active program, including toe raises, inversion and eversion exercises with weights or other resistance devices, jogging on flat and even terrain, and skipping rope. Many of these therapeutic modalities can be monitored by the physical therapist and, of course, are limited by the amount of pain the patient experiences. Nearly all physical rehabilitation centers have an ankle/soft tissue injury protocol designed to promote healing, maintain conditioning, and reduce disability.

In more severe sprains, the first 3 to 4 days after injury should allow adequate time for swelling and pain reduction and for the follow-up physician to conduct a more reliable examination. At this follow-up, the patient may have physical therapy prescribed if needed. Being more severe, grade III injuries may require operative repair by an orthopedic surgeon, especially if the patient's livelihood depends on a strong stable ankle (ie, the young active patient, professional and semi-professional athletes, construction workers). Operative management may be necessary, but does not have to be done immediately (operative criteria are discussed by Boruta et al.[25]). Many institutions choose conservative treatment for a period of time with immobilization, physical therapy, and reevaluation with stress radiography, MRI, or contrast studies prior to operating. Late repair can be achieved after conservative treatment without added morbidity. The immediacy of orthopedic attention seems to vary from institution to institution. It is helpful for the physician to be familiar with the recommendations of one's colleagues in orthopedics, sports medicine, and physical medicine.

**Complications.** Most lateral ankle sprains are benign, but many can be associated with chronic disability. In fact, 20% to 40% of patients with ankle ligament injuries have some degree of ankle instability, depending on the severity of the initial insult.[18] The etiology of this instability is due primarily to an abnormal glissading motion, an increase in subtalar motion, and internal rotation of the tibiotalar junction.[18] The patient basically has a "weak ankle," leading to repeated sprains. Other noted problems include stiffness during activity, chronic pain, and peroneal muscle weakness. This weakness is usually temporary, but without adequate follow-up therapy, it can become permanent. The common peroneal nerve and the posterior tibial nerve can be injured as well, leading to another major contributor to reinjury—loss of proprioception.[26] With diminished afferent feedback, functional instability will remain, and this deficit must be addressed during rehabilitation using agility, balance, and coordination exercises.

A case of compartment syndrome in the foot as a complication of severe inversion ankle injury has been reported.[27] The cause of the syndrome was postulated to be a concomitant "vascular injury." This complication of inversion ankle injury is extremely rare but should be considered by the emergency physician in patients presenting with signs and symptoms suggestive of compartment syndrome.

All ankle injuries may be complicated by reflex sympathetic dystrophy, which is characterized by persistent pain that is disproportionate to the injury, hyperesthesis, swelling, and muscle atrophy. The skin is shiny, cool and erythematous, and osteopenia may be seen on radiography. It is more prevalent in patients on prolonged immobilization or in those in whom the functional anatomy was not restored during treatment. Reflex sympathetic dystrophy can be a perplexing complication when not recognized. Patients may suffer for up to 4 to 5 years with symptoms before the diagnosis is realized.[28] Analgesics and nonsteroidal anti-inflammatory drugs are usually of little benefit, and local injections and nerve blockades are also of limited value. Once the diagnosis is suspected, the patient should be referred to an orthopedist for further evaluation, aggressive rehabilitation, and pain control.

## Medial ankle sprains

Approximately 5% to 15% of ankle sprains involve the medial ankle.[2,19] Because of the strength and thickness of the medial (deltoid) ligament, and because eversion is somewhat limited due to ankle design, medial ankle sprains are usually mild and relatively infrequent. Partial tears are more common than a complete rupture. (The grading system for these sprains is similar to that of lateral ankle sprains.)

**Mechanism of injury.** Injuries to the deltoid ligament are generally associated with eversion stresses or external rotation of the ankle. Dorsiflexion may also play a role in eliciting these injuries. However, a small number of inversion injuries may have an accompanying deltoid ligament injury.

**Clinical presentation, physical findings, and diagnostic evaluation.** The patient may give a history of stepping into a hole or off a curb just prior to twisting the ankle, or he or she may have been engaged in a running or jumping activity. If the mechanism of injury can be defined, generally eversion and dorsiflexion have occurred. The patient will have swelling and pain at the medial and anteromedial ankle (over the deltoid ligament).

Examination of the ankle should be carried out in a systematic fashion as previously described to include inspection, as well as palpation of the deltoid ligament, bony elements, and pulses. Any bony crepitus should be noted, and passive range of motion without stress should be checked.

When there are findings significant enough to justify radiography, the films should be carefully reviewed for any asymmetry of the mortise and any associated fractures. A widening of the mortise at the tibiotalar aspect suggests significant tearing or rupture of the deltoid ligament. Because a significantly larger amount of force is required to rupture the deltoid ligament compared with the lateral ligaments, concomitant tibial fractures, syndesmotic ligament tears, and occasionally lateral malleolar fractures can occur. Once it is established that the patient does not have a fracture, and the emergency physician needs further confirmation of a deltoid ligament rupture, stress films may be obtained. The patient should be allowed to relax and should be given adequate pain relief through local anesthesia before these maneuvers are applied.

**Management and referral.** Once the diagnosis of deltoid ligament injury is determined, treatment of mild and moderate sprains to this ligament is essentially the same as discussed for inversion injuries (ie, RICE). The young active patient or professional athlete or dancer with a grade III injury or complete rupture should be referred to an orthopedist for consideration of surgical repair. As with lateral ligament ruptures, good supportive splinting done in the emergency department, along with instructions for non–weight-bearing, elevation, and ice application will suffice until the patient is evaluated by an orthopedist. The timing of such a referral varies from institution to institution; however, prudent referral (ie, within 3 to 7 days) would be wise for the emergency physician. Patients with milder injuries may be referred in 1 to 2 weeks to physical and sports medicine clinics, or at least given home therapy instructions and listings of future precautions.

**Complications.** Complications associated with medial sprains include an unstable ankle after complete rupture of the ligament, leading to chronic disability and recurrent injury. The patient may have recurrent swelling and pain and may present repeatedly to the emergency department with another sprain to the same ankle.

**Rehabilitation.** The first step toward rehabilitation is education, which begins in the emergency department. The timing of start to finish for rehabilitation varies from patient to patient. A well-planned program, consisting of a healing period followed by range-of-motion, strengthening, agility, and proprioceptive exercises, can return the patient to a satisfying functional lifestyle in 1 to 2 weeks for mild injuries, 2 to 4 weeks for moderate injuries, and 6 to 8 weeks for severe injuries; this conservative approach must be followed religiously by the patient. It should be remembered and communicated to the patient that complete healing of the mildly sprained ligament may take 4 to 6 weeks. Complete healing of grade II injuries can require 2 to 3 months; and sports-minded individuals may wish to take this into account before returning prematurely to a full level of activity.

### Syndesmotic ligament injury

The syndesmotic ligaments (anterior and posterior tibiofibular ligaments and the interosseous membrane) may also be injured either singly or in combination with other ankle ligaments, depending on the mechanism of injury. Injuries to these particular ligaments may be seen in as many as 10% of all ankle injuries and, if torn, will require almost twice the healing time as other ligaments of the ankle.[29,30] A higher percentage of syndesmotic ligament injuries is seen in sports like football, hockey, downhill skiing, and soccer, and these usually occur during competition, not during practice sessions.

**Mechanism of injury.** The mechanism leading to tibiofibular syndesmosis injury tends to be external rotation of the ankle in the neutral position. However, patients may report simple inversion, hyperdorsiflexion, or extreme plantar flexion leading to their injury.[30] It is thought that a considerable amount of force is required to produce these injuries, thereby explaining the preponderance of injuries occurring during competition as opposed to during practice. There seems to be no correlation with the type of playing surface, footwear, or player position to this specific injury.

**Clinical presentation and diagnostic evaluation.** Injuries to the anterior tibiofibular ligament may be misdiagnosed or confused with injuries to the ATFL due to the location of the two ligaments. The squeeze test is used in diagnosing syndesmosis injuries, and is performed by squeezing the fibula to the tibia just above the midpoint of

the leg. If the patient complains of pain distally when pressure is applied proximally, the test is positive. An external rotation stress test also may also support a suspicion of a syndesmotic ligament tear (Fig. 21-10). This test is performed by externally rotating the injured ankle and foot in a neutral position with the knee flexed at 90°. If the patient experiences pain over the tibiofibular ligament and interosseous membrane, the test is positive.

Radiographic examination of this injury may reveal widening or diastasis of the mortise (Fig. 21-11). On the ideal mortise view, the ankle joint space medially, superiorly, and laterally should be symmetric. Discrepancy in these spaces should raise suspicion of a syndesmotic ligament tear. The clear space, 1 cm above the tibial plafond between the fibula and tibia, should measure less than 6 mm on the AP and mortise views. If diastasis beyond this width is present, the syndesmotic ligament is suspect for rupture. Concomitant deltoid injury was previously reported to be common, but recent reviews have failed to support this finding.[29,30]

**Management and referral.** It is important for the emergency physician to consider the diagnosis of syndesmotic ankle sprain and to refer for appropriate therapy. Initial therapy of this injury includes application of a rigid ankle splint consisting of casting material and, in more

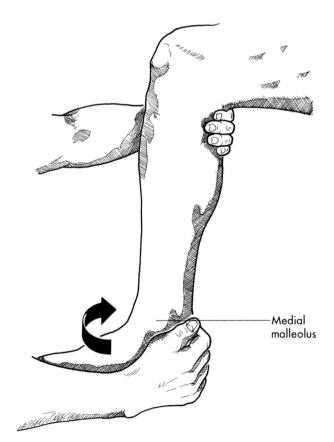

**Fig. 21-10.** External rotation stress test to assist in the diagnosis of syndesmotic ligament injuries.

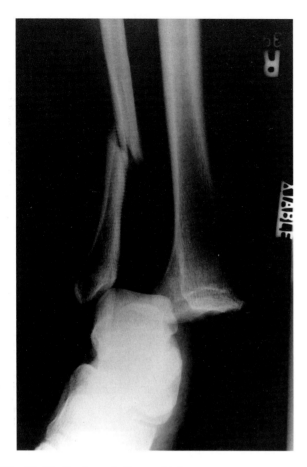

**Fig. 21-11.** Syndesmotic ligament injury.

severe injuries, non–weight-bearing for at least 4 to 7 days, until further evaluation by an orthopedist or sports medicine specialist. There is no consensus regarding the best management of these injuries. Surgical fixation may be the preferred subacute or late management of tibiofibular ligament tears and ruptures, especially when significant lateral displacement of the talus exists.

**Prognosis and complications.** Prolonged disability is a common result of this type of injury, as are degenerative joint changes and ligamentous calcification. The presence of interosseous calcification has been said to support the diagnosis if seen on follow-up radiographs.[30] Fracture of the lateral malleolus is probably the most common associated injury and carries high morbidity.

## FRACTURES AND DISLOCATIONS

Ankle fractures generally result from the same mechanism as ankle sprains, with the only difference being which element fails (ligament or bone). The structures involved can be the malleoli (lateral, medial, or posterior), either singly or in combination, and the talus. Overall, approximately 30% of ankle injuries will involve a malleolar fracture.[19]

There are two primary classification systems for ankle fractures with which the emergency physician should be

---

**Lauge-Hansen classification of ankle injuries**

*Supination-adduction*

*Stage I*
Transverse fracture of lateral malleolus at or below joint or lateral collateral ligament tear
*Stage II*
Steep oblique fracture of medial malleolus

*Supination–lateral rotation*

*Stage I*
Rupture of anterior tibiofibular ligaments
*Stage II*
Spiral fracture of distal fibula near or at joint
*Stage III*
Disruption of posterior tibiofibular ligaments with or without avulsion of lip of bone from posterior malleolus
*Stage IV*
Oblique fracture of medial malleolus

*Pronation-abduction*

*Stage I*
Transverse fracture of medial malleolus or tear of deltoid ligament
*Stage II*
Disruption of the posterior and anterior tibiofibular ligaments with or without avulsion of lip of bone from the posterior malleolus
*Stage III*
Oblique fracture of distal fibula at level of joint

*Pronation–lateral rotation*

*Stage I*
Transverse fracture of medial malleolus or tear of deltoid ligament
*Stage II*
Disruption of anterior tibiofibular ligament complex and interosseous membrane
*Stage III*
High fracture of the fibula (≥6 cm) above joint level
*Stage IV*
Disruption of posterior tibiofibular ligament with or without avulsion of lip of bone from posterior malleolus

Adapted from Daffner RH: Radiol Clin North Am 28:395, 1990

---

familiar: the Lauge-Hansen (see the box on this page) and the Danis-Weber systems (see the box on page 532). The Lauge-Hansen system was developed through cadaver study and is based on the position of the foot when the injury occurs and the direction of the forces producing the injury (Fig. 21-12): supination-adduction (inversion), supination with lateral rotation, pronation-abduction (eversion), and pronation with lateral rotation. Several subcategories exist within each of these four broad groups of fractures. In

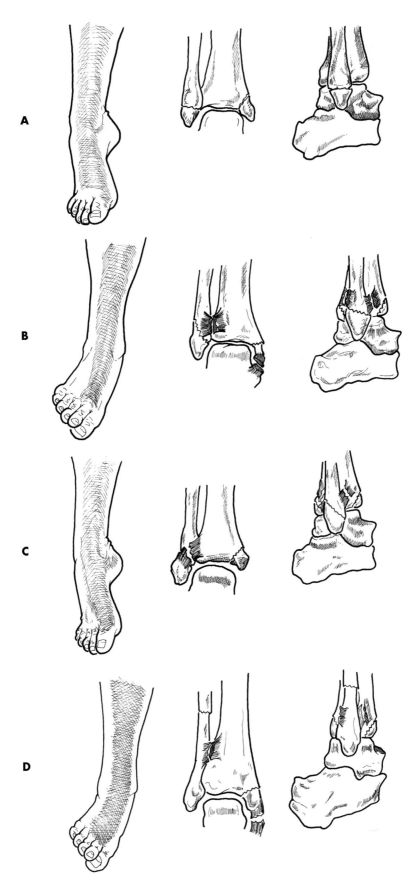

**Fig. 21-12.** The Lauge-Hansen classification of ankle fractures. Shown are supination-adduction (**A**), supination–lateral rotation (**B**), pronation-abduction (**C**), and pronation–lateral rotation (**D**). See the box on page 530 for description of stages.

---

### Danis-Weber classification of ankle injuries

*Type A*

Transverse fibular avulsion fracture at or below joint level with a possible oblique fracture of the medial malleolus; internal rotation and adduction

*Type B*

Oblique fracture of the lateral malleolus at level of the joint line with or without rupture of the tibiofibular syndesmosis, and associated medial injury (medial malleolus fracture or deltoid rupture); external rotation

*Type C*

High fibular fracture with rupture of the tibiofibular ligament and transverse avulsion fracture of the medial malleolus; a more extensive syndesmotic injury usually exists; adduction or abduction with external rotation

Adapted from Daffner RH: Radiol Clin North Am 28:395, 1990.

---

the Lauge-Hansen classification systems it is principally the appearance of the fibular fracture that aids in determining the mechanism of injury. Although it continues to be used by some orthopedists, this system is confusing to many emergency physicians and radiologists because of its terminology and multiple stages.

The Danis-Weber classification system is more simplified, and describes three types of injury: types A, B, and C (Fig. 21-13). These fracture types are based on the anatomic location and appearance of the fibular fracture rather than mechanism of injury. Type A injury is analogous to the Lauge-Hansen supination-adduction injury and is associated with an oblique fracture of the medial malleolus. These injuries may also be accompanied by rupture of the lateral collateral complex. Type B injuries produce a spiral or oblique fracture of the lateral malleolus and approximately half will also have an injury to the tibiofibular syndesmotic ligament as well as a transverse fracture of the medial malleolus. The mortise will be asymmetric. Type C injuries involve a more proximal fracture of the fibula in association with the anterior and posterior tibiofibular ligaments. Either the deltoid ligament is torn or there is a transverse fracture of the medial malleolus. These injuries will require anatomic reduction and internal fixation and screw stabilization of the tibiofibular ligament.

The emergency physician should be able to describe the fracture in language that enables the orthopedist to understand the extent of injury. Many orthopedists use these radiologic classification systems to determine management of the fracture. It may be necessary at times for the emergency physician to review the classification system used by his or her institution. As with any fracture, important points to relay should include fracture location, degree of angulation, amount of displacement, whether the fracture is open or closed, and whether the fracture is transverse, spiral, or comminuted. It would seem somewhat difficult to memorize the various classification systems unless such fractures were encountered and managed daily, but having some familiarity and understanding of the injury severity will enable the emergency physician to communicate more effectively with the orthopedic consultant.

Ankle dislocations are associated with a high-energy insult. Commonly associated ligament ruptures and avulsion fractures are involved. Although dislocation can occur without fracture, this tends to be the exception rather than the rule.

### Isolated lateral malleolus fractures

The most commonly fractured area of the ankle is the lateral malleolus. Fractures here vary from a simple chip or avulsion fracture (Fig. 21-14) to severe comminution and fragment displacement.

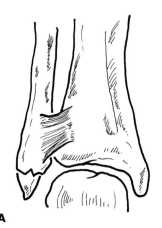 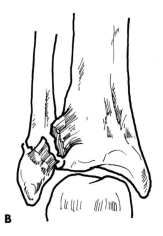 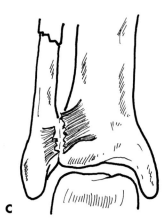

**A**          **B**          **C**

**Fig. 21-13.** The Weber classification of ankle fractures: **A,** Type A, **B,** Type B, **C,** Type C. See the box on this page for description.

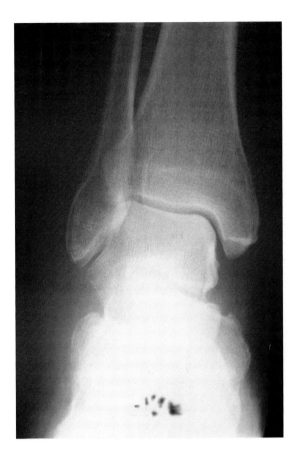

**Fig. 21-14.** Small chip or avulsion fractures of the lateral malleolus.

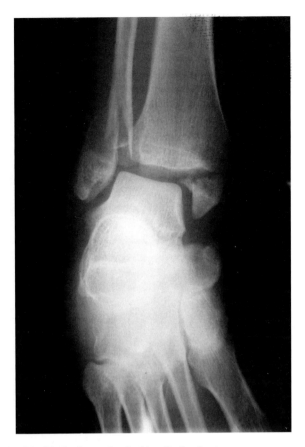

**Fig. 21-15.** Radiograph of a bimalleolar fracture.

**Mechanism of injury.** In any fracture, an understanding of the forces leading to injury and the mechanism of injury helps to raise the clinical suspicion of associated injuries. The usual mechanism involved in simple lateral malleolar fractures is inversion of the foot for avulsion fractures. Internal rotation and direct trauma to the lateral ankle can be forceful enough to cause a similar fracture in this area. When severe enough, eversion injuries can cause the talus to impart enough force to fracture the lateral malleolus. In the majority of cases, when there is rupture of one collateral ligament complex, there is fracture of the malleolus on the opposite side. However, in some injuries, the lateral malleolus can be fractured with lateral ligament rupture.[31]

**Clinical presentation.** Patients often present with signs and symptoms similar to those of an ankle sprain. It is the emergency physician's responsibility to determine whether a fracture exists. When the patient states that he or she is unable to bear weight on the extremity, and this is accompanied by swelling, bony tenderness over the lateral malleolus, and ecchymosis, a fracture should be suspected. Obviously, if there is bony deformity, a fracture is strongly suggested. As previously discussed, sprains may present with swelling and tenderness over the ligament. Perimalleolar swelling may be a clue to possible fracture. Ecchymo-

sis can appear in both types of injuries. Radiographs of the ankle should be obtained whenever a fracture is suspected.

**Management.** The initial treatment in the emergency department of small chip fractures will be to apply a rigid short-leg splint of casting material and to keep the patient non–weight-bearing until he or she is seen by the orthopedist in 1 week. During the interim, the patient should be instructed to elevate the extremity, apply ice packs, and avoid keeping the leg in the dependent position for extended periods of time. These instructions, if followed, will help reduce swelling and pain and will allow the orthopedist to obtain a more meaningful examination.

More severe lateral malleolar fractures should be referred immediately to the orthopedic consultant once the diagnosis is realized. The application of a rigid short-leg splint with sufficient padding is warranted to stabilize the joint until the patient is seen. If the mortise is disrupted or there is widening of the tibiofibular joint, immediate referral is recommended.

### Isolated medial malleolus fractures

Medial malleolar fractures are generally discussed in combination with bimalleolar (Fig. 21-15) and trimalleolar (Fig. 21-16) ankle fractures. Isolated medial malleolus fractures can occur singly with a significant eversion or inversion injury. A direct blow can also lead to this type of fracture.

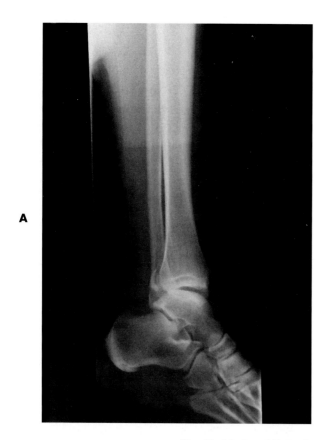
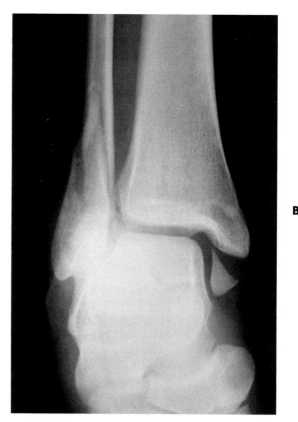

**Fig. 21-16. A** and **B,** Radiographs of a trimalleolar fracture.

The patient presents with medial ankle pain and swelling accompanied by ecchymosis and limited range of motion. The patient may be unable to bear weight on the foot. Tenderness over the medial malleolus is present. AP, lateral, and mortise views should be obtained.

Simple avulsion fractures may be treated initially by the emergency physician with a stirrup splint with moderate or bulky padding. Fractures involving the medial articulation (or the joint space) may require operative fixation, and consultation with an orthopedic surgeon is warranted. The injuries should be maintained in a bulky splint and the patient should be instructed not to bear weight until evaluation by the orthopedic surgeon. The prognosis of medial malleolar fractures is typically worse than that of an isolated lateral malleolar fractures. The prognosis is also worse when a medial malleolar fracture is part of a bimalleolar or trimalleolar fracture.[32]

**Other fractures of the ankle**

**Talar-dome fractures.** Talar-dome fractures are often referred to as osteochondritis dissecans of the talus, osteochondral fractures, transchondral fractures, or flake fractures. These lesions are typically small and may be overlooked on initial radiographs. The emergency physician must be familiar with the terminology and must have a high index of suspicion for this type of injury. The two most common locations of talar-dome fractures are the supero-

---

**Classification of talar-dome fractures[31]**

*Stage I*

The subchondral bone and articular cartilage is compressed

*Stage II*

The osteochondral fragment is partially avulsed

*Stage III*

The fragment is completely detached but remains in its anatomic location

*Stage IV*

The fragment is avulsed and is rotated out of its anatomic location

Adapted from Whitelaw GP et al: J Bone Joint Surg 71-A: 1396, 1989

---

lateral and superomedial margins of the dome. The staging of the fracture is described in the box on this page and in Fig. 21-17. Fracture displacement forms the basis for classifying or staging this injury.[33]

Lateral osteochrondral fractures of the talus can occur with dorsiflexion and forceful inversion of the foot. Medial

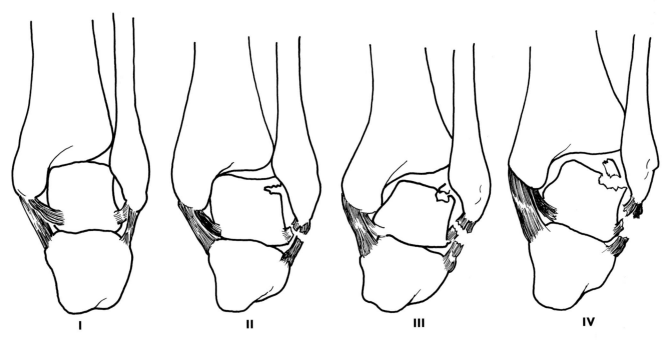

**Fig. 21-17.** Transchondral fractures in stages I to IV.

osteochondral fractures occur with supination leading to osteochondral impaction. Lateral lesions are generally anterior on the dome, while medial lesions are posterior.

Classically, the patient presents with a history of an ankle sprain that will not heal. Prolonged swelling, pain after excessive walking, ankle weakness, and crepitation should raise suspicion of a transchondral talar-dome fracture. Other complaints may include locking of the ankle and relief of pain after a period of rest from routine activities.

Clinical findings are minute in that there is little or no tenderness over the malleoli or the ankle ligaments. To elicit point tenderness at the talar dome, the emergency physician must palpate the dome with the foot plantar-flexed. Radiographs are generally not helpful in diagnosing a stage I injury. If a stage I fracture is suspected, and radiographs are nondiagnostic or equivocal, bone scan may be helpful. With the higher stages, CT or MRI is probably the most helpful in defining the fragment or stage of the fracture.

The lower grades, stage I and stage II, have less symptoms and are easily missed clinically, but may be managed conservatively without surgery. The higher grades of injury, stages III and IV, will have more severe symptoms causing the patient to return to the emergency department for reevaluation and pain relief. Stage III medial lesions may or may not require surgery, depending on the radiographic appearance and severity of symptoms. Conservative treatment of the medial fractures consists of casting and non–weight-bearing for up to 6 months. Stage III lateral lesions respond best to arthroscopic surgical management. Stage IV lesions should receive operative management to remove the loose body and crater debridement

should be performed. The arthroscopic approach has less morbidity, can be done as an outpatient procedure, and the patient may return to full activity in 6 to 8 weeks.[34]

**Trimalleolar fractures.** Trimalleolar fractures are sometimes confused with pilon fractures (discussed below), but the mechanisms of injury differ and the fracture fragments of trimalleolar fractures are displaced from their anatomic position. As the name suggests, all three ankle malleoli (lateral, medial, and posterior) are fractured. The ankle sustains a significant amount of multidirectional forces to produce this injury.

The patient will present with severe pain and swelling acutely with very limited range of motion of the ankle. On examination there is usually swelling, tenderness, and ecchymosis around the Achilles tendon to indicate the posterior malleolar fracture. At least three views (AP, lateral, and mortise) of the ankle generally will assist in making the diagnosis of a trimalleolar fracture. The examining physician should inspect and palpate the leg and foot, as well as the dorsalis pedis and posterior tibial pulses, during the emergency department evaluation.

In cases in which there is displacement, the joint should be reduced in the emergency department with the patient under sufficient analgesia, and stabilized in bulky splinting material until the orthopedist sees the patient in the emergency department or on the ward. Early reduction of these injuries has been shown to reduce morbidity significantly, especially ischemic necrosis.[11] These injuries require consideration for operative treatment with internal fixation, particularly when displaced.

**Pilon fractures.** Ankle fractures resulting from axial compression are referred to as *pilon* (or *pylon*) *fractures.*

The forces are directed vertically, driving the talus forcefully into the tibial plafond (hence the name "pilon," which is French for "pile driver"), leading to a severely comminuted fracture of the tibia and distal fibula. Typically, the malleoli maintain their usual anatomic positions. These fractures have been classified by severity into types I, II, and III (Fig. 21-18). In type I fractures, there is little or no displacement of the comminuted fragments and the articular surface appears to be maintained. In type II, the articular surface is disrupted, and in type III, there is severe comminution with significant separation of the fragments.

Computed tomography of the ankle may be necessary to differentiate the pilon fracture from a trimalleolar fracture. Once diagnosed in the emergency department, it is obvious that such injuries require operative intervention to regain joint stability. The orthopedist should be consulted while the patient is in the emergency department. Rarely will such a fracture not be operated on. When nonoperative reduction and immobilization are used, generally poor results are seen.[35] The patient is left with limited range of motion after an extended period of immobilization. The ankle neurovascular complex is usually not compromised in pilon fractures because of the lack of angular forces.[36] Although there may be marked swelling, compartment syndrome is usually not a major concern.

**Maisonneuve injury complex.** The Maisonneuve injury complex is a relatively common fracture complex (Fig. 21-19), seen in as many as 5% to 7% of ankle fractures.[37,38] If the emergency physician does not have a high index of suspicion, this fracture can be missed. It is classically defined as a combination of an oblique fracture of the proximal fibula, disruption of the tibiofibular ligament distally, and a medial malleolar fracture or deltoid ligament tear. The interosseous membrane may also be torn, in which case partial or complete diastasis is observed on radiography.

The mechanism of injury producing the Maisonneuve injury complex is typically external rotation of the inverted or adducted foot. The sequence of events producing this complex most likely involves five stages: 1) rupture of the anterior-inferior tibiofibular ligament, 2) fracture of the posterior malleolus of the tibia or rupture of the posterior tibiofibular ligament, 3) rupture of the anteromedial capsule, 4) oblique fracture of the proximal fibula, and 5) fracture of the medial malleolus or rupture of the deltoid ligament.[38]

Clinical presentation varies depending on the severity of injury. The patient may state that he or she sprained the ankle but that the entire leg hurts. Perimalleolar swelling and tenderness may be noted with ecchymosis at the ankle. Usually the patient is unable to bear weight. After an examination of the ankle's neurovascular status, ligaments, and bones, attention should be directed to the proximal fibula. Inspection and palpation of this area of the leg may prompt the emergency physician to radiograph the ankle and the proximal fibula. A missed Maisonneuve injury complex teaches the emergency physician to examine, or at least inquire about, symptoms at the proximal fibula. By diagnosing this injury early rather than days later, when the patient is likely to return with continued severe pain, definitive therapy can be started.

Management in ankle injuries is directed toward maintaining the anatomic integrity of the ankle mortise. In general, when there is a fracture of the medial malleolus and/or the medial joint space is widened, open reduction of the fracture and involved ruptured ligaments is followed by casting. When there is no associated medial malleolar fracture and the medial joint space is within normal limits on radiography, the patient may expect to be immobilized in a long-leg cast for 6 to 12 weeks.[37]

**Tillaux fractures.** An avulsion fracture of the anterolateral aspect of the distal tibia was described by Tillaux in

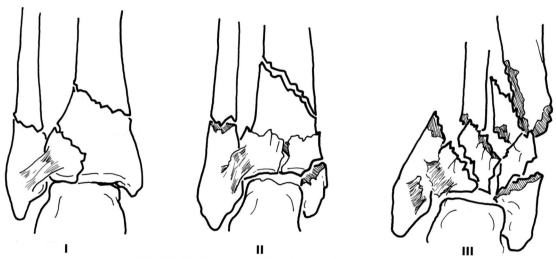

I            II            III

**Fig. 21-18.** Drawings of pilon fractures in types I to III.

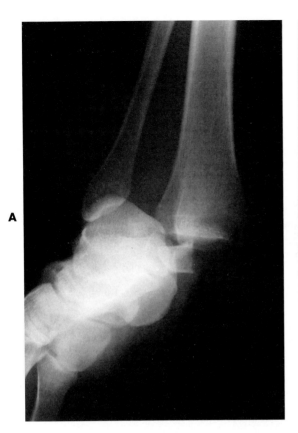

**Fig. 21-19.** Radiographs of Maisonneuve injury. **A,** The ankle component. **B,** The proximal fibular component.

1872. Starting at the joint, the fracture line extends vertically to the fused epiphyseal plate, then becomes horizontal or oblique through the distal tibia.[39] The usual mechanism for this injury is external rotation and abduction leading to avulsion of the bony element by the anterior tibiofibular ligament. Closed reduction may be attempted in this injury, but open reduction and internal fixation may be necessary to obtain optimum anatomic restoration. Prognosis is usually good if this is accomplished. Otherwise, the patient can anticipate chronic pain and stiffness of the ankle.

**Triplane (marmor-lynn) fractures.** These fractures consist of three components involving the lateral aspect of the tibial epiphysis and extend into the metaphysis. The coronal plane of the metaphysis and sagittal plane of the epiphysis contain a vertical fracture, and the axial plane has a horizontal fracture.[16] The CT scan is probably the best diagnostic modality to evaluate this fracture and its reduction because of the need to obtain adequate reduction and joint alignment.

### Open fractures of the ankle

Puncture wounds and lacerations over the lateral malleolus may suggest an open fracture, in which case the disposition and management will be altered. These fractures occur with much less frequency[40] and are considered an orthopedic emergency that should be handled aggressively. They are generally the result of high-energy trauma from motor vehicle accidents and gunshot wounds. The soft tissue wound overlying the fracture is caused by the sharp edge or point of the fracture fragment. There is a tendency for these wound to ooze dark red blood with small globules of fat.

These wounds may be typed as to the degree of contamination. Type I open fractures are less than 1 cm long without gross contamination; type II wounds are longer than 1 cm and have minimal or no gross contamination; and type III open wounds are longer than 3 cm with extensive soft tissue damage and significant gross contamination.[16,41] These fractures carry a high infection rate. In the emergency department, the injured area should be cleared of obvious contaminants as soon as possible, and parenteral antibiotics administered. Cephalosporin is given for type I and type II wounds, and double antibiotic therapy of cephalosporin and gentamicin is used for type III wounds.[16] It should be remembered that antibiotics do not replace timely débridement, wound irrigation, and definitive wound care.[41]

### Ankle dislocations

Ankle dislocations without fractures are rarely seen in the emergency department. Since the first radiographic demonstration of this injury in 1913, less than 100 cases have been reported.[42] Such dislocations without fracture are extremely

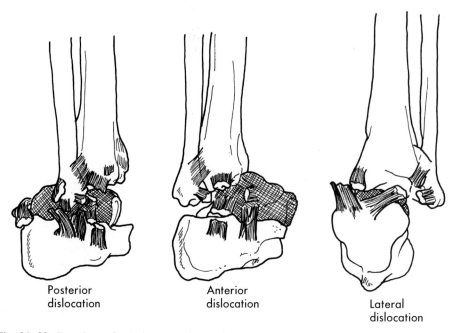

Posterior
dislocation

Anterior
dislocation

Lateral
dislocation

**Fig. 21-20.** Drawings of anterior, posterior, and lateral ankle dislocations.

uncommon because of the mechanical stability of the mortise and the relatively high degree of stress required to disrupt the ligaments.

Ankle dislocations are of three types: anterior, posterior, and lateral (Fig. 21-20), with posterior dislocations being the most common. These injuries occur most often in the young and are frequently associated with sports activities, falls, and vehicular accidents, when sudden excessive and unexpected rotational forces are applied to the joint, and there is inadequate muscle resistance (because of weakness or relaxation). The classic mechanism for a posterior dislocation is when the foot is maximally plantar-flexed with axial loading, followed by inversion stress at the ankle; the talus is anteriorly extruded, resulting in a posterior dislocation (Fig. 21-21). The structural damage to the supporting elements of the ankle includes disruption of the anterolateral capsule, the ATFL, and the calcaneofibular ligament, as well as the extensor and peroneal retinaculi. In more severe dislocations, the PTFL may also be ruptured.

The most important management priority is to determine whether there is neurovascular compromise. If compromise is noted, reduction should be accomplished as soon as possible, if not immediately (before prereduction radiographs are obtained). If the patient is neurovascularly stable, radiographs should be obtained prior to reduction to determine the presence and severity of fractures. Reduction is accomplished by administering adequate analgesic and sedation to the patient and having the patient flex the knee prior to manipulation of the ankle joint. An assistant is required to stabilize the lower leg while the foot and heel are grasped as if the physician is removing a boot, ie, the foot is plantar-flexed and pulled forward. Once reduction has been achieved, the pulses of the foot and ankle should

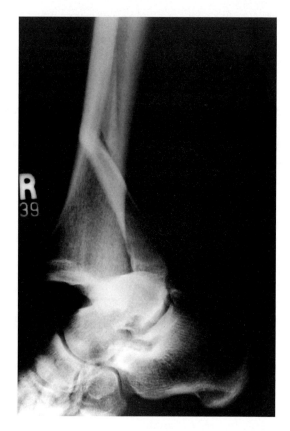

**Fig. 21-21.** Radiography of a posterior dislocation of ankle.

be palpated again and compared with those of the uninjured side. If there is no neurovascular compromise, a Robert Jones splint should then be applied to maintain stability until the patient receives postreduction radiographs and can be seen by the orthopedic consultant in the emergency department.

Most of these injuries are associated with fractures of the medial and lateral malleoli, either singly or in combination. Many of these injuries are open and carry a high morbidity. Even though a fracture is present, emergency reduction of the dislocation can be done by the emergency physician. Again, if there is no neurovascular compromise, radiographs should be obtained to rule out the possibility of an intra-articular fracture fragment that could complicate relocation. Postreduction radiographs should always be obtained to assess the results and rule out an intra-articular foreign body. The patient can be maintained in a splint and referred for surgical stabilization.

Anterior ankle dislocations are usually the result of extreme plantar flexion with posterior displacement of the tibia on the fixed foot ("luxatio pedis cum talo"). This mechanism is exemplified by the position of the foot in aviators and motorcyclists as the foot rests on the rudder bar or foot peg, respectively.[43] Fracture of the malleoli is normally seen with anterior dislocation. Neurovascular status should be assessed carefully and radiographs obtained if there is no neurovascular compromise. To reduce the injury in the emergency department, the patient should be properly sedated and pretreated with sufficient analgesia (or regional anesthesia if time permits) prior to manipulation. The foot should be plantar-flexed slightly with downward traction to disengage the talus, then pushed posteriorly to relocate the talus to its normal position. A bulky splint can then be applied while the patient awaits orthopedic evaluation in the emergency department.

Lateral dislocations of the ankle present with gross deformity and always are associated with a malleolar fracture, either lateral malleolus or both medial and lateral malleoli. Reducing this type of dislocation is usually relatively simple. The author's perferred method is with the patient supine, and the knee and hip flexed. Axial traction is applied to the ankle by the physician grasping the patient's heel in one hand and the dorsum of the foot in the other hand, while an assistant holds the patient's leg and applies countertraction. Sedation and regional anesthesia are required to relax the patient and allow a smooth reduction without adding to the patient's discomfort.

## PERONEAL TENDON SUBLUXATION

The peroneal tendons are the main lateral dynamic stabilizers of the ankle. They function as strong everters of the ankle. They also have limited function as a plantar flexor of the ankle and lie in a shallow groove at the posterior lateral fibula. The shallowness of the groove may be the primary factor for the occurrence of peroneal tendon subluxation. This injury occurs infrequently and may be misdiagnosed and mistreated as an ankle sprain. Although most commonly seen in skiers, this injury can occur in other sports. It was initially described in a ballet dancer by Monteggia.[17]

The violent contraction of the peroneal tendons associated with forceful dorsiflexion and slight inversion of the ankle is the usual mechanism of injury. A tear in the superior peroneal retinaculum can occur and lead to a peroneal tendon subluxation. Considerable retromalleolar swelling and ecchymosis will be present and anatomic landmarks are indistinct. This should raise the physician's index of suspicion for a retinaculum injury and tendon subluxation.[44] A small vertical fibular avulsion fracture may be the only radiographic sign found on emergency department evaluation to assist in making the diagnosis. If this avulsion is seen in conjunction with a talar, calcaneal, or other ankle fracture, it is nearly pathognomonic of retinacular injury. A more useful imaging study to define this injury acutely is the CT scan or MRI. Obtaining these radiologic studies from the emergency department setting, however, is impractical for most institutions.

If this injury is suspected in the emergency department, the patient should be treated with non–weight-bearing and a stirrup splint of casting material, with the malleoli adequately padded. Timely referral to an orthopedist is necessary to prevent chronic pain and instability of the ankle. A short-leg cast or surgical repair are the primary treatment options. Generally, conservative treatment involving non–weight-bearing and casting for 4 weeks is the initial management, but some orthopedists prefer operative management to reduce chronic ankle pain and instability. This decision should be left to the orthopedist. A bulky splint should be placed and the patient instructed to ambulate with crutches until the referral evaluation date.

## DISCUSSION

Ankle injuries are common in the emergency department and can be associated with a number of complications from chronic pain and instability to subsequent partial loss of the limb. It is extremely important for the emergency physician to be able to recognize and provide initial management of the various types of ankle injuries. There are obviously other types of ankle injuries that occur less frequently and are not covered in this chapter. Recognizing the severity of the injury and recognizing one's own limitations will assist the physician in providing appropriate care for the patient. In my opinion, emergency physicians should be proficient in the application of various splints, and should not forget to educate the patient regarding his or her injury. Providing appropriate referral to rehabilitation clinics and timely follow-up with orthopedics, sports medicine, or occupational medicine clinics helps reduce the morbidity associated with many ankle injuries. The specific referral clinic will depend on the type of injury, the patient's occupation, and the clinic's capabilities.

## REFERENCES

1. Ankle injuries: In Bukata WR, Hoffman JR, eds: *Emergency medicine and acute care essays,* vol 14, no 2, Harleysville, PA, 1990, Emergency Medical Abstracts.
2. Wilkerson LA: Ankle injuries in athletes, *Prim Care* 19: 377-392, 1992.
3. Auletta AG, Conway WF, Hayes CW, et al: Role of radiography in ankle trauma, *AJR* 157:789-791, 1991.

4. Stiell IG, Greenberg GH, NcKnight RD, et al: A study to develop clinical decision rules for use of radiography in acute ankle injuries, *Ann Emerg Med* 21:384-390, 1992.

5. Hergenroeder AC: Diagnosis and treatment of ankle sprains, *Am J Dis Child* 144:809-814, 1990.

6. Cockshott WP, Jenkin JK, and Pui M: Limiting the use of routine radiography for acute ankle injuries, *Can Med Assoc J* 129:129-131, 1983.

7. deLacey GJ, Bradbrooke S: Rationalizing requests for x-ray examination of acute ankle injury, *BMJ* 1:1597-1598, 1979.

8. Dunlop MG, Beattie TF, White GK, et al: Guidelines for selective radiological assessment of inversion ankle injuries, *BMJ* 293:603-605, 1986.

9. Sujitkumar P, Hadfield JM, and Yates DW: Sprain or fracture? Analysis of 2000 ankle injuries, *Arch Emerg Med* 3:101-106, 1986.

10. Vargish T, Clarke WR, Young RA, et al: The ankle injury: indications for the selective use of x-rays, *Injury* 14:507-512, 1983.

11. Wallis MG: Are three views necessary to examine acute ankle injuries? *Clin Radiol* 40:424-425, 1989.

12. West A: Assessing the injured ankle without x-rays, *Br J Clin Pract* 43:360-362, 1989.

13. Harris JH Jr, Harris, WH: *The radiology of emergency medicine,* ed 2, Baltimore, 1981, Williams and Wilkins, pp. 593-635.

14. Freed H, Shields NN: Most frequently overlooked radiographically apparent fractures in a teaching hospital emergency department, *Ann Emerg Med* 13:900-904, 1984.

15. Schneck CD, Mesgarzadeh M, and Bonakdarpour A: MR imaging of the most commonly injured ankle ligaments, *Radiology* 184:507-512, 1992.

16. Daffner RH: Ankle trauma, *Radiol Clin North Am* 28:395-421, 1990.

17. Scheller AD, Kasser JR, and Quigley TB: Tendon injuries about the ankle, *Orthop Clin North Am* 11:801-811, 1980.

18. Lassiter TE Jr, Malone TR, and Garrett WE Jr: Injuries to the lateral ligaments of the ankle, *Orthop Clin NorthAm* 20:629-640, 1989.

19. Mayeda DV: Ankle and foot. In Rosen P, Baker II FJ, Braen GR, et al, eds: *Emergency medicine: concepts and clinical practice,* ed 2, vol 1, St Louis, 1987, CV Mosby: pp. 897-909.

20. Attarian DE, McCrackin HJ, DeVito DP, et al: Biomechanical characteristics of human ankle ligaments, *Foot Ankle* 4:54-58, 1985.

21. Farry PJ: Ice treatment of injured ligaments: an experimental model, *N Z Med J* 91:12-15, 1980.

22. Lindenfeld TN: The differentiation and treatment of ankle sprains, *Orthopedics* 2:203-206, 1988.

23. Karlsson J, Lansinger O: Lateral instability of the ankle joint, *Clin Orthop* 276:253-261, 1992.

24. Linde F, Hvass I, Jurgensen U, et al: Early mobilization treatment in lateral ankle sprains, *Scand J Rehab Med* 18:17-21, 1986.

25. Boruta PM, Bishop JO, Braly WG, et al: Acute lateral ankle ligament injuries: a literature review, *Foot Ankle* 11:107-113, 1990.

26. Torg JS, Vegso JJ, and Torg E: *Rehabilitation of athletic injuries: an atlas of therapeutic exercises,* Chicago, 1987, Year Book Medical Publishers, pp. 26-68.

27. Kym MR, Worsing RA Jr: Compartment syndrome in the foot after an inversion injury to the ankle, *J Bone Joint Surg* 72A:138-139, 1990.

28. Stanton RP, Malcolm JR, Wesdock KA, et al: Reflex sympathetic dystrophy in children: an orthopedic perspective, *Orthopedics* 16:773-779, 1993.

29. Boytim JM, Fischer DA, and Neuman L: Syndesmotic ankle sprains, *Am J Sports Med* 19:294-298, 1991.

30. Hopkinson WJ, St. Pierre P, Ryan JB, et al: Syndesmosis sprains of the ankle, *Foot Ankle* 10:325-330, 1990.

31. Whitelaw GP, Sawka MW, Wetzler M, et al: Unrecognized injuries of the lateral ligaments associated with lateral malleolar fractures of the ankle, *J Bone Joint Surg* 71-A:1396-1399, 1989.

32. Broos PLO, Bisschop APG: Operative treatment of ankle fractures in adults: correlation between types of fracture and final results, *Injury* 22:403-406, 1991.

33. Whitelaw GP, Getelman MH, and Corbett M: Painful ankle: differential diagnosis, *Hosp Med* 27(6):47-58.

34. Ewing JW: Arthroscopic management of transchondral talar dome (osteochondritis dissecans) and anterior impingement lesions of the ankle joint, *Clin Sports Med* 10:677-685, 1991.

35. Bourne RB, Rorabeck CH, and MacNab J: Intra-articular fractures of the distal tibia: the pilon fracture, *J Trauma* 23:591-595, 1983.

36. Kennedy JP: Fractures of the tibia/fibula shaft and pilon fracture. In Kennedy JP, Blaisdell FW, eds: *Extremity trauma,* vol 6 of Blaisdell FW, Trunkey DD, series eds: *Trauma management,* New York, 1992, Thieme, pp. 322-329.

37. Lock TR, Schaffer JJ, and Manoli A II: Masonneuve fracture: case report of a missed diagnosis, *Ann Emerg Med* 16:805-807, 1987.

38. Pankovich AM: Maisonneuve fracture of the fibula, *J Bone Joint Surg* 58-A:337-342, 1976.

39. Protas JM, Kornblatt BA: Fractures of the lateral margin of the distal tibia: the Tillaux fracture, *Radiology* 138:55-57, 1981.

40. Bray TJ, Endicott M, and Capra SE: Treatment of open ankle fractures, *Clin Orthop* 240:47-52, 1989.

41. Gustilo RB, Anderson JT: Prevention of infection in the treatment of 1025 open fractures of long bones, *J Bone Joint Surg* 58-A:453-458, 1976.

42. Greenbaum MA, Pupp GR: Ankle dislocation without fracture: an unusual case report, *J Foot Surg* 31:238-240, 1992.

43. Segal LS, Lynch CJ, and Stauffer ES: Anterior ankle dislocation with associated trigonal process fracture: a case report and literature review, *Clin Orthop* 278:171-176, 1992.

44. Ebraheim NA, Zeiss J, Skie MC, et al: Marginal fractures of the lateral malleolus in association with other fractures in the ankle region, *Foot Ankle* 13:171-175, 1992.

# CHAPTER 22

# Foot and Toes

*Louis J. Ling*

The foot is frequently taken for granted, until through some injury or mishap it is unable to function. The foot acts as a shock absorber when the heel strikes the ground, balances the body, and pushes off to propel the body forward. The contour structure of the foot with its 28 bones and soft-tissue structure make it remarkably able to fulfill its function.

## ANATOMY

Structurally, the foot has three parts—the hindfoot, midfoot, and forefoot (Figs. 22-1 and 22-2). The hindfoot is comprised of the calcaneus and the talus. The talus, otherwise known as the *astragalus,* has three parts. The body rests on the anterior part of the calcaneus and beneath the tibia. The lateral and medial malleoli of the tibia project down and around the talus on either side. Posteriorly, there is a medial and lateral tubercle. The flexor hallucis longus tendon lies in the groove between the two tubercles. On the inferior surface of the body is the sulcus tali. The neck is the narrow constriction just ahead of the body and behind the head, which is the round anterior articulation with the navicular and the most anterior part of the calcaneus.

The calcaneus, known to the layman as the heel bone, is the largest bone in the foot. The body of the posterior third of the calcaneus projects posteriorly. The anterior surface of the calcaneus holds the talus and on the medial side, there is a shelf to hold the head of the talus called the *sustentaculum tali.* The flexor hallucis longus tendon continues to extend below the sustentaculum. On the anterior surface, there is a groove corresponding to the sulcus tali. The combination of these two grooves forms the sinus tarsi. This area can be palpated just inferior to the lateral malleolus.

The midfoot consists of the navicular, a boat shaped bone on the medial side, which articulates with the head of the talus. Distal to the navicular are the three wedge-shaped bones known as either the medial, intermediate, and lateral or first and second cuneiforms, which transmit the force of the foot from the navicular to the metatarsals. Lateral to the lateral cuneiform and the navicular is the cuboid that forms the direct connection between the calcaneus and the fourth and fifth metatarsals.

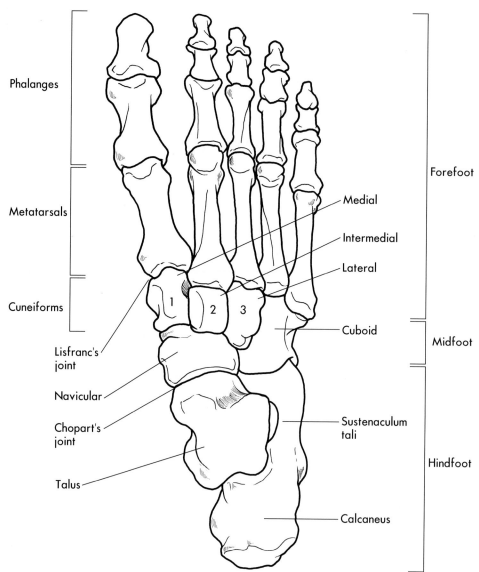

**Fig. 22-1.** Dorsal view of the bones of the right foot.

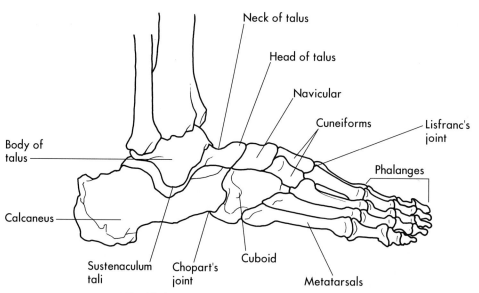

**Fig. 22-2.** Lateral view of the right foot.

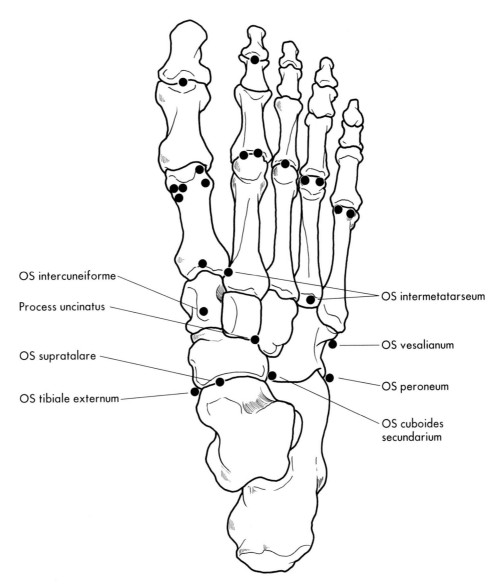

OS intercuneiforme

Process uncinatus

OS supratalare

OS tibiale externum

OS intermetatarseum

OS vesalianum

OS peroneum

OS cuboides
secundarium

**Fig. 22-3.** Dorsal view of the foot showing sesamoid and accessory bones.

The proximal portion of the forefoot is the five metatarsals numbered from medial to lateral. Each metatarsal consists of a base at the proximal end that articulates with the tarsal bones and the bases of the adjoining metatarsals. The relatively thin body ends in a head that articulates with the proximal phalanx. The fifth metatarsal has a posterior projection that forms the insertion of the peroneus brevis muscle and is a frequent site of injuries. The first metatarsal is the shortest but thickest of the metatarsals and has two sesamoid bones at the plantar surface of the distal end (Figs. 22-3 and 22-4). Each of the metatarsals accounts for approximately one sixth of the body weight, except for the first metatarsal, which makes up one-third of the body weight. The foot ends with the fourteen phalanges, two for the large toe and three for the remaining toes.

The large number of bones in the foot allow for both great mobility and the capacity to absorb a great deal of shock. The many bones, especially in the toes, are important in balance, running, and climbing.

The foot is not flat, but consists of two arches that allow for maximum shock absorption and flexibility (Fig. 22-5). The posterior calcaneus forms the posterior arch's that progresses anteriorly through the longitudinal arch medial and lateral column. The medial column starts with the calcaneus and talus and, transmitted through the navicular to the medial three toes, bears most of the body weight. The lateral column consists of the calcaneus and, transmitted through the two lateral toes, functions to balance the weight. There is also a transverse arch that helps the first and fifth metatarsals, as well as the first cuneiform and the cuboid, to have the firmest contact with the ground. The bones of the midfoot are wedge-shaped (Fig. 22-5). This arch adds stability as well as flexibility, to better serve as a shock absorber and springboard. The plantar ligaments and

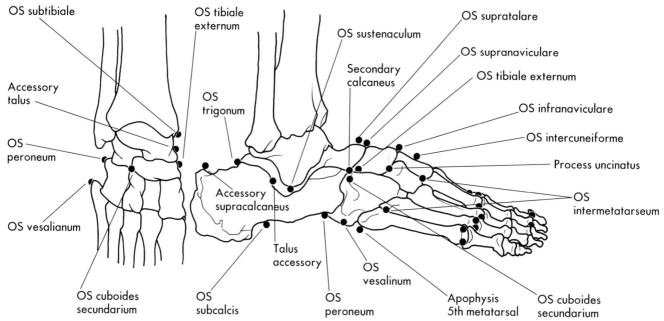

**Fig. 22-4.** Anterior and lateral projection of the foot showing sesamoid and accessory bones.

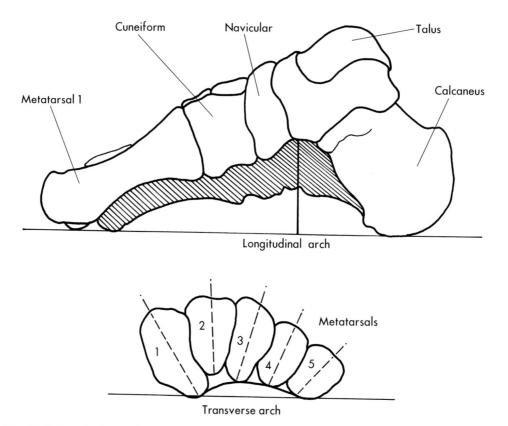

**Fig. 22-5.** Longitudinal and transverse arches of the foot that flatten with weight-bearing to absorb shock and provide a spring on pushoff.

plantar fascia keep tension on these arches like a bowstring and, with weight-bearing, absorb 80% of the stress to the foot. The other 20% of the stress is absorbed by muscles and tendons of the plantar foot. During weight bearing, the longitudinal arch distributes the weight so that 50% is placed on the calcaneus and 50% is transmitted to the head of the metatarsals, as the two areas of the foot that actually make contact with the ground.

Under the thick sole of the foot, the plantar aponeurosis is the thick deep fascia extending from the tuberosity of the calcaneus to the skin over the heads of the metatarsals and the flexor tendon sheaths. The posterior tibial artery courses behind the medial malleolus around the dorsum of the foot and separates into two branches. The medial plantar branch follows the medial side of the foot and border of the first toe. The lateral branch of the posterior tibial artery crosses diagonally to the base of the fifth metatarsal before coursing medially to join the deep branch or the dorsalis pedis artery to form the plantar arch. Arteries from the plantar arch send branches to the digital arteries and also perforating branches to the dorsum.

The tibial nerve accompanies the posterior tibial artery and ends with branches that detect sensation on the heel of the foot. The saphenous nerve, an extension of the femoral nerve, enervates a small portion of the medial arch. The majority of the anterior two-thirds of the sole are supplied by the medial and lateral plantar nerves. The *sural nerve,* with branches from the tibial and peroneal nerves, ener-

vates a very small portion on the most lateral surface of the fifth metatarsal (Figs. 22-6 and 22-7).

The plantar surface of the foot has four layers of muscles and tendons that are involved in plantar flexion, abduction, and adduction of the toes as well as fine tuning the balance of the body. On the dorsum of the foot there are fewer muscles, but many extensor tendons held in place by the extensor retinaculum. The dorsalis pedis artery extends straight down the foot between the first and second toes branching off to form the arcuate artery, eventually ending as the arteries to each metatarsal. The saphenous nerve enervates the medial and proximal one third of the dorsum and the sural nerve provides sensation to the lateral surface of the fifth toe. The majority of the dorsum of the foot is enervated by the superficial peroneal nerve, except for the webbed space between the first and second toes which is enervated by the deep peroneal nerve. Although the dorsum of the foot has a number of extensors and interossei, the names and functions of the individual muscles are not of clinical significance to the practicing emergency physician.

The movement of the foot is complex and may be difficult to describe. Plantar flexion is flexion toward the plantar surface or the sole and dorsiflexion is movement toward the head. Inversion refers to inward rotation about the long axis of the foot and eversion is external rotation. Adduction refers to inward rotation about the vertical axis and abduction refers to external rotation about the vertical axis. Inversion when the foot is on the ground, forcing the

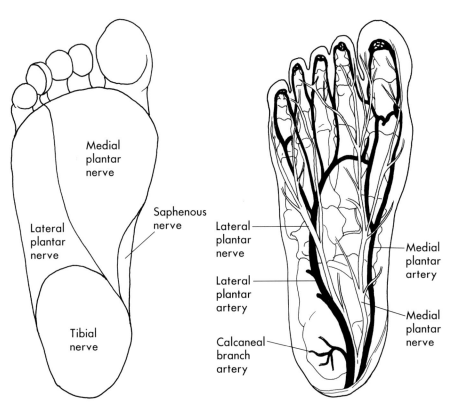

**Fig. 22-6.** Nerves and arteries of the plantar foot.

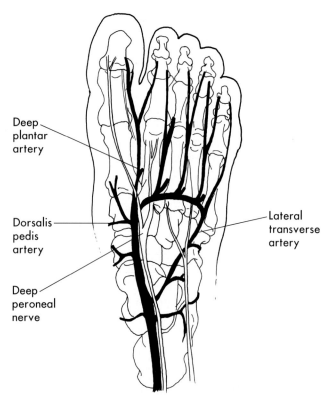

Deep
plantar
artery

Dorsalis
pedis
artery

Deep
peroneal
nerve

Lateral
transverse
artery

**Fig. 22-7.** Nerves and arteries of the dorsum of the foot.

great toe closer to the ground, is called pronation and eversion with the foot on the ground is called supination.

## HINDFOOT
### Fractures of the talus

The talus is at considerable risk for fractures because it supports the entire body weight. The talus distributes that weight by forming a right angle to the foot so the foot can serve as a springboard. Because of the particular function and articulations of the talus, 60% of the surface area is covered by articular cartilage and there are no muscle connections to the bone. This limits the vascular supply to a very small area that may be easily compromised during injury.[1] This places the talus at a risk for avascular necrosis as a complication of fractures or dislocations. Most of the superior surface of the talus is covered with articular cartilage that supports the tibia. Slightly anterior to this joint is the neck of the talus, which is the area of the bone most likely to fracture. Anterior to the neck is the head, which is rounded and supplies the anterior articulations with the navicular and the odontoid ligament medially. The lateral process that projects laterally and rests below the tip of the fibula may be fractured. The posterior process has two tubercles. The lateral tubercle is positioned directly posterior to the talus, and the medial tubercle is positioned to the medial side. They are separated by a groove where the flexor halluces longus resides. The posterior talofibular ligament inserts on the lateral tubercle and the posterior

deltoid ligament inserts on the medial tubercle. Because the lateral tubercle projects posteriorly, it may be fractured, although the presence of the os grigonum, a common accessory bone, is frequently confused with the fracture. The os grigonum is present in approximately 50% of feet.[2]

### Fractures of the talar neck

This fracture was commonly seen in pilots of World War I, which resulted in the name *Aviator's Astragalus*.[3] At that time, the sole of the foot was placed on the rudder bar of the aircraft and when the aircraft struck the ground, the impact was transmitted to the foot, resulting in a hyperdorsal flexion of the foot on the leg. In modern times, this mechanism is recreated during motor vehicle accidents when the feet are pushed firmly down against the floorboards, which are compressed in a frontal accident, or in a fall from a significant height, again where the foot is dorsal flexed. With this injury, the posterior ligaments encapsulate, and the subtalar joints with the calcaneus are torn, and the talus is rotated so that the neck is forced against the anterior edge of the distal tibia. The tibia is then forced like a wedge into the neck, causing the fracture.[9] With extreme dorsal flexion, the ligament attachment to the calcaneus is torn away completely, resulting in a subluxation or dislocation of the subtalar joint (Fig. 22-8).[4] In an extreme case, the ligament structures to the tibia are also disrupted, resulting in displacement of the talus from both the calcaneus and the tibia and fibula. These are commonly called type I, type II, and type III fractures, respectively. Because medial malleolar fractures are frequently associated with talar neck fractures, all patients presenting with a malleolar fracture should have particular attention paid to the talar neck.[5]

Ankle and foot radiographs may both be scrutinized (Figs. 22-9, 22-10). The fracture itself is best seen on the lateral view, as well as displacement of the calcaneus and talus. The oblique view of the ankle should be examined for displacement of the ankle joint.

**Treatment.** Typically, best results are achieved with an anatomic reduction of the talar neck fracture performed in a timely manner. Fractures with no displacement and no disruption of the subtalar joint should be immobilized with a short leg cast for 8 to 12 weeks, usually with an initial period of nonweight bearing. Any displacement requires reduction. Closed reduction is successful approximately 50% of the time; otherwise open reduction is necessary.

Emergency physicians should be aware that displacement may cause pressure on the skin with the possibility of converting a closed fracture into an open fracture.[6] If this appears to be true, the dislocation should be reduced with gentle traction and splinting to take pressure off of the skin until more definitive treatment. Because of the high degree of nonunion and other complications, an orthopedic consultant should promptly evaluate every patient with a fracture of the neck of the talus soon after presentation.

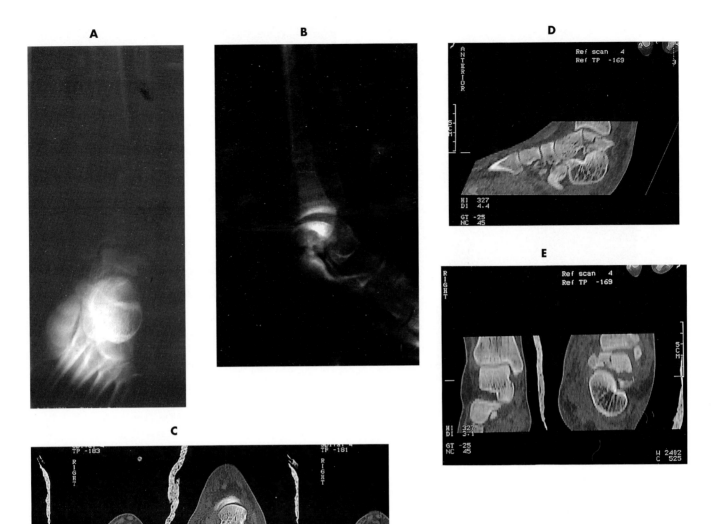

Fig. 22-8. A, B, C, D, E Comminuted fracture of the talus with fracture extending to the superior articular surface of the dome of the talus (A). There is loss of height of the talus, seen best on the lateral projection (B). There is extensive soft-tissue swelling along the medial aspect of the talus. Axial (C), coronal (D), and sagittal (E) CT images better demonstrate the extensive comminuted fracture of the talus with better delineation of the displacement, location, and number of fragments.

### Fractures of the talar body

This fracture is rare, compared with fractures of the talar neck, and shares with the common trait of having a high complication rate (Figs. 22-9 and 22-11). Typically, these fractures occur with compression between the tibia and calcaneus as a result of a fall without dorsal flexion. Because these are high-impact injuries, there is usually considerable displacement of fracture fragments along with dislocation of both the ankle and subtalar joint.

**Treatment.** Similar to fractures of the talar neck, these injuries require a prompt evaluation by an orthopedic surgeon and frequently require open reduction and internal fixation.

### Fractures of the talar head

This is another rare fracture thought to result from force transmitted longitudinally through the metatarsal and navicular, compressing the head directly.[7] This fracture usually results in an intra-articular fracture that may be missed on physical examination but is typically visible on radiograph (Figs. 22-11 and 22-12).

**Treatment.** Although nondisplaced fractures may be treated with splinting, ice, elevation, and immobilization, displaced fractures should be reduced.[8] Because of the unusual nature of this fracture, an orthopedic consultation should be sought, but without the urgency that other talar fractures require.

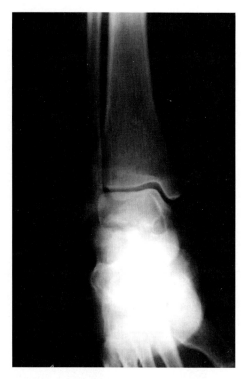

**Fig. 22-9.** Fracture of the body of the talus is seen as a horizontal lucency through the body of the talus, seen best along its lateral margin on this AP ankle view.

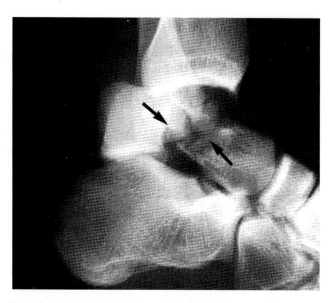

**Fig. 22-10.** Comminuted fracture of body of the talus (arrows), lateral view. (From Rosen et al: Diagnostic Radiology in Emergency Medicine. St. Louis: Mosby–Year Book, 1992; p 204.)

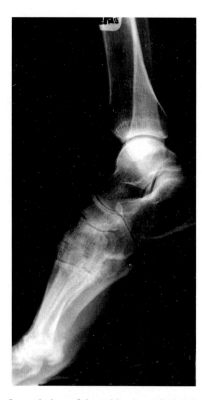

**Fig. 22-11.** Lateral view of the ankle. A small chip fracture off of the dorsal aspect of the anterior talus is seen on this lateral ankle view. Note the small sesamoid seen along the anterior inferior aspect of the calcaneus area.

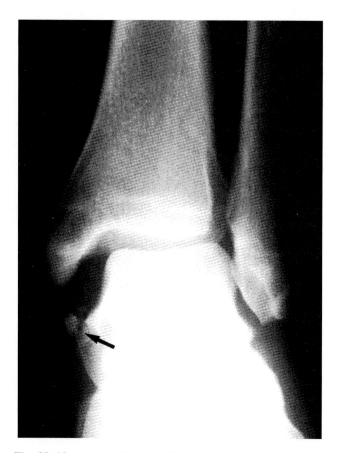

**Fig. 22-12.** Avulsion fracture of talus (arrow), AP view. (From Rosen et al: Diagnostic Radiology in Emergency Medicine. St. Louis: Mosby–Year Book, 1992; p 204.)

### Fractures of the calcaneus

The calcaneus absorbs the weight of the body and as such is a frequently fractured bone. Because of its importance in supporting the body weight, injuries often have a long-term impact.[9,10]

The calcaneus articulates to the cuboid anteriorly and the talus on the superior surface. The articulations for the talus are on the anterior and lateral surface. The lateral process of the talus projects down into the calcaneus at the crucial angle of Gissane. This arrangement forces the talus to act as a wedge, splitting the calcaneus during impact after a fall from a significant height.[9] Bilateral calcaneus fractures also occur frequently with falls, as well as compression fractures of the lumbar spine.

Standard calcaneal radiograph views include: 1) a lateral view; 2) an anterior posterior view shooting down on the foot; and 3) an axial calcaneal view shooting down on the posterior half of the calcaneus.[12] Because the calcaneus has a very thin cortex, the body is comprised of trabecula that radiate throughout the calcaneus. This trabecular pattern should be closely scrutinized to make sure there is no disruption that may indicate a subtle fracture. Bohler's angle is viewed on the lateral film and consists of the angle between lines connecting the three highest points on the calcaneus (Fig. 22-13).

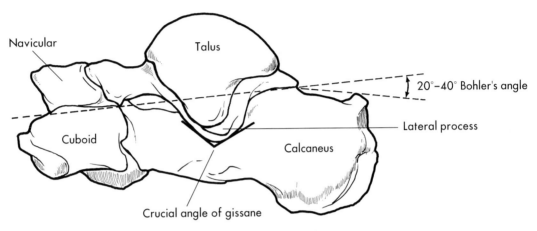

Fig. 22-13. Bohler's angle.

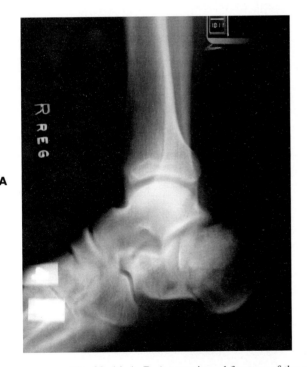
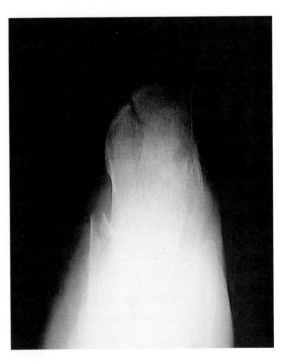

Fig. 22-14. **A, B** A comminuted fracture of the calcaneus with a vertically oriented main fracture extending to both the superior and inferior articular surfaces, and an additional longitudinally oriented fracture toward the posterior margin of the calcaneus. There is flattening of Bohler's angle with loss of height of the calcaneus seen on the lateral projection (**A**).

Bohler's angle varies between 25° and 40° and for its greatest use should be compared with the contralateral foot. Because of the overlapping shadows, it may be difficult to evaluate a comminuted fracture. Therefore, a CT scan may be necessary to fully evaluate the severity and involvement with the joint (Fig. 22-14).

### Fractures of the calcaneus involving the subtalar joint

When a patient falls landing with his full weight on the calcaneus, the talus is forced into the weak area of the calcaneus. This usually causes it to fracture into two main fragments—the first fragment is the anterior medial and the second, the posterior lateral. These two main fragments may remain intact or may be comminuted, and the posterior lateral fragment is most likely displaced (Fig. 22-14). On lateral radiograph, these fractures are easily seen and are usually associated with a flattening of Bohler's angle. Because of the overlap, it is very difficult to precisely define the fragments. The orthopedic surgeon may require a CT scan to fully define the extent of the fracture. An axial view of the calcaneus may show a widening of the heel as well as crowding of the lateral malleolus. Oblique views may be helpful to fully assess the subtalar joint (Fig. 22-15).

**Treatment.** Calcaneus fractures frequently result in an unhappy outcome for the patient. There are several methods of treatment with variations between the amount of reduc-tion, type of reduction (ie, closed or open), and the method of fixation. Because of the variability in treatment methods, orthopedic surgeons must assess each and every patient with a calcaneus fracture in hospital to determine the preferred treatment.

### Isolated fracture not involving the subtalar joint

The primary reason for complications is injury to the sub-talar joint. In extra-articular fractures, the result is usually improved. The fractures may be simple or comminuted but, because of the thick padding, are most commonly closed fractures. Although the subtalar joint is spared, Bohler's angle can still be decreased and should be measured on the lateral radiograph. On an axial view, the calcaneus has typi-cally widened. Because the treatment is quite different from fractures involving the subtalar joint, a CT scan is usually obtained to ensure that fractures are truly extra-articular.

**Treatment.** These fractures do not require anatomic reduction and are most commonly treated with elevation and compression. Immobilization should be added after swelling subsides. Reduction in fracture displacement may be attempted by lateral compression on both sides of the heel to decrease the width of the heel. Occasionally, in certain young athletically motivated patients, K-wire fixa-tion has been advocated after a restoration of Bohler's angle. Another fracture can occur with avulsion of the Achilles tendon from the tuberosity of the calcaneus,

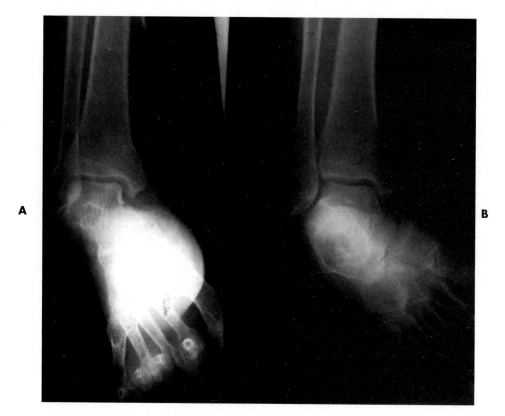

**Fig. 22-15. A, B** Subtalar dislocation. Dislocation of both the talar calcaneal and talar navicular (Chopart's) joints. The calcaneus, navicular, and remainder of the foot are displaced medially with respect to the talus, which remains normally aligned with the distal tibia and fibula. There is no visible fracture.

although females with some degree of osteoporosis are at most risk for this injury. Usually immobilization in a slight equinus will be adequate for healing of this fracture. If there is displacement, open reduction may be necessary to lengthen the Achilles tendon to its full length. The medial process of the tuberosity can rarely be fractured and is seen on the axial radiograph view of the calcaneus. There may be some displacement and these fractures may be treated with elevation and compression with appropriate follow-up with an orthopedic surgeon.

### The sustentaculum tali

The sustentaculum tali is a process on the medial surface of calcaneus that usually presents as an inversion injury of the ankle. Although the pain is below the medial malleolus, extension of the great toe stretches the flexor hallux longus as it courses under the sustentaculum tali. This fracture should be seen on the axial radiograph view of the calcaneus.

**Treatment.** Typically, immobilization with elevation is adequate treatment for this isolated fracture. The fracture may be reduced with direct pressure below the medial malleolus.

## MIDFOOT
### Fractures of the cuneiforms

The joints of the midfoot are lacking in flexibility, more so on the lateral side than the mobile medial side. The three cuneiform bones are uncommonly fractured but fracture may result from direct trauma on the dorsum of the foot (Figs. 22-16 and 22-17). There is usually a direct tenderness to palpation and swelling and frequently two or three of the bones are fractured (Fig. 22-18). It is important for the physician to look for associated injury if a fracture is found (Fig. 22-19). Because of unfamiliarity with the foot radiographs and overlap of the structures, this area is particularly difficult to interpret. When looking at an anterior-posterior (AP) view, the navicular should overlap all three cuneiforms equally. The metatarsal should be checked to ensure that there is no increased gap between any of them and that the metatarsal shafts are parallel (Fig. 22-20).

**Treatment.** Because these fractures are usually nondisplaced (Fig. 22-18), patients usually do not require reduction and may be placed in a short leg nonweight-bearing cast in the emergency department with follow-up.

**A**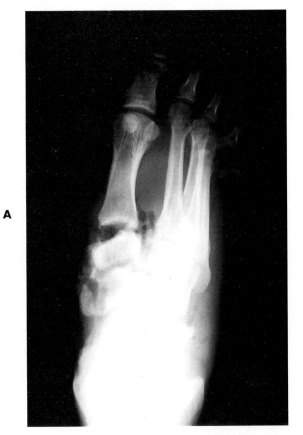

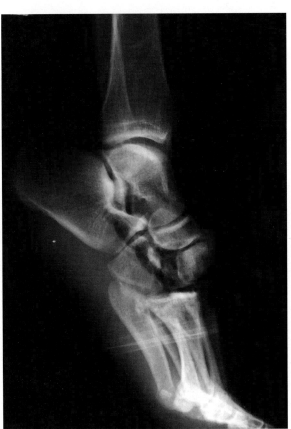 **B**

**Fig. 22-16. A, B** Extensive comminuted fracture of the medial aspect of the navicular and first cuneiform with dislocation of the first tarsal metatarsal joint. There is extensive soft-tissue deformity and subcutaneous emphysema. Additionally, there is dislocation of the fourth and fifth metatarsal phalangeal joints with medial displacement of the fourth and fifth metatarsal heads with respect to the proximal phalanges, which appear to be in relatively normal position.

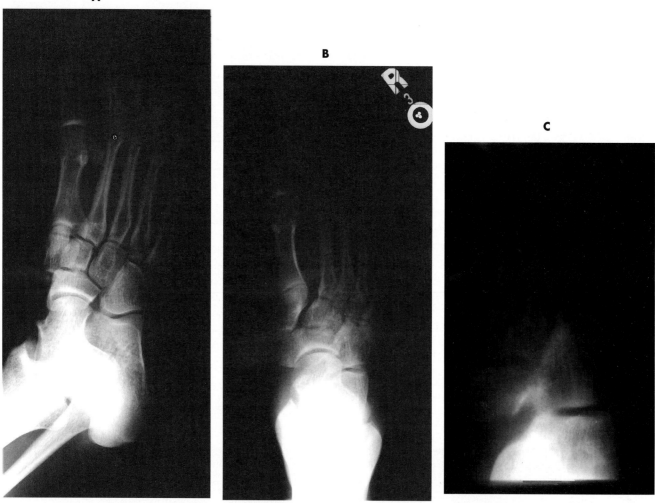

**Fig. 22-17. A, B, C** Fracture and ligamentous injury of cuneiforms. There is separation of the first and second cuneiforms. There is a linear calcification along the medial aspect of the first cuneiform suggesting a tiny avulsion fracture. The medial aspect of the second metatarsal continues to be normally aligned with the second cuneiform. A small calcification along the medial aspect of the navicular on the oblique view is a navicular fracture. AP tomograms (**C**) show much clearly a larger fracture fragment seen between the first and second cuneiforms.

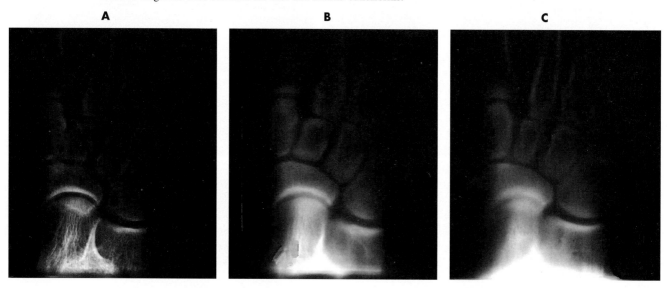

**Fig. 22-18. A, B, C** On the AP view (**A**) of the midfoot there is no fracture identified. Tomograms (**B** and **C**) demonstrate a minimally displaced fracture along the anterior lateral aspect of the third cuneiform and an undisplaced fracture through the lateral aspect of the base of the fourth metatarsal.

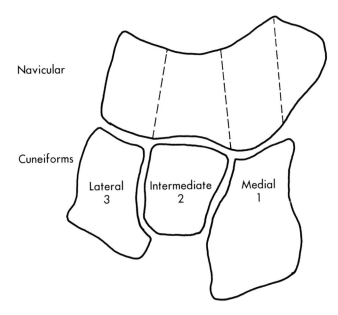

**Fig. 22-19.** Lines of force between the cuneiforms that result in common navicular fractures.

## Fractures of the cuboid

The cuboid is the most lateral bone in the midfoot. It may be fractured either by direct trauma or rarely by inversion of the foot (Fig. 22-21). These fractures may be missed because they are relatively undisplaced and may be best seen on an oblique film. A nonweight-bearing short leg cast is adequate emergency department treatment.

## Fractures of the navicular (Fig. 22-22)

A cortical avulsion fracture usually results when a ligament is stretched during an eversion injury. This results in an avulsion of the dorsal anterior element of the navicular. Initial treatment includes casting for 4 to 6 weeks with follow-up unless over 20% of the articular surface is affected. In those cases, fixation with a K-wire will hold the fragment to allow anatomic healing of the joint.

The navicular tuberosity may be fractured again with eversion of the foot (Figs. 22-11 and 22-23). This is best seen on an AP view as a small cortical irregularity situated laterally. This fracture is also treated with a short leg walking cast.

The body of the navicular may be fractured often in association with other midfoot flexors (Figs. 22-24 and 22-25). These are difficult to see on radiographs. The navicular fracture may occur in line with the joints between the cuneiforms when the cuneiforms have some flexibility, but the naviciular is too rigid and fractures instead (Fig. 22-19).

## Lisfranc dislocation (Figs. 22-26 and 22-27)

**Treatment.** Prompt manipulation and reduction is indicated to relieve pain and to minimize the danger of gangrene to the forefoot. Plaster immobilization may be

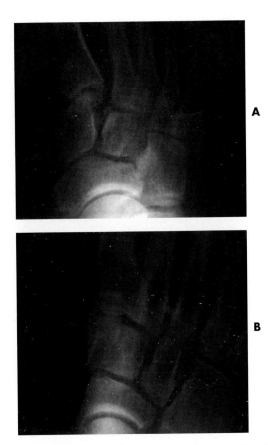

**Fig. 22-20. A, B** A tiny fracture of the medial aspect of the base of the first metatarsal and the oblique view demonstrates a tiny fracture along the medial distal aspect of the first cuneiform.

adequate but for those fractures where disruption of the base of the second metatarsal has precluded accurate reduction, and where the diagnosis is delayed, open fixation is necessary. Immobilization for three to five weeks may be adequate for a ligamentous strain with normal radiologic findings.

## FOREFOOT
## Fractures of the toes

Because of their location, the phalanges of the toes are frequently injured by direct trauma (Figs. 22-28 and 22-29). The injury is usually from a heavy object that falls on the toes (Fig. 22-30) or by a swing of the toes (usually the fifth toe) against a wall or piece of furniture. Typically, there is swelling and tenderness of the toes, making it difficult to determine if there is an actual fracture. When the fifth toe has been fractured by catching it against furniture, it is frequently angulated laterally and, in comparison with the other foot, the fifth toe may not tuck in as close against the neighboring fourth toe. If this angulation is not reduced, the fifth toe will always be more vulnerable to re-injury of the same nature. Routine radiographs easily diagnose these toe fractures and should be obtained, especially when angulation is suspected. If this is an isolated injury, it is not necessary to radiograph the entire foot and the radiograph can be limited to the involved toe(s).

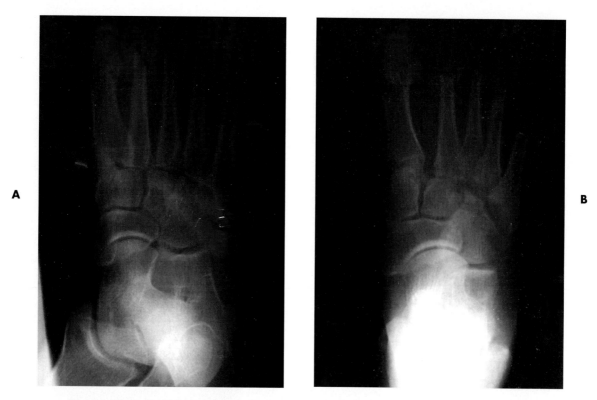

**Fig. 22-21. A, B** Oblique fractures through the distal shafts of the second, third, and fourth metatarsals are slightly comminuted. The metatarsal heads are displaced laterally with respect to the shafts. There is a comminuted fracture of the cuboid with separation between the cuboid and fourth and fifth metatarsals. A curvilinear calcification on the medial aspect of the first cuneiform on the oblique view (**A**) suggests a nondisplaced fracture that is not seen on the AP view (**B**).

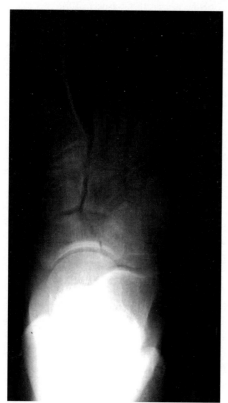

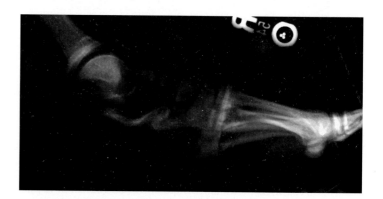

**Fig. 22-22.** A nondisplaced linear fracture through the lateral third of the navicular extends to both proximal distal articular surfaces.

**Fig. 22-23.** Fracture of the navicular. The navicular is impacted against the anterior margin of the talus with a fracture line visualized running vertically through the navicular.

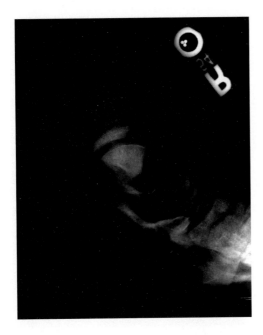

**Fig. 22-24.** Fracture dislocation of the talar navicular joint. The navicular appears impacted and the proximal navicular overlaps the distal aspect of the talus with the fracture seen along the dorsal aspect of the navicular. The navicular is displaced dorsally with respect to the talus. There is an additional longitudinal fracture line at the inferior aspect of the navicular extending to the anterior articular surface. The entire navicular is dislocated proximally and dorsally with respect to the talus.

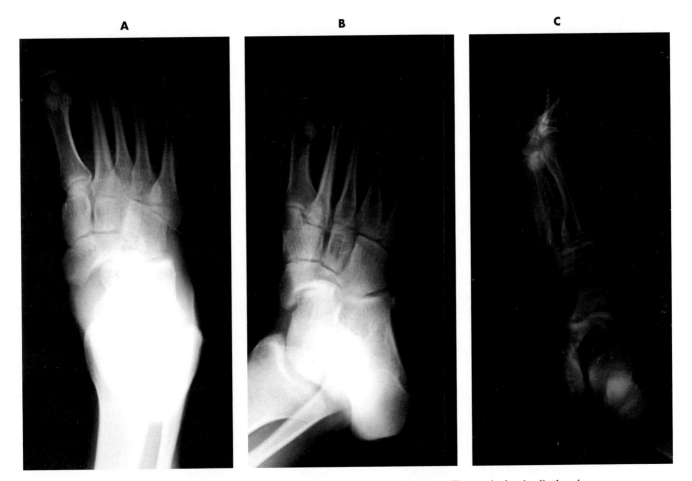

**Fig. 22-25. A, B, C** Fracture dislocation of talar navicular joint. The navicular is displaced medially with respect to the talus. There is an impaction fracture of the lateral aspect of the navicular into the medial aspect of the distal talus. This is seen on the AP (**A**) and oblique (**B**) views, and is seen as overlap of the distal talus and proximal navicular on the lateral projection (**C**).

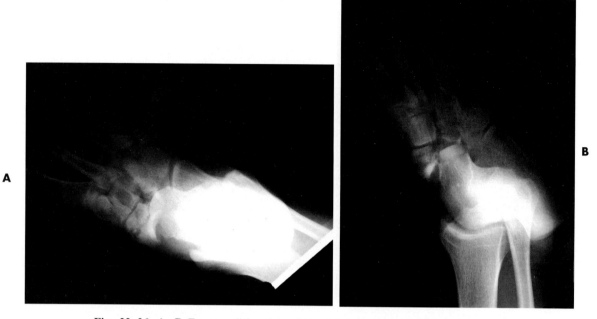

**Fig. 22-26. A, B** Fracture dislocation of the third, fourth, and fifth tarsal metatarsal joints consistent with a Lisfranc fracture dislocation. The third, fourth, and fifth metatarsal are displaced laterally with respect to the third cuneiform, and cuboid and fracture fragments are identified between the bases of the second and third metatarsals. There is a fracture dislocation of the talar navicular joint with a medial and dorsal displacement of the navicular with respect to the distal talus and transverse fracture of the navicular. On the oblique view (**B**), there is a small fragment at the proximal and medial aspect of the third cuneiform originating from the cuneiform.

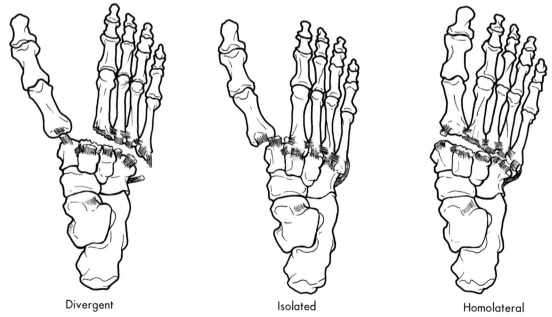

Divergent                    Isolated                    Homolateral

**Fig. 22-27.** Common patterns of Lisfranc dislocations.

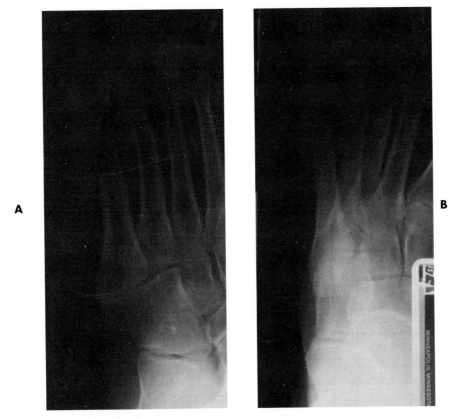

**Fig. 22-28. A, B** A nondisplaced oblique fracture through the fourth proximal phalange. Adjacent subcutaneous emphysema in the soft tissues is noted with soft-tissue swelling.

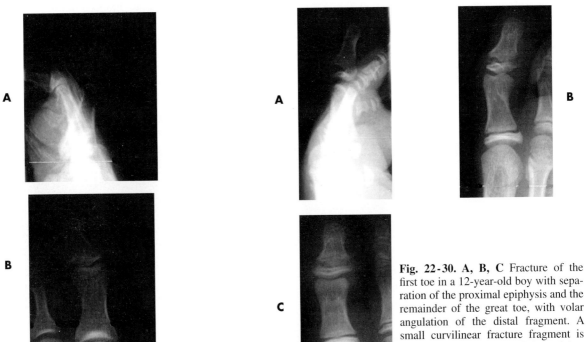

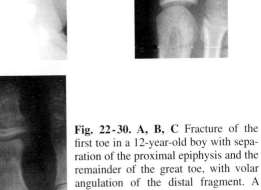

**Fig. 22-29. A, B** Oblique fracture along the lateral aspect of the base of the first distal phalange that extends to the proximal articular surface with 2 to 3 ml of anterior displacement of the lateral fragment.

**Fig. 22-30. A, B, C** Fracture of the first toe in a 12-year-old boy with separation of the proximal epiphysis and the remainder of the great toe, with volar angulation of the distal fragment. A small curvilinear fracture fragment is identified in the region of the epiphyseal plate originating from the metaphysis or less likely, the proximal epiphysis. This is probably a Salter II fracture, but could also be a Salter III.

**Treatment.** Most commonly, the fractures are nondisplaced or may involve a comminuted distal phalanx. With these types of injuries, buddy taping usually provides sufficient support with cotton padding between the toes to prevent maceration and skin breakdown. If there is angulation, this fracture must be reduced. Although direct longitudinal traction may be sufficient, it is an easy matter to flex the toe at 90° at the interphalangeal (IP) joint, forming a slight lever arm. Rotation of this lever arm medially would typically cause a click correction of any angulation. Another option is traction by fingertraps that provide a longer period of more general traction. This again is followed by buddy taping. In general, buddy taping should be continued for 4 to 6 weeks. Because these injuries are painful, patients should wear a hard-soled shoe with an open-toe box that does not impinge on the injured toes. The patient should be encouraged to elevate their foot and may require analgesics for 1 to 2 weeks.

### Dislocations of the interphalangeal joints

Dislocation of these joints is very rare. They are usually diagnosed by displacement during the physical exam and confirmed by radiograph results. Longitudinal traction, ideally after a digital block, will result in a stable reduction that should be buddy taped for 2 weeks to allow the capsule to heal.

### Fracture of the sesamoid bones

There are two sesamoid bones below the first metatarsal head. These may be fractured with direct trauma such as jumping. The medial sesamoid is fractured more frequently than the other (Fig. 22-31). Because the sesamoid bones are enclosed in the flexor hallucis brevis tendon, passive hyperextension of the toe at the metatarsal phalangeal (MTP) joint will exacerbate the pain. This fracture typically appears on a radiograph; however, the fracture must be differentiated from a bipartite sesamoid bone, which normally has a smooth edge. Bipartite sesamoids

occur in 8% to 33% of people and are bilateral 85% of the time.[16]

**Treatment.** Because of the pain, the patient should be nonweight-bearing initially with progression as tolerated. Follow-up should be arranged, because a small number of patients will have continued pain that may benefit from excision of this bone.[17]

### Metatarsal fractures

Because of the length of the metatarsals, these bones are frequently fractured when a weight falls across the top of the foot. These are usually transverse fractures. Twisting of the foot will result in a torque that can produce spiral fractures of the shaft—usually of the second, third, and fourth metatarsals (Figs. 22-21, 22-32, and 22-33). The second and third metatarsals are particularly vulnerable to stress fractures, although these fractures can occur in any of the metatarsals. Because the foot may be fairly swollen, radiographs are usually necessary to demonstrate these fractures. If the patient is seen immediately before the swelling sets in, there will be point tenderness over the dorsum of the foot and palpation along the metatarsal heads will produce pain when the involved metatarsal head is palpated. Axial compression down the length of the toe can also produce pain at the fracture site. Although the fractures are easily diagnosed on AP films, the lateral radiograph is important to identify plantar displacement of the fracture segments that may not be visible on an AP film. These fractures may be at the base, within the shaft itself or at the neck of the metatarsal. There may be point tenderness without radiographic findings until a transverse lucency appears seven to ten days later, followed by a periosteal reaction. Persistent pain after initially normal X-rays should bring this diagnosis to mind.[13]

**Treatment.** Most of these fractures are nondisplaced and may be managed with a hard shoe with partial weight-bearing or a short leg walking cast for 2 to 4 weeks (Fig. 22-32). Candidates for more aggressive treatment are frac-

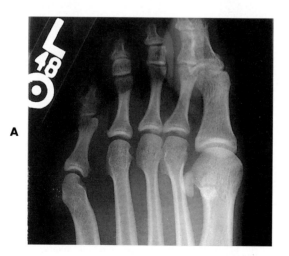
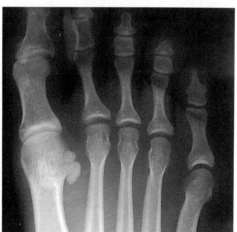

**Fig. 22-31. A, B** Transverse lucency through the medial sesamoid on the left foot is a nondisplaced fracture of the more medial sesamoid (A). The right foot (B) has a bipartite appearing sesamoid with smooth margins along the proximal and distal segments of the lateral sesamoid.

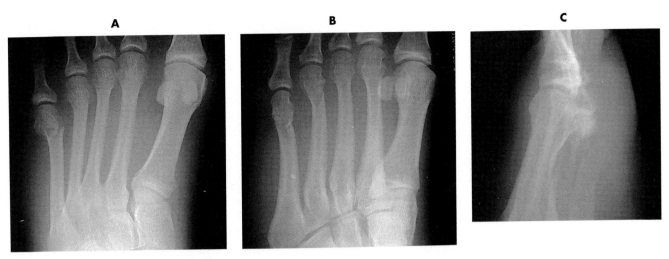

**Fig. 22-32. A, B, C** An oblique nondisplaced fracture through the fourth and fifth metatarsal necks. There is minimal lateral angulation of the fifth metatarsal head with respect to the shaft.

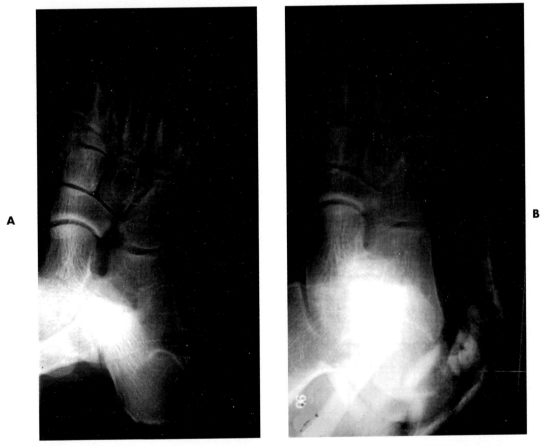

**Fig. 22-33. A, B** Oblique fractures through the distal shafts of the second, third, and fourth metatarsals with slight lateral displacement of the metatarsal heads with respect to the shafts. Fracture of the second metatarsal appears incomplete. Closed reduction views, after hanging from fingertraps, and posterior mold demonstrate improved alignment.

tures of the metatarsal necks with plantar rotation of the metatarsal head. If the head is left in this position, the metatarsal head forms a prominence that causes increased pressure on the soft tissue, resulting in an underlying callous and long-term pain. This fracture may be reduced in the emergency department by hanging the involved toes in Chinese fingertraps and then applying direct pressure against the involved metatarsal head in a dorsal direction. After this, the foot should be placed in a short leg cast and sent for close follow-up. When this closed reduction fails, there is usually a need for open reduction and fixation with a K-wire.

### Fifth metatarsal fractures

The base of the fifth metatarsal is fractured either through direct trauma or more commonly through an inversion of the foot, causing the peroneus brevis muscle to suddenly contract. It is commonly but incorrectly called a Jones fracture.[14] The tendon for this muscle inserts at the base of the fifth metatarsal and this contraction may result in an avulsion of a bone segment from the fifth metatarsal (Fig. 22-34). This injury may be missed with the history of inversion, because the examiner may only search for ankle sprain. It is important to palpate for tenderness over the base of the metatarsal in all cases of ankle sprains, and radiographs should be obtained if this tenderness exists. The true Jones fracture is 1.5 cm.

**Treatment.** Patients with an avulsion fracture may be treated with an Ace wrap for compression and comfort and crutches for partial weight-bearing with progression over 2 to 3 weeks. Alternatively, patients may be placed in a cast that may allow for earlier weight-bearing, although at added expense. Although an avulsion fracture is more frequent, the true Jones fracture is actually a transverse fracture across the proximal diaphysis of the metatarsal within 1.5 cm of the tuberosity (Fig. 22-35).[14] Because the segment is larger and there is greater force on this fracture, the rate of nonunion or refracture is increased.[15] These patients should be placed in a short leg walking cast with close follow-up. Internal fixation may be necessary in those who continue on to nonunion.

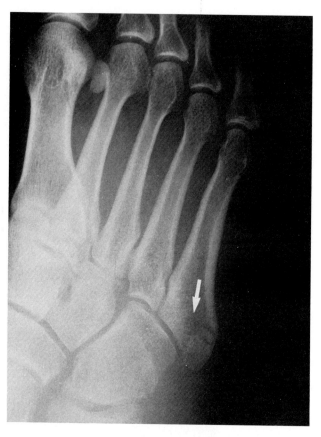

**Fig. 22-34.** Avulsion fracture of the fifth metatarsal base, AP view. Note the transverse fracture line (arrow). (From Rosen et al: Diagnostic Radiology in Emergency Medicine, St. Louis: Mosby–Year Book, 1992; p 208.)

### REFERENCES

1. Kelly PJ, Sullivan CR: Blood supply of the talus, *Clin Orthop,* 30:37-44, 1963.
2. Ihle CL, Cochran RM: Fracture of the fused os trigonum, *Am J Sport Med* 10:47-50, 1982.
3. Collart WD: Aviator's astragalus, *J Bone Joint Surg,* 34B:545-566, 1952.
4. Blair HC: Comminuted fractures and fracture dislocation of the body of the astragalus, *Am J Surg,* 59:37-43, 1943.
5. Lorentzen JE, Christensen SB, Krogsoe O et al: Fractures of the neck of the talus, *Acta Orthop Scand,* 48:115-120, 1977.
6. Barber JR, Bricker JD, and Haliburton RA: Peritalar dislocation of the foot, *Can J Surg,* 4:205-210, 1961.
7. Dimon JH: Isolated displaced fracture of the posterior facet of the talus, *J Bone Joint Surg,* 43A:275-281, 1961.
8. Straus DC: Subtalus dislocation of the foot, *Am J Surg,* 30:427-434, 1935.
9. Essex-Lopresti P: The mechanism, reduction techniques, and results in fractures of the os calcis, *Br J Surg,* 39:395-419, 1952.
10. Lance EM, Carey EJ, and Wade PA: Fractures of the os calcis: A follow-up study, *J Trauma,* 4:15-56, 1964.
11. DeLee JC, Curtis R: Subtalar dislocation of the foot, *J Bone Joint Surg,* 64A:433-437, 1982.
12. Isherwood I: A radiological approach to the subtalar joint, *J Bone Joint Surg,* 43:566-574, 1961.
13. Solomon CD: The inadequacy of initial radiographs in the diagnosis of foot fractures, *J Am Podiatric Assoc,* 68:659-663, 1978.
14. Dameron TB: Fractures and anatomic variations of the proximal portion of the fifth metatarsal, *J Bone Joint Surg,* 57:788-792, 1975.
15. Torg JS, Balduini FC, Zelko RR: Fractures of the base of the fifth metatarsal distal to the tuberosity. *J Bone Joint Surg,* 66:209-214, 1984.
16. Jahss MH: The sesamoids of the hallucis, *Clinical Orthopedics,* 157:88-97, 1981.
17. Val Hal ME, Keene JS, Lange TA: Stress fractures of the great sesamoids, *Am J Sports Med,* 11:249-253, 1983.

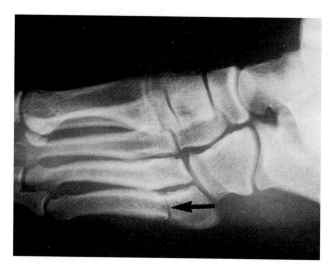

**Fig. 22-35.** Fracture of proximal shaft of the fifth metatarsal (arrow). (From Rosen et al: Diagnostic Radiology in Emergency Medicine, St. Louis: Mosby–Year Book, 1992; p 208.)

# INDEX